NUTRITION IN AGING

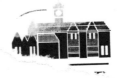

NUTRITION IN AGING

ELEANOR D. SCHLENKER, Ph.D., R.D.

Professor and Department Head
Department of Human Nutrition and Foods
College of Human Resources
Virginia Polytechnic Institute & State University
Blacksburg, Virginia

SECOND EDITION

With 45 illustrations

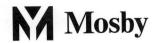 **Mosby**

St. Louis Baltimore Boston Chicago London Philadelphia Sydney Toronto

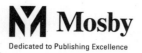

Mosby

Dedicated to Publishing Excellence

Editor-in-Chief: James M. Smith
Acquisitions Editor: Victoria E. Malinee
Developmental Editors: Gina Gay Chan, Wendy Schiff
Project Manager: Gayle May Morris
Production Editor: Donna L. Walls
Designer: Gail Morey Hudson
Manufacturing Supervisor: Kathy Grone
Cover illustration: Molly Babich

SECOND EDITION

Printed in the United States of America

Mosby–Year Book, Inc.
11830 Westline Industrial Drive, St. Louis, Missouri 63146

Library of Congress Cataloging in Publication Data

Schlenker, Eleanor D.
    Nutrition in aging / Eleanor D. Schlenker.—2nd ed.
      p. cm.
    Includes index.
    1. Aging—Nutritional aspects. 2. Aged—Nutrition. 3. Nutrition
disorders in the aged. I. Title.
  QP86.S35 1993
  613.2'084'6—dc20
                                        93-20261
                                        CIP

International Standard Book Number   0-8016-6568-X

93 94 95 96 97 CL/MY 9 8 7 6 5 4 3 2 1

Contributors

MARIE FANELLI KUCZMARSKI, PH.D., R.D., L.D.

Associate Professor
Department of Nutrition and Dietetics
University of Delaware
Newark, Delaware

ROBERT J. KUCZMARSKI, DR.P.H., R.D., L.D.

Nutritionist, National Center for Health Statistics,
Centers for Disease Control and Prevention
United States Public Health Service
Hyattsville, Maryland

MARSHA READ, PH.D., R.D.

Professor
Department of Nutrition
University of Nevada
Reno, Nevada

CONNIE E. VICKERY, PH.D., R.D.

Associate Professor
Department of Nutrition and Dietetics
University of Delaware
Newark, Delaware

TO
my father
who throughout his 81 years
continued to learn and to grow
and be a role model for those around him.

Preface

Over the past decade the older population has expanded rapidly and become increasingly diverse. Older adults have a broad spectrum of nutrition needs that depends on their health status and living arrangement. Those who are physically active need reliable sources of health education and health promotion; homebound individuals need the development and delivery of appropriate shelf-stable and easily prepared foods; and chronically ill, institutionalized individuals need nutrient-dense, easily swallowed foods. All these groups provide a unique challenge to the professional who is providing their nutritional care. Students now entering the field of health care will deliver services to significant numbers of each of these groups in their future professional role. New knowledge has become available that provides greater insights about the nutrition requirements of the aging and the role of nutrition in promoting health and delaying the development of chronic disease. In addressing these new perspectives, this second edition of *Nutrition in Aging* is virtually a new book with current research information, expanded topic areas, and new features.

Older adults are a growing segment of the population using nutrition services in health care facilities and community-based programs. This textbook is designed to provide the nutrition professional with the knowledge necessary to make appropriate decisions regarding the specific food and nutrition needs of older people and provide helpful advice to the client and caregiver regarding food selection. Every older person is unique, and I have emphasized evaluating each as an individual and seeking alternative solutions to best meet his or her needs.

THE SECOND EDITION

Certain features have been retained and updated from the first edition.

Comprehensive Coverage of Topics

Preparation for working with older people requires a knowledge of the diversity within older groups and the ability to anticipate future changes. The opening chapters provide an overview of this population and their social, economic, and health characteristics. Biologic and physiologic changes related to the aging process affect nutrient requirements and digestion, absorption, metabolism, and excretion. These changes are described in detail to provide a background for understanding and predicting nutrient needs in older people in various states of health. The relationships between lifelong nutrition practices and the enhancement of physical well-being, the prevention of morbidity, and the slowing of the aging process are interpreted in light of current health promotion and nutrition intervention efforts.

The middle chapters focus on current research that evaluates the older population's requirements for macronutrients, vitamins, and minerals. Many nutrients are included for which there was no available research in aging when the first edition was prepared. The reader is alerted to the particular subgroups within the aging population, who, because of their ethnic and socioeconomic backgrounds or food selection patterns, are especially vulnerable to inadequate nutrient intakes. Patterns of both prescription and over-the-counter drug use by older adults and the interactions of nutrients and foods with drugs are discussed in relation to nutritional status. The causes of nutrition-related chronic disorders common among this population, including osteoporosis, osteomalacia, anemias, underweight and overweight, and osteoarthritis, are described along with current prevention and intervention strategies.

The later chapters focus on the application of principles in nutrition practice. Tools for evaluating nutritional status in various clinical and community settings are presented for future application. The student is introduced to the emerging role of nutrition within the continuum of health care and is given recommendations for implementing nutrition services in both community and institutionalized populations. Factors influencing the food choices of older people and food programs supporting independent living are evaluated in the context of maintaining or achieving nutritional well being.

Recognition of Controversy

Despite the increasing emphasis on research in nutrition and aging, many questions remain unanswered, including those about the nutrient requirements and metabolism of older people, and those about the relationship of particular nutrients and nonnutrients to the development of chronic and nutrition-related disorders. Alternative points of view and their supporting experimental evidence are presented to encourage the student to analyze available data and develop his or her own conclusions.

Balance of Theory and Clinical Practice

Working with older adults demands a clear understanding of nutrition theory as well as the skills to translate these principles into nutrition care plans that are both practical and appropriate in various settings. The nutrition and health professional must understand why a problem exists, identify alternative solutions, and work with the older client or caregiver to decide on the most realistic plan of action. Meeting the food and nutrition needs of older individuals may require a compromise between what is ideal and what is possible in the situation presented.

New directions and features of the second edition include the following.

Focus on Diversity

Since my preparation of the first edition, increasing information has become available describing the socioeconomic, health, and nutritional characteristics of many ethnic and cultural groups, including black, Mexican-American, Hispanic, and Asian-American older people. A new chapter focusing on the nutritional status of older people has been added to highlight findings of recent national surveys that provide new information on ethnic groups residing in the United States. Available data are presented throughout this edition to allow comparison of the young-old (ages 65-74) with the oldest-old (ages 85 +), who often differ in health status, functional ability, nutrient needs, and the types of nutrition services required.

Health Issues and Long-Term Care

As older persons are and will continue to be the largest users of health care services, positive nutrition practices and health promotion strategies to reduce or delay degenerative diseases are a constant theme throughout this text. A chapter focusing on nutrition services within the continuum of health care builds awareness of nutrition opportunities, challenges, and creative approaches for delivering quality food and nutrition education within congregate, home delivered, and institutional meal programs. Coverage of current trends in polypharmacy and drug use in the treatment of older people has been expanded.

Resources for Future Use

To maximize the usefulness of this text when the student has moved on to professional responsibilities, an extensive bibliography is provided with each chapter that includes both current and classical references. Screening tools and dietary assessment materials found in Chapter 11 and in the Appendices can be adapted to various community and clinical situations. The resource lists for nutrition education and program development have been updated and expanded, and a section on audiovisual resources has been added.

New Pedagogical Aids

Several chapter features have been added to facilitate use of the book by both educators and students.

- **Learning Objectives** direct the student's attention to specific subject areas and outcomes to be achieved by studying the chapter.
- **Review Questions** aid in the study and discussion of the material. These questions are designed to reinforce the important content to be retained from the chapter.
- **Suggested Learning Activities** provide opportunities for students to apply the theories and principles learned to professional situations and case studies. In addition, students are encouraged to interact with older people in various facilities and thus develop communication skills with this client group. Current controversies in the field are defined for further study or evaluation.
- **Key Words** help students become familiar with specific terms and definitions that are critical to an understanding of the material presented.
- **Glossary** has been expanded to include key words and terms noted in each chapter.

ACKNOWLEDGEMENTS

I am indebted to the many people who made possible the preparation of this new edition. Both the content and organization of this edition were improved immeasurably by the following reviewers who gave time and effort to evaluating the first edition and offering many helpful suggestions: Diane Veale Jones, College of St. Benedict; Margaret E. Briley, The University of Texas at Austin; Christine Rosenbloom, Georgia State University; Diane Arnold, Foothill College; Judith C. Byrne, Indiana State University; Sarah E. Burroughs, California Polytechnic State University; and Marie Fanelli Kuczmarski, University of Delaware.

I would also like to recognize the contributors to this edition, who shared their expertise in providing new and expanded coverage of important topics: Marie Fanelli Kuczmarski, Robert Kuczmarski, Connie E. Vickery, and Marsha Read. Christine Rosenbloom developed the pedagogical aids for each chapter. The resourcefulness and encouragement of Gina Gay Chan and later, Wendy Schiff, my developmental editors at Mosby–Year Book, kept us moving toward the goal.

Others who contributed to this effort included Joseph Carlin, Nutritionist, Region 1, Administration on Aging, Boston, MA, who provided helpful materials and statistics for Chapter 13; Christopher Adamson and Rita Lugogo, who worked tirelessly tracking down references that I didn't know existed; Mary Taylor, whose unlimited patience and computer skills turned my material into readable manuscript; Sherry Saville, who produced the illustrations and was always willing to try something new; the faculty, students, and staff of the Department of Human Nutrition and Foods, who provided continued encouragement and answered questions in their areas of expertise; and Dean S.J. Ritchey of the College of Human Resources, who supported this endeavor. A source of constant encouragement and optimism in my preparation of the first edition was my late father, Harold Schlenker. His ongoing support was greatly missed this time.

Eleanor D. Schlenker

Contents

Contents

1

Demographic and Biologic Aspects of Aging

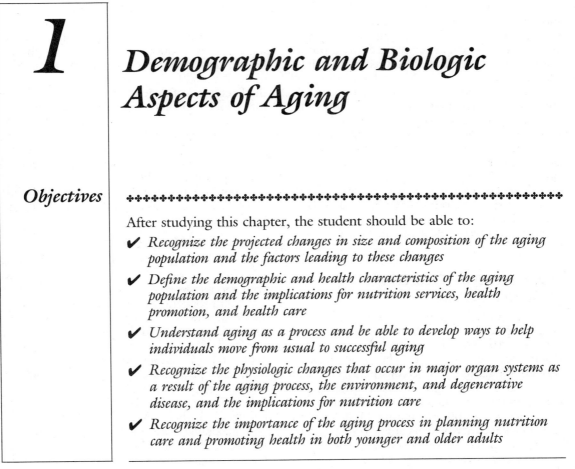

Objectives

✱✱

After studying this chapter, the student should be able to:

✔ *Recognize the projected changes in size and composition of the aging population and the factors leading to these changes*

✔ *Define the demographic and health characteristics of the aging population and the implications for nutrition services, health promotion, and health care*

✔ *Understand aging as a process and be able to develop ways to help individuals move from usual to successful aging*

✔ *Recognize the physiologic changes that occur in major organ systems as a result of the aging process, the environment, and degenerative disease, and the implications for nutrition care*

✔ *Recognize the importance of the aging process in planning nutrition care and promoting health in both younger and older adults*

Introduction

America is getting older. One in eight individuals is now age 65 or older, and by the year 2030, it will be one in five.[52] One of the fastest growing segments of the population is the 85 and older age group. These shifts in population have far-reaching implications for many aspects of our society, from public policy on health care to increasing efforts by food manufacturers to develop products that will be attractive to the older consumer. The increasing number of older individuals presents both a challenge and

a responsibility for the health professional. In the coming years the number of older workers reaching retirement age will exceed the number of younger individuals entering the work force. As a result, older workers in good health will be encouraged to continue working, and nutrition and health education, which promote physical well-being, will be priorities.[37] Older individuals in declining health will require specialized nutrition services designed to maintain the highest level of independence and functional capacity possible. As pointed out in the

Surgeon General's Workshop on Health Promotion and Aging,[1] the projections describing the increases in the older population are more than mere numbers. They represent real people with particular needs and resources who will be old and will require health and nutrition services that are not even understood today. At this time we have limited knowledge about the nutrient needs, nutrition problems, and socioeconomic and health factors that influence the food choices of older people; furthermore, we do not completely understand the biologic and physiologic changes that occur as part of the aging process. Our challenge is to begin developing nutrition recommendations and services that will meet the changing nutrient needs of tomorrow's diverse older population.

POPULATION TRENDS
Definition of Age

In legal matters age is defined on the basis of **chronologic age,** or the number of years a person has lived. Reaching a particular age usually determines eligibility for benefits or services, although standards are not consistent. One can participate in the congregate meal program and other services mandated under the **Older Americans Act** at age 60 and receive **Medicare** and full **Social Security** benefits at age 65; laws protecting the older worker against age discrimination become effective at age 55. In the United States, age 65, the typical age of retirement, is viewed as the benchmark of the older population.

When older people were few in number, census and health statistics grouped all individuals over the age of 64, failing to recognize the physical and socioeconomic changes that occur in older people as they continue to age. For example, those age 65 and recently retired are likely to be in good health; **functional** disability and the need for assistance with housekeeping or transportation are more common in those age 75 or older. Most women ages 65 to 74 live with a spouse; most of those over age 84 live alone.[50] So that we might evaluate these differences and recognize when they occur, current census statistics categorize people ages 65

to 74 as the **young-old** and those age 85 or older as the **oldest-old.**[51]

Although usually easy to determine, chronologic age is a poor measure of the physical health, mental alertness, or vitality of an older individual. Although advancing age increases the likelihood of degenerative physical changes, many older people entering their eighth or ninth decade have independent, active life-styles that include household chores, regular walking, and visiting with friends. Conversely, young people sometimes lose their zest for life. A health professional should never form an opinion about the needs or physical or mental status of an older client solely on the basis of chronologic age.

Increase in Numbers

During this century older age groups have increased in size far more rapidly than have younger age groups, both in absolute numbers and as a proportion of the total population. In 1900, statistically fewer than one in 10 Americans was age 55 or older, and only one in 25 was age 65 or older. According to census reports of 1987, one in five Americans, or about 52 million people, are at least 55 years old, and one in eight, or about 30 million people, are at least 65 years old. More than 25,000 people have reached their 100th birthday.[58]

It generally is assumed that this increase in the number of older people is the result of increased **longevity**. In fact, increased life span is only part of the explanation. Another primary cause is the dramatic increase in the annual number of births before 1920 and between 1946 and 1964. The aging of people born before 1920 has resulted in the rising number of individuals now in their 80s and 90s. The aging of the **baby boom generation,** born between the mid-1940s and the mid-1960s, will lead to the rapid increase in the number of older people that is expected to begin about 2010. By the year 2030 the United States will have more than 65 million people over age 64, accounting for 21% of the population.[58] Also, because the precipitous decline in the birth rate after 1964 has slowed the growth of younger age groups, the **median** age of the U.S. population in 2030 will be 44 years.[58] Those now entering health and social service professions will deal with the impact of these **demographic** changes on the client groups they serve throughout their careers.

Composition of the Older Population

Age. The projected increase in the number of older people will not be equal across all age groups and will result in changes in the age pattern within the older population (Fig. 1-1). Currently most older people are among the young-old (ages 65 to 74). By the year 2000 half of the older population will be age 75 or older, and 100,000 people will be 100 years of age or older. The 85 and older age group is one of the fastest growing age groups in the country and will triple in size by the year 2030.[52] This speaks to the major advances in disease prevention and health care that have been made in recent years. It also raises important issues about allocation of health and community resources, since people of this age are likely to require extended health and social services.

Race. Older age groups will also increase in ethnicity. Currently the older population is predominantly white. The black and Hispanic populations have smaller proportions of older people than does the white population. Only 8% of blacks and Hispanics are age 65 or older, compared to 13% of whites.[58] This difference is partly related to the higher fertility rates among the black and Hispanic populations, resulting in greater proportions of children and young people. Also, minority populations have a lower **life expectancy.** In the future, however, the proportion of older people in the black and Hispanic populations will increase as life expectancy continues to rise in those groups. The older minority population now accounts for 10% of the total population age 65 or older; this will increase to 17% within this decade.[58]

Sex. The ratio of women to men varies dramatically among different age groups. At younger ages the numbers of women and men are about equal, but at older ages women outnumber men 3 to 2. This disparity becomes even greater as individuals age. Between ages 65 and 69, there are 83 men for every 100 women. However, by age 85, there are only 39 men for every 100 women.[51] These numbers reflect the increasing life expectancy of women compared to men. Because women on the average live longer than men, they have a longer period of retirement and are more likely to live alone or with nonrelatives in their later years. These factors also increase their vulnerability to economic insecurity at advanced ages.

Implications of Current Trends

The projected increases in the number and proportion of older people have implications for both the family and our society as a whole. The decline in the birth rate implies that aged parents will have fewer children and grandchildren to provide economic and emotional support or to assist with shopping, transportation, and household tasks. Currently one third of older women with some functional disability receive their primary care from their children, whereas disabled older men are more likely to be cared for by their wives.[58] Unmarried older people or those with no children are more likely to be institutionalized. In the coming years support services usually provided by family members may have to be provided by government or private agencies for the rising number of

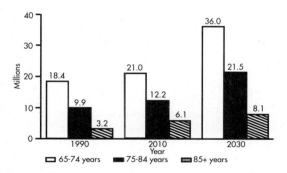

FIG. 1-1 Projected increases in the U.S. population age 65 and older. Although the over-65 population will almost double between 1990 and 2030, the fastest growing segment will be those age 85 and older.

(Data from US Bureau of the Census: Projections of the population of the United States by age, sex, and race: 1988 to 2080, Curr Pop Reports Series P-25, No 1018, Washington, DC, 1989, US Government Printing Office.).

older people who have no close family members.

Older people are the largest users of health services, including visits to physicians, hospital stays, and prescription drugs. Although people over age 65 represent 12% of the population, they account for more than one third of all health care expenditures.[56] As their number increases, they will require an ever-growing share of both public and private health insurance resources. Health promotion activities focusing on appropriate diet, exercise, and life-style patterns should be directed toward young and middle-aged segments of the population to ensure continuing good health at older ages.

An increase in the number of older people in good health coupled with a decrease in the number of younger workers will result in more older people remaining in the work force beyond the usual age of retirement. Current policies of compulsory retirement have led to the loss of individuals from industry, government, and service agencies who have unique skills and in some cases the desire to continue working. The growing number of older people in the general population will reinforce positive attitudes toward aging in our society, which in recent years has been youth oriented. As the number of older consumers with buying power continues to increase, more products, services, and advertising will be targeted toward this market. Nutrition professionals should be teaming with food industry specialists and social service providers to develop unique food products and nutrition services that will meet the needs of tomorrow's older population.

TRENDS IN MORTALITY AND MORBIDITY

Life expectancy, **mortality rates,** and the prevalence of chronic disease have all changed dramatically during this century. Medical advances in the treatment of diseases, as well as alterations in life-style, have contributed to the changes observed. For the most part the effects of these changes have been positive. However, the increased use of cigarettes by women has led to a rapid rise in the mortality rate from lung cancer among women.[9] Because all major causes of death in middle age and beyond are influenced by modifiable risk factors, efforts toward promoting health and reducing disease could further increase life expectancy.

Changes in Life Expectancy

Basis of changes in life expectancy. Life expectancy, the average remaining years of life for a person of a given age, has increased in all age groups since 1900. The most striking increases occurred during the first half of this century as a result of reduced infant mortality and the development of antibiotics to control pneumonia, influenza, and other infectious diseases.[58] Decreased mortality from heart disease and **cerebral hemorrhage,** achieved through improved management of hypertension and an emphasis on appropriate diet, exercise, and life-style patterns, has contributed to the increase in life expectancy in recent years. Overall life expectancy at birth increased from a mean of 47 years in 1900 to about 75 years in 1990.[56] Although gains in life expectancy at birth have been substantial, gains in life expectancy at age 65 have been relatively small, especially in men. Since 1900, life expectancy at age 65 has increased by 3.3 years for men and 6.5 years for women. A 65-year-old in the United States can expect on the average to live another 17 years. Currently 20% of the U.S. population will live to age 85 or older.[46] If current trends continue, by 2010 half of the population will survive to at least age 85. This has important implications for both health care institutions and community service agencies, since individuals over age 85 are more likely to have some functional disability or to require specialized health care.

Differences in life expectancy among population groups. Gains in the average life span have not been uniform among all populations (Fig. 1-2). Women have made increasing strides in life expectancy compared to men. In 1900 women could expect to live 2 years longer than men of similar age; women now live about 7 years longer. The **gender gap in life expectancy** has been decreasing, however, with men making greater gains. The current difference in

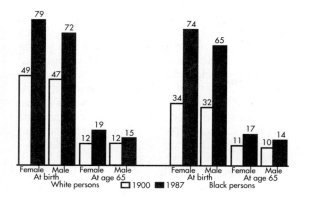

FIG. 1-2   Life expectancy at birth according to sex and race. Females have a longer life expectancy than males, and whites have a longer life expectancy than blacks.

(Data from US Senate Special Committee on Aging: Aging America: trends and projections [annotated], Serial No 101-J, Washington, DC, 1990, US Government Printing Office.)

life expectancy at birth between men and women is 6.8 years, compared to 7.7 years in 1970.[58]

The basis for the increased life span of women as compared to men has received much attention. The increased life span of females observed in experimental animals is believed to relate to genetic factors. The difference in life span between men and women could be influenced by genetic factors or environmental factors or a combination of both. An early study that attempted to control for environment was performed by Madigan,[33] who examined the mortality records and life spans of 10,000 men and 32,000 women living in Catholic teaching orders over a 50-year period. In those groups women lived longer. Since the living situations (and presumably the environmental stress) were believed to be similar, Madigan concluded that women had a biologic resistance to the degenerative diseases that led to earlier death in men. Although this study had major limitations (e.g., possible use of tobacco or alcohol by men or sex differences in adjustment to life in a religious order), it represented a beginning effort

to account for environmental influences when evaluating human life expectancy.

Life-style behaviors influence mortality patterns in both sexes. Cigarette smoking has brought about changes in mortality patterns among women. In the early 1970s it was concluded that two thirds of the difference in life span between men and women at middle age and beyond could be explained by differences in smoking habits. In the first half of this century, smoking was uncommon among women. The increased use of cigarettes in recent decades by women of all ages has caused lung cancer to surpass breast cancer as the leading cause of cancer deaths among women[5] and has added to their risk of heart disease.

A major influence on the mortality differential between men and women is the incidence of heart disease; the mortality rate for men is twice that for women.[17] A biologic component of this difference in deaths from heart disease is the female sex hormone estrogen, which until menopause provides some protection against this disease. Estrogen is known to increase the blood levels of **high-density lipoproteins** (**HDL** cholesterol), which reduce cardiovascular risk, and decrease blood levels of **low-density lipoproteins** (**LDL** cholesterol), which increase the risk. Although after menopause the serum LDL cholesterol levels in women closely approximate those of men, HDL cholesterol levels remain consistently higher.[16] In addition, estrogen controls the distribution of body fat and promotes **fat deposition** about the hips (lower body fat), resulting in a pear shape, rather than about the abdomen and trunk (upper body fat), resulting in an apple shape. Upper body fat, deposited above the umbilicus, is characteristic of weight gain in men and increases the risk of heart disease. Women of all ages also have a heightened immune response, providing more resistance to infections and malignancies.[17]

The accelerated movement of women into the work force led to speculation that stress, considered a major contributor to premature mortality in men, would exert a similar influence in women. An effect of stress per se has yet to be documented; however, other factors that may be job related such as increased cigarette smoking or reduced levels of exercise may in time lead to increased mortality rates in working women.[17]

Race and income also influence life expectancy. As described in Fig. 1-2, blacks have decreased life expectancies compared to whites.[23] Blacks have a lower mean income, which can result in poor quality diets, poor quality medical care, and inferior living conditions. Blacks also are more likely to live in neighborhoods characterized by high rates of crime and victimization.

Mortality rates differed between the black adults and white adults, ages 35 to 77, who participated in the First National Health and Nutrition Examination Survey (NHANES I).[38] About 70% of the higher mortality observed among the black participants was related to smoking habits, a high rate of diabetes, elevated systolic blood pressure (160 mg Hg or higher), high body mass index, and low family income. Otten and colleagues also pointed to racial inequalities in the use of medical intervention procedures to treat coronary heart disease; whites are more likely to receive surgical intervention procedures. Inadequate medical supervision and lack of nutrition counseling for appropriate management of obesity, diabetes, and hypertension very likely contributed to the higher death rate observed among the black participants.

Leading Causes of Death

The leading causes of death in the United States are heart disease, cancer, and **cerebrovascular disease.** These three conditions are responsible for three of every four deaths in people age 65 or older. The number of deaths caused by cancer, especially lung cancer, continues to rise in comparison to the number of deaths caused by heart disease. However, eliminating deaths caused by cancer would have relatively little effect on life expectancy, increasing the average life span by only 2 years. Eliminating deaths from heart disease would add an average of 5 years to life expectancy in the over 65 group.[58]

The current leading causes of death are in sharp contrast to the causes of death common at the turn of the century. At that time infant mortality and infectious diseases such as pneumonia and tuberculosis were the primary causes of death, and many individuals died at a young age. People now survive to an older age and over time develop **chronic** diseases. The increasing vulnerability of the older individual to infection and life-threatening events associated with chronic disease is evident in the dramatic increase in mortality rates between those ages 65 to 74 and those age 85 or older (Table 1-1).

The number of deaths associated with chronic diseases has declined significantly in recent years. Since 1970 death rates from **ischemic heart disease** and cerebrovascular disease have dropped by more than 40%.[55] This decline has been attributed to the implementation of preventive health measures, including reduced dietary fat, regular physical exercise, and avoidance of smoking and excessive use of alcohol. At the same time an increasing number of middle-aged and older adults are rating their health as good to excellent rather than fair to poor.[56] This would suggest that older people who enjoy an increased life span are actually healthier. However, declines in mortality rates could come about through heroic medical inter-

TABLE 1-1   *Leading Causes of Death According to Age*

Cause of Death (Rates/100,000 in Age Group)	65-74	75-84	85+
All causes	2,764	6,266	15,406
Diseases of the heart	1,020	2,556	7,122
Malignant neoplasms	846	1,283	1,632
Cerebrovascular diseases	153	563	1,734
Chronic obstructive pulmonary disease	146	306	363
Pneumonia and influenza	57	235	1,029
Diabetes	60	122	207

Modified from US Senate Special Committee on Aging: *Aging America: trends and projections (annotated),* Serial No 101-J, Washington, DC, 1990, US Government Printing Office.

ventions that rescue frail or debilitated persons from death. These survivors will continue to suffer from serious disease and disability.

According to Verbrugge,[59] prevalence rates for heart disease, **hypertension,** and arthritis have actually increased in recent years as has use of health services and physicians visits. This suggests a greater burden of illness among older people. However, an increased awareness of health issues and more honest reporting, rather than an actual increase in disease prevalence and disability, may account for the observed trends in these latter statistics. Nevertheless, measures promoting good health should be implemented in all age groups to ensure the highest possible level of physical well-being among older adults.

Future Trends

Cigarette smoking is considered the greatest single preventable cause of illness and premature death in the United States.[55] Smokers have a 70% greater risk of death from all causes than nonsmokers, and it is believed that coronary deaths would decrease by 30% if all Americans stopped smoking. Chronic obstructive pulmonary disease is now the fifth leading cause of death in older age groups. Environmental smoke, however, appears to carry less risk for adults than for children.[21] Although smoking continues to decline among adults, each day about 3,000 young people, many of them teenagers, begin smoking.[39]

The report **Healthy People 2000: National Health Promotion and Disease Prevention Objectives** [57] addresses many other health-related factors besides smoking that now contribute to the risk of disease among Americans. About 30% of adults have high blood pressure (above 140/90 mm Hg), and fewer than one fourth of these have it under control. Excess weight is a problem for about one quarter of Americans, and most people in this group are not following sound practices for weight reduction. Fewer than half of adult Americans exercise three or more times per week. Dietary fats, both saturated and unsaturated, account for more than 37% of total kilocalories in the American diet. All of these factors contribute measurably to the development of chronic disease and should be prime targets for health and nutrition education.

SOCIOECONOMIC CHARACTERISTICS OF THE OLDER POPULATION

Living Arrangements

Most older people (95%) live in the community with their spouse, with other family members, with nonrelatives, or alone; only 5% of older people are institutionalized.[50] The living arrangements of those age 65 or older are influenced by sex, marital status, and age (Fig. 1-3). Although most older men remain married until they die, most older women are widowed. Because women have a longer life expectancy, they tend to outlive their husbands. Thus 75% of all

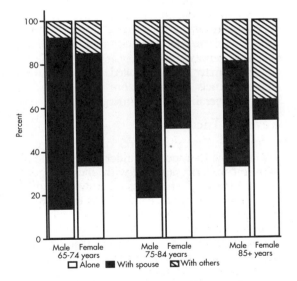

FIG. 1-3   Living arrangements of men and women age 65 and older. Older men are more likely to live with a spouse, whereas older women, especially those over age 74, are more likely to live alone.

(Data from US Bureau of the Census: Marital status and living arrangements, March 1989, Curr Pop Reports Series P-20, No 445, Washington, DC, 1990, US Government Printing Office.)

older men are married and living with their spouses, whereas only 40% of older women are living with their spouses. Nearly half of older women are widowed.

This difference in marital status becomes even more pronounced at older ages. Two thirds of men age 75 or older still live with a spouse, whereas only one fourth of women that age do. More than half of women over age 74 live alone.[50] Although widowed white women tend to maintain individual households, widowed black and Hispanic women are more likely to live with family members.[34] This may relate to the fact that minority older women are more likely to have incomes below the **poverty level**. More older people live in rural or suburban locations than in densely populated areas. Less than one third live in the center of cities.

Living arrangements influence the food intake of older people. The older person who lives alone and has some limitation in physical activity may rely on preprepared items. An aged widow who lives in a rural area and can no longer drive is dependent on friends or relatives for transportation to a food store. Although older people in the inner city may have greater access to services, they may not be visible and therefore may be overlooked. Those living in shabby hotels (single room occupancy) are highly vulnerable to malnutrition.

Level of Income

In general people age 65 or older have less cash income than people under age 65. The median income of families with older heads is about 61% that of younger families; for older individuals, the median income is only 48% of those younger.[53] To a great extent this decrease in cash income is related to retirement, when people lose their former earnings and become dependent on Social Security or other pensions. Social Security payments, which are based on one's income when working, are the principal source of income for most older Americans. Since 1975 Social Security benefits have increased annually according to the increase in the **Consumer Price Index (CPI)** for the previous year.

Since many older people are limited in their ability to increase their income by working,

they become vulnerable to economic uncertainty. The loss of a husband is critical for a wife who depended on his pension and is eligible for very limited Social Security or pension benefits in her own right. A deterioration in health, resulting in continuing medical costs that may not be covered by Medicare or private health insurance can deplete the older person's savings, creating financial anxiety. Costly prescription drugs often divert money from the food budget. Although it is commonly believed that older persons have other financial resources to supplement their cash income, this is not true for many older individuals.[58] As a result, older adults are more likely to fall below the poverty level than younger adults, and they are less able through marriage or employment to increase their income above this level.

Despite the effort through Social Security to provide some income for older people, particular segments of the older population are especially vulnerable to financial insecurity (Fig. 1-4). The oldest-old (those age 85 or older) are the most likely to be poor, with a poverty rate about twice that of the 65 to 74 age group (19% versus 10%).[58] The increased prevalence of poverty in the oldest age group is related in part to marital status. Most women this age are

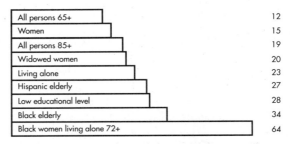

All persons 65+	12
Women	15
All persons 85+	19
Widowed women	20
Living alone	23
Hispanic elderly	27
Low educational level	28
Black elderly	34
Black women living alone 72+	64

Data for persons age 65+ unless noted otherwise

FIG. 1-4 Percentage of typical groups of older people with incomes below the poverty level. Age, sex, race, and marital status influence poverty status in older people.

(From US Senate Special Committee on Aging: Aging America: trends and projections [annotated], Serial No 101-J, Washington, DC, 1990, US Government Printing Office.)

widows and are likely to have been dependent on their husband's income.

Black and Hispanic elderly have lower incomes than do white elderly.[53] Blacks and Hispanics are more likely to have low incomes as younger adults and therefore receive lower Social Security or pension benefits. As described in Fig. 1-4, those with several of these characteristics have an even greater chance of being poor. As more women are entering the work force and establishing Social Security and pension accounts in their own right, this increased prevalence of poverty among older women may decline in future decades.

Older people spend a larger proportion of their income on food, utilities, and health care than do younger people.[58] Conversely, younger households spend proportionately more on clothing, transportation, and entertainment. Both groups spend about the same amount on housing. Out-of-pocket costs for health care are the greatest threat to the economic security of the older individual. Such costs consume 9% of the income of those ages 65 to 74 and 15% of the income of those age 75 years or older, compared to only 4% of the income of younger age groups.[58] The dilemma of who will pay the ever-increasing health care costs of the elderly is far from resolved as government planners seek to shift more of the costs to private insurance companies and the elderly consumers themselves. The relationship between income, food expenditures, and nutritional status in older people is discussed in Chapter 12.

BIOLOGIC ASPECTS OF AGING

The progression of biologic and physiologic events that occur over the life span has been observed for centuries, but only in recent years has the study of aging begun to emerge as a science. Investigators have tried to separate those changes that occur in all people, and are therefore considered to represent normal aging, from the changes associated with the development of chronic disease. However, this approach to the study of aging, using age-related versus disease-related changes, does have serious limitations in that it neglects the extreme heterogenicity that exists among older people

who are relatively free of chronic disease.[42] In recent years the study of aging has focused on the cell and those internal mechanisms that trigger the age-related changes observed in organs, tissues, and functions. Identifying the biologic mechanisms responsible for these age-related events will allow us to develop strategies to retard or minimize their effects.

The Aging Process

In broad terms the definition of aging includes all of the structural and functional changes that occur throughout the life span from embryonic development through maturation and **senescence**.[44] **Gerontology,** or the study of aging, encompasses not only the physiologic or behavioral changes observed but also the environmental factors—biologic, sociologic, or psychologic—that influence these changes. The *sequence* of age-related changes tends to be the same in all members of a particular species, although the *rate* at which changes occur differs widely from one individual to another. **Geriatrics,** in contrast to gerontology, is the study of the medical problems of the aged. Unfortunately, research in aging has tended to emphasize age-related losses and the time-dependent changes that increase one's vulnerability to disease.

Usual versus Successful Aging

The study of **normal aging** has allowed us to evaluate the physical and psychological differences between adults of different ages. At the same time the emphasis on normal aging has implied that such changes are natural and therefore unresponsive to modification. Rowe and Kahn[42] have introduced the concept of **"usual"** versus **"successful" aging.** According to these authors, the portrayal of the aging process as unpreventable or irreversible has been exaggerated and the potential modifying effect of life-style factors has been underestimated. Usual aging refers to the changes occurring in older people that represent the aging process exacerbated by disease and adverse environmental and life-style factors. Successful aging is demonstrated in individuals in whom age-related changes have not been augmented or accelerated as a result of disease, environmental influences, or life-style.

Positive intervention and health promotion strategies have in fact reduced or delayed age-related changes in body composition, glucose tolerance, and cardiovascular function. The goal of nutrition intervention in both younger and older adults is to facilitate the transition from usual to successful aging. Examples of positive intervention will be presented in succeeding chapters.

Factors Influencing the Aging Process

Intrinsic factors. In his treatise on how to live three score and 10 years, Oliver Wendell Holmes facetiously recommended that individuals advertise for parents from families whose members survived to age 80 or 90.[44] The genetic material combined at the moment of fertilization, along with environmental influences, determines the rate of aging and the ultimate life span. One very obvious genetic characteristic influencing longevity is one's sex; in most species, including humans, females live longer than males. People who live to age 70 or beyond are more likely to have had parents who also survived to that age.[44] Although it is generally recognized that genetic inheritance exerts a major influence on the length of life, the mechanism of genetic control is poorly understood. Genetic control of the rate of aging could be exerted through the regulation of protein synthesis. Atherosclerotic damage to major coronary arteries increases one's risk of a cardiovascular attack. As pointed out by Weksler,[63] the individual with an increased ability to produce HDL cholesterol may enjoy increased protection against coronary heart disease.

The immune system and the body's defense mechanisms are under genetic control. **Centenarians** have a well-preserved immune system compared to other older people.[11] They produce a greater number of lymphocytes in response to an antigenic stimulus, but fewer of those cell types capable of producing **autoimmune** reactions and cellular injury. The study of centenarians who have "something special" as far as their genetic makeup is concerned could help shed light on the genetic mechanism controlling the rate of aging.

Extrinsic factors. Environmental factors can modify the genetic program in both animal models and humans. In animals exposed to irradiation, aging is accelerated as a result of genetic mutation and the subsequent replication of imperfect proteins.[7] Chronic exposure to sunlight or an ultraviolet lamp increases the rate of change in skin collagen that results in characteristic skin wrinkling. Excessive exposure to sunlight is associated with an increased incidence of skin cancer. Nutrient intake, both qualitatively and quantitatively, appears to have the greatest potential for positive alteration of the genetic program. Dietary intervention can not only extend the life span but also promote successful aging and an enhanced quality of life. The influence of nutrition on the life span and the development of chronic disease is discussed in Chapter 2.

Aging at the Cellular Level

The classic work in cellular aging was performed by Hayflick,[15] who used undifferentiated cells obtained from connective tissue and cultured on a nutrient medium. These experiments revealed that all normal cells are limited to a finite number of divisions. The number of divisions reflects the life span of that particular species. Cells taken from a mouse with a life expectancy of 3½ years will divide about 21 times; cells taken from a human with a life expectancy of 70 years will divide about 50 times. The number of cell divisions is also related to the donor's age; 60% of the cells obtained from young men divided at least eight times over a 2-week period, but this was true for only 2% of the cells obtained from older men.[54]

Although these studies provide a conceptual framework for understanding the aging process at the cellular level, the limited **proliferative capacity** of cells is not generally considered to be the basis of age-related changes in organs and tissues. Highly differentiated cells in muscle or neural tissues lose their mitotic ability early in life. Liver and kidney cells retain the ability to divide, but do not do so under normal circumstances. Organs made up of highly specialized cells lose tissue as a result of cell death or functional changes in remaining cells.

Currently the molecular mechanisms leading to cell death are not understood. Senescent cells do lose their ability to synthesize deoxyribonucleic acid (DNA). Concentrations of normal cellular proteins decrease, and abnormal cellular proteins increase. In light of these changes, current research on aging mechanisms is directed toward protein synthesis and genetic regulation.[18]

Theories of Aging

Aging does not have a single cause, and no adequate theory has emerged to explain it.[7] Historically researchers have viewed aging as "a thing that happens" rather than as a period in the life of an individual that begins at maturity and continues for the remainder of the life span. Our view of aging should be the same as our view of development. In both development and aging, numerous changes occur, some caused by the environment and others directed from within the body. From these processes have developed two major theories of aging, the **environmental theory** and the **developmental-genetic theory.**[7]

Environmental theory. The environmental theory suggests that aging is the result of random insults that cause mutations in the genetic material and the synthesis of abnormal proteins. The proteins produced from faulty DNA do not perform as expected, leaving the cell impaired in its ability to carry on essential functions, and eventually death ensues. This theory was studied using irradiation as the insult leading to genetic mutation. Although irradiation does shorten the life span, the mechanism involved does not bear any relationship to normal mechanisms of aging. The notion that environmental influences on genetic material lead to the accumulation of nonfunctional proteins is not supported by direct evidence indicating the synthesis of altered proteins. Although abnormal proteins are found in aging cells, their presence could be explained by the inability of an older cell to remove unusable proteins.[7,18]

Developmental-genetic theory. The developmental-genetic theory proposes that aging is a continuation of development and is under genetic control. The mechanism by which the genetic program unfolds is still unclear. The master timekeeper could be the hypothalamus, which exerts its influence on major organ systems through the pituitary and adrenal hormones. Genetic control of the aging process could also be exerted through the immune system. Reduced T-cell function and reduced resistance to infection have been related to a reduced life span in both humans and animal models.[3,7] As noted earlier, centenarians have a level of immune function more like healthy young adults than older adults.

The most compelling evidence to support a genetic involvement in the aging process comes from the fact that monozygotic twins with an identical genetic inheritance are markedly similar in life span, whereas dizygotic twins or other siblings are not.[44] Nevertheless, environmental and life-style factors may act to hasten or retard the genetic effect. Genetic control of the life span is likely to be related to a predisposition to a potentially fatal disease (e.g., diabetes, hypercholesterolemia).

PHYSIOLOGIC ASPECTS OF AGING

Physical Health

Functional assessment. Changes in physical appearance (graying of the hair or use of a cane for walking) may provide clues to chronologic age; however, an individual's functional ability to continue independent living in the community or personal care is less easily defined. In **acute** conditions such as diabetic coma, the medical diagnosis and the ability to function are closely linked. This is not true for chronic diseases. An older individual with compensated cardiac failure or well-controlled diabetes mellitus may function quite well and lead an active, independent life. Thus disease-oriented models are limited in their power to identify those who require help with personal or household tasks. Two indices that have been developed to measure functional status as related to the ability to live independently or the need for care are the **activities of daily living** and the **instrumental activities of daily living.**[28]

Activities of daily living (ADLs) relate to personal care:
- Bathing
- Dressing
- Feeding oneself

- Using the toilet
- Transferring between bed and chair

The instrumental activities of daily living (IADLs) involve the ability to perform household and social tasks:

- Meal preparation
- House cleaning
- Handling money
- Shopping
- Getting around in the community

Inability to walk is not always a predictor of dependence, since individuals may overcome the problem by relying on canes, walkers, or wheelchairs.

In a recent national survey[28] nearly 13% of noninstitutionalized people age 65 or older had difficulty with at least one ADL task or with walking, and most had had the problem for longer than 3 months. Bathing (9%) and walking (8%) were the most common problems. A greater number of elderly (18%) had difficulty with at least one IADL task, and getting about the community (14%) and shopping (11%) were mentioned most frequently. Functional difficulties also increase with age. Only 6% of people ages 65 to 69 had difficulty with at least one ADL, compared to 34% of those ages 80 to 84, more than a fivefold difference. The effect of advancing age is even more pronounced when evaluating difficulties with household tasks. More than half of those ages 80 to 84 reported difficulty with at least one IADL. The proportion of black elderly reporting problems with IADL tasks was higher than for white or Hispanic elderly. Among older people living alone, nearly one in four reported difficulty with at least one IADL task.

Older people who report difficulty with at least one IADL could have a compromised nutrient intake. Some older individuals cannot shop for food and are dependent on family or friends, who may deliver food somewhat infrequently; these older people are forced to rely on shelf-stable items, and they consume fewer dairy products and fresh fruits and vegetables. If freezer space is limited, the diet may include many canned or dehydrated vegetables, fruits, soups, or main dishes, which can be high in sodium and fat and limited in important vitamins and minerals. For the older person who has difficulty preparing meals, preprepared items may make up the majority of foods eaten. Helping older people with limited functional capacity make appropriate food choices from those available and making them aware of available nutrition services (e.g., home-delivered meals) should be an important component of home care.

Presence of chronic disease. Chronic incurable diseases are uncommon in younger people but increase in frequency through middle age. At least four of every five individuals age 65 or older have one chronic condition, and many have several.[58] Watkin[61] quoted a survey of congregate meal participants in which 60% had one to six chronic disorders. The most common chronic conditions among older people are arthritis (48%), heart disease (44%), hypertension (37%), impaired hearing (30%), orthopedic problems (16%), and cataracts (16%). Impaired mobility caused by arthritis or poor vision hinders the older person in both food shopping and meal preparation. Failing eyesight precludes driving or walking to a food store. At least 40% of older people have heart disease, hypertension, or arthritis, conditions that require a reduction in dietary fat or sodium and weight control as part of their treatment.

Health status. Most older people consider themselves to be in good health despite the presence of chronic disease. In a national health survey of more than 27,000 noninstitutionalized elderly,[58] 69% of the participants described their health as excellent, very good, or good as compared with others their age; only 31% considered their health to be fair or poor. A person's perception of his or her health, however, is directly related to income. Only 11% of those with the lowest income reported their health to be excellent, and 15% reported their health to be poor. Conversely, 26% of those with the highest income considered their health to be excellent, and only 6% considered it to be poor.

Despite generally positive attitudes toward their health, depression and mental health problems play a significant role in the health status of older people. Depression may adversely affect the course of an illness in an older person. Poor self-rated health has been shown to be a significant predictor of hospital stays and nursing home placement among lower income elderly.[62] Among older participants in NHANES I, however, health behaviors (e.g., smoking) and demographic characteristics (e.g., age, race, marital status) were stronger predictors of mortality over a 12-year period than poor self-rated health.[20] Older people are at particular risk for depression because of physical illness and their high use of prescription drugs that can alter mental function. Mental health services must be made available to older people on a more consistent basis. (Cognitive disorders resulting from organic brain syndrome are discussed later in this chapter.)

Use of health services. Use of health services is related to sex and income level as well as age. Because older women live longer, they continue to develop chronic physical problems that require medical attention. Low-income elderly and black and Hispanic elderly are less likely to have private health insurance[14] and may not seek medical care even when it is necessary because they are unable to pay for the service. On the average people age 65 or older visit a physician eight times a year, compared to five visits per year by the general population.[56] Older people are three times more likely than younger ones to be hospitalized during the year.[58] Most of these hospital admissions are for acute episodes related to a chronic condition such as heart disease or respiratory disease. When admitted to the hospital, older people stay longer than younger persons. People over age 75 make up only 5% of the population but account for 23% of all hospital days.[58] The need for health care is greatest among the oldest-old. Individuals age 85 or older are seven times more likely to enter a nursing home than those ages 65 to 74.[58]

Integration of Physiologic Systems

Changes in physiologic function. One characteristic of physiologic aging is a decrease in the ability to respond to changes in either the internal or external environment. The rate of recovery or return to homeostasis is slowed in the older individual. This altered response could stem from a decrease in the sensitivity of control receptors or from actual changes in tissue

and organ function. Fig. 1-5 shows the age-related decline in physiologic systems observed among men ages 30 to 80.[54] The age-related loss in function is shown as a percentage of the level of function observed at age 30. These data were obtained from the **Baltimore Longitudinal Study of Aging (BLSA)** being conducted by the National Institute on Aging. Although these values represent **cross-sectional** comparisons of the level of function of different age groups, the long-range goal of the BLSA is to record the changes occurring within individuals over their adult lives.

Physiologic responses differ in their level of change according to the degree of coordination required among organ systems. The fasting blood glucose level exhibits little change under resting conditions. Nerve conduction velocity, a function involving one organ system, decreases by about 15%. Resting cardiac output, which requires both neural and muscular coordination, declines by 30%. When the desired response involves many organ systems (e.g., maximum work rate) the age-related decline is substantial (70%).[54]

In general, changes in physiologic function are most evident when simple behaviors are

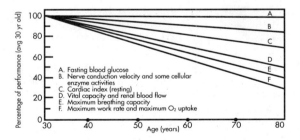

FIG. 1-5   Degree of loss in physiologic functions between ages 30 and 80. Major organ systems, including the heart, lungs, and kidneys, undergo a loss in function as a result of normal aging (e.g., by age 80, nerve conduction velocity is only 85% of its level at age 30). These changes were observed in men in the Baltimore Longitudinal Study of Aging.

(Data from US Department of Health and Human Services: Normal human aging: the Baltimore Longitudinal Study of Aging, NIH Publication No 84-2450, Washington, DC, 1984, US Government Printing Office.)

compared to more complex ones. An older person may walk with comparative ease on a level surface, whereas climbing stairs, which demands more complicated muscular motions and compensation for a greater oxygen expenditure, may require heavy effort and lead to **tachycardia** and labored breathing. Food preparation that requires both visual and motor coordination, such as peeling vegetables, may become difficult. Loss of neuromuscular control is believed to contribute significantly to the loss of muscle coordination.

Despite changes in physiologic capacity, most older people function quite well on a day-to-day basis under normal conditions. For most organ systems the level of maximum functional performance is seven to 11 times the average physiologic demand[54]; thus some degree of loss can occur with no noticeable change in function. However, when extreme demands are placed on the system or when functional losses are excessive, problems become evident. As described in a later section, physiologic considerations such as reduced kidney function enter into dietary recommendations for older people.

Variability among individuals. Normal aging results in functional changes in the same direction in most people, but the *rate* of change is unique to each individual. In fact, the variability among individuals of the same age may actually exceed the variability among people of different ages.[44] Both genetic constitution and lifelong experiences that influence physical well-being exert an effect. Since no two people experience the same combination or intensity of influences, by age 60 all individuals are remarkably different. On this basis older people differ more from one another than do younger persons. Such differences underscore the need to assess each older person as an individual.

AGING AND NEUROENDOCRINE FUNCTION
Mental Function

Neither the changes in mental function associated with normal aging nor the age when such changes occur have been defined. Yet ascertaining the degree of loss of mental function in a particular individual can be of practical importance. When to relinquish one's driver's license often is an excruciating decision for the older person or for the family of an older driver whose reaction time has deteriorated below a safe level.[60] The results of a test of **cognitive** skills developed to measure response time, memory, and reasoning suggest that mental capacity begins to decline about age 45, but greater changes occur after age 65.[47] However, not all people experience the same degree of change. Those beyond the usual retirement age of 65 whose test scores were similar to those of younger subjects were most likely to be working, whereas those scoring lower than younger subjects were in many instances retired. This finding leaves us with a dilemma: do people stop working because they realize they are no longer able to function at the same level, or do people lose mental acuity because they no longer have the mental stimulation associated with work responsibilities? Continuing research on both behavioral and biologic aspects of neural function may provide an answer to this question.

Brain and Neural Tissue

Structural aspects. The central nervous system is composed of neurons, or structural cells, and glia, or supporting cells. Neurons lose the capacity to divide after cell differentiation; glial cells continue to divide throughout life. The functional significance of the resulting change in proportion of neurons to glia is not yet understood.[48] At one time it was believed that normal aging was characterized by brain atrophy and a significant loss of neurons. Recent work suggests that some degree of neuronal loss occurs after age 50; however, massive losses of neurons occur only in those suffering from brain diseases such as **senile dementia of the Alzheimer type (SDAT)**.[19,22] In normal older people neither brain size nor cell number is related to mental function.

The aging brain also appears to be capable of some degree of regeneration not heretofore recognized.[22] As some nerve cells deteriorate and die, accounting for the decreased number of neurons, one special type of neuron is preserved and in healthy older people may actually increase in number. These neurons, found in the regions of the brain associated with higher thought processes, contain acetylcholinesterase, the enzyme required for the metabolism of acetylcholine. **Acetylcholine** is the neurotransmitter required for normal neuronal function in this region of the brain.

The aging brain also retains the ability to form additional **dendrites** in the remaining neurons.[47] This increase in dendrites, the treelike branches that transmit impulses to and from the nerve cell body, makes new connections possible and may compensate for the loss in number of nerve cells. This growth in dendrites also allows the formation of new pathways for neural transmission and may explain why some older people maintain a high level of cognitive function despite some neuronal loss.

Biochemical aspects. Biochemical as well as structural changes take place in the brains of older people even in the absence of neurologic diseases. Conduction of neural impulses requires the release of a chemical transmitter (e.g., **dopamine,** serotonin, or acetylcholine) by the neuron. Sufficient numbers of transmitter molecules must be present in the synapse (the space between the neural cells) to activate the adjoining cell. Normal aging is associated with reduced levels of neurotransmitters in brain tissues. This decreased level of neurotransmitters could result from a decrease in synthesis. Two common neurotransmitters, dopamine and norepinephrine, are derived from tyrosine; serotonin is derived from tryptophan. The enzymes required for these biochemical conversions, tyrosine hydroxylase and aromatic amino acid decarboxylase, are also reduced in the neurons of older people.[41] Whether these differences relate to the changing proportions of neurons and glia or to changes in the synthesis of neurotransmitters within existing cells is not clear.

It is known, however, that the production of neurotransmitters by nerve cells can fall by 20% to 30% with no significant change in brain function.[35] Thus normal physiologic aging would not appear to exceed the functional reserve capacity of the normal brain. However, when neurotransmitter synthesis falls below 50% of that observed in young adults, some degree of dementia ensues.[35]

Age-Related Disorders of the Nervous System

Of all the age-related changes that can present difficulties for older individuals and their families, none causes greater anxiety than the loss of mental function. In most healthy older people, occasional forgetfulness may be the only obvious change in mental function. In about 10% of older persons, forgetfulness progresses to mild or moderate confusion. About 15% of older people have severe dementia, or so-called senile **dementia,** with loss of cognitive function and disturbances in behavior and mood.[48]

Age is the single most important risk factor for dementia in older people.[48] SDAT is the most common cause of dementia in older people and accounts for more than half of all cases. Loss of brain cells resulting from a cerebral hemorrhage or interruption of the blood supply to a particular region of the brain accounts for 20% to 30% of all cases.[48] Delirium or severe dementia can arise from acute electrolyte disturbances involving changes in sodium or potassium levels, thyroid dysfunction, drug toxicity, or illnesses that decrease the oxygen supply to the brain, as occurs in pneumonia or cardiac failure. Dementia occurring for the latter reasons usually is reversible following amelioration of the metabolic disturbance or infection (see Chapter 9). Changes in cognitive function stemming from SDAT or other excessive loss of brain cells are irreversible.

Senile dementia of the Alzheimer type. Two million Americans have SDAT and the associated costs of long-term care exceed $40 billion a year.[6] SDAT is characterized by (1) a loss of cells from the cerebral cortex and other areas of the brain that control higher level function, and (2) the appearance in brain tissue of senile plaques (nerve cells surrounding a protein core) and neurofibrillary tangles of helical filaments. Although senile plaques and neurofibrillary tangles occur in normal aging, they are fewer in number. In SDAT the levels of all neurotransmitters are markedly reduced.

SDAT is more common among women; however, this may be because women live longer than men. Nevertheless, female gender might be a risk factor, since family history is involved in about half of SDAT patients.[48] The roles of viruses or environmental contaminants, particularly aluminum, are being studied, but at this time no specific involvement has been identified. Trauma to the head earlier in life does appear to be related to the development of SDAT.

In the early stages people with SDAT experience recent memory loss, personality changes, and increasing difficulty with daily activities, including finding their way around or preparing meals. In the latter stages these patients cannot perform any activity of daily living, and they become totally dependent on family care givers or are admitted to a long-term care facility. (Problems related to feeding the SDAT patient are discussed in Chapter 12.)

Parkinson's disease. About 1 million Americans have **Parkinson's disease.**[65] Although this disorder is uncommon among people under age 50, the incidence increases with age and peaks about age 75. Parkinson's disease is caused by a loss of neurons from the base of the brain whose function is production of the neurotransmitter dopamine. Dopamine is important in the control of muscle movement. When dopamine is no longer produced in sufficient quantities, the characteristic symptoms of Parkinson's disease—muscular rigidity, tremors, difficulty with balance, and a shuffling gait—become evident.

The usual treatment has been administration of the drug levodopa to supplement the body's natural supply of dopamine.[65] As more neurons are lost, the patient is forced to take ever-increasing levels of the drug to keep symptoms in check. Such levels of levodopa can cause undesirable side effects such as mental confusion and gastrointestinal distress. Unfortunately, administered levodopa becomes less effective over time. Current research is directed toward drugs that will slow the rate of neuronal loss, thereby reducing the amount of levodopa required for control.

Endocrine System

Many components of the endocrine system undergo changes in the aging individual, but these changes do not proceed in a uniform direction (Table 1-2).[45] Some endocrine organs

TABLE 1-2   *Age-Related Changes in Serum Hormone Levels in Older People*

Increased Levels	Decreased Levels	No Change
Norepinephrine	Triiodothyronine	Epinephrine
Antidiuretic hormone (vasopressin)	Estradiol (in women)	Cortisol
Insulin	Testosterone (in men)	Thyroxin
Parathyroid hormone		Growth hormone
		Aldosterone

Modified from Solomon DH: Introduction. Organs systems: metabolic and endocrine disorders. In Abrams WB, Berkow R, editors: *Merck manual of geriatrics,* Rahway, NJ, 1990, Merck Sharp & Dohme Research Laboratories.

become hypoactive as a result of disease or reduced hormone utilization or excretion. For example, a reduction in lean body mass and hormone utilization is thought to be the basis for the age-related decline in the secretion of triiodothyronine and its metabolic conversion to thyroid hormone. (This is discussed further in Chapter 3.) Age-associated increases in vasopressin (antidiuretic hormone) and norepinephrine are thought to reflect a compensatory response of the **hypothalamic-neurohypophyseal axis** to the decreased number of hormone receptors in target tissues. Serum hormone levels are the end result of all structural and metabolic changes in endocrine-related tissues.

Nutritional status can influence endocrine activity.[36] Changes in the synthesis of plasma proteins that serve as transport molecules for hormones influence not only blood hormone concentrations but also the rates of conversion to active forms. At the same time, endocrine function has an important influence on nutritional status. Mild decreases in the secretion of growth hormone and changes in serum testosterone levels may contribute to the decline in nitrogen retention observed in some older people.[36] The role of insulin in protein utilization and storage could be especially critical in aged individuals with borderline intakes or excessive losses of protein.[36] Altered endocrine function could contribute to impaired ability to adapt to changes in nutrient intake. Current research on endocrine function in aging is directed toward the hypothalamic-neurohypophyseal axis, which regulates hormone secretion, and possible changes in sensitivity to messages received in both the hypothalamus and target tissues.

AGING IN ORGAN SYSTEMS
Cardiovascular System

Cardiac structure and function in older individuals are the result of age-related changes complicated by life-style factors and disease. **Occult** forms of disease can exaggerate the functional changes in the heart assumed to be due to aging, leading to an erroneous conclusion about the age effect.[26] This problem is complicated further by difficulties in diagnosis. Although half of all individuals age 60 or older have severe coronary artery disease, only half of these exhibit clinical symptoms.[26] Coronary artery disease, along with age-related changes, contributes to the considerable decline in cardiovascular performance observed among some older people.

Structural changes in the cardiovascular system. The aging heart can atrophy, exhibit moderate or marked hypertrophy, or remain unchanged, depending on the particular individual.[26] Cardiac atrophy occurs only with severe wasting disease and does not represent normal aging; neither does marked cardiac hypertrophy, which usually is the result of severe hypertension. Mean heart weight when related to body surface area or body size does not change with age in healthy older men.[25] In women heart weight increased slightly between the ages of 40 and 70.[25] This increase in women may be related to the small rise in blood pressure sometimes associated with menopause. Modest increases in the thickness of the left ventricular wall occur in normotensive individuals who are free of disease. This change in thickness is believed to result from an increase in cardiac cell size, not from an increase in fatty or fibrous tissue. Fat deposition in the human heart is related to total body fat and not to age.[26]

Changes caused by aging take place in the major arteries independent of atherosclerotic disease. The aorta increases in diameter and length, and the arterial walls stiffen and lose their elasticity. Increases in elastin and collagen and the deposition of calcium contribute to these changes. Whether any changes take place in the smooth muscle of the major arteries is not known.[26]

Changes in cardiovascular function. For most healthy older people, cardiac function at low or moderate levels of activity is sufficient to meet physiologic needs. Resting heart rate does not change with age. **Cardiac output** at resting levels does not decline in physically active older people who have no heart disease. Although cardiac output need not change as a function of age, it does so in many elderly individuals as a result of coronary artery disease or hypertension. A reduction in lean body mass, resulting in a lower tissue demand for oxygen, can also lead to lower cardiac output.[27]

Age-related changes in cardiovascular function become most obvious under conditions of strenuous exercise, when the workload of the heart increases fourfold to fivefold above resting levels. Although older individuals cannot increase their heart rate to the extent that younger individuals can, older people can increase their **stroke volume,** or the amount of blood delivered with each beat of the heart, thereby increasing cardiac output. In younger people added adrenergic stimulation increases the strength of the contraction of the cardiac muscle but decreases the duration of the contraction, thus increasing the heart rate. Plasma epinephrine and norepinephrine levels are higher in older adults than in younger adults under conditions of vigorous exercise, suggesting an increase in adrenergic activity; however, the aging cardiovascular system is less responsive to adrenergic stimulation and less able to react to excessive physiologic demands.[26]

The ability to perform physical work or vigorous exercise depends on a constant and sufficient supply of oxygen to working muscles and tissues. This places demands on both the respiratory and cardiovascular systems, since sufficient oxygen must be taken into the body and delivered to the cells and tissues. Maximum body oxygen consumption, along with maximum work capacity, declines with age, although to a variable extent. The maximum oxygen consumption of older people who exercise regularly exceeds that of sedentary younger people. This suggests that physical conditioning retards the age-related decline in cardiovascular performance or, conversely, that a lack of physical activity rather than the aging process itself brings about cardiovascular decline.[26]

The decrease in maximum oxygen consumption observed in healthy older people may be caused by changes in the **peripheral** tissues rather than by changes in cardiovascular function. A loss in lean body mass reduces the maximum amount of work performed and in proportion the level of oxygen required. In fact, when maximum oxygen consumption is evaluated on the basis of creatinine excretion, an indicator of lean body mass, the differences between older and younger groups are greatly diminished.[27] Regular physical exercise is an important factor in maintaining cardiovascular function and promoting successful aging.

The older person with advanced coronary artery disease poorly tolerates stress arising from either physiologic or emotional causes. These individuals may function well under ordinary conditions but develop tachycardia with emotional stress, fever, or exercise. This points to the importance of medical evaluation of an older person before he or she starts an exercise program. Also, those who have been sedentary must take a gradual approach to increasing the length and intensity of exercise.

If cardiac function is impaired, the reduced cardiac output will compromise the function of other organ systems. In those with cardiovascular disease, cerebral blood flow can be decreased by 20% and renal blood flow by as much as 60%.[24] A diminished supply of blood and oxygen to the brain has been implicated in the loss of mental function in some older people. Removal of waste products is less efficient when the glomerular filtration rate is reduced. A decline in cardiovascular performance has far-reaching consequences for the functional capability of the aged individual. Therefore efforts

throughout adulthood to decrease the risk of coronary artery disease and maintain a high level of fitness should be a priority.

Hypertension. In western societies both systolic and diastolic blood pressures tend to rise until about age 60. Beyond that age systolic blood pressure may continue to rise, whereas diastolic blood pressure remains the same or may actually decline. When defined on the basis of a systolic pressure of 140 mm Hg or higher and a diastolic pressure of 90 mm Hg or higher, 64% of those between the ages of 65 and 74 have hypertension.[13] Aged blacks have a higher incidence of hypertension than aged whites. Eighty-three percent of older black women, compared to 66% of older white women, have elevated blood pressure. Comparable values for older black men and older white men are 67% and 59%, respectively.[64] Hypertension carries with it a high risk of cardiovascular mortality, and the high prevalence of elevated blood pressure among older blacks no doubt contributes to the increased number of deaths from **stroke** among blacks.[4] Controlled studies of antihypertensive therapy among older people have demonstrated a 38% reduction in cardiovascular mortality.[64] In general, elevated systolic blood pressure is a stronger predictor of cardiovascular complications than is elevated diastolic pressure.[13]

The widespread prevalence of hypertension among older people has led to the belief that a rise in arterial blood pressure is associated with normal aging. Evidence to suggest that this rise is environmental or cultural rather than biologic comes from the observation that in primitive societies, neither systolic nor diastolic blood pressure rises with age.[26] Hypertension can have many causes in older people. Atherosclerotic disease increases the rigidity and decreases the distensibility of the large arteries. Reduced distensibility of the aorta to the volume of blood delivered from the left ventricle is a major factor in the development of isolated systolic hypertension in older people. Enhanced activity of the renin-angiotensin system, which increases vascular resistance, or decreased activity of the prostaglandin system, which normally reduces vascular resistance and blood pressure levels, can contribute to the development of hypertension. Hyperthyroidism, thiamin deficiency with clinical or subclinical beriberi, and fever bring about a rise in systolic blood pressure.[13]

A study comparing urban and rural communities in China[2] suggests that age-related changes in blood pressure may be prevented, at least in part, by reducing sodium consumption. Arterial blood pressure and arterial distensibility were measured in 524 people ranging in age from 2 months to 94 years from two communities with a low and high sodium intake, respectively. Measurements of the arterial pulse wave velocity (pulse waves travel more rapidly along the blood vessel if it is less distensible) indicated a difference in the two groups independent of arterial blood pressure. The arterial walls were more rigid and less distensible in individuals from the community in which salt intakes were traditionally high. Lowering the intake of sodium may help delay the onset of age-related changes in blood pressure.

Hypertension is a significant medical and nutritional problem among older people. Unabated hypertension brings about hypertrophy of the left ventricle of the heart and eventually cardiac failure with impaired kidney function. The prevention of and appropriate treatment for hypertension is discussed in subsequent chapters.

Renal System

Changes in renal function. Kidney function can deteriorate with age as a result of both the loss of nephrons and changes in blood flow. The pathophysiology of these changes, however, is open to question. The long-held notion that aging led to an inevitable loss of nephrons and deterioration in renal function is not supported by findings from the BLSA based on 254 men who have been followed for 24 years.[31] One third of the men demonstrated no change in renal function based on a measurement of the **glomerular filtration rate (GFR)**. In fact, a small group showed an actual increase in glomerular filtration rate over time.

Despite these findings among the generally healthy BLSA men, it must be recognized that degenerative changes in renal structure and function do take place in some individuals beginning about age 40. Kidney mass can decrease by as much as 30% by age 90, with primary losses occurring in the capillary bed where filtration occurs. These structural changes contribute to an age-related decline in GFR of about 1 ml per minute per year after age 30. In the BLSA the GFR fell from 140 ml per minute in men ages 25 to 34 to 97 ml per minute in those ages 75 to 84.[54]

The aged kidney is also less able to increase the urine flow rate or increase urine osmolality.[54] These changes reduce the capacity to excrete waste products and can become critical in older individuals who have low fluid intakes and high intakes of protein or electrolytes. The ability to form a concentrated urine after 12 hours of restricted fluid intake was significantly less in older versus younger or middle-aged people. Older people remain sensitive to vasopressin but are less able to transport solute into the renal tubule.[29]

Hyperperfusion and hyperfiltration. The wide variation in kidney function among older people supports the idea that detrimental changes may result from disease or pathologic processes rather than from normal aging. When the number of functioning nephrons is reduced because of disease or infection or when the filtration load of the kidney is increased, the kidney responds with an "adaptive" hyperperfusion and hyperfiltration.[30] The filtration load of the kidney can increase with hypertension, in uncontrolled diabetes when blood glucose levels become excessive, or when protein intake is high, leading to increased levels of urea or other nitrogenous waste. Under such conditions the renal cells increase in size by means of hypertrophy. The GFR increases through vasodilation of the arterioles that deliver blood to the nephron. These responses appear in situations of stress and are discontinued when the need to increase both blood flow and filtration is removed.[30] For example, the GFR is known to rise after a meal containing 80 g of protein and then return to normal.[29] However, when this adaptive increase in the GFR is long in duration as a result of continued high protein intake, systemic hypertension, or infection, the capillary membranes are damaged and deposition of connective tissue and mineral salts ensues.

The inability of many older people to increase their GFR suggests that they are already in a state of hyperperfusion and hyperfiltration and no longer have a renal reserve. Limiting protein intake in older people with compromised kidney function might restore some degree of renal reserve and slow the progression of renal deterioration. Controlling high blood pressure also offers some protection to the aging kidney.[29]

Any loss in kidney function has implications for both the conservation of nutrients and the excretion of potentially harmful waste products. Important molecules actively reabsorbed in the kidney tubule include glucose, amino acids, ascorbic acid, and plasma proteins. An excessive protein intake that produces high levels of nitrogenous waste and hydrogen ions may burden a less efficient kidney. It has been suggested that protein intake not exceed two times the Recommended Dietary Allowance in people of all ages.[10] Megadoses of vitamins, taken on the assumption that what is not needed can be readily excreted, may accumulate at high levels while awaiting excretion. Drug dosages may also need to be adjusted in light of altered excretion rates.

Pulmonary System

Aging changes can interfere with the functions of the lungs, including ventilation of the **alveoli** and the exchange of oxygen and carbon dioxide across the alveolar membrane. Inflammatory injuries to the lungs resulting from smoking or oxidation reactions with environmental toxins or smoke can lead to obstruction of airways and can interfere with tissue repair.[49]

Structural changes in the lung cause a decrease in elasticity and loss of alveolar surface area. Alveolar membranes weaken and stretch, and air sacs become larger with the collapse of small airways. The surface area for gas exchange can decline by as much as 30% in advanced age.[49] Gas exchange is also less efficient because of the thickening and reduced permeability of the alveolar membranes and the reduced flow of blood through the alveolar capillaries. As a result, oxygen partial pressure in arterial blood

decreases; oxyhemoglobin saturation is about 90% in older people, compared to 96% in younger people.[24] Because the chest wall stiffens and is less easily expanded, the work of breathing is increased. Total lung capacity does not change, although the proportion of alveolar space that is ventilated with each breath decreases and **residual volume** increases. Even when corrected for sex, height, and weight, the volume of air moved in and out of the lung with each breath decreases with age.[49]

Healthy older people who are relatively free of lung disease can still be vulnerable to complications with diseases such as pneumonia that lead to reduced oxygen levels. Age-associated alterations in the central nervous system appear to decrease the sensitivity of the chemoreceptors to changes in the blood and tissue levels of oxygen and carbon dioxide. In younger people **hypoxia** and **hypercapnia** usually bring about an increase in the breathing and heart rates, which increases the supply of oxygen or removes the excessive levels of carbon dioxide. In older people response rates are about half those in younger persons and are independent of changes in the lung itself. Older people in whom lung function is compromised are especially limited in their ability to respond to a decreased oxygen supply because of their diminished capacity to ventilate the lungs as well as their reduced neural drive to breathe.[49]

Internal Environment

Body cells require a fluid environment maintained within narrow limits of pH, oxygen content, and electrolyte composition. Blood plasma constituents exhibit little variation on the basis of age. The return to resting levels after the addition of acid or base, however, is slowed in advanced age as a result of altered lung and kidney function.[32] Because older individuals are less able to increase their breathing rate, even under stress, carbon dioxide is less easily removed. Reduced renal blood flow also contributes to the increased time required to achieve homeostasis after an alteration in pH. Excessive use of self-prescribed drugs that add significant amounts of hydrogen or bicarbonate ions to the internal environment puts added stress on the homeostatic mechanisms in the older adult.

Perspective on Aging—Biologic or Medical?

The association of the aging process with changes in organ systems and the development of chronic disease has led to the consideration of aging as a medical problem. This biomedical approach emphasizes illness and disability rather than the overall biologic, social, and behavioral aspects of the aging process.[8] Our society will soon experience a rapid increase in the number of older people, including the oldest-old who are likely to have chronic diseases and require medical services. These projections have raised concern among health care providers[43] about the number of older people who, because of muscular weakness, bone fractures, or SDAT, will require a high level of care. It is possible, however, through health promotion strategies to reduce or postpone at least some of these causes of disability.[40] Fries[12] reminds us that 99 of every 100 people below age 75 are living independently, and 80 of every 100 people above age 85 are still living in the community. Half of those who are now in nursing homes have conditions that could have been prevented through healthy life-styles and risk reduction.

We should not lose sight of the complex issues that affect the health status and quality of life of all older people. Adequate housing, income, and social services and a sense of physical and emotional well-being are all important in determining appropriate food intake and other positive life-style choices. A scientific model for the study of aging that incorporates all of these issues will allow us to develop innovative approaches that will best serve our older people.

Summary

America is getting older, and this trend will continue. The high birth rate extending from the mid-1940s to the mid-1960s will contribute to the significant increase in the over-65 population in the next decades. By the year 2030 one in five people will be at least age 65. A growing segment of the older population will be those age 85 or older who will require an increasing share of health and other support services. Currently the individual over age 65 is most likely to be a white woman. The preponderance of women in older age groups is a reflection of the increased life expectancy of women compared to men. In this century the discovery of drugs to control infectious diseases has led to a significant decline in the mortality rates of younger people. At present the major causes of death are heart disease, cancer, and cerebrovascular disease, chronic problems that develop with advancing age and for which we have no cures. Although the aging process is associated with degenerative changes, an appropriate life-style can retard these changes and support successful aging with a minimum decline in physiologic function. Comparisons of older and younger individuals in respect to cognitive, renal, pulmonary, and cardiovascular functions suggest that some older people retain the level of performance observed in those much younger. An important goal for future research should be the study of these older individuals and their life-style patterns to determine those factors that support continuing physical and mental well-being.

REVIEW QUESTIONS

1. What factors will contribute to the projected increase in both the number and proportion of older people in the general population? Will all segments of the 65 and older population increase to the same extent? Explain. What are the implications for nutrition and health service providers?
2. What are the activities of daily living (ADLs) and the instrumental activities of daily living (IADLs)? How are they used? How would you as a nutrition professional use the ADLs and IADLs in evaluating an older individual and planning appropriate nutrition services?
3. How are an older person's food choices or need for nutrition services influenced by the following demographic characteristics: (1) age; (2) sex; (3) marital status; (4) living arrangement; (5) income; and (6) race.
4. What is the difference between usual and successful aging? What are some intervention strategies that would promote successful aging? Using the cardiovascular system as an example, explain the differences between usual and successful aging within a major organ system.
5. What are major age-related changes in the (1) cardiovascular, (2) renal, (3) pulmonary, and (4) endocrine systems? Discuss the nutritional implications of these changes.

LEARNING ACTIVITIES

1. Visit a local library, and review current census statistics for your community. Determine the relative proportion of older people in your geographic area and their demographic characteristics. How do they compare to your state or the United States as a whole?
2. Visit a senior center or congregate meal program and an adult day care center and interview the directors of each program about their participants. Compare the groups on the basis of ADLs, IADLs, and general health.
3. Determine the current amount of money allotted for a single older woman under the US Department of Agriculture's (USDA) Thrifty Food Plan. Develop a 3-day menu that is adequate in nutrient intake and stays within this budget allotment.
4. Make a list of community agencies that provide services to older people, and determine what food- and nutrition-related services are available.

Key Terms

Provided here for review is a list of the major terms in this chapter. The definitions can be found in the Glossary, which begins on p. 336. To help you understand how these terms are applied, the page number is given for the first mention of each term in the chapter.

acetylcholine, 15
activities of daily living (ADLs), 11
acute, 11
alveoli, 20
autoimmune, 10
baby boom generation, 2
Baltimore Longitudinal Study of Aging (BLSA), 13
cardiac output, 17
centenarian, 10
cerebral hemorrhage, 4
cerebrovascular disease, 6
chronic, 6
chronologic age, 2
cognitive, 14
Consumer Price Index (CPI), 8
cross-sectional, 13
dementia, 15
demographic, 3
dendrites, 15
dopamine, 15

fat deposition, 5
functional, 2
gender gap in life expectancy, 4
geriatrics, 9
gerontology, 9
glomerular filtration rate (GFR), 19
Healthy People 2000: National Health Promotion and Disease Prevention Objectives, 7
high-density lipoproteins (HDL), 5
low-density lipoproteins (LDL), 5
hypercapnia, 20
hypertension, 7
hypothalamic-neurohypophyseal axis, 16
hypoxia, 20
instrumental activities of daily living (IADLs), 11
ischemic heart disease, 6
life expectancy, 3
longevity, 2
median, 2
mortality rates, 4
occult, 17
Older Americans Act, 2
Parkinson's disease, 16
peripheral, 18
poverty level, 8
proliferative capacity, 10
residual volume, 20
senile dementia of the Alzheimer type (SDAT), 14
senescence, 9
Social Security, 2
stroke volume, 17
stroke, 18
tachycardia, 14
young-old, 2
oldest-old, 2
usual versus successful aging, 9

REFERENCES

1. Abdellah FG, Moore SR, editors: Proceedings of the Surgeon General's workshop: health promotion and aging, Washington, DC, 1988, US Department of Health and Human Services.
2. Avolio AP and others: Effects of aging on arterial distensibility in populations with high and low prevalence of hypertension: comparison be-

tween urban and rural communities in China, *Circulation* 71(2):202, 1985.

3. Barinaga M: How long is the human life span? *Science* 254:936, 1991.
4. Berkman L, Singer B, Manton K: Black/white differences in health status and mortality among the elderly, *Demography* 26(4):625, 1989.
5. Brown CC, Kessler LG: Projections of lung cancer mortality in the United States: 1985-2025, *J Natl Cancer Inst* 80(1):43, 1988.
6. Butler RN: Senile dementia of the Alzheimer type (SDAT). In Abrams WB, Berkow R, editors: *Merck manual of geriatrics*, Rahway, NJ, 1990, Merck Sharp & Dohme Research Laboratories.
7. Cristofalo VJ: Overview of biological mechanism of aging, *Annu Rev Gerontol Geriatr* 10:1, 1990.
8. Estes CL, Binney EA: The biomedicalization of aging: dangers and dilemmas, *Gerontologist* 29(5):587, 1989.
9. Fiore MC and others: Trends in cigarette smoking in the United States: the changing influence of gender and race, *JAMA* 261(1):49, 1989.
10. Food and Nutrition Board: Improving America's diet and health. From recommendations to action, Washington, DC, 1991, National Academy Press.
11. Franceschi C and others: Aging, longevity, and cancer: studies in Down's syndrome and centenarians, *Ann NY Acad Sci* 621:428, 1991.
12. Fries JF: The sunny side of aging, *JAMA* 263(17):2354, 1990.
13. Frohlich ED: Hypertension. In Abrams WB, Berkow R, editors: *Merck manual of geriatrics*, Rahway, NJ, 1990, Merck Sharp & Dohme Research Laboratories.
14. Gilford DM, editor: The aging population in the twenty-first century: statistics for health policy, Washington, DC, 1988, National Academy Press.
15. Hayflick L: The cell biology of human aging, *Sci Am* 242(1):58, 1980.
16. Hazzard WR: Atherosclerosis and aging: a scenario in flux, *Am J Cardiol* 63:20H, 1989.
17. Holden C: Why do women live longer than men? *Science* 238:158, 1987.
18. Holliday R: The limited proliferation of cultured human diploid cells: regulation or senescence, *J Gerontol* 45(2):B36, 1990.
19. Hyman BT and others: Alzheimer's disease, *Annu Rev Public Health* 10:115, 1989.
20. Idler EL, Angel RJ: Self-rated health and mortality in the NHANES-I epidemiologic follow-up study, *Am J Public Health* 80:446, 1990.
21. Janerich DT and others: Lung cancer and exposure to tobacco smoke in the household, *N Engl J Med* 323:632, 1990.
22. Joynt RJ: Normal aging and patterns of neurologic disease. In Abrams WB, Berkow R, editors: *Merck manual of geriatrics*, Rahway, NJ, 1990, Merck Sharp & Dohme Research Laboratories.
23. Keith VM, Smith DP: The current differential in black and white life expectancy, *Demography* 25(4):625, 1988.
24. Kenney RA: *Physiology of aging: a synopsis*, Chicago, 1982, Yearbook.
25. Kitzman DW, Edwards WD: Minireview: age-related changes in the anatomy of the normal human heart, *J Gerontol* 45(2):M33, 1990.
26. Lakatta EG: Normal changes of aging. In Abrams WB, Berkow R, editors: *Merck manual of geriatrics*, Rahway, NJ, 1990, Merck Sharp & Dohme Research Laboratories.
27. Lakatta EG: The aging heart: aging, life-style, and disease, *Ann Intern Med* 113:456, 1990.
28. Leon J, Lair T: Functional status of the noninstitutionalized elderly: estimates of ADL and IADL difficulties, DHHS Publication No (PHS) 90-3462, National Medical Expenditure Survey Research Findings 4, Rockville, Md, 1990, US Department of Health and Human Services.
29. Lindeman RD: The aging renal system. In Chernoff R, editor: *Geriatric nutrition: the health professional's handbook*, Gaithersburg, Md., 1991, Aspen.
30. Lindeman RD, and Goldman R: Anatomic and physiologic age changes in the kidney, *Exp Gerontol* 21:379, 1986.
31. Lindeman RD, Tobin J, Shock NW: Longitudinal studies on the rate of decline in renal function with age, *J Am Geriatr Soc* 33:278, 1985.
32. Lye MDW: The milieu interieur and aging. In Brocklehurst JC, editor: *Textbook of geriatric medicine and gerontology*, London, 1985, Churchill Livingstone.
33. Madigan FC: Are sex mortality differentials biologically caused? *Milbank Mem Fund Q* 35:203, 1957.
34. Markides KS: Consequences of gender differentials in life expectancy for black and Hispanic Americans, *Int J Aging Hum Dev* 29(2):95, 1989.
35. Meier-Ruge W, Hunziker O, Iwangoff P: Senile dementia: a threshold phenomenon of normal aging, *Ann NY Acad Sci* 621:104, 1991.
36. Morley JE, Glick Z: Endocrine aspects of nutrition and aging. In Chernoff R, editor: *Geriatric*

nutrition: the health professional's handbook, Gaithersburg, Md, 1991, Aspen.

37. Nestle M, Gilbride JA: Nutrition policies for health promotion in older adults: education priorities for the 1990s, *J Nutr Educ* 22(6):314, 1990.
38. Otten MW and others: The effect of known risk factors on the excess mortality of black adults in the United States, *JAMA* 263(6):845, 1990.
39. Pierce JP and others: Trends in cigarette smoking in the United States, *JAMA* 261(1):61, 1989.
40. Powell KE and others: Physical activity and chronic diseases, *Am J Clin Nutr* 49:999, 1989.
41. Rossor MN: The central nervous system: neurochemistry of the aging brain and dementia. In Brocklehurst JC, editor: *Textbook of geriatric medicine and gerontology,* London, 1985, Churchill Livingstone.
42. Rowe JW, Khan RL: Human aging: usual and successful, *Science* 237:143, 1987.
43. Schneider EL, Guralnik JM: The aging of America: impact on health care costs, *JAMA* 263(17):2335, 1990.
44. Shock NW: Biologic concepts of aging, *Psych Res Rep* 23:1, 1968.
45. Solomon DH: Introduction. Organ systems: metabolic and endocrine disorders. In Abrams WB, Berkow R, editors: *Merck manual of geriatrics,* Rahway, NJ, 1990, Merck Sharp & Dohme Research Laboratories.
46. Sutherland JE, Persky VW, Brody JA: Proportionate mortality trends: 1950 through 1986, *JAMA* 264(24):3178, 1990.
47. Thomas P: Aging and the brain: stopping the brain drain, *Harvard Health Letter* 16(12):6, 1991.
48. Timiras PS: Alzheimer disease compared with normal aging of the brain, *Ann Intern Med* 113:461, 1990.
49. Tockman MS: The effects of age on the lung. In Abrams WB, Berkow R, editors: *Merck manual of geriatrics,* Rahway, NJ, 1990, Merck Sharp & Dohme Research Laboratories.
50. US Bureau of the Census: Marital status and living arrangements, March 1989, Curr Pop Reports Series P-20, No 445, Washington, DC, 1990, US Government Printing Office.
51. US Bureau of the Census: Population profile of the United States: 1989, Curr Pop Reports Series P-23, No 159, Washington, DC, 1989, US Government Printing Office.
52. US Bureau of the Census: Projections of the population of the United States, by age, sex, and race: 1988 to 2080, Curr Pop Reports Series P-25, No 1018, Washington, DC, 1989, US Government Printing Office.
53. US Bureau of the Census: Poverty in the United States: 1990, Curr Pop Reports Series P-60, No 175, Washington, DC, 1991, US Government Office.
54. US Department of Health and Human Services: The Baltimore longitudinal study of aging, NIH Publication No 84-2450, Washington, DC, 1984, US Government Printing Office.
55. US Department of Health and Human Services: The Surgeon General's report on nutrition and health, DHHS Publication No (PHS) 88-50210, Washington, DC, 1988, US Government Printing Office.
56. US Department of Health and Human Services: Health: United States, 1990, DHHS Publication No (PHS) 91-1232, Hyattsville, Md, 1991, US Government Printing Office.
57. US Department of Health and Human Services: Healthy people 2000: national health promotion and disease prevention objectives, DHHS Publication No (PHS) 91-50212, Washington, DC, 1991, US Government Printing Office.
58. US Senate Special Committee on Aging: Aging America: trends and projections (annotated), Serial No 101-J, Washington, DC, 1990, US Government Printing Office.
59. Verbrugge LM: Recent, present, and future health of American adults, *Annu Rev Public Health* 10:333, 1989.
60. Walser N: When to hang up the keys, *Harvard Health Letter* 17(1):1, 1991.
61. Watkin DM: The physiology of aging, *Am J Clin Nutr* 36:750, 1982.
62. Weinberger M and others: Self-rated health as a predictor of hospital admission and nursing home placement in elderly public housing tenants, *Am J Public Health* 76:457, 1986.
63. Weksler ME: Genetic and immunologic determinants of aging. In Haynes SG, Feinleib M, editors: Epidemiology of aging, DHHS Publication No (NIH) 80-969, Washington, DC, 1980, US Government Printing Office.
64. Working Group on Hypertension in the Elderly: Statement on hypertension in the elderly, *JAMA* 256(1):70, 1986.
65. Yahr MD, Pang SWH: Movement disorders. In Abrams WB, Berkow R, editors: *Merck manual of geriatrics,* Rahway, NJ, 1990, Merck Sharp & Dohme Research Laboratories.

2 Nutrition and the Life Span

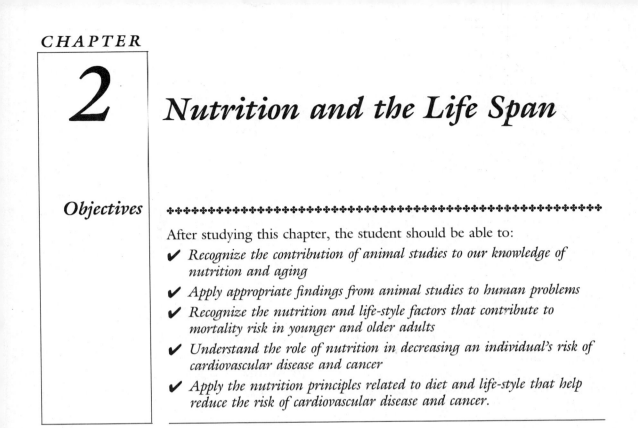

Objectives

❋❋

After studying this chapter, the student should be able to:

✔ *Recognize the contribution of animal studies to our knowledge of nutrition and aging*

✔ *Apply appropriate findings from animal studies to human problems*

✔ *Recognize the nutrition and life-style factors that contribute to mortality risk in younger and older adults*

✔ *Understand the role of nutrition in decreasing an individual's risk of cardiovascular disease and cancer*

✔ *Apply the nutrition principles related to diet and life-style that help reduce the risk of cardiovascular disease and cancer.*

Introduction

Since antiquity people have been searching for magical potions to preserve youth and prolong life. Early explorers came to the New World seeking the "fountain of youth." Today hormonal and herbal preparations that promise to retard aging or restore physical health receive widespread attention. Long-lived individuals are sought after for their advice on food choices and life-style habits. Studies that have followed individuals over several years to obtain information on daily diet, state of health, and years of life have focused primarily on cardiovascular disease or other chronic problems and have recorded intakes of particular nutrients such as types and amounts of dietary fat rather than overall dietary intake. Much of what is now known about the influence of nutrition on the aging process has come from animal studies that have examined the effects of both quantitative and qualitative dietary changes. The relationship between lifelong dietary patterns and physical well-being is an urgent issue for future research.

HISTORICAL PERSPECTIVE

Historical writings contain many directives for maintaining good health and prolonging life. Cornaro, whose book, *The Art of Living Long,* was published in 1558,[13] became an ardent advocate of a temperate diet after becoming ill with fever, pains in the stomach, and perpetual thirst.[1] Previously given to excessive food and drink, from that time on he ate sparingly of bread, meat, milk, egg yolk, and soup and at the age of 95 wrote his final treatise on the wisdom of a moderate diet. Cornaro suggested that one needs less food as the body grows older. He limited himself to 12 ounces of food and 14 ounces of wine a day and exhorted younger people to avoid overindulgence.

Francis Bacon (1561-1626) was the first author to recommend a scientific approach to the evaluation of diet and longevity.[3] He advocated a frugal diet and encouraged the study of people living in different climates and eating different diets to determine those characteristics that influence the life span. In his opinion, diet was the most important component in prolonging life. Unfortunately, Bacon's recommendation to evaluate the influence of diet and life-style on mortality has only recently begun to receive attention. Suggested practices regarding food and health were popular reading in colonial America. Benjamin Franklin's *Poor Richard's Almanac,* published in 1733, advised readers to limit the amount they ate.[13] Franklin urged his followers to "eat to live and not live to eat."

Early writings also stressed a prudent diet for the elderly. A physician living in A.D. 1000 urged his older patients to eat only small amounts of food at a time and to avoid foods that could lead to digestive upset, such as spiced and pickled items.[3] A treatise on geriatric medicine that appeared in 1796 advised older people to avoid sugar and confectionery foods, to consume liberal amounts of vegetables, to limit the amount of meat they ate, and to eat only sparingly at night.[3] A paper titled "Food and Hygiene of Old Age," which appeared in the *Journal of the American Medical Association* in 1892, suggested that errors in food selection are less serious in the young, who can recover from such mistakes.[4]

In this century Metchnikoff, a Russian physiologist, proposed the theory of autointoxication, suggesting that death occurred as a result of toxins that were produced in the large intestine by fecal waste and then absorbed into the body. Yogurt and other fermented milk products containing lactic acid–producing bacilli were recommended to destroy the intestinal microbes responsible for the poisonous waste.

The first study evaluating the relationship between body weight and mortality was reported in 1913,[69] as life insurance companies began to recognize that policyholders with higher body weights in proportion to their heights had shorter lives. It was important to the company to be able to predict how long a policyholder might live or, conversely, how soon the company would have to pay the life insurance claim. Life insurance statistics have continued to be a source of both information and controversy about the relationship between nutrition and the life span. It is rather interesting to note that throughout history, writers have emphasized limiting one's intake of food. Current issues relating to energy intake, obesity, and longevity will be discussed in this chapter.

CALORIC RESTRICTION AND AGING IN ANIMAL MODELS
Caloric Restriction and Length of Life in Animal Models

Studies over the past 60 years using experimental animals have confirmed that caloric restriction increases the life span. The classic studies of McCay and coworkers[46] in the 1930s revealed that energy intake controls not only the rate of growth but also the rate of development and aging. Those researchers demonstrated that laboratory rats fed diets adequate in protein, vitamins, and minerals but limited in kilocalories could be maintained at their weaning stage and weight for several years. When additional kilocalories were provided, the animals would begin to grow and mature. The life span of these animals was nearly twice as long as the life span of those given the usual amount of food throughout their lives. This work established the principle that caloric intake controls fundamental metabolic processes that influence the life span. This relationship between caloric intake and the life span has provided the foundation for current research directed toward identifying the site and mechanism of metabolic control.

Current studies[25,26,38,44] using caloric restriction in animal models provide a level of kilocalories that supports the growth and maturation of that species. Restricted animals are fed 60% of the kilocalories consumed by the control animals, who have free access to food (**ad libitum fed**). It is important to recognize that the caloric-restricted diets are formulated to provide adequate amounts of protein, vitamins, and minerals; only kilocalories are kept below the usual level.

The profound effect of such restriction is evident when comparing the median and maximum length of life in restricted and ad libitum—fed rats. Those given free access to food had a median life span of 701 days, compared to 956 days for the restricted animals; the maximum life span was 941 days for the unrestricted and 1,295 days for the restricted animals, respectively. More than half of the restricted animals were still alive when the last ad libitum—fed animal died.[44] Length of life provides an acceptable measure of outcome when evaluating the effect of caloric restriction in animal models. In humans, qualitative assessments of health and well-being are also important measures of outcome in the study of nutrition and the life span.

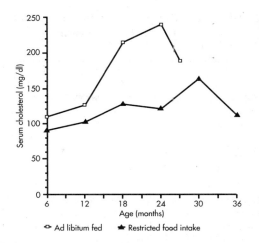

FIG. 2-1　Energy intake and serum cholesterol in aging rats. Age-related increases in serum cholesterol are delayed in animals whose caloric intake is restricted.

(From Liepa GV and others: Food restriction as a modulator of age-related changes in serum lipids, *Am J Physiol* 238:E253, 1980.)

Physiologic Effects of Caloric Restriction in Animal Models

In animals caloric restriction delays the appearance and reduces the magnitude of age-related changes in physiologic functions. One example of this effect is the time of appearance and level of age-related increase in serum cholesterol in restricted and ad libitum—fed animals (Fig. 2-1).[38] At 6 months of age, the serum cholesterol levels were similar in both groups; however, serum cholesterol in ad libitum—fed animals was markedly higher at 12 months of age and reached a peak at 18 months of age. In restricted animals serum levels peaked about 18 months later, and the magnitude of the change was markedly less. Motor coordination and learning ability as tested in a complex maze did not decline in older caloric-restricted animals compared to younger ones, whereas older unrestricted animals made more errors than younger unrestricted animals.[25] Other physiologic changes associated with aging in

which this pattern of delay has been observed in animals include changes in the proteins in skeletal muscle, loss of dopamine receptors in the central nervous system, and changes in the structure of the eye's lens.[72]

Disease Processes in Animal Models

In animals caloric restriction may delay aging changes in physiologic systems by slowing the development of chronic disease. Laboratory rats develop both heart disease and kidney disease in advancing age. As described in Table 2-1, the incidence and severity of both diseases are reduced in restricted animals.[44] Caloric restriction also influences the cause of death in experimental animals. Kidney disease is a major cause of death among ad libitum—fed animals; the major causes of death among caloric-restricted animals are tumors and leukemia. Caloric restriction does delay the development of tumors, and tumor growth is not increased at younger ages in restricted animals; older restricted animals show a greater prevalence of tumors because

TABLE 2-1   Energy Intake and Incidence of Age-Related Disease in Older Rats

	Caloric Restricted	Ad Libitum Fed
Kidney disease		
Absent or minimal	93%	18%
Severe	7%	82%
Heart disease		
Absent or minimal	75%	41%
Severe	25%	59%

Modified from Masoro EJ, Shimokawa I, Yu BP: Retardation of the aging processes in rats by food restriction, *Ann NY Acad Sci* 621:337, 1991.

they live longer and have additional time to develop tumors.

Caloric restriction acts in two ways to extend the life span: (1) by delaying age-related physiologic changes, and (2) by retarding the development of chronic disease. The effect of calorie restriction in delaying physiologic changes such as the increase in serum cholesterol or the loss of neural dopamine receptors occurs much earlier in life, long before age-related diseases become evident. Because it occurs earlier in life, the effect of caloric restriction in delaying physiologic changes is likely to be the major way it increases the length of life. [43]Nevertheless, the influence of caloric restriction on the development of chronic disease may also be important, depending on the particular organ system involved.

Composition of the Diet and the Life Span in Animal Models

The relative proportions of protein, fat, and carbohydrate in the diet can influence when degenerative changes appear and the length of life. In experimental animals high-protein intake results in rapid growth, increased body weight, and a shorter life span.[72] Restricting the protein component of the diet or substituting soy protein for casein reduces the incidence of severe kidney disease but has little effect on

the life span unless caloric intake is also restricted.[26] The association of high-protein intake and rapid growth with decreased life span in animal models may have implications for growth patterns in humans. Children today are both taller and heavier than in previous generations, and girls reach puberty at an earlier age.

Animal studies have examined the influence of the type and level of dietary fat and its degree of saturation on longevity. High intake of fat, regardless of the type of fat, has been associated with a decreased life span.[72] However, the caloric density of the high-fat diet and the excessive weight gain that results, in addition to the properties of the fat itself, may contribute to the decreased life span. Recent work suggests that substituting carbohydrate for fat does not increase the life span unless kilocalories are also restricted.[44] An area for further study is the influence of dietary carbohydrate on length of life. A diet high in fat is likely to be low in carbohydrate. Decreased dietary carbohydrate (and fiber) rather than increased dietary fat could contribute to the reduced life span associated with a high-fat diet.[44]

Calorie Restriction and Metabolic Outcome

The influence of caloric intake on the rate of aging and the length of life in animal models is well recognized. What is still to be determined is the mechanism by which caloric restriction exerts its effect. Many explanations have been presented, but no single theory has withstood careful scrutiny. An enhanced growth rate and a higher level of body fat have been suggested as factors that accelerate the aging process.[43] Animals restricted in caloric intake grow more slowly and have a lower content of body fat per gram of body weight. In restricted animals the level of body fat is positively related to the length of life. Ad libitum–fed animals have a higher body weight and level of body fat than restricted animals, but these measurements do not always correlate with their length of life. One piece of evidence suggesting that factors other than growth rate and maximum body weight influence the life span is that food restriction begun in mature animals later in life leads to gains in life span similar to those achieved when restriction is begun at weaning.

A decrease in the **metabolic rate,** or slowing of the "rate of living," as a result of caloric restriction has been proposed to explain the observed increase in life span.[44] The metabolic rate per unit of body mass does decline in animals when caloric restriction is first initiated, but it returns to normal shortly thereafter. Also, the proportion of energy intake used for growth or essential physiologic functions versus that expended as heat appears to increase in caloric-restricted animals. This increase in **metabolic efficiency** makes sense, since fewer kilocalories are available to the organism, and therefore available kilocalories are more likely to be directed toward essential functions. However, how an increase in metabolic efficiency might retard the aging process is not known. In humans an increase in metabolic efficiency appears to have the opposite effect; individuals who have greater metabolic efficiency and are less able to expend unneeded kilocalories as heat are more likely to have a higher level of body fat and become more vulnerable to chronic disease.

Antioxidants and Aging in Animal Models

The free radical theory of aging, first proposed in 1956, suggested that highly charged particles with an unpaired electron (free radicals) caused **peroxidation** reactions at the site of the double bond in unsaturated fatty acids.[44] Because cell membranes are high in polyunsaturated fatty acids, they are particularly vulnerable to peroxidation damage and degenerative changes. Efforts to increase the life span by feeding animals higher amounts of vitamins (e.g., vitamin E, ascorbic acid) or other compounds (e.g., mercaptoethylamine hydrochloride) with **antioxidant** functions were unsuccessful. Although animals fed antioxidants appeared to have a reduced level of lipid peroxidation reactions in their tissues, their life span was not increased. However, caloric-restricted animals who do have longer life spans synthesize higher levels of the enzymes and molecules that act as antioxidants and increase the body's defenses against such age-related damage.[32] (In-

creased intake of vitamins with antioxidant functions appears to offer some protection against diseases in humans and is discussed later in this chapter.)

Caloric Intake and Hormonal Mechanisms in Animal Models

In recent years attention has been directed toward neural or hormonal pathways that may link reduced caloric intake with increased longevity. One hypothesis involves the **glucocorticoid hormones** secreted by the adrenal cortex.[43] According to this theory, a high level of food intake leads to sustained hyperadrenocorticism. Excessive levels of glucocorticoids lead to physiologic changes associated with aging. High levels of glucocorticoids bring about sustained reductions in antibody production, with increased vulnerability to infection. Glucocorticoids increase the urinary excretion of calcium, and over time, inappropriately high levels of these hormones can promote the development of osteoporosis in humans.

Another theory involving a hormonal pathway proposes that the glucose-insulin response mediates aging changes.[43] High-caloric intakes could result in higher serum glucose levels and reduced sensitivity to insulin. High serum glucose levels might increase the number of **glycosylation** reactions occurring between the aldehyde group of the glucose molecule and the amino group of a protein molecule. The resulting glucoproteins will not function in the usual way and could lead to degenerative changes. The glycosylation reaction produces the glycosylated hemoglobin molecules associated with uncontrolled diabetes in humans.

Each of the theories described above relating caloric intake to the aging process may be in fact a partial explanation. Although weak experimental evidence supports each idea, none offers a complete explanation for the extensive physiologic changes observed. All of these mechanisms may combine to control the aging process.

Animal Studies and Human Aging

Research findings from animal models cannot be applied directly to human aging, although some comparisons are possible. Limiting caloric intake to prevent excessive accumulation of body fat can influence human life span. Increasing **adiposity** increases an individual's vulnerability to many physiologic changes, including elevated blood pressure, elevated serum cholesterol, and glucose intolerance. In animals caloric restriction initiated in adulthood still retards physiologic aging, suggesting that reducing an inappropriately high caloric intake at any point in the life span will be of some benefit. The finding in animals that the source of kilocalories is less important than the total amount consumed requires further definition for humans. Both the amount and type of fat consumed is related to the onset of chronic disease in humans. The following section explores these issues in developing positive nutrition strategies.

NUTRIENT INTAKE AND HUMAN LIFE SPAN
Scope of the Problem

Limited information is available to evaluate the influence of lifelong dietary habits on health and longevity. The Baltimore Longitudinal Study of Aging (BLSA) has not emphasized food habits, and few data have been collected on women. Major **epidemiologic** studies evaluating the impact of diet and life-style on the incidence of heart disease and cancer examined key nutrients but not the diet as a whole. A longitudinal approach that follows the same individual over time provides information on not only the rate of change but also the periods when aging changes occur. Such an evaluation of the influence of diet on physiologic and biochemical aging is urgently needed. The data obtained could provide the basis for comprehensive recommendations on diet and health. The major causes of death for Americans in middle or advanced age are heart disease, cancer, and stroke. Nutrition is a factor in preventing each of these problems.

Nutrition and Cardiovascular Disease

A major health initiative in recent decades has been public education defining the risk factors for coronary heart disease and their possi-

ble modification. The early 1960s marked the beginning of a significant decline in mortality from coronary heart disease. Changes in food consumption that contributed to this decline, the substitution of vegetable fats for animal fats, and the movement toward foods lower in total fat, began in the late 1940s and accelerated from that time on.[60] Food patterns indicating reduced consumption of total fat and saturated fat became evident 10 to 15 years before the downward trend in mortality from coronary heart disease became apparent.[60] This interval of 10 to 15 years between the initiation of positive dietary behavior and the reduction in the incidence of disease points to our need to encourage life-style changes among young and middle-aged individuals to ensure their successful aging.

Cardiovascular risk in the aged. It is commonly believed that the risk factors known to predispose middle-aged people to heart disease do not apply to older people. In fact, elevated blood pressure, inappropriate blood lipid patterns, obesity, smoking, and glucose intolerance are also strong predictors of coronary risk in the elderly.[27] When examined singularly, some risk factors decrease in importance. Current evidence suggests that after age 65, stopping smoking does not measurably decrease cardiovascular risk, because the incidence of stroke increases among both smokers and nonsmokers after that age.[54] In contrast, elevated blood pressure and an undesirable serum lipid profile remain powerful predictors of cardiovascular risk, regardless of age. Elevated systolic or diastolic blood pressure multiplies the risk of heart disease in all individuals beyond age 45.[27] A follow-up after 6 years of men participating in a dietary intervention study designed to lower serum lipid levels suggested that elevated blood pressure increases an individual's risk of stroke despite an appropriate blood lipid profile.[54] Total serum cholesterol levels have less influence at older ages; however, the ratio of low-density lipoprotein (**LDL**) **cholesterol** to high-density lipoprotein (**HDL**) **cholesterol** is closely associated with the risk of heart disease.[27]

Older men and women with several risk factors are especially vulnerable to heart attack or stroke. Results from the Framingham Heart

Study indicate that the risk of coronary heart disease is about doubled in older people with three risk factors compared to those with one (Fig. 2-2).[66] Elevated blood pressure and abnormal glucose tolerance, if associated with obesity, increase the risk of coronary heart disease and stroke in women even before menopause. Dietary modification plays a prominent role in reducing the risk of cardiovascular disease and is appropriate regardless of age.

Dietary fat. The average American diet, high in total fat (37%) and saturated fat (13%), has long been associated with high serum cholesterol and the development of **atherosclerotic** plaques in the coronary arteries.[12] Clinical trials have demonstrated that reducing serum cholesterol decreases cardiovascular risk. The National Cholesterol Education Program (NCEP)[15] has been established to develop public awareness of inappropriately high serum cholesterol levels and the associated risk and to implement strategies for improvement. For individuals whose serum cholesterol levels are too high, dietary intervention is the first step. NCEP guidelines indicate that dietary fat should provide no more than 30% of total kilocalories. A clinical trial to lower serum lipid levels in men ages 40 to 59 has suggested that dietary fat provide no more than 27.5% of total kilocalories.[7] Men whose fat intake did not exceed that level developed no new atherosclerotic lesions in their coronary arteries. Those men increased their dietary protein while decreasing dietary fat by substituting lower fat meats and dairy products for the higher fat versions.

Clinical trials demonstrating the successful use of dietary changes to lower serum cholesterol have focused primarily on middle-aged men. At this time we have little information on the success of dietary intervention in lowering serum lipid levels in men and women over age 60. Another issue involved in implementing a low-fat diet is the diet's fatty acid composition. The NCEP recommends that fat be divided as follows:[15]

Type of fat	Percentage of total kilocalories
Saturated fatty acids	less than 10%
Polyunsaturated fatty acids	10% or less
Monounsaturated fatty acids	10% to 15%

Recent work evaluating the specific abilities of individual fatty acids to raise or lower total serum cholesterol has complicated this issue. Although saturated fatty acids are generally expected to raise total serum cholesterol, stearic acid does not have this effect. Linoleic acid decreases LDL cholesterol but decreases HDL cholesterol as well. Oleic acid, a monounsaturated fatty acid, is receiving increasing attention, because it appears to lower LDL cholesterol to the same degree as polyunsaturated fatty acids do without also lowering HDL cholesterol.[18]

The major issue surrounding the development of a low-fat diet is its acceptance by the public. In light of the positive effect of oleic acid on serum **lipoprotein** levels, Grundy[19] has suggested that increased use of oleic acid or other monounsaturated fatty acids might allow total dietary fat content to reach 30% to 35% of total kilocalories and still achieve reasonable control of total serum cholesterol. Although a diet containing this level of fat may not be as

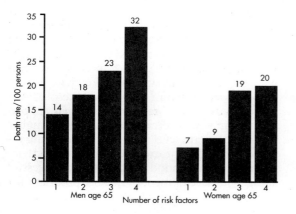

FIG. 2-2 Probability of developing coronary heart disease according to number of risk factors. The risk of coronary heart disease rises progressively in both older men and older women as the number of risk factors increases. Risk factors include obesity, elevated blood pressure, abnormal glucose tolerance, elevated serum lipids, and smoking.

(Data from Castelli WP and others: Cardiovascular risk factors in the elderly, *Am J Cardiol* 63:124, 1989.)

desirable as one lower in both fat and energy, it may be better accepted for lifelong use.

Blood lipid levels. The gender difference in the incidence of coronary heart disease in younger age groups relates at least in part to the differences in serum lipoprotein levels between men and women. The female sex hormones impart to women about 10 years of relative immunity to coronary heart disease, compared to men. The mortality rate from heart disease for women ages 65 to 74 is about that for men ages 55 to 64. Between puberty and menopause, LDL cholesterol is lower in women than in men. At the time of menopause LDL cholesterol begins to rise, and in time it equals or exceeds the level in men of comparable age. HDL cholesterol remains lower in men than in women throughout adulthood. As a result, the LDL-to-HDL ratio is higher in men at all ages, although the gap between men and women tends to narrow as LDL cholesterol rises in women at older ages.[21]

A common characteristic among older people who remain free of cardiovascular disease is a relatively high level of HDL cholesterol.[58,63,75] In the Framingham Heart Study,[58] the mean plasma LDL and HDL cholesterol levels of 163 octogenarians (mean age of 83 years) with no evidence of cardiovascular disease did not differ from those of octogenarians with diagnosed cardiovascular disease. However, none of the 57 healthy men and only one of the 106 healthy women had an HDL cholesterol level in the lowest percentile. Extremely low HDL cholesterol levels and extremely high LDL cholesterol levels are uncommon in healthy people over age 80.[63]

The Framingham Heart Study has suggested that the LDL-to-HDL ratio, rather than the total serum cholesterol, indicates cardiovascular risk in older people.[27] On this basis one could question the value to older people of screening programs that measure only total serum cholesterol. A report from the Honolulu Heart Program[5] after 12 years of followup has indicated that the incidence of coronary heart disease among 1,480 men age 65 or older increased proportionately as total serum cholesterol increased. This would suggest that the current NCEP guidelines can effectively identify cardiovascular risk at older as well as younger ages;

those guidelines call for determination of LDL and HDL cholesterol levels in individuals with other risk factors when total serum cholesterol reaches 200 mg/dl or higher.

Physical activity. Increasing physical activity can improve fitness and reduce mortality from cardiovascular disease in men and women at middle and older ages. Among nearly 17,000 Harvard alumni between the ages of 35 and 84, groups who reported walking, stair climbing, or sports activity had fewer deaths from cardiovascular or respiratory causes.[53] Individuals who walked 1 to 1 ½ miles each day had a 20% decrease in risk compared to those who were less active. Among the sedentary men ages 70 to 84, twice as many died of heart attack or stroke compared to active men of similar age. A brisk walk of 30 to 60 minutes each day was found to lower the risk of death from any cause in both older men and older women.[6] In fact, older people may benefit more from exercise than younger people, who have a lower risk of death regardless of their level of physical activity.

Physical activity may act in several ways to decrease mortality and improve an individual's functional capacity. Those who continue to exercise as they get older have lower resting heart rates and lower **waist-to-hip ratios** than those of similar age who do not exercise.[17,55] Although regular exercise does not always lower the serum LDL cholesterol level, older men and women who engage in regular physical activity have a higher level of serum HDL cholesterol. Postmenopausal women receiving **estrogen** supplementation who exercise have an even higher HDL cholesterol level than women receiving estrogen who do not exercise.[55] Physical activity throughout adulthood contributes to successful aging. The development of exercise programs for older people is discussed in Chapter 3.

Body Measurements and Cardiovascular Risk

The influence of body weight on mortality, first examined by life insurance companies nearly 100 years ago, is still an issue of considerable debate.[69] Based on the heights and weights of policyholders who lived the longest, insurance companies have derived tables listing appropriate body weights for people of a particular sex and height. Although these tables are widely used by insurance companies and health professionals, they have many limitations.

Limitations of height and weight tables. The body weights given as standards in height and weight tables are presumed to represent an appropriate proportion of lean body mass and body fat, and deviations from these weights are presumed to be a gain or loss of body fat. However, for a person participating in an exercise program, body weight could remain unchanged despite an increase in fitness as body fat is replaced by lean body mass. An individual may have a low lean body mass and an excessive amount of body fat, yet meet the suggested weight for height. Height and weight tables do not always allow for variations in body build.

Use of height and weight tables also requires an accurate measurement of body height. A height measurement can be difficult to obtain from an older person with curvature of the spine who is unable to stand straight. A loss of height, as often occurs with increasing age, raises questions about the appropriate height measurement to be used in evaluation. Another issue relates to the appropriateness of weight gain throughout adulthood. Tables derived from life insurance statistics present an appropriate body weight for a person of a given height and sex that is applicable to all adults regardless of age. In fact many people do gain weight throughout adulthood. Some gerontologists have proposed the use of age-specific height and weight tables that would reflect this age-associated weight gain.[69] Most health professionals consider age-related weight gain to be unhealthy and a significant risk factor for cardiovascular disease and other chronic problems.

Finally, height and weight tables derived from life insurance statistics are not representative of the general population. Whites and individuals from middle and upper socioeconomic groups are more likely to buy life insurance than are low-income or minority groups. Despite these problems, appropriate body weights derived from life insurance records are used to evaluate mortality risk.

Body weight and mortality. The most recent compilation of life insurance data is the 1979 Build Study,[62] which traces the mortality of 4.2 million policyholders between 1954 and 1972. These individuals were considered to be in good health, although about 10% were overweight or underweight to some extent. In general, the greater the deviation from average weight, the greater the mortality risk (Table 2-2).[69] Among both older men and older women, mortality ratios, or the risk of death, increased sharply for those 25% to 35% underweight. These **mortality ratios** represent a decrease in life expectancy of about 2 years in men and 1 ½ years in women. Among the men op-

TABLE 2-2 *Mortality Risk and Body Weight in Older People*

Classification	Mortality Risk* (Ratio of Expected to Actual Mortality)	
	Men	Women
25% to 35% underweight	137	143
15% to 25% underweight	120	108
5% to 15% underweight	100	91
Average weight	96	99
5% to 15% overweight	98	100
25% to 35% overweight	103	107
35% to 45% overweight	148	128

*Average risk is 100 (mortality ratios above 100 indicate a higher risk of death; mortality ratios below 100 indicate a lower risk of death.)
Modified from Van Itallie TB, Lew EA: Health implications of overweight in the elderly. In Prinsley D, Sandstead HH, editors: *Nutrition and aging*, New York, 1990, Alan R Liss.

timum mortality ratios (100 or below) occur at about average weight, whereas among women mortality ratios are most favorable at a body weight 5% to 15% below average. Mortality ratios increase sharply at a weight 35% or more above average, with a decrease in life expectancy of 1 to 1 ½ years. These findings suggest that overweight, unless 35% or more above average, carries somewhat less risk than underweight, particularly in women.

Issues in evaluating body weight and mortality. Although life insurance statistics point to the increased vulnerability of overweight and underweight individuals, it has been suggested that underweight rather than overweight is more dangerous at older ages. Manson and co-workers[39] suggest that four major biases can minimize the deleterious effect of overweight and exaggerate the deleterious effect of underweight in studies of body weight and mortality.

1. Smoking is more prevalent among people with low body weight. In the Framingham Heart Study, only 55% of those in the highest overweight category reported smoking, compared to 80% of those in the lowest weight category. Because smoking itself increases mortality risk and is also associated with reduced body fat, failure to control for this effect will lead to calculation of an inappropriately high rate of mortality in lean subjects.

2. The mortality risk of obese individuals is less apparent when glucose intolerance, hypertension, and hyperlipidemia, chronic physiologic problems linked to obesity, are removed from the statistical analysis. Removing these variables from the equation provides an estimate of the independent effect of obesity apart from associated chronic diseases. If, however, the goal is to determine the extent to which obesity adversely affects health and longevity, it is important to include variables that can result from obesity and negatively influence health.

3. High mortality rates associated with underweight can be caused by underlying clinical disease that was present when the study began. In that case weight loss resulting from cancer or respiratory disease is a signal of serious disease rather than a cause of early death. This bias can be avoided by carefully screening subjects for a **prospective** study or by disregarding data collected during the first few years of follow-up when weight loss from underlying disease will be most evident.

4. Whether a long-term or a short-term study was done influences the conclusion reached about the impact of body weight on mortality. Short-term evaluations are influenced by underlying disease and often suggest that underweight per se carries a high mortality risk. Obesity, on the other hand, may appear to have less effect when evaluated over the short term, since the mortality rates of the most obese may be similar to those of average-weight individuals. Over the long term, however, the risk of death can be one third higher for the most obese compared to those of average weight. This is because the risk factors associated with obesity, hypertension, glucose intolerance, or hyperlipidemia, develop slowly over several years. The longer the period of overweight, the more likely are these conditions to develop.

Body mass index and mortality. The relationships described above were evident among 1,723 nonsmokers over age 65 who were part of the Framingham Heart Study.[20] In this study body mass index (BMI) was used to evaluate the relationship between body weight and mortality. The BMI (body weight in kilograms divided by height in meters squared) provides a useful estimate of body fatness and is a better evaluation tool than height and weight tables. Mortality was highest in the early years of follow-up among those with the lowest BMI. For those with the greatest BMI, mortality risk remained high throughout the follow-up period (Fig. 2-3). The increased risk of mortality among the most obese was still evident after adjustment for other associated risk factors. The importance of the length of time that an individual was overweight was also apparent. The risk of death was doubled for men who were overweight both at ages 55 and 65, compared to those who became overweight after age 55. Despite the general perception that increasing adiposity carries less risk for women, risk at age 65 for both men and women with the highest BMI was about twice that of individuals with an average BMI.

Obesity in middle age significantly increases mortality risk at older ages, and well-supervised

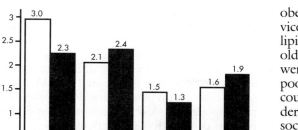

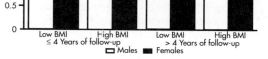

FIG. 2-3 Body mass index and mortality risk of older people. Underweight carries a higher risk among men, and overweight carries a higher risk among women. Overweight continues to carry risk on a long-term basis.

(Data from Harris T and others: Body mass index and mortality among nonsmoking older persons, *JAMA* 259 (10):1520, 1988.)

weight reduction programs should be considered at younger ages. At the same time, unintentional weight loss or substantial losses achieved by weight loss regimens lacking in required nutrients adversely affect nutritional status and general health.

In contrast to the findings of the Framingham Heart Study, in which excessive adiposity increased mortality risk beyond age 65, an 8-year follow-up of 4,710 older participants in the First National Health and Nutrition Examination Survey (NHANES I)[67] reported only moderate changes in risk with increasing BMI, even among the most overweight. Conversely, mortality risk was highest among those most underweight. The NHANES I study did not control for smoking and underlying illness and represented a shorter period of follow-up than the Framingham Heart Study, facts that no doubt contributed to the differences in findings.

An important observation from the NHANES I follow-up was the increased mortality risk of those with the lowest and highest BMI who also had incomes below the poverty level.[67] The increased risk associated with a low income and

obesity could result from a lack of medical services for control of high blood pressure or hyperlipidemia associated with the obesity. Among older women the mortality risk of those who were severely underweight was twofold in the poor versus the nonpoor. This poverty effect could represent poor nutritional status and underlying illness. In any case, the increased risk associated with poverty in the elderly requires further scrutiny.

The influence of race on the relationship between BMI and mortality was evaluated in a 15-year study of more than 5,000 blacks between the ages of 30 and 70.[73] Because these individuals were members of a prepaid health maintenance organization, information about possible underlying disease was available for review. When controlling for smoking and the early years of follow-up, no relationship between BMI and mortality was evident in women across the entire range of severe underweight to severe overweight. In men relative risk increased significantly with overt obesity. Thinness, when unrelated to cigarette smoking, did not increase risk.

Despite the fact that in this evaluation BMI was not associated with mortality risk in black women, these researchers were hesitant to suggest that obesity carries less risk for black women compared to white women. The access to medical services enjoyed by this group no doubt contributed to the control of chronic health problems, such as diabetes mellitus and hypertension, that are associated with obesity and are prevalent among blacks. The incidence of diabetes is one third higher among blacks than among whites, and mortality rates are doubled among blacks with diabetes.

Waist-to-hip ratio and cardiovascular risk. The waist-to-hip ratio, or proportion of abdominal to **gluteal** fat, is associated with the risk of cardiovascular disease in both younger and older age groups. Individuals with more abdominal or upper body fat (which produces a larger waist-to-hip ratio) are more likely to develop hypertension or diabetes and have a greater risk of stroke regardless of their total body fat.[16] Women with a greater proportion of lower body fat (more typical of females) have less risk.

There are several mechanisms by which increased abdominal fat could lead to metabolic changes that influence cardiovascular risk. Increased abdominal fat is associated with higher serum insulin and decreases in insulin sensitivity. Abdominal fat cells have relatively high rates of lipolysis, and the free fatty acids released flow directly into the portal circulation, providing the liver with a constant supply of fatty acids for lipoprotein synthesis. It has been suggested that the sex steroid hormones estrogen and **testosterone** are responsible for the fat patterning as well as the lipoprotein profiles of males and females.[17] In both men and women over age 60, the plasma HDL cholesterol level is inversely related to the waist-to-hip ratio.[52]

Heart Disease in Women

The incidence of heart disease in women lags far behind that of men until the age of menopause. Because men are younger when coronary heart disease becomes evident, this disorder traditionally has been viewed as a man's disease, and clinical trials have focused on reducing risk factors in men but not in women. Although women develop a risk for heart disease about 10 years later than men, the average 55-year-old woman can have the same risk of heart attack as the average 55-year-old man.[76] If significant risk factors are present—smoking, elevated serum cholesterol, and elevated blood pressure—her risk can be even higher than for a man with similar risk factors.

Age, race, obesity, lack of physical activity, and diabetes are risk factors in women as they are in men. Black women are at greater risk of heart disease than white women up to the age of 74; beyond that age white women have a greater risk. Women who smoke have a threefold risk of myocardial infarction compared to nonsmokers.[57] However, those who stop smoking can significantly decrease their risk. After 3 years of nonsmoking, the risk of former smokers was no different than that of those who had never smoked.

Obesity as determined by BMI was a significant risk factor for coronary heart disease in a study of nearly 116,000 nurses between the ages of 30 and 55.[40] After 8 years it was apparent that even mild to moderate overweight increased the risk of heart disease twofold to threefold in women of middle age or older. Age-adjusted risk was higher in those who gained more than 10 kg after age 18 than in those who gained 3 kg or less. Dietary intake of energy and fat were not related to BMI or coronary risk. Hypertension and inappropriate serum lipoprotein levels accounted for a major portion of the effect of overweight.

Estrogen imparts some protection against cardiovascular disease through its effect on serum lipoprotein levels. After menopause, however, LDL cholesterol begins to rise. In menopausal women receiving estrogen or hormone replacement therapy, LDL cholesterol remains at its former level, although plasma triglyceride levels increase significantly.[2,10] Natural menopause does not appear to affect plasma glucose or insulin levels or body weight. Clinical trials to examine the long-term effect of hormone replacement therapy on coronary heart disease in women are urgently needed.[2]

Heart Disease in Ethnic Groups

Black Americans, Hispanic people, and Native Americans appear to be at particular risk for conditions contributing to the development of coronary heart disease.[34,42] Hypertension and subsequent renal failure or stroke are more prevalent among black Americans than among white Americans. The causes of increased hypertension among blacks are likely to be both genetic and environmental. Hypertension is prevalent among black populations in Africa, suggesting a genetic link. Dietary factors, including excessive intakes of kilocalories or sodium or alcohol, may also be involved. Black women are more likely to be obese than white women and have a higher risk of hypertension.

Native Americans and Mexican Americans have the same degree of obesity as black Americans but are not as likely to develop hypertension.[34] In spite of their obesity, their blood pressure and serum cholesterol remain low. However, obese Native Americans and Mexican Americans do have a higher incidence of diabetes. Blood pressure levels are lower in Asian Americans and Pacific Islanders compared to white Americans.[42] Hypertension is prevalent in Cuban and Puerto Rican men and women, although data are limited. Minority group approaches to intervention should be implemented in clinical trials.

Preventing Heart Disease

Current opinions differ as to the efficacy or appropriateness of particular strategies for preventing coronary heart disease. Several large-scale clinical trials tested the effect of dietary and drug intervention on lowering serum cholesterol and blood pressure and reducing the number of deaths from coronary heart disease, but the outcomes remain controversial. An evaluation of six primary prevention trials[47] suggested that although deaths from coronary heart disease were lower among men receiving aggressive therapy to lower their serum cholesterol, total mortality did not differ between those who received the therapy and those who did not. Groups receiving treatment to lower their serum cholesterol showed an increase in deaths unrelated to illness (deaths from accidents or suicide). Those authors concluded that efforts to lower serum cholesterol should be confined to people at high risk rather than directed toward the general population.

In contrast, a recent report from the Multiple Risk Factor Intervention Trial,[48] which followed 7,000 men for 10½ years, noted that the mortality rates among those receiving dietary treatment were about 11% lower for coronary heart disease and 8% lower for all causes compared to mortality rates among those not receiving dietary treatment. This effect was observed 4 years after completion of the treatment program. It appears that the benefits of intervention are ongoing and may not become evident until years after the program. In fact, the full benefit of treatment may not be apparent for 10 to 20 years.

Current research in coronary heart disease is directed toward dietary and life-style changes that can prevent the formation of atherosclerotic plaques or even lead to the regression of existing plaques. One dietary habit that may pay dividends in reducing one's risk of coronary heart disease is eating fish several times a week. Eicosapentaenoic acid (an omega-3 fatty acid), found in fatty fish, has been reported to lower LDL cholesterol, raise HDL cholesterol, and

reduce blood clotting factors in certain individuals. Supplementation with fish oil also has been found to lower systolic blood pressure in men and women with systolic blood pressure between 141 and 180 mm Hg.[9] In nearly one third of the subjects, systolic blood pressure decreased more than 10 mm Hg. A significant change in blood pressure following supplementation was more likely to occur in individuals who ate little fish before the study. Cod, herring, mackerel, and other fatty fish are good sources of omega-3 fatty acids.

Recent reports have suggested that regular use of aspirin at low doses can prevent myocardial infarction in middle-aged men and women.[1,41,64] The protective effect of one aspirin tablet (325 mg) each day or one aspirin tablet every other day has been attributed to aspirin's ability to prevent the formation of blood clots that can block the passage of blood through a coronary artery.[41,64] However, larger amounts of aspirin (650 mg per day or more) have been associated with a risk of hemorrhagic stroke and resulting disability.[1] In light of the serious side effects associated with inappropriate use of aspirin, individuals of all ages should consult a health professional before beginning regular use of aspirin for preventing coronary attack.

A comprehensive regimen consisting of a low-fat vegetarian diet, stress management techniques, prescribed exercise, and regular group sessions to provide social support has proven successful in reducing the size of existing atherosclerotic lesions in middle-aged men and women.[51,56] The reduction in size tended to be greater in women, suggesting that gender influences the progression of atherosclerosis. The prescribed diet contained 70% to 75% complex carbohydrates, 15% to 20% protein, and 10% fat. It provided the recommended levels of all nutrients with the exception of vitamin B_{12}, which was given in the form of supplements. Following this test diet without constant nutrition monitoring would be unwise, but the study provides evidence that through changes in diet and exercise, people can reduce existing atherosclerotic plaques and coronary risk. A less stringent diet that would allow sufficient animal protein to meet the requirement for vitamin B_{12} and a higher intake of essential fatty acids could also be beneficial in reducing coronary risk.

Cancer

Cancer is the second leading cause of death among people over age 65 and by the year 2000 is expected to replace heart disease as the leading cause of death in the United States.[50] The anticipated emergence of cancer over heart disease as the leading cause of death is related to the consistent decline in deaths from heart disease over the past 40 years. This decline was brought about in part by public education and life-style modification designed to reduce the prevalence of risk factors that lead to coronary heart disease.

Incidence. Unfortunately, the life-style factors associated with cancer (except for cigarette smoking) are just beginning to receive attention. As pointed out by Nissinen and Stanley,[50] cancer research is now at the stage where cardiovascular research was 30 years ago. Epidemiologic studies have revealed some indication of associations between diet and cancer, but the evidence is not strong and often is conflicting.[12] This has led to considerable debate over whether there is sufficient evidence to make specific dietary recommendations.

Breast cancer has increased in incidence over the past 15 years, and its association with dietary fat remains an issue.[22] The decline in reported cases of stomach cancer has been attributed to the increased use of refrigeration in food storage and lower consumption of salted and pickled foods.[22] The incidence of colon cancer has remained relatively unchanged despite public education about eating foods high in fiber.[22] Dietary components being evaluated in relation to cancer incidence include total kilocalories, fat, fiber, iron, selenium, calcium, ascorbic acid, beta carotene, and vitamins E and A.

Development. The sequence of events that transform a normal cell into cancerous tissue includes three steps: **initiation, promotion,** and progression.[71] Dietary influences may interact in any of these steps. The initiation step in carcinogenesis is an irreversible genetic alteration that gives a normal cell the potential for uncontrolled growth. This genetic damage may result from an environmental toxin, a free radical molecule, or unknown causes. In the promotion step the abnormal cell is stimulated to grow and produce a cancer. Nutrients that act as antioxidants and thus can prevent cellular damage by free radical molecules may offer some protection against cancer initiation or promotion. The last and most serious step in cancer development is the progression step in which the tumor cells **metastasize** and colonize new cancer sites in the body.

Genetic and environmental factors, including diet, appear to be involved in the development of cancer. In animal models high-fat diets promote tumor growth; however, both the total caloric intake and the type of fat influence this response.[71] In certain animals diets high in energy that lead to rapid growth and enhanced cell proliferation increase tumor development, whereas in other animals with similar caloric intakes, no tumors develop. This evidence supports the concept of a genetic influence on cancer development.

Dietary fat. Ongoing human epidemiologic studies evaluating dietary fat intake and cancer incidence have produced inconclusive results.[12] Although some studies suggest that an increased fat intake leads to an increased risk of cancer, others have found no relationship. Many factors contribute to these differences in findings among studies.[12] The food records obtained may not be valid representations of actual food intake or the particular type of fat consumed. Food patterns may have changed between the time of the initial survey and the intervening years of follow-up. A further complicating factor is that high-fat diets are likely to be high in energy as well. Little work has been done on dietary intake at older ages and cancer incidence.

Dietary fat has been most closely associated with cancers of the breast and colon. A study of more than 89,000 nurses ages 34 to 59[33] revealed no significant association between total dietary fat or type of dietary fat and breast cancer, after 4 years of follow-up. Fat consumption by these women ranged from 32% to 44% of total energy. Similarly, the risk of breast cancer was not related to the intake of meat, eggs, cheese, and milk among more than 27,500 Seventh Day Adventist women in California studied between 1960 and 1980.[61] Although Seventh Day Adventists are less likely to eat meat (on the average, 55% had meat less than once a week), most of the women ate cheese and eggs at least one to three times a week and drank one or two glasses of milk a day. Mean fat intake was 38% of total energy; saturated and polyunsaturated fats contributed 11% and 18%, respectively, of total kilocalories.

Findings differed among a group of Israeli women over age 50.[12] Those who had a high-fat, low-fiber diet had double the risk of breast cancer of those who had a low-fat, high-fiber diet. The differences in the results of these studies may relate to the amount of dietary fat consumed by the various groups. It has been suggested that dietary fat intake must fall below 20% of total energy before an impact on the incidence of breast cancer can be demonstrated.[33] Both the nurses and the Seventh Day Adventist women were well above that level.

Colon and rectal cancer have also been associated with high intakes of dietary fat, particularly animal fat.[12] In the group of nurses described above, dietary intake of animal fat was significantly related to incidence of colon cancer.[74] Women who ate beef, pork, or lamb five to six times a week had a risk nearly twice that of women who ate chicken with the skin removed or fish. Energy intake was unrelated to the incidence of colon cancer. A low intake of fiber from fruit appeared to contribute to risk, but this association was not statistically significant. Among the Seventh-day Adventist men and women,[61] consumption of animal foods, including dairy products and eggs, was unrelated to colon cancer. The use of low-fat dairy products by this group may have contributed to this finding.

Dietary fiber. Dietary fiber has been promoted as a means of reducing the risk of colorectal cancer.[12] Possible mechanisms by which dietary fiber may exert a protective effect include (1) reducing exposure to carcinogens by acting as a diluent and increasing fecal bulk, (2) reducing exposure to carcinogens by decreasing transit time, or (3) increasing the excretion of fecal bile acids that enhance the risk of cancer. Certain fiber components such as pectin decrease intestinal cell proliferation and thereby reduce risk. It appears, however, that fiber-rich foods, rather than fiber per se, provide a more consistent protective effect against colorectal cancer, suggesting that factors other than the fiber (e.g., carotenoids or ascorbic acid) also may be involved.[12]

Dietary minerals. Epidemiologic studies have examined dietary intakes of calcium, iron, and selenium in relation to cancer risk. A high intake of calcium reduces the loss of surface epithelial cells in the gastrointestinal tract and thereby reduces compensatory cell proliferation; however, further work is needed to determine the physiologic importance of this reaction.[12] International comparisons of calcium availability and colorectal cancer have been complicated by the fat present in the milk products supplying calcium.

Iron can catalyze the production of high-energy oxygen molecules considered to be potential carcinogens; consequently, iron status has been evaluated in respect to cancer risk.[65] Individuals with high body stores of iron may be at greater risk, but there is no association between dietary iron levels and the development of cancer.[65] The role of selenium in human cancer is not understood. Cancer patients tend to have low serum selenium compared to healthy people, but this may be a consequence rather than an antecedent of the disease. Tissue selenium levels are unrelated to the incidence of breast cancer.[24]

Dietary vitamins. Increasing evidence suggests that ascorbic acid, vitamin E, and the carotenoids decrease the risk of cancer. All can function as antioxidants and protect tissues against oxidative damage from highly reactive free radicals. Ascorbic acid is the primary antioxidant in blood plasma; it protects vitamin E in cell membranes and complements the action of the carotenoids. Apart from its role as a precursor of vitamin A, beta carotene can interfere with carcinogenesis at both the initiation and promotion steps. Low intake of vegetables and fruits and low plasma levels of beta carotene have been associated with subsequent development of lung cancer.[12]

A study of 872 men ages 40 to 59 who were followed for 25 years revealed an inverse relationship between intake of ascorbic acid and the incidence of lung cancer.[8] Ascorbic acid taken in amounts of 70 mg or more appeared to offer some protection against the risk of cancer, even among those who smoked. Ascorbic acid also has been shown to exert a significant protective effect against breast, gastric, cervical, and rectal cancer. Serum vitamin E is higher in individuals who remain free of lung cancer compared to those with similar risk factors who develop the disease.[12]

Because the intake of both carotenoids and ascorbic acid has been related to cancer mortality, one research approach has been to develop a fruit and vegetable score for study participants. This also recognizes the possibility that other compounds present in these foods may contribute to reducing the risk of cancer. The fruit and vegetable scores of 1,271 people over age 65 who live in the community suggested that daily consumption of carotenoid-containing fruits and vegetables can lower the risk of cancer even at older ages.[11] After 5 years, individuals who ate an average of less than one serving daily of deep yellow fruits and vegetables had three times the risk of dying of cancer than those who ate more than two servings daily. Another possible explanation for this finding is that people who eat more servings of fruits and vegetables eat lesser amounts of other foods that may contribute to risk. In this group neither age nor smoking status was related to cancer mortality. Eating fruits and vegetables daily appears to be a practical way to decrease the risk of cancer for people of all ages.

Evaluation of International Populations

Long-lived populations. Over the years attention has been directed toward populations who appear to enjoy long lives with a minimum of chronic disease and disability. Three isolated locations thought to have an above-average number of older residents were (1) the village of Vilcabamba, high in the Andes Mountains of Ecuador[14]; (2) the Hunza, a small territory in the Himalayas of Pakistan[36]; and (3) the republic of Georgia in the Caucasus Mountains of the former Soviet Union.[36] Although it was learned that residents systematically exaggerated their ages by at least a decade,[45] so that so-called centenarians were actually 80 to 90 years old, the fact remains that these communities have individuals of advanced age who remain physically active. Examining their diet and activity patterns may provide clues to health practices that promote successful aging.

The dietary patterns of these communities are outlined in Table 2-3.[35,36] The Vilcabambians and Hunzas are primarily vegetarians, whereas the Georgians have a mixed diet containing meat and dairy foods. In Vilcabamba the primary source of energy is carbohydrates, including grains, corn, beans, potatoes, oranges, and bananas. Meat is eaten an average of less than once a week, and the total protein obtained from animal sources is estimated to be about 12 g daily. What little milk is available is made into cheese. Hunza is primarily an agrarian society that raises barley, wheat, millet, vegetables, fruits, and nuts. The rough terrain prohibits the

TABLE 2-3   Estimated Daily Nutrient Intake of Long-Lived Populations

	Vilcabambians	Hunzas	Georgians
Energy (kcal)	1,200-1,700	1,900	1,700-1,900
Total protein (g)	35-38	50	70-90
Animal protein (g)	12	<1	(predominantly animal)
Fat (g)	12-19	35	40-60
Carbohydrates (g)	200-360	350	250-300

Modified from Davies D: A Shangri-la in Ecuador, *New Scient* 57:236, 1973; Leaf A: The aging process: lessons from observations in man, *Nutr Rev* 46:40, 1988; Leaf A: *Youth in old age*, New York, 1975, McGraw Hill.

raising of livestock, and less than 1% of total kilocalories is obtained from meat or dairy foods. Meat, usually mutton, is eaten only once or twice a year on special days. Oil derived from apricot seeds is used in cooking.

In contrast, animal foods are used frequently by the Georgians. Dairy products are eaten at each meal and are the major source of protein, although meat is served frequently. Bread and corn meal mush are the major carbohydrate foods. In general, diets in these communities are low to moderate in energy. Although the intakes of protein and saturated fat differ considerably, the primary source of kilocalories in all three groups is complex carbohydrates, suggesting a generous intake of fiber.

A general characteristic of these populations is a high degree of physical activity continuing into advanced age, particularly for those who work in agriculture. Among 25 older Hunzas, serum cholesterol ranged from 150 to 180 mg/dl.[68] In these communities low to moderate intakes of energy and fat and continued physical activity appear to contribute to survival to advanced ages.

The China study. A comprehensive study of diet and disease in more than 6,000 adults in China[37] is providing additional perspective on the role of nutrition in preventing disease. China is one of the few places in the world where it is possible to find a group of individuals who are genetically homogeneous and who have lived in the same place and eaten the same foods throughout their lives. At the same time, there are large regional differences in China that allow comparison of different eating patterns and the development of degenerative diseases. Researchers collected information on what and how much individuals ate by spending 3 days in each household and observing dietary practices.

The average Chinese diet contains 2,600 kcal, 75% from carbohydrate, 15% from fat, and 10% from protein (93% comes from plant protein).

Rice is an important staple food and is eaten at almost every meal. Vegetables are eaten in season, and large amounts of tubers, such as sweet potatoes, are also consumed. In some regions fish is a daily part of the diet, but in other areas fish is seldom available. Eggs, pork, and chicken are eaten infrequently. In most areas milk products are unknown, and for most of the country the major sources of calcium are vegetables.

The Chinese eat about one third less protein than Americans, and only 15% of their energy is supplied by fat. In general the incidence of heart disease is significantly lower than in the United States; however, Chinese living in more affluent urban locations who consume diets higher in animal protein have the highest rates of heart disease and cancer. The Chinese diet contains about three times more fiber than the typical American diet and is rich in carotenoids. The rate of colon cancer among the Chinese is only two thirds that observed in the United States. The Chinese consume about 20% more kilocalories than the typical American, but obesity is rare. High levels of physical activity are common among most people in China.

Serum cholesterol levels among the Chinese indicate a life-style that includes a low-fat diet, a high level of physical exercise, and an appropriate body weight. Among urban Chinese between the ages of 25 and 64, the mean serum cholesterol level was 158 mg/dl, compared to 216 mg/dl in the United States.[70] Only 12% of the Chinese people had a serum cholesterol level above 200 mg/dl. In the United States 60% of the adult population have such levels.

Although analysis of data from the China study continues, these reports suggest that diets in which most of the kilocalories are obtained from plant foods reduce the incidence of chronic diseases. This supports the recent recommendation of the National Research Council[12] that Americans obtain at least 55% of their total kilocalories from plant foods.

Nutrient Intake and Life Span

Longitudinal dietary studies. Longitudinal studies evaluating the overall dietary pattern of individuals and their subsequent **morbidity** and mortality have been few in number. A longitudinal study of 103 older Michigan women evaluated over a 24-year period suggested that the nutrient quality of the diet influenced both physical well-being and the length of life.[59] After 7 years[29] mortality was higher in those women consuming diets containing less than 40% of the Recommended Dietary Allowance (RDA) for one or more nutrients. The nutrients most frequently deficient were calcium, vitamin A, and ascorbic acid.

A follow-up after 24 years revealed that the survivors, who ranged in age from 64 to 90 years, had reduced the quantity and improved the quality of the food they ate.[59] Caloric intake decreased from 1,683 to 1,297 kcal and fat from 74 to 51 g. Protein intake did not change. Foods such as sweet baked items that are high in simple carbohydrates and fat but low in other nutrients were eaten less frequently. Fruits, vegetables, breads and cereals, and low-fat rather than high-fat dairy products were emphasized. Fat as a percentage of total kilocalories decreased from 40% to 35%; carbohydrates supplied 47% of total kilocalories. Reducing dietary fat to 30% of total caloric intake and increasing complex carbohydrates to 55% to 60% of total caloric intake can be a model for successful aging.

Health Practices and Mortality

The Alameda Health Study. A longitudinal study begun in 1965 is examining behavioral, social, and demographic influences on the incidence of disease and mortality in nearly 7,000 residents of Alameda County, California.[28] A recent follow-up conducted 17 years after the study began examined factors related to mortality in people who were 60 to 94 years of age when they were first interviewed.[28] In both men and women, four health-related factors decreased one's risk of death:

- not smoking
- regular physical activity
- appropriate **relative weight** (not more than 10% under or 30% over average weight for height)
- regularly eating breakfast

These patterns were particularly consistent among individuals age 70 or older.

In the Alameda study, factors shown to increase the mortality risk in people of middle age also increased the risk in people of older ages. Current smokers had a mortality risk 1½ times that of nonsmokers or past smokers of similar age. The increased risk associated with inappro-

priate relative weight and low physical activity was similar for those age 70 or older and those ages 50 to 59. In contrast, eating breakfast regularly, which positively influenced the length of life in the oldest age group, had no impact on risk in those of middle age. Unfortunately, information on specific food intake was not available; however, one might expect that individuals who consider breakfast important also attach importance to other aspects of their diet.

The Alameda study suggests that patterns of mortality and morbidity, even among the elderly, are not a random process. Life-style choices over which the individual has some control play a role in exacerbating or reducing risk. Behavior in later life is at least partly responsible for an individual's health status, regardless of genetic influences. In pairs of male identical twins, an increase in systolic and diastolic blood pressure and a 50 mg/dl increase in serum triglyceride occurred only in the twin who had a significant weight gain between young adulthood and middle age.[49] These findings emphasize the need for and the potential benefits of intervention strategies directed toward individuals at both younger and older ages. Improving health practices can have a positive effect even among those in poor health by preventing further decline. Nutrition education should be an integral part of such a program.

What can we learn from centenarians? In the United States about 1 in 10,000 people lives to be at least 100 years old. It is likely that both genetic and life-style habits contribute to this accomplishment. A recent study of 30 Kentucky centenarians, 19 women and 11 men, indicated that most had parents who survived to age 70 or older.[30] But the most striking characteristic common to these individuals was their history regarding use of cigarettes and alcohol. None was a current smoker, and only one had ever smoked. Eighteen of the 30 had never used alcohol, and the remaining 12 had no excessive alcohol use. Four of these centenarians lived alone, 11 lived with family members or others, and 15 lived in long-term care facilities. About half had hypertension and one third were being treated for heart disease. Despite some chronic disease, more than half of these older people were moderately active and frequently left their homes, although some required assistance. Only two were totally dependent on others for their care. It would appear that hypertension is not inconsistent with an extended life span if other compelling risk factors are not present.

An evaluation of autopsy records obtained from centenarians[31] indicated that infection was the leading cause of death, followed by cancer and cardiovascular disease. Disorders that were conspicuously absent from these records were diabetes mellitus, obesity, and hypertension. It is interesting to note that two of the characteristics associated with centenarians, reasonable weight for height and not smoking, were also predictors of longevity in the Alameda study described earlier. The reduced prevalence of chronic diseases observed in these centenarians should be the goal for health promotion efforts designed to reach all age and ethnic groups.

Need for Continued Research

Although an appropriate nutrient intake, regular physical activity, and an appropriate body weight extend physical well-being and delay physiologic deterioration, the mechanisms by which this is accomplished are not understood. Furthermore, the literature on which these conclusions are based is fragmentary, involving only small numbers of people observed over short periods of time.

In their comprehensive review of nutrition and aging published more than 20 years ago, Howell and Loeb[23] called for studies that evaluate the lifelong food intake of individuals in relation to their physical health and chronic disease in later years. Theoretically such a study should begin in childhood, as animal work suggests that food habits early in life influence biochemical processes and the development of chronic disease. Obviously such an evaluation would be a mammoth undertaking from the standpoint of funding and the level of organization required. We could begin by expanding the nutritional component of the BLSA now being carried on by the National Institute on Aging. Although this study has focused on the stages of life beyond adolescence, younger individuals might be added to the ongoing age **cohorts**. Another major need is longitudinal studies with women and ethnic minorities, who have different patterns of disease risk. Only by such a strategy will we learn what dietary and life-style patterns are necessary to ensure optimum health throughout the life cycle.

Summary

Both qualitative and quantitative aspects of the diet influence physical well-being, the incidence of disease, and length of life. A nutritionally adequate diet, restricted only in energy, increases the life span and delays the appearance of age-related physiologic and biochemical changes in experimental animals. Caloric restriction retards the appearance of both normal, age-related changes and degenerative diseases, although the neural or hormonal mechanisms by which this is accomplished are not understood.

The major causes of death in older people are cardiovascular diseases and cancer, and both are influenced by nutritional factors. Contrary to popular opinion, the factors that increase cardiovascular risk in younger people (smoking, inappropriate serum lipoprotein levels, obesity, limited physical activity, elevated blood pressure, and glucose intolerance) continue to do so at older ages. Obesity, both as an independent risk factor and because of its association with other risk factors, represents a significant health hazard at middle and advanced ages. Programs designed to adjust dietary energy and fat levels to appropriately modify serum lipoprotein levels can improve physical well-being and decrease the risk of heart attack or stroke in people of all ages. Limiting dietary fat and increasing consumption of fruits and vegetables rich in carotenoids and ascorbic acid appears to offer some protection against the development of cancer. Although longitudinal studies of humans have been limited in number, the evidence suggests that diets with moderate levels of energy and fat but generous servings of fruits, vegetables, and unrefined grain products promote the continuation of good health throughout adulthood.

REVIEW QUESTIONS

1. How does caloric restriction influence (1) life span, (2) incidence of degenerative disease, and (3) age-related biochemical changes in animal models? Discuss possible hormonal mechanisms by which caloric restriction may bring about these changes.
2. What are the major risk factors for cardiovascular disease in people age 65 or older? Do risk factors differ for older people compared to middle-aged people? How might these risk factors be reduced or modified?
3. How does obesity contribute to mortality risk in older people? What are possible biases in research studies that may obscure the risk associated with obesity?
4. What are the three steps in the development of cancer? What are the nutrients associated with increased and decreased risk of cancer? How do they relate to cancer development?
5. List several health practices associated with increased length of life in older people. How might these practices retard the development of degenerative disease?

LEARNING ACTIVITIES

1. Review the health practices associated with increased life span in the Alameda Health Study. Visit a congregate meal site or senior citizens center, and interview 10 older people about their general health habits.
2. Plan an activity program for an older person that will allow him or her to expend 200 to 250 kcal a day.
3. Develop a nutrition education program for a senior citizens center that will help participants decrease their cardiovascular risk.
4. Plan a 3-day menu for an older woman living alone that will help her reduce her risk of cancer.

Key Terms

Provided here for review is a list of the major terms in this chapter. The definitions can be found in the Glossary, which begins on p. 336. To help you understand how these terms are applied, the page number is given for the first mention of each term in the chapter.

REFERENCES

1. Appel LJ, Bush T: Preventing heart disease in women: another role for aspirin, *JAMA* 266:565, 1991.
2. Barrett-Connor E, Bush TL: Estrogen and coronary heart disease in women, *JAMA* 265(14): 1861, 1991.
3. Beeuwkes AM: Early speculations on diet and longevity. I, *J Am Diet Assoc* 28:628, 1952.
4. Beeuwkes, AM: Early speculations on diet and longevity. II, *J Am Diet Assoc* 28:707, 1952.
5. Benfante R, Reed D: Is elevated serum cholesterol level a risk factor for coronary heart disease in the elderly? *JAMA* 263(3):393, 1990.
6. Blair SN and others: Physical fitness and all-cause mortality: a prospective study of healthy men and women, *JAMA* 262(17):2395, 1989.
7. Blankenhorn DH and others: The influence of diet on the appearance of new lesions in human coronary arteries, *JAMA* 263:1646, 1990.
8. Bloch G: Epidemiologic evidence regarding vitamin C and cancer, *Am J Clin Nutr* 54:1310S, 1991.
9. Bonaa KH and others: Effect of eicosapen-

taenoic and docosahexaenoic acids on blood pressure in hypertension: a population-based intervention trial from the Tromso study, *N Engl J Med* 322:795, 1990.

10. Campos H and others: Differences in apolipoproteins and low-density lipoprotein subfractions in postmenopausal women on and off estrogen therapy: results from the Framingham offspring study, *Metabolism* 39(10):1033, 1990.

11. Colditz GA and others: Increased green and yellow vegetable intake and lowered cancer deaths in an elderly population, *Am J Clin Nutr* 41:32, 1985.

12. Committee on Diet and Health, Food and Nutrition Board: Diet and health: Implications for reducing chronic disease risk, Washington, DC, 1989, National Academy Press.

13. Darby WJ: Early concepts on the role of nutrition, diet, and longevity. In Prinsley DM, Sandstead HH, editors: *Nutrition and aging,* New York, 1990, Alan R Liss.

14. Davies D: A Shangri-la in Ecuador, *New Scient* 57:236, 1973.

15. Expert Panel: Report of the national cholesterol education program expert panel on detection, evaluation, and treatment of high blood cholesterol in adults, *Arch Intern Med* 148:36, 1988.

16. Folsom AR and others: Incidence of hypertension and stroke in relation to body fat distribution and other risk factors in older women, *Stroke* 21:701, 1990.

17. Freedman DS and others: Body fat distribution and male/female differences in lipids and lipoproteins, *Circulation* 81:1498, 1990.

18. Ginsberg HN and others: Reduction of plasma cholesterol levels in normal men on an American Heart Association step 1 diet with added monounsaturated fat, *N Engl J Med* 322:574, 1990.

19. Grundy SM: Cholesterol and coronary heart disease, *JAMA* 264:3053, 1990.

20. Harris T and others: Body mass index and mortality among nonsmoking older persons, *JAMA* 259(10):1520, 1988.

21. Hazzard WR: Atherosclerosis and aging: a scenario in flux, *Am J Cardiol* 63:20H, 1989.

22. Henderson BE, Ross RK, Pike MC: Toward the primary prevention of cancer, *Science* 254:1131, 1991.

23. Howell SC, Loeb MB: Nutrition and aging: a monograph for practitioners, *Gerontologist* 9(suppl):1, 1969.

24. Hunter DJ and others: A prospective study of selenium status and breast cancer risk, *JAMA* 264(9):1128, 1990.

25. Ingram DK and others: Dietary restriction benefits learning and motor performance of aged mice, *J Gerontol* 42:78, 1987.

26. Iwasaki K and others: The influence of dietary protein source on longevity and age-related disease processes of Fischer rats, *J Gerontol* 43:B5, 1988.

27. Kannel WB: Nutrition and the occurrence and prevention of cardiovascular disease in the elderly, *Nutr Rev* 46(2):68, 1988.

28. Kaplan GA and others: Mortality among the elderly in the Alameda County study: behavioral and demographic risk factors, *Am J Public Health* 77:307, 1987.

29. Kelley L, Ohlson MA, Harper LJ: Food selection and well-being of aging women, *J Am Diet Assoc* 33:466, 1957.

30. Kinzel T, Wekstein D, Kirkpatrick C: A social and clinical evaluation of centenarians, *Exp Aging Res* 12:173, 1986.

31. Klatt E, Meyer PR: Geriatric autopsy pathology in centenarians, *Arch Pathol Lab Med* 111:367, 1987.

32. Koizumi A, Weindruch R, Walford RL: Influences of dietary restriction and age on liver enzyme activities and lipid peroxidation in mice, *J Nutr* 117:361, 1987.

33. Kolata G: Dietary fat–breast cancer link questioned, *Science* 235:436, 1987.

34. Kuller LH: Overview: cardiovascular diseases and stroke in African-Americans and other racial minorities in the United States, *Circulation* 83:1462, 1991.

35. Leaf A: The aging process: lessons from observations in man, *Nutr Rev* 46:40, 1988.

36. Leaf A: *Youth in old age,* New York, 1975, McGraw Hill.

37. Liebman B: Lessons from China: interview with T Colin Campbell, *Nutr Action Health Letter* 17:10, 1990.

38. Liepa GU and others: Food restriction as a modulator of age-related changes in serum lipids, *Am J Physiol* 238:E253, 1980.

39. Manson JE and others: Body weight and longevity, *JAMA* 257:353, 1987.

40. Manson JE and others: A prospective study of obesity and risk of coronary heart disease in women, *N Engl J Med* 322:882, 1990.

41. Manson JE and others: A prospective study of aspirin use and primary prevention of cardiovascular disease in women, *JAMA* 266:521, 1991.

42. Martinez-Maldonado M: Hypertension in Hispanics, Asians, Pacific-Islanders, and Native Americans, *Circulation* 83:1467, 1991.

43. Masoro EJ, McCarter RJM: Dietary restriction as a probe of mechanisms of senescence, *Ann Rev Gerontol Geriatr* 10:183, 1990.

44. Masoro EJ, Shimokawa I, Yu BP: Retardation of the aging processes in rats by food restriction, *Ann NY Acad Sci* 621:337, 1991.

45. Mazess RB, Forman SH: Longevity and age exaggeration in Vilcabamba, Ecuador, *J Gerontol* 34:94, 1979.

46. McCay CM and others: Retarded growth, life span, ultimate body size, and age changes in the albino rat after feeding diets restricted in calories, *J Nutr* 18:1, 1939.

47. Muldoon MF, Manuck SB, Matthews KA: Lowering cholesterol concentrations and mortality: a quantitative review of primary prevention trials, *Br Med J* 301:309, 1990.

48. Multiple Risk Factor Intervention Trial Research Group: Mortality rates after 10.5 years for participants in the multiple risk factor intervention trial, *JAMA* 263(13):1795, 1990.

49. Newman B and others: Nongenetic influences of obesity on other cardiovascular disease risk factors: an analysis of identical twins, *Am J Public Health* 80:675, 1990.

50. Nissinen A, Stanley K: Unbalanced diets as a cause of chronic diseases, *Am J Clin Nutr* 49:993, 1989.

51. Ornish D and others: Can lifestyle changes reverse coronary heart disease?: the lifestyle heart trial, *Lancet* 336:129, 1990.

52. Ostlund RE and others: The ratio of waist-to-hip circumference, plasma insulin level, and glucose intolerance as independent predictors of the HDL_2 cholesterol level in older adults, *N Engl J Med* 322(4):229, 1990.

53. Paffenbarger RS and others: Physical activity, all-cause mortality, and longevity of college alumni, *N Engl J Med* 314(10):605, 1986.

54. Psaty BM and others: Risk ratios and risk differences in estimating the effect of risk factors for cardiovascular disease in the elderly, *J Clin Epidemiol* 43(9):961, 1990.

55. Reaven PD and others: Leisure time exercise and lipid and lipoprotein levels in an older population, *J Am Geriatr Soc* 38:847, 1990.

56. Reversing heart disease through diet, exercise, and stress management: an interview with Dean Ornish, *J Am Diet Assoc* 91:162, 1991.

57. Rosenberg L, Palmer JR, Shapiro S: Decline in the risk of myocardial infarction among women who stop smoking, *N Engl J Med* 322(4):213, 1990.

58. Schaefer EJ and others: Plasma lipoproteins in healthy octogenarians: lack of reduced high-density lipoprotein cholesterol levels: results from the Framingham Heart Study, *Metabolism* 38:293, 1989.

59. Schlenker ED: Nutritional status of older women, doctoral dissertation, East Lansing, Mich, 1976, Michigan State University.

60. Slattery ML, Randall DE: Trends in coronary heart disease mortality and food consumption in the United States between 1909 and 1980, *Am J Clin Nutr* 47:1060, 1988.

61. Snowdon DA: Animal product consumption and mortality because of all causes combined, coronary heart disease, stroke, diabetes, and cancer in Seventh-day Adventists, *Am J Clin Nutr* 48:739, 1988.

62. Society of Actuaries: Build study: 1979, Chicago, 1980, The Society.

63. Stavenow L and others: Eighty-year-old men without cardiovascular disease in the community of Malmo. I. Social and medical factors, with special reference to the lipoprotein pattern, *J Intern Med* 228:9, 1990.

64. Steering Committee of the Physicians Health Study Research Group: Final report on the aspirin component of the ongoing physicians health study, *N Engl J Med* 321:129, 1989.

65. Stevens RG and others: Body iron stores and the risk of cancer, *N Engl J Med* 319(16):1047, 1988.

66. Sytkowski PA, Kannel WB, D'Agostino RB: Changes in risk factors and the decline in mortality from cardiovascular disease: the Framingham Heart Study, *N Engl J Med* 322:1635, 1990.

67. Tayback M, Kumanyika S, Chee E: Body weight as a risk factor in the elderly, *Arch Intern Med* 150:1065, 1990.

68. Toomey EG, White PD: A brief survey of the health of aged Hunzas, *Am Heart J* 68:841, 1964.

69. Van Itallie TB, Lew EA: Health implications of overweight in the elderly. In Prinsley D, Sandstead HH, editors: *Nutrition and aging*, New York, 1990, Alan R Liss.

70. Vartiainen E and others: Mortality, cardiovascular risk factors, and diet in China, Finland, and the United States, *Public Health Rep* 106:41, 1991.

71. Visek WJ: Diet and cancer. In Prinsley DM, Sandstead HH, editors: *Nutrition and aging*, New York, 1990, Alan R Liss.

72. Weindruch R, Walford RL: *The retardation of aging and disease by dietary restriction*, Springfield, Ill, 1988, Charles G Thomas.

73. Wienpahl J, Ragland DR, Sidney S: Body mass index and 15-year mortality in a cohort of black men and women, *J Clin Epidemiol* 43(9):949, 1990.
74. Willett WC and others: Relation of meat, fat, and liver intake to the risk of colon cancer in a prospective study among women, *N Engl J Med* 323(24):1664, 1990.
75. Wilson PWF, Abbott RD, Castelli WP: High-density lipoprotein cholesterol and mortality: the Framingham Heart Study, *Arteriosclerosis* 8:737, 1988.
76. Women and heart disease: an equal opportunity, *the Johns Hopkins Medical Letter* 2(6):4, 1990.

3

Body Composition, Energy, and Physical Activity

✦✦

After studying this chapter, the student should be able to:

✔ *Recognize the influence of aging on body composition*

✔ *Understand the limitations of existing methods of measuring body composition*

✔ *Recognize the factors affecting body composition in older people*

✔ *Understand the effect of physical activity on body composition in older people*

✔ *Determine appropriate methods of estimating energy expenditure*

Introduction

An issue of concern to both health professionals and the public is the amount of fat and muscle tissue in our bodies. Early workers also recognized the relationship of body constituents to health and disease and examined cadavers to determine the size and content of various body compartments. In the nineteenth century, as the chemical elements were being identified, many were found to be present in body tissues and fluids. The discovery of naturally occurring isotopes and the development of electrical conductivity measurements in recent years have made it possible to evaluate body compartments in living people. Body composition can provide an indication of nutritional status and level of physical fitness, and point to changes that reflect disease processes rather than normal

aging. Changes in body composition and body fat content contribute to the decrease in caloric requirements observed in many older people. Energy balance in older age groups is complicated further by the age-related decline in physical activity. These relationships are important clinically in helping the older individual achieve or maintain an appropriate body weight.

BODY COMPARTMENTS
Definitions

To evaluate body composition, we must divide the body into compartments according to chemical, anatomic, or fluid characteristics.[39] The chemical model used to evaluate body composition organizes the body compartments according to their water, mineral, and organic components. The major organic components of the body by weight are protein and fat. Another approach to the study of body composition divides the body into metabolically active tissues and relatively inactive tissues. These two tissues are contained in two compartments: the fat-free mass, which contains the metabolically active tissues, and body fat, which contains the relatively inactive energy stores.

Current work is focusing on a four compartment model that would include (1) body protein, (2) body fat, (3) **total body water,** and (4) total body mineral.[39] The advantage of this model is that total body water, fat, and mineral can be measured directly using new methods that do not depend on established formulas. Body nitrogen can be measured directly, and this value multiplied by 6.25 determines total body protein. Direct measurements are preferred, since formulas established in healthy young adults can be inappropriate for the malnourished or reasonably healthy older adult. Both the absolute and relative sizes of the body compartments are influenced by the aging process and by disease.

Fat-Free Mass

The body's **fat-free mass (FFM)** is equal to the total body weight minus the weight of body fat.[31] Body components included in the FFM are water, protein, and minerals. The intracellular and extracellular fluids, muscle tissue, vital organs, protein components of adipose cells, and the skeleton are included in the FFM. Another frequently used term is **"lean body mass" (LBM).** LBM designates the compartment remaining when the ether-extractable fat from the adipose tissue is subtracted from body weight. LBM is considered synonymous with FFM.[31] LBM does include the structural lipids in cell membranes and nerves, although this lipid is rather insignificant in amount compared to the amount of triglyceride stored in adipose tissue. FFM is a rather heterogeneous tissue and is determined by using both direct and indirect measurements. Total body water and total body potassium can be measured directly in living individuals, and the values obtained are used to calculate body fat.

Body Cell Mass

Body cell mass (BCM) is the term used to describe the body compartment that includes the active energy-using cells of the body but not the less metabolically active cells in the supporting structures.[82] BCM includes the cells in the muscle, vital organs, blood, and brain. Cells in bone or connective tissues, which have slower turnover rates, are excluded. BCM is calculated on the basis of total body potassium and includes the tissues that account for most of the body's oxygen consumption and its potassium content. BCM is a useful concept, because it involves tissues that are directly influenced and altered by nutrient intake and physical activity over days or weeks.[82]

Total Body Water

On a weight basis, water is the most abundant constituent in the body, making up about 60% of body weight in young adult men. About 55% of total body water (TBW) is intracellular, and about 45% is extracellular.[54] Extracellular water consists of plasma, lymph, and the interstitial fluid bathing the cells. Sodium is the primary electrolyte in the extracellular fluid, and potassium is the primary electrolyte in the intracellular fluid. Eighty-five percent of the sodium in the body is found in the extracellular compartment; 98% of the potassium in the body is found within the cell.[30]

TBW is relatively easy to measure, since a radioactively labeled tracer dose of water will reach equilibrium with both intracellular and extracellular water in several hours. TBW can be calculated according to the volume of labeled water given and the final equilibrium concentration. Specific isotopes or dyes can be used to provide an estimation of total extracellular fluid volume, which allows the intracellular fluid volume to be calculated by difference.[31]

Body Fat

The human body has an unlimited capacity to store fat. Fat is stored in the adipose tissue in the form of triglycerides (neutral fat) and can account for as much as one half of total body weight. Adipose tissue consists of about 83% triglyceride, 2% protein, and 15% water.[36] Total body fat can be measured directly through the uptake of fat-soluble gases, **anthropometric measurements, computed tomography** (CT), and **neutron activation** systems. Total body fat can also be calculated using equations derived from direct measurement of FFM and BCM.

Influences on Body Compartments

Body compartments are constantly subject to changes in volume as a result of external or internal influences. External influences, such as increases or decreases in calorie intake or exercise, lead to changes in body FFM and body fat. Internal influences include the aging process or pathologic processes related to disease.

A shift in the size of one compartment effects a change in the size of another. TBW will be altered if FFM decreases or increases. Since adipose tissue contains less water than does FFM, an increase in fat at the expense of lean tissue decreases total body water. A loss of bone mineral as a consequence of aging decreases the size of the FFM but not that of the BCM, which is made up solely of highly metabolically active cells.[30] In the following section we review current methods for evaluating body composition and consider the appropriateness of each for use with the older adult.

METHODS FOR EVALUATING BODY COMPOSITION
Limitations of Existing Methods

Early researchers studied body composition by chemically analyzing human cadavers for water, fat, nitrogen, and specific minerals.[30] Highly specialized methods have since been developed to evaluate body composition as a function of age, sex, level of nutrition, or state of health. Unfortunately, because many of these methods are based on relationships between body water and body electrolyte content in young adults, they may not hold true in older adults. Methods based on physical measurements do not take into account the possible age-related movement of body fat from one location to another, nor do external dimensions accurately reflect internal changes in tissue composition caused by normal aging or chronic disease. Research methods that assess the size and

composition of body compartments need to be validated in healthy older adults. Methods to assess body composition that are reasonably accurate, inexpensive, and noninvasive are urgently needed for clinical evaluation of older people in both community and health care settings.

Methods now being used to evaluate body composition, as well as their limitations when used with older people, are described in Table 3-1. Except for anthropometric and body density measurements, none of these methods have been used with large numbers of older people, and reference standards for older age groups have not been developed. Many of these methods are either invasive to the individual or require highly specialized, expensive equipment available in relatively few locations. Because of the effort and travel required of the individuals who have participated in these studies, only fairly healthy older people have been examined, and there is little information about those over age 85.[14] For frail elderly people, methods that involve intense cooperation from the participant (e.g., determination of body density by underwater weighing) are both stressful and difficult.

In general, the methods that provide direct measurement of a body compartment or constituent are more likely to yield appropriate estimates of body composition in older people. These methods include dilution measurements, whole body counting, computed tomography, **dual photon absorption,** and neutron activation analysis. Body water, mineral, fat, and nitrogen can be directly measured using one or a combination of these methods, which provide data that allow estimation of compartment size without using established formulas that may not be valid in older people.[5,40]

Overestimation and Underestimation of Body Compartments

Body composition methods that rely on standard formulas describing the density and hydration of body tissues appear to underestimate FFM and overestimate body fat in older people.[5] Measuring body density by underwater weighing provides information on only two

TABLE 3-1   *Methods for Evaluating Body Composition in Older People*

Method	Basis of Measurement	Usefulness With Older People
Dilution methods	Estimates body fluid volumes using stable isotope tracers such as O^{18} or Br^{82} or Evans blue dye; calculation based on assumption that FFM is 73.2% water	Fat-free tissue will vary in water content in fatter individuals, and fat will be underestimated; method is inappropriate for older people who are dehydrated or edematous
K^{40} counting	Uses whole body scintillation counter to measure the naturally occurring radioactive isotope K^{40}; lean tissue is believed to have a relatively constant potassium concentration	Potassium concentration is higher in muscle than in connective tissue; older people have less muscle mass and more connective tissue; whole body potassium concentration often is lower in older people, presenting problems with interpretation
Excretion of muscle metabolites (creatinine)	**Urinary creatinine** derived from creatine phosphate is a valid index of lean body mass using height as a standard for body size	Age-related changes in height and kidney function influence creatinine-height index; requires 24-hour urine collection
Neutron activation	Individual is exposed to a carefully controlled flow of neutron irradiation raising the activity level of nitrogen, calcium, sodium, potassium and chloride, which can then be quantified in a whole body scintillation counter	Only minimal assumptions are required (protein = nitrogen value $\times$ 6.25); not influenced by edema or reduced bone calcium; requires expensive equipment
Dual photon absorptiometry	Photons directed into the body pass through different tissues at different rates of speed, and changes in speed are recorded by the system's detectors; will differentiate bone mineral, fat, water, and fat-free, mineral-free tissue	Low level of radiation allows repeated measurements; provides correct analysis for people with differing bone densities and muscle mass; can serve as a reference standard for new clinical techniques; requires expensive equipment
Computed tomography	An x-ray technique than can quantify total volumes of muscle, fat, and specific organs based on the assumption that potassium content of fat-free tissue is 66 mmol/kg in men and 60 mmol/kg in women	Requires fair amount of radiation; not adversely affected by level of hydration, mineral density, or muscle wasting in older people; black women have higher body potassium than white women; obese have less potassium per unit weight than nonobese
Density measurement	Body density is determined by weighing an individual first in air and then completely submerged in water to obtain an estimate of water displacement; equations are based on standard densities (fat = 0.9 g/ml; FFM = 1.1 g/ml)	Can be unsuitable for frail older people; older person may be dehydrated or edematous, leading to inappropriate calculations; standard value used for proportion of bone mineral is inaccurate for older women with bone loss

Continued.

TABLE 3-1   Methods for Evaluating Body Composition in Older People—cont'd

Method	Basis of Measurement	Usefulness With Older People
Whole body electrical conductivity (TOBEC)	Lean tissues with a high water content conduct electricity better than fat tissue; measures the change in electrical conductivity pattern when person is placed in a chamber with oscillating electromagnetic waves	Can overestimate LBM in person with considerable body fat; estimate is improved by including an accurate height measurement in calculations; no radiation exposure; expensive apparatus required
Bioelectrical impedance	A weak electrical current is passed through the body (between right hand and right foot); the resistance to the current flow is proportional to total body water and lean body mass	Problems similar to those noted with TOBEC; no radiation exposure; fairly inexpensive apparatus; offers promise for routine use if specific equations can be developed for use with older people
Anthropometric measurements	Direct measurement of body height, weight, skinfold thicknesses, and circumferences allows calculation of body fat using available formulas	Does not provide valid estimate of internal fat; assumptions and equations may not hold true for older person in whom the regional fat pattern is individualized; equipment is inexpensive and portable

body compartments, body fat and FFM, and neither compartment is measured directly. Dilution and dual photon absorption methods, on the other hand, directly measure body water, mineral, fat, and lean tissue. Estimates of body fat and FFM obtained by body density, dilution, and dual photon absorption measurements were compared in 98 people ranging in age from 65 to 94 years.[5] The percentage of body fat in both the men and the women was 2% higher when calculated by body density measurement equations than when measured directly by dual photon absorption. The percentage of body fat was 25% and 23% in men and 33% and 31% in women, respectively, using the two methods. Differences within individuals were even more striking. In three women the percentage of body fat as calculated from the density measurement was 6% higher than by the other methods; for several men it was 8% higher. Conversely, the FFM was higher by 1 kg in both sexes when measured by dual photon absorption than when calculated from body density measurements.

The difference in percentages for body fat obtained by these methods relates in part to the standard values of the equations used to predict body density.[21] Based on research with young adults, the FFM is believed to have a density of 1.10 g/ml. It appeared in this study that the density of the FFM was lower in both the older men and the older women.[21] Several factors could effect this decrease in density.[5] An increase in total body water, which has a density of 1 g/ml, would lower the overall density of the FFM. An increase in adipose tissue, as occurs with aging, effectively increases the relative water content of the FFM. This is because adipose cells, when the fat has been removed, have a water content of 98%, since the only other remaining constituent in the cell is a small amount of protein (2%); other cells that make up the fat-free tissue are about 73% water, since their protein content is higher. Even a small change in the density of the FFM will lead to significant errors in calculating the volume of body fat. A variation of 0.02 g/ml from the established value of 1.10 g/ml will result in a 5% error in the calculation of percentage of body fat. The density of the FFM will also be decreased if bone mineral or body protein is lost. It is likely that all these factors contribute to the decrease in the density of the FFM observed in older people.

Gains or losses in body water, potassium, and protein in particular body compartments become especially important when estimating body composition in individuals who have metabolic disorders. Cohn and coworkers[19] recommend that in these individuals, body nitrogen and calcium be used to measure body compartments rather than body potassium or total body water. In patients with electrolyte disturbances or severe renal disease, body water can shift to other body compartments, and body potassium may be lost. Thus estimates based on these constituents have a high degree of error.

Body Composition Methods for Nutrition Screening

There is a need for rapid, inexpensive body composition methods for use in nutrition screening and clinical intervention. In this direction efforts are being made to improve the estimates of body compartments obtained by the **bioelectrical impedance** technique and anthropometric measurements.[7] Several studies[40,50,75,83,86] have compared results obtained by dual photon absorption, neutron activation analysis, and density measurements with these less expensive methods. Estimates of body fat in people over age 60, as determined by bioelectrical impedance, were highly correlated with values obtained by the more expensive methods; however, the prediction equations developed for use with younger age groups overestimated the FFM in the older people by about 6 kg.[23] Nevertheless, bioelectrical impedance measurements, which require only a few minutes and involve no effort or discomfort to the client, hold promise for use in clinical settings. Using both bioelectrical impedance and anthropometric measurements improved the estimates of body compartments in cancer patients evaluated in a hospital setting.[33]

Bioelectrical impedance has particular potential for the assessment of older people who are paraplegic or confined to a bed or a chair. Measurement of a body segment such as an arm or a leg might still provide an estimate of degree of hydration, body water distribution, and level of fatness.[15] Before such use is possible, however, standards must be established that are consistent with age-related changes in body compartments, and new techniques must be validated in relation to these standards.

Anthropometric Measurements

Body measurements to evaluate relative leanness or obesity usually are included in physical examinations and nutrition assessments; body weight, height, circumferences, and **skinfold thicknesses** are most commonly used. Unfortunately, these measurements, which are simple, inexpensive, and require relatively little cooperation from the patient, have only limited value for estimating body fatness. Estimates of body fatness obtained by newer, more reliable methods such as dual photon absorption or neutron activation analysis do not correspond with those derived from a simple anthropometric measurement or equations incorporating several measurements from a variety of body locations.

Body weight. Body weight is one of the least reliable estimates of body fat, even if corrected for height, sex, and age. Body weights normally are not distributed about the mean but rather skew to the right, since more people are heavier in weight.[79] Thus an average weight usually is above the median weight of the group being evaluated. Moreover, because body weight among adults in the United States is constantly increasing, the average weight derived from the most recent compilation of life insurance data is actually 20% higher than that considered desirable in earlier evaluations.[94] (The limitations of desirable or relative weight standards developed by life insurance companies are discussed in Chapter 2.)

The biggest problem associated with body weight measurements is the oversimplification of the obesity question. The term "obesity" implies that an individual has an excess of body fat, not merely a body weight above the average for his or her height or sex. When an individual is overweight, the extra weight could represent bone, fluid, muscle, or a combination of these. Nevertheless, the terms "obesity" and "overweight" are related, since an obese individual very likely will be overweight; the overweight individual, however, may not be obese. Most older people are somewhat obese relative to younger people of the same sex and similar height and weight. In older people fluctuations in body water content, caused by fluid retention or dehydration, can result in significant changes in body weight (remember, 2 cups of water weighs 1 pound).

Body build, or the proportion of muscle tissue to fat tissue, differs among older individuals as well as between older and younger individuals. The older man who did hard physical labor before retirement will differ in body composition from the retired sedentary executive who had limited physical activity. Seltzer and co-workers[76] evaluated relative body weight and obesity as determined by skinfold thickness measurements in more than 1,700 healthy men ages 25 to 64. Among those who were 15% above their suggested weight (relative weight was 115) only one third were actually obese. Among the men who were 25% above their suggested weight, about half were obese. The overweight men who were not obese had a large body frame, a large skeletal mass, and heavy muscular development.

Body mass index. The reliability of height and weight measurements in assessing relative fatness has been strengthened by the development of the body mass index (weight in kilograms divided by height in meters squared) originally developed by Quetelet. An index of relative weight should be equally reliable with tall or short individuals and should provide a reasonable estimate of body fat.[53] In younger people the **body mass index (BMI)** is more strongly correlated with body fat estimates from body density measurements and whole body counting than is relative weight as derived from height and weight tables.[12] On this basis the BMI is believed to provide a better estimate of body fat than does relative weight.

Unfortunately, recent work suggests that the BMI may not provide an appropriate estimate of body fat in older adults. A BMI of 25 to 25.9, considered to represent normal weight or only a minor degree of overweight in younger people, is associated with a high proportion of body fat in some older people.[22] Among 75

Dutch elderly between the ages of 60 and 83, a BMI of 25 in men was associated with a mean body fat of 31% derived from body density measurements. The women with a BMI of 25.9 had a body fat level of 44%.

The relationship between BMI and body fat percentage may be population specific even among older people of similar age. In a group of healthy 75-year-olds,[86] the mean BMIs in both men and women were the same as those observed in the Dutch elderly (25 in men and 25.9 in women). However, the proportions of body fat as determined by dual photon absorption were lower, 21% in men and 34% in women, a difference of 10 percentage points from the previously described study. If BMI is to be used to estimate relative fatness in older adults, research to establish appropriate criteria for the definition of overweight will be required.

Skinfold measurements. The use of skinfold thicknesses as an indicator of body fatness evolved from the physiologic finding that about half of all body fat is **subcutaneous,** or found directly under the skin.[78] Standard methods of measurement were developed using specific **skinfold calipers** at constant pressure. The most commonly used caliper is the Lange skinfold caliper with a pressure of 10 g/mm. Estimations of body fat based on skinfold measurements at various anatomic sites have been found to compare favorably with values obtained by body density, whole body counting, and dilution techniques, although much of this work was performed on young adults.[14,17] Because individuals have different patterns of body fat distribution, estimations of body fat content based on several skinfold thicknesses at various anatomic sites are more closely related to values obtained by density measurements than are estimations based on a single skinfold thickness. Skinfold thicknesses provide better estimates of total body fat in women than in men.[30]

The most common skinfold thickness measurements taken are the triceps (upper arm), subscapular area (upper back), and abdomen. The triceps skinfold is widely used, since the individual does not have to disrobe. A circumference of the upper arm taken at the same location as the triceps skinfold thickness permits calculation of the total arm muscle area and fat area. The upper arm fat and muscle areas have been recommended as simple yet effective indicators of excessive body fatness or protein energy malnutrition. Chumlea and coworkers[15] pointed to the usefulness of arm measurements with edematous individuals for whom body weight is not a valid measure of nutritional status. However, this method requires further evaluation with older people, since recent work with computed tomography has indicated a high degree of error.[32] This is because the relative proportion of fat and muscle differ significantly at various sites around the bone in the upper arm. Moreover, the upper arm is not a true circle, which leads to further errors in calculation. Nevertheless, upper arm fat and muscle areas may provide some estimate of an individual's nutritional status.

Limitations of skinfold measurements. Although simple and inexpensive, skinfold measurements have many limitations with older people. Although subcutaneous fat is believed to be proportional to total body fat in younger age groups, this may not be true in older age groups.[17,78] Fat changes location as a function of age; body fat moves in a centripetal direction from the limbs to the trunk as a person grows older. Less fat is deposited in subcutaneous locations, and more fat is deposited as internal fat about the abdomen and hips. Equations that estimate percentage of total body fat based on the triceps skinfold thickness are sometimes inaccurate when used with older adults. On the basis of an equation using an upper arm skinfold measurement, a healthy, 74-year-old woman, free of edema, who weighed 197 pounds (relative weight was 144) was found to have a body fat content of 27%; women of similar weight and age have been reported to have a body fat content of 45%.[69]

General patterns of fat distribution are influenced by sex, age, and nutritional status, but fat patterns are also a highly individual characteristic. Body fat is not gained or lost equally at all locations on the limbs or trunk. A recent study[17] involving 30 cadavers of persons over age 55 and 40 older people of similar age living in the community has raised several issues relating to the use of skinfold thicknesses. Although

it generally is recognized that **skinfold compressibility** differs between individuals, it appears that compressibility also differs among anatomic sites in the same individual. In those with similar body fat content, the sum of seven skinfold thicknesses from various sites differed by over twofold (59 versus 116 mm) as a result of differences in skinfold compressibility. Skinfold compressibility decreases with age and could result from an increase in connective tissue, a decrease in the elasticity of the skin, or retention of fluid in the tissues. Skinfolds with identical thicknesses may also differ in fat content. Adipose tissue from individuals who are more obese is likely to have a decreased water content and an increased fat content. Those authors[17] suggested using skinfold thicknesses on the legs, where there is less variability, or using circumference measurements to estimate fat stores.

Before skinfold thicknesses and other anthropometric measurements can be used with confidence in a clinical facility or nutrition survey, it is necessary to establish reliability among the examiners. In elderly patients, triceps skinfold measurements varied by 150% if taken 1 cm above or below the designated location.[85] This has serious implications for patient care if repeated measurements are being used to monitor a patient's progress or nutritional status. Repeated measurements on patients with little subcutaneous fat are more precise than on patients who are more obese.

Body circumference measurements. Body circumference or **envelope measurements** may be a useful alternative for assessing body fat. Body circumferences provide a reliable estimate of fatness in older individuals. Among 62 healthy women over age 60, the hip circumference at the level of the umbilicus was highly correlated (r = 0.717) with body density determined by underwater weighing.[98] Moreover, circumference measurements are not subject to the errors associated with individual and anatomic site differences in tissue compressibility. Abdominal and hip circumferences would appear to have particular value for assessing health status in light of the association of waist-to-hip ratio and physical health. Kuczmarski[48] has emphasized the need to establish normal values and evaluation standards for these measurements. The use of anthropometric measurements will be expanded in the third National Health and Nutrition Examination Survey (NHANES III).

Standards for evaluation. Evaluation and interpretation of anthropometric measurements require a set of reference values against which to compare individual values. Measurements obtained from older people need to be compared with reference values developed from people of similar age, since both the level and distribution of fat and muscle differ from those of younger age groups.[14] Because of the limited information available, reference standards based on an older population usually are the average values obtained from that age group and may not represent the ideal. However, the mere survival of these individuals suggests that even average values present a reasonable basis for comparison.

FACTORS AFFECTING BODY COMPOSITION
Genetic Influence

The relative proportion of body fat in an individual is controlled to some extent by genetic factors. Bouchard and coworkers[10] suggested that deposition of internal fat is influenced more by genetic factors than is deposition of subcutaneous fat. Females at all ages have a higher percentage of body fat than males and a smaller proportion of FFM. Among 700 healthy men and women ages 23 to 30,[4] body fat determined by body density measurements was 17% in men and 29% in women, respectively. By age 66 body fat had risen to 29% in the men and 38% in the women. Women have a greater amount of body fat regardless of their level of physical activity, although women characterized as physically fit have less fat. Increases in body fat from youth to middle age were reported in women even before the advent of laborsaving devices, when housekeeping and farm chores required heavy physical labor. In a study conducted with rural women nearly 30 years ago,[78] body fat evaluated by density and anthropometric techniques rose from 26% to 39% between the ages of 18 and 67 years. Body fat increased from 32% to 39% between middle age and older age despite the fact that body weight was unchanged, suggesting that nonfat tissue was lost over this period.

Physical Activity

Physical exercise influences the accumulation of body fat in individuals of all ages. As determined by underwater weighing, physically active older men had less body fat (24% versus 27%) and more lean body mass (62 kg versus 57 kg) than inactive men of similar age and body weight.[30] In fact, the physically active older men, some of whom were long-distance runners, had a lower percentage of body fat than inactive younger men. Older women employed in positions requiring physical labor are more muscular and less fat than sedentary women of the same age. Physical activity also brings about changes in fat pattern or distribution. In an adult physical fitness program, participants who exercised regularly showed a decrease in abdominal fat and **waist-to-hip ratio,** although total body fat was unchanged.[74]

Nutrient Intake

At one time it was believed that a gain in body weight or body fat represented a simple excess of caloric intake over caloric expenditure. We have come to realize that many factors relating to the type of calories consumed and the physiologic status of the individual influence the gain or loss of body fat. Consumption of kilocalories in the form of fat rather than carbohydrate may accelerate the accretion of body fat.[88] The conversion of dietary carbohydrate to storage fat through the synthesis of fatty acids requires 23 of every 100 kcal consumed; in contrast, dietary fatty acids can be converted to triglycerides and deposited directly in adipose tissue at a cost of only 3 kcal per 100 kcal consumed.[6,12]

An individual's history of obesity or weight reduction can influence both the rate of gain of body fat and the pattern of deposition. Individuals who lose weight through very-low-calorie diets and with no accompanying exercise are very likely to lose muscle tissue as well as body fat. This loss of muscle tissue results in a lower basal energy requirement, which encourages weight gain when normal eating is resumed.[6] Individuals with repeated cycles of weight gain and weight loss have increased deposition of abdominal fat and higher waist-to-hip ratios. In the very obese, weight loss causes an increase in the **lipoprotein lipase** enzymes in adipose tissue. This enzyme hydrolyzes the triglycerides taken up from the circulating lipoproteins and enhances their esterification and storage in the adipose cells. Thus any future weight loss becomes more difficult.[47] An individual's body weight history significantly influences not only the level of body fat but also the ability to change weight in advanced age.[65]

AGE-RELATED CHANGES IN BODY COMPOSITION
Longitudinal Versus Cross-Sectional Studies

Advances in methodology that allow us to evaluate precisely the size and composition of body compartments have begun to provide information about the changes in these compartments that occur throughout adulthood.[18,27] There is general agreement that body compartments change as a function of age, although the degree of change in a particular individual varies considerably. A major limitation is the lack of longitudinal evaluations that would enable us to relate changes in body composition to diet, exercise, or life-style patterns.

The cross-sectional comparison of the size of body compartments among individuals of different ages is complicated by secular as well as age-related changes. Each succeeding generation is taller and heavier; thus older people tend to be shorter and may weigh less than younger people regardless of age-related changes. Ideally, the effect of the aging process on body composition should be evaluated on the basis of longitudinal changes observed in the same individual. These data are being recorded in the Baltimore Longitudinal Study of Aging (BLSA) and will allow such evaluations in the future.

Changes in Body Compartments

The relative sizes of body compartments change with age even if body weight remains unchanged. A general characteristic of these age-related changes is a loss of FFM and a gain in fat. Cohn and coworkers[18] evaluated body composition in 135 healthy adults between the ages of 20 and 80, using whole body counting and neutron activation techniques. Fig. 3-1 compares the size of the body compartments of the men ages 20 to 29 with those of the men ages 70 to 79. Mean body weights were about equal; however, fat made up 14 kg (17%) of

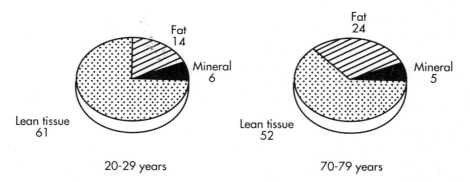

FIG. 3-1 Body compartments in men ages 20 to 29 and 70 to 79. Lean body mass decreases and body fat increases as a result of normal aging.

(Data from Cohn SH and others: Compartmental body composition based on total body nitrogen, potassium, and calcium, *Am J Physiol* 239:E523, 1980.)

total body weight in the younger group, compared to 24 kg (30%) in the older group. Total body protein decreased by almost 2 kg over this age range. The decline in body mineral from 5.9 to 5.3 kg could represent a loss of bone mass with increasing age, or the fact that the older men were shorter in stature and thus had less bone. The decline in total body water is to be expected when muscle tissue is replaced with adipose tissue, which is substantially lower in water content (adipose tissue is 15% water, muscle is 73% water).

In the general population, mean body weight continues to increase throughout middle age and declines only in the oldest age groups.[56] Because an increase in body weight usually results from a gain in fat rather than a gain in muscle, the percentage of body fat may rise even higher than suggested in Fig. 3-1.

Loss of Lean Body Mass

The age-related decreases in body potassium and body nitrogen observed in both men and women parallel the loss of muscle tissue described above. In an 18-year longitudinal evaluation[27] of more than 600 university faculty members who ranged in age from 28 to 60 years when the study began, body potassium declined progressively with increasing age (Fig. 3-2). Women have less body potassium than men (about 63% that of men) but lose it less rapidly. In this study the men lost about 5 g of potassium per decade until age 60, whereas women lost only 1 to 2 g per decade. Beyond age 60 losses accelerated in both sexes.

The highest concentration of body potassium is in the muscle, and the loss of body potassium with advancing age indicates a substantial loss of muscle mass. Cohn and coworkers[18] reported that both muscle mass and total muscle protein decreased by nearly one half among the men and women in their study over the age range from 20 to 80 years (Table 3-2). In contrast, relatively little protein was lost from nonmuscle tissues, which included internal organs, blood, and bone; body fat increased. Further evidence confirming an age-related loss of muscle tissue comes from the BLSA.[91] In that group urinary creatinine excretion, a measure of muscle mass, decreased from 1,790 mg per 24 hours in those ages 17 to 24 to 1,259 mg per

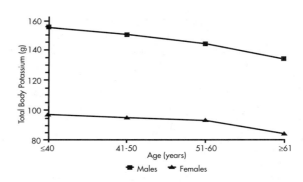

FIG. 3-2 Body potassium according to age and sex. Body potassium decreases with age, although men have a higher level of body potassium than women regardless of age.

Data from Flynn MA and others: Total body potassium in aging humans: a longitudinal study, *Am J Clin Nutr* 50:713, 1989.

TABLE 3-2 *Changes in Body Fat and Body Protein With Age*

Age (yrs)	Muscle Protein (kg)	Nonmuscle Protein (kg)	Fat (kg)
Men			
20-29	4.54	8.32	15.3
40-49	3.80	8.20	19.3
70-79	2.50	8.60	24.6
Women			
20-29	1.85	7.23	16.0
40-49	1.94	6.53	21.2
70-79	1.11	6.10	23.0

(Data from Cohn SH and others: Compartmental body composition based on total body nitrogen, potassium, and calcium, *Am J Physiol* 239:E523, 1980.)

24 hours in those ages 75 to 84, a decline of about 30%. This loss of muscle and protein has serious implications for protein metabolism and nutritional adaptation in the older adult; it is discussed further in Chapter 5.

Losses of body tissue and changes in body

compartments continue well into advanced age. A longitudinal study of nine Swedish men and 14 Swedish women[81] who were examined four times between the ages of 70 and 81 indicated that the type of tissues lost differs between men and women. In the men body cell mass declined from 30 to 28 kg over the 11-year period, but in the women BCM remained stable at 20 kg. On the other hand, the women appeared to lose a small amount of body fat. The major component of the weight lost by these older people (7 kg in the men and 6 kg in the women) was extracellular water.

Body water decreases continuously as people age. A newborn child is about 80% water, and this has decreased to 60% by the time the individual reaches adulthood.[54] By age 80, the Swedish elderly had a body water content of less than 50% of body weight.[81] This decrease in body water is influenced by the loss of muscle tissue, which has a high water content, and by the loss of extracellular fluid, as reported in the Swedish elderly. Losses in total body water over adulthood contribute to the risk of dehydration in older people (dehydration is discussed further in Chapter 7).

Hormone Secretion and Changes in Body Compartments

Sex steroid hormones. Both hormonal and life-style changes have been implicated in the age-related loss of tissues high in potassium and water and the gain in body fat. Secretion patterns of the sex steroid hormones, estrogen and testosterone, are changed at older ages. The decline in testosterone in older men has been associated with the decreased ability of older men to maintain positive protein status. The loss of estrogen at menopause leads to changes in calcium absorption and bone metabolism and may contribute to the accelerated loss of skeletal muscle observed in postmenopausal women.[2] The rate of loss of body potassium is greatest during the first 3 years after menopause, similar to the accelerated loss of bone mineral that occurs immediately after estrogen withdrawal. Beyond that time potassium and calcium losses continue, although at a slower rate. Aloia and coworkers[2] suggest that lean body mass may be lost first and that this contributes to the loss of

bone mineral through reduced mechanical stress on the skeleton. Currently data are not available to determine whether the loss of muscle mass occurs before or concurrently with the loss of mineral mass, but this issue deserves additional scrutiny. Hormone replacement therapy designed to maintain favorable serum lipoprotein patterns and decrease cardiovascular risk might also prevent postmenopausal loss of both muscle tissue and bone.

Growth hormone. Growth hormone levels decrease in both aging men and women. Growth hormone controls the production and release by the liver of **somatomedin C,** an insulin-like growth factor. Plasma levels of somatomedin C decline with age even in healthy older adults.[68] Although fewer than 5% of healthy men under age 40 have somatomedin C levels below the average, more than 30% of healthy men over age 60 have plasma values below this level. A decline in growth hormone and somatomedin C in younger people leads to atrophy of the lean body mass and an increase in adipose tissue. Thus, it has been suggested that the characteristic changes in body composition associated with aging may relate to diminished secretion of these hormones in later life.

The administration of growth hormone to older men not only increased their plasma growth hormone levels but also led to significant changes in their body composition.[68] After 6 months of hormone treatment, lean body mass had increased by 9% and adipose tissue had decreased by 15%. Mean body weight increased by about 1 kg over this period, whereas lean body mass increased by almost 5 kg and body fat decreased by about 3.5 kg. Body composition was unchanged in control subjects of similar age who did not receive the hormone therapy. The researchers noted that 6 months of growth hormone administration reversed the changes that occur over 10 to 20 years of aging.

Despite the successful reversal of aging changes through short-term use of growth hormone, many questions remain about the appropriateness of this treatment.[55] On a short-term basis growth hormone may prove beneficial for older individuals with catabolic illnesses, shortening the duration of protein loss and supporting recovery. At the same time, growth hormone can have adverse effects on carbohydrate metabolism, causing hyperinsulinemia, deterioration of glucose tolerance, and eventually diabetes mellitus. High levels of growth hormone lead to edema and congestive heart failure, as seen in acromegaly. Such issues must be resolved before considering long-term treatment to restore or prevent the loss of lean body mass.

Physical Activity and Changes in Body Compartments

Inactivity and loss of muscle fibers. The loss of muscle in older adults has been documented by computed tomography and by counting individual muscle fibers at autopsy. One report[24] noted that older men (ages 70 to 73) had 23% fewer muscle fibers than younger men (ages 19 to 37). Computed tomography indicated a reduced cross-section of muscle area as well as a decrease in the density of muscle fibers and an increase in intramuscular fat. One explanation for this decrease in muscle mass is the sedentary life-style common in our society and muscle atrophy related to a lack of use. Similar changes—atrophy of the skeletal muscle and loss of muscle strength—occur in young people when muscular activity is significantly reduced because of bed rest or immobilization.[67] Another contributing factor may be age-related changes in the nervous system that result in reduced neural input to the muscle and consequent tissue atrophy. It is likely that both of these processes influence muscle losses in older people.

A gradual and selective loss of muscle fibers leads to muscle atrophy.[25] The muscles that maintain posture and control the low-intensity movements required in day-to-day activities **(type I fibers)** are fairly well preserved into advanced age. On the other hand the muscle fibers required for high-intensity or sprinting movements **(type II fibers)** decrease markedly in number. Sedentary young men have only 60% of the number of type II fibers as active young men; men over age 80 have only 30% of the number of sedentary young men. In older people the loss of type II fibers is directly related to a decrease in muscle strength.

Endurance training and muscle fibers. Endurance training involves prolonged, rhythmic exercise; strength training involves lifting or lowering heavy weights. These two types of training have very different effects on body composition in older people.[24] Endurance training lowers body fat but does not increase muscle mass. Older endurance-trained athletes have a lower proportion of body fat than sedentary men of similar age but not an increased muscle mass. This effect of endurance training on body composition is also true in women. Among endurance-trained and sedentary postmenopausal women,[57] lean body mass as determined by body density measurements was similar in both groups; however, the mean body weight of the sedentary women was 10 kg higher than that of the endurance-trained women. The difference in body weight was explained by the difference in body fat. The physically active women had a body content of 36% fat, whereas the sedentary women were 41% fat.

Strength training and muscle fibers. Strength training, on the other hand, leads to hypertrophy of both type I and type II muscle fibers and an increase in muscle mass. This occurs in both younger and older adults who begin a strength training regimen. An 8-week program of weight training enhanced both muscle size and muscle strength in nursing home residents up to 96 years of age.[26] The absolute weight that could be lifted by the knee extensor muscles more than doubled in both the men and the women over the period of training. Computed tomography measurements indicated that muscle area increased by 11%, although subcutaneous and intramuscular fat levels did not change. Functional mobility and ease in walking improved as muscle strength and size increased. The researchers concluded that the muscle strength of older people depends strongly on the preservation of muscle mass.

Some reversal of muscle atrophy appears to be possible with regular exercise despite advanced age or poor functional status. The need to continue regular training to maintain the gains in muscle is emphasized by the fact that 4 weeks after the older people resumed a sedentary life-style, the muscle strength described above again began to deteriorate.[26] The fact that muscle status could be improved in frail elderly people emphasizes the potential for reversing or preventing the age-related loss of muscle mass in middle age adults or those recently retired.

Preventing muscle fiber loss. Although endurance training will not restore muscle tissue that has been lost, it may help to prevent further loss. Sidney and coworkers[77] reported a small but significant increase (4%) in body potassium in 38 older people enrolled in an exercise program for 1 year. Exercise sessions were 4 hours per week and emphasized vigorous walking or jogging if possible. These researchers considered this gain in body potassium an indication of muscle building, albeit proceeding at a slow rate. Even this slight increase was adequate to support an observable improvement in general conditioning and fitness.

Further evidence suggesting that age-related changes in body compartments can be prevented comes from a study of Swedish women[59] between the ages of 50 and 66 who were studied for 6 years. These women showed no increase in body fat, and mean body weight changed by less than 1 kg. Although clinical records did not indicate an increase in physical exercise among these women, their general interest in diet and health could have been heightened by the ongoing national health campaigns in Sweden.

Life-style, Aging, and Body Fat

Normal aging is associated with a loss in muscle mass and a gain in body fat, although life-style factors rather than biologic factors may be the cause. People from regions of the world where intense physical activity is a daily pattern and high-calorie foods are less available do not exhibit these age-related increases in body weight or body fat. Biologic and life-style factors were evaluated in a comparison of Cape Verdean Islanders who remained at home with Cape Verdeans who had moved to New England (the Cape Verde Islands are 400 miles off the coast of West Africa).[1] All groups were similar in body height, and BMI was used to estimate the degree of fatness.

As described in Fig. 3-3, not only did the Is-

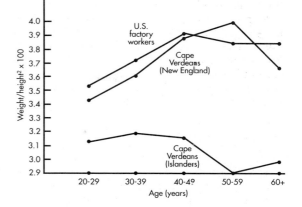

FIG. 3-3 Body mass index (BMI) according to age and population. Body mass index tends to increase with age only in groups with high caloric intake and little physical activity.

(Data from Albrink MJ, Meigs JW: Serum lipids, skinfold thickness, body bulk, and body weight of native Cape Verdeans, New England Cape Verdeans, and United States factory workers, *Am J Clin Nutr* 24:344. 1971.)

landers have less body fat at younger ages, they also gained relatively little fat throughout adulthood.[1] Among the New England Cape Verdeans, BMI continued to increase until age 59 and then declined. The Islanders were characterized by extreme leanness, whereas the New England Cape Verdeans resembled U.S. factory workers in their degree of adiposity. As the genetic background of both groups of Cape Verdeans was similar, life-style and caloric intake would appear to have influenced these differences. The Islanders maintained a high degree of physical activity, and on the Islands the food supply was limited.

A 6-year longitudinal study of the Tristan da Cunba Islanders,[51] who also live off the coast of Africa, revealed that increases in body weight and skinfold thicknesses accompanied a change in life-style. Over the period of study, the island changed from an economy in which agriculture predominated to an economy based on fishing. Food became more plentiful, and physical exercise decreased, particularly among the women, who had planted and harvested the crops. The men who combined paid employment with maintaining their property continued some strenuous physical activity but still had a mean weight gain of 4 kg; the women who discontinued their intense physical exercise had a mean weight gain of 11 kg. Before these changes in occupation, the mean body weight within all age groups had been stable, changing by 1 kg or less over 25 years.

The evaluations presented above indicate that age-related increases in body weight and body fat result from a positive calorie balance rather than normal aging. In Western societies continued consumption of concentrated sources of calories as physical activity declines leads to weight gain; this does not occur in cultures where food is less plentiful and physical exercise is intense. A question still to be answered, however, is whether people who continue a high degree of physical exercise can prevent or retard the age-related loss of lean body mass observed in sedentary populations. A longitudinal evaluation of people with different but consistent levels of physical activity would provide needed information about body changes and preventive measures required for successful aging.

CURRENT TRENDS IN BODY MEASUREMENTS

Changes in Body Stature

Age versus secular influences. Older age groups are shorter in stature than younger age groups as a result of actual losses in height by older people as well as **secular changes.**[14] Secular changes refer to changes occurring over time as each succeeding generation increases in height. The classic work evaluating the relative influence of age changes versus secular changes on body height involved measuring the length of the long bones (the femur and tibia) in 855 cadavers.[89] Bone length does not change as a result of the aging process; therefore, differences in bone length between generations result from secular influences. Age-related losses in height are caused by the vertical shrinking and collapse of the vertebrae and curvature of the spine, as seen in **lordosis** or **kyphosis.**

Both secular and age-related factors contributed to the differences in stature among age cohorts.[89] Age-related changes were most prominent among white women, who lost 7.8 cm in

height over adulthood. Black women and white and black men lost 2.6 to 3.5 cm in height. The average rate of loss across all groups was 0.6 cm per decade between ages 20 and 90; however, losses occurred most rapidly after age 50, with only slight losses occurring before age 40. Within specific age and sex groups, individuals will differ in their loss of height. A 10-year longitudinal study[60] of 11 women between the ages of 48 and 77 revealed no change in height in two of the participants (ages 56 and 77) and losses of 0.5 to 2 cm in the other nine.

An ongoing longitudinal study of 220 older people over age 65[16] suggests that actual losses in height may be greater than previously reported. Based on 6 years of observation, the rate of decline in this population is about 0.5 cm per year and is constant in all age and sex groups. If continued, these losses will translate to 4 to 5 cm per decade. A continual loss in stature has serious implications for the selection of an appropriate body weight standard for an older individual.

Stature of U.S. adults. According to measurements obtained in NHANES II,[90,92] both sex and age influence standing height. Men are taller than women of the corresponding age. Standing height decreases by 2.2 inches between the ages of 18 and 74 in both black men and white men.[92] In white women standing height decreases by 2.1 inches and in black women by 1.8 inches over this age range. An individual's ethnic group appears to have little influence on standing height at any age. Black women do have a greater bone mineral mass than white women at all ages, and they have less risk of osteoporosis and damage to the vertebrae. Loss of bone in the vertebrae contributes to the loss of height in older men and older women.

Changes in Body Weight

All adult age groups in the United States are becoming both larger and heavier. In men mean body weight increases until age 54 and then declines.[90,92] In women trends in body weight are influenced by ethnic group. In white women body weight peaks between the ages of 45 and 64. Black women are heavier than white women at all ages, but in black women body weight peaks at ages 45 to 54 and then declines.[92] The decline in body weight in older age groups could represent an actual loss of weight by individuals or the earlier death of those with higher body weights. In either case people at older ages are leaner.

The percentage of adults in NHANES II and Hispanic HANES who were classified as overweight differed on the basis of age, sex, and ethnic group.[90,92] Overweight in these surveys was defined as a BMI greater than or equal to 27.8 kg/m^2 for men and 27.3 kg/m^2 for women. Among men the highest percentage of overweight individuals occurred in the 45- to 54-year-old group, with 30% of the white men and 41% of the black men classified as overweight. In black men the proportion overweight dropped substantially after age 54, reaching a level of 26% in the oldest age group. In white women the greatest number of those overweight (36%) was found in ages 65 to 74; in black women ages 45 or older more than 61% were overweight. Eight percent to 12% of white men, white women, and black men over age 64 were severely overweight, compared to 26% of black women this age.

In Hispanic men the prevalence of overweight was similar for those of Mexican American, Cuban, and Puerto Rican origin. After age 44, about one third of Hispanic men were overweight. Mexican American and Puerto Rican women are more likely to be overweight than are Cuban women. By age 35 nearly 40% of the women of Mexican American and Puerto Rican origin were overweight, and this rose to 50% to 60% by age 65. Nearly one fifth of Mexican American and Puerto Rican women are severely overweight, compared to about one tenth of Cuban women. Women appear to survive to older ages despite an excessive amount of body fat. (The prevalence of overweight in specific population groups over age 50 is discussed in Chapter 10.)

CALORIC REQUIREMENTS AND ENERGY EXPENDITURE
Approaches to Defining the Caloric Requirement

Defining the caloric requirement of an older individual is complicated at best. Loss of meta-bolically active tissue and a decrease in physical activity lower the calorie requirement, and caloric intake may have to be sharply reduced to prevent unwanted weight gain. At the same time protein, vitamin, and mineral needs remain the same or may even increase in certain situations. The continuing need for other nutrients at former levels coupled with the declining need for energy emphasizes the importance of nutrient density in food selection for older adults.

One approach to defining the caloric needs of the older adult has been to survey apparently healthy older people and determine their intake of kilocalories.[46] This approach assumes that the intakes of the individuals surveyed are appropriate for maintaining health and well-being, and recommendations are developed based on those intakes. Alternatively, James[44] suggests a proactive approach to the development of calorie requirements for older adults. This would entail defining what the energy expenditure of a healthy, active older person of appropriate size and body composition *should be*. The appropriate energy expenditure of that individual or population then becomes the recommended level of kilocalories to be consumed.

Components of the Energy Requirement

The components of the caloric requirement of adults can be described as biologic, social, and medical (see the box on page 64).[46] The biologic components of energy expenditure include the support of normal body functions, the maintenance of tissues, and the energy cost associated with digesting and metabolizing food and nutrients. The energy required for digestion and metabolism usually is defined as the **thermic effect of food.**

Another major component of energy expenditure is physical activity, and this component, in contrast to the energy expended for biologic functions, is under voluntary control. Thus an individual may increase physical activity as a means of achieving energy balance. The energy expended in physical activity can involve essential needs, gainful employment, food preparation, household chores, or personal care. En-

❖

COMPONENTS OF ENERGY EXPENDITURE

- *Biologic*
Basal requirements
Thermic effect of food
- *Physical activity*
Occupational (economic)
Socially desirable activities
  Household chores
  Personal chores
  Recreational activities
- *Medically desirable*
High-intensity exercise for cardiovascular fitness

Adapted from James WPT, Ralph A, Ferro-Luzzi A: Energy needs of the elderly, a new approach. In Munro HN, Danford DE, editors: *Nutrition, aging, and the elderly,* New York, 1989, Plenum Press.

ergy expenditure sometimes is associated with social interaction or recreation that enhances a person's sense of well-being. The third component of the caloric requirement is health related and refers to the prescriptive high-intensity exercise and conditioning required for cardiovascular fitness and maintenance of muscle mass.

Despite the influence of a variety of factors on energy expenditure (including smoking,[42] which appears to increase energy expenditure, diet-induced thermogenesis resulting from overfeeding,[45] or the ingestion of caffeine,[61]) the energy expenditure of adults is remarkably stable. The major variables are the biologic differences between individuals, which reflect differences in body composition and metabolic efficiency, and patterns of physical activity. Unfortunately, we know very little about the influence of the aging process on energy metabolism.

Resting Energy Expenditure

Resting energy expenditure and basal metabolism. The largest portion of energy expenditure in most older individuals is the **resting energy expenditure (REE)**. In an older, sedentary adult, the REE usually represents 60% to 75% of the total energy expenditure.[29] The REE is measured on an individual at rest and under conditions of thermal neutrality, which means the person is neither perspiring nor shivering. The REE is the energy required to

(1) Carry on the vital processes of the body, including renal, cardiovascular, pulmonary, and neural function
(2) Maintain electrolyte gradients and body temperature
(3) Support necessary chemical reactions in the body under resting conditions[46]

The REE is more commonly used as an estimate of the involuntary energy expenditure than the **basal metabolism,** although the terms are interchangeable. An individual's basal metabolism is measured immediately upon awakening in the morning and 12 hours after the last meal. Thus basal metabolism is measured after digestion and absorption have been completed and does not include any energy expenditure related to the thermic effect of food. The REE, although measured with the individual at rest, may include energy expenditure resulting from the thermic effect of food from the last meal; however, the basal metabolism and the REE of an adult usually differ by less than 10%.[29]

Factors influencing the resting energy expenditure. The REE is influenced by age, sex, body size, body composition, thyroid status, and prior exercise. Thyroid hormones are to a great extent responsible for regulation of the REE.[61] Both age and sex differences in REE relate to body composition. Women have lower resting energy needs per unit of height and weight than men of similar age because women have a higher proportion of body fat and a lower proportion of muscle mass than men. Individuals with a larger body size and a greater surface area for heat loss have a higher REE. Studies with twins[11] suggest that genetic influences can account for 40% to 50% of the individual variability in the REE and may contribute to the tendency to develop obesity that exists within families. Among American Indian families in Arizona, the resting energy metabolism varied by about 500 kcal per day in individuals from different families who were of similar age, sex, and build, but varied by only 60 kcal in similar individuals from the same families.[9]

Age and resting energy expenditure. It has long been recognized that the REE declines with age. Records from the BLSA suggest that basal metabolic needs decline by 3% to 4% per decade after age 40.[91] James and coworkers,[46] after reviewing available data, concluded that basal needs expressed on the basis of body weight decline by 24% in men and 15% in women between the ages of 20 and 60 years. These age-related decreases in basal requirements are believed to result from the loss of muscle tissue and the increase in body fat that occur over adulthood. REE when calculated on the basis of FFM, total body water, or total body potassium is remarkably similar in younger and older individuals. Among healthy, physically active older men,[13] basal metabolism was 13% lower than in younger men when calculated on the basis of body weight. When expressed per unit of body potassium, however, values were similar. In that study the total body potassium was 12% lower in the older compared to the younger men.

A recent evaluation[96] suggests that factors other than changes in body composition may lead to a lower REE in older versus younger individuals of the same sex. The basal metabolic rate and 24-hour energy expenditure of 64 young adults with a mean age of 24 years, and 38 older adults with a mean age of 71 years were studied using a **total body respiratory chamber.** (A total body respiratory chamber is an environmentally controlled walk-in room with a constant temperature that allows continuous measurement of the oxygen consumption and carbon dioxide production of the person inside.[64] The chamber has a sleeping and a sitting area and toilet facilities so that a person can remain inside for 24 hours or more. Meals are passed through a special airlock system.) The chamber allows measurement of the 24-hour energy expenditure, including spontaneous physical activity (i.e., fidgeting).

The 24-hour caloric intake and 24-hour energy expenditure were 2,145 and 2,150 kcal in the younger group and 1,861 and 1,914 kcal in the older group.[96] Although the 24-hour energy expenditure was higher in the younger group on an absolute basis, when adjusted for FFM, total body fat, and sex, the 24-hour energy expenditure was similar in both groups. As shown in Fig. 3-4, the same line explains the relationship between the 24-hour energy expenditure and the FFM in both age groups. The basal metabolic rate, however, was still lower in the older age group after adjustments for sex

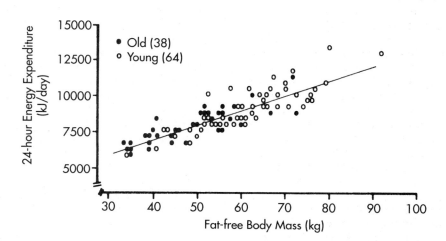

FIG. 3-4 Relationship of 24-hour energy expenditure and fat-free mass in younger and older adults. This relationship was similar in both age groups.

(From Vaughan L, Zurlo F, Ravussin E: Aging and energy expenditure, *Am J Clin Nutr* 53:821, 1991.)

and body composition, whereas the sleeping metabolic rate was the same in both groups. In other words, the younger individuals increased their energy expenditure (by 12%) from the sleeping to the basal state (awake but resting), whereas the older individuals did not.

It is generally assumed that older people are less physically active than younger ones; however, there was no difference in spontaneous physical activity between age groups in the respiratory chamber. That 24-hour period, however, most likely did not reflect the normal activity or usual living situation of either age group. In the respiratory chamber physical activity is limited to restless sleep patterns or daytime pacing in the confined area.

Sympathetic nervous system and resting energy expenditure. The age-related decrease in basal metabolic rate observed in the respiratory chamber may be associated with the change in sympathetic nervous system activity observed in older adults. Plasma norepinephrine concentrations are elevated in older persons as a result of the enhanced secretion of norepinephrine by the neural tissues. It is suggested that this enhanced secretion is caused by the increased levels of abdominal and visceral fat in older people; the percentage of body fat is a predictor of plasma norepinephrine levels independent of age.[41,61] Despite their higher plasma levels of norepinephrine, older adults still have a lower response to sympathetic nervous system stimulation.

Cell loss and resting energy expenditure. The age-related decline in basal metabolism was first described in the 1930s; however, the basis for this change was unclear. A decrease in basal energy expenditure could represent a decline in the number of functioning cells, reduced metabolic activity in existing cells, or a combination of the two.[91] It has since been observed that changes in basal oxygen consumption closely parallel age-related changes in body water and body potassium. This is consistent with the explanation that the aging process leads to a loss of cells, because total body water is closely related to total lean body mass. Measurements of body composition and basal metabolism in the BLSA[91] indicate that losses of skeletal muscle can account for the decrease in basal energy ex-

penditure. The metabolic activity of remaining cells is unchanged.

Longitudinal studies[91] have identified older adults in whom basal oxygen consumption did not decline with advancing age. A logical question is how the loss of body cells or expected decline in basal energy expenditure was prevented. It has since been learned that in these individuals, the metabolic rate of nonmuscle tissues increased and so compensated for the decrease in basal metabolism brought about by the loss of muscle mass. Increased oxygen consumption in nonmuscle tissues is often a sign of elevated metabolic work associated with cardiovascular disorders or malignancy. Energy expenditure for basal needs can be expected to decline each decade beyond age 40 regardless of sex or body size.

Thyroid hormone and resting energy expenditure. Thyroid hormone controls the rate of oxygen consumption in the cell, although age-related decreases in basal energy expenditure do not reflect a deficiency of **thyroxin.** Gregerman and coworkers[37] evaluated thyroid function in 73 euthyroid men ages 18 to 91. Although they observed a 50% decrease in the thyroxin degradation rate in the older men, this appeared to result from a reduction in tissue utilization and metabolism of thyroxin. The decrease in secretion of thyroid hormone is a homeostatic response to the loss of metabolically active muscle tissue. In normal older people serum levels of thyroxin are not reduced[80]; if the thyroid gland was dysfunctional, thyroxin levels would drop accordingly. If stimulated by the administration of **thyroid-stimulating hormone (TSH),** the aging thyroid gland can respond with increased production and release of thyroid hormone.

Hypothyroidism and **hyperthyroidism** are serious conditions in older people. Both conditions are more commonly found in women and among institutionalized elderly people. The incidence of hypothyroidism increases with age. Among 258 healthy older adults,[66] 13% had elevated serum TSH levels, an early indicator of hypothyroidism and thyroid failure. Within 4 years one third of those with elevated serum TSH became overtly hypothyroid. Unfortunately, mild hypothyroidism is not always recognized in older people because many of the characteristic symptoms—lethargy, constipation, or limited tolerance to cold—often are assumed to be typical of older people.

Hyperthyroidism is an equally serious condition in the aged, since excessive thyroid hormone increases the work of the heart with tachycardia and arrhythmias. Weight loss, tremors, and muscle weakness, first noticed when climbing stairs, occur frequently. In contrast to younger hyperthyroid individuals, older people with hyperthyroidism do not always have increased appetites, and they may be apathetic or withdrawn. Because the signs and symptoms of thyroid disorders may be overlooked in clinical evaluations, older individuals should undergo periodic screening of blood thyroxin levels.[87]

Predicting Basal Energy Needs

Simple prediction equations use body height, body weight, age, and sex to estimate basal or resting energy expenditure.[29] Such equations have been found to overestimate or underestimate the resting energy expenditure of older people, depending on the particular group being studied. Among 40 healthy older people between the ages of 51 and 82,[34] the actual REE was significantly different from the predicted REE (1,512 versus 1,420 kcal). Although the mean REE for the group was underestimated by only about 6%, the REE of particular individuals was overestimated or underestimated by 10% to 20%. The researchers emphasized the stability of the REE in their older subjects, since individual measurements taken 6 months apart differed by less than 20 kcal.

Of major concern is the reliability of prediction equations in a malnourished patient. The major difficulty in using prediction equations with a malnourished adult lies in the estimate of the body cell mass. In a normally nourished individual, the body cell mass is directly related to the body size. In a malnourished individual, both body fat and body cell mass are lost; however, it is the muscle component of the body cell mass that is preferentially lost, whereas visceral organs remain relatively intact. Because the visceral component of the body cell mass is responsible for 60% to 70% of the REE, pre-

diction equations based on body weight will underestimate the REE of a malnourished individual by as much as 18%.[33] Compiled data from several sources suggest that older men and women have a basal energy need of about 20 kcal/kg per day.[46] The basal energy expenditure of an individual who is lighter in weight may be somewhat higher per kilogram of body weight, since visceral tissues with a higher level of metabolic activity will constitute a greater proportion of the fat-free mass.

Thermic Effect of Food

The **thermic effect of food (TEF)** is the increase in energy expenditure above the REE that occurs for several hours after a meal is eaten.[61] The TEF represents the energy expended in digesting, transporting, metabolizing, and storing food and nutrients. Although the TEF accounts for about 10% of the total daily energy expenditure, this will vary according to the energy source being fed and its metabolic fate. Protein brings about the greatest increase in energy expenditure, carbohydrate brings about a moderate increase, and fat brings about little or none.

The influence of age on the TEF is not well understood. Meals containing up to 60 g of protein led to similar increases in energy expenditure in younger and older adults, and the magnitude of the response was proportional to the amount of protein fed.[35,70] The increment in energy expenditure in response to 75 g of glucose was less in older men than in younger men when expressed as total kilocalories per minute but was not different when expressed on the basis of body FFM.[8] An evaluation of the TEF in younger and older men with a high or low level of fitness suggested that increasing age, as well as a poor level of fitness, decreases the response.[58, 62]

Schwartz and coworkers[72] propose that the decrement in the TEF observed in some older adults is caused by decreased sympathetic nervous system response. The TEF includes a meal-induced thermogenesis, which is controlled by the action of the sympathetic nervous system. Although this decrement in the TEF would at most amount to 2% to 5% of the total energy expenditure, it could over time contribute to the increase in adiposity that occurs with advancing age.

Physical Activity

Benefits of physical activity. In developing the energy requirement of an older adult, two benefits can be realized from including appropriate amounts of physical activity. First, the increased energy expenditure contributes to overall nutritional status by allowing the intake of additional food supplying important protein, vitamins, and minerals without unwanted weight gain. It has been suggested that caloric intakes of at least 1,600 to 1,800 kcal are necessary to ensure adequate intake of other important nutrients unless intake of sugar, fat, and alcohol is severely restricted.[28] Secondly, physical training contributes to cardiovascular fitness, the maintenance of muscle mass, and improved functional capacity to carry on household duties and personal care.

Supervised physical exercise improves the response and recovery of the cardiovascular and respiratory systems and positively alters body composition and serum lipoprotein levels in older men and women. Exercise programs consisting of three to five 1-hour sessions each week that include walking, calisthenics, or jogging improve **aerobic capacity,** strength, and endurance. Such programs also lead to a decrease in body fat as measured by body density, skinfold thickness, or computed tomography.[43,71,74,77]

Schwartz and coworkers[74] evaluated improvements in aerobic capacity and body composition in older men ages 60 to 82 and younger men ages 24 to 31 enrolled in a 6-month endurance training program. The older men began their program exercising at only 50% to 60% of their maximum heart rate, but after 4 months all were able to exercise for 45 minutes at 85% of their maximum heart rate. The older men also began with a lower aerobic capacity but achieved a 20% increase in their maximum aerobic capacity, about the same degree of increase as the younger men. In contrast, only the older men demonstrated changes in body composition, with a 2.5 kg loss in body weight, a 2.4 kg loss in body fat, and a 2.3% loss in total body fat. These changes in body fat content become physiolog-

ically significant when evaluated according to the change in fat distribution. It was evident by computed tomography that fat was preferentially lost from abdominal and chest fat deposits; thus a rather small loss in body weight and body fat still may have contributed to a reduction in cardiovascular risk. Although total FFM did not change in the older men, thigh muscle mass increased significantly. The length of an exercise program may be an important consideration, since changes in body composition were not observed after 3 months of training but became evident by the end of 6 months.

Endurance training also leads to metabolic changes in skeletal muscle that diminish the risk of chronic disease. After 12 weeks of walking, jogging, and calisthenics, older men had higher levels of muscle glycogen, which suggests an increased sensitivity of tissues to insulin, and a greater ability to metabolize glucose.[52]

The increased functional capacity and muscle strength resulting from an exercise program can contribute immeasurably to the older adult's ability to continue household and personal care and remain independent. Older women ages 57 to 77 who participated in a low-impact aerobics program increased their cardiorespiratory endurance and muscle strength by more than 50% compared to control women of similar age.[43] Regular physical activity increases aerobic capacity and decreases fatigue, increases mental alertness and effectiveness, and increases bone strength (see Chapter 8). Even moderate consistent exercise can lead to improved cardiorespiratory fitness in an older person. Through continued physical activity, a 70-year-old person can achieve an aerobic capacity equal to that of a sedentary 30-year-old.[38] However, no strenuous exercise regimen should be undertaken without a medical evaluation beforehand and professional supervision.

Developing an exercise program. The older person must enjoy the exercise planned or the program is likely to be abandoned.[38] For those with muscular or skeletal problems, walking at a comfortable pace with a cane or walker for support, if needed, is appropriate exercise. Abrupt, overly strenuous activity for those who have been sedentary is dangerous for both the heart and the large muscles. Allowing for individual differences and gradually increasing activity when conducting a group exercise program will increase the probability of success.[55] Although some older people enjoy doing exercises or walking and jogging in a group, others prefer to exercise by themselves. The sedentary older individual with stiff joints and awkward movements might find group activities embarrassing but may attend sessions to hear about exercises that could be done at home. The cost of equipment must be considered when planning exercise activities. Although a stationary bicycle or other equipment offers the advantage of exercising indoors and allows the individual to stop and rest when necessary, such a purchase is prohibitive for many. Activities requiring no financial expenditure are more likely to be adopted by older clients.

Arm and hand exercises are possible for individuals who can no longer walk. Flexing the arm and finger muscles can reduce and retard stiffness and promote self-feeding and recreational pursuits such as arts or crafts or playing a musical instrument. These activities can be presented in the context of nutrition education or as a group social activity.

Physical activity counseling. Healthy older people are more likely to begin and continue regular exercise than less healthy people of similar age. With this in mind, Harris and coworkers[38] recommend physical activity counseling with older adults. The obvious health benefit of even a moderate level of physical activity is not always presented to an older person who could benefit from an increased energy expenditure of even 500 kcal per week. Safety is an important consideration when working with someone who is considering an exercise program. Most injuries among those exercising for health reasons are caused by excessive activity after a long period of muscle disuse. Such risk is minimized by selecting an appropriate activity and gradually increasing the intensity and duration. Activities perceived as requiring a high level of exertion and carrying possible risk of injury are less likely to be adopted or, if adopted, continued on a regular basis.

Physical activities are more likely to be continued if they are easy to perform, convenient, and associated with social support.

Walking programs fulfill all of these requirements and are a safe way to begin exercise for an individual who has had a very low level of physical activity. Walking can be done alone or with a senior citizens group or indoor mall walking club and demands no particular time schedule. It does not cause excessive discomfort and, when begun on a gradual basis, carries little risk. Walking 4 hours a week (about 30 minutes a day)[3] has been shown to measurably increase lean body mass and bone mineral and decrease body fat. Physical activity counseling should be incorporated into nutrition counseling.

Developing the Caloric Requirement

Age and energy needs. If caloric consumption continues at former levels as the REE and physical activity decline, a slow but continual gain in body fat will ensue. Diaries of food intake and physical activity patterns from 252 men from the BLSA were analyzed according to caloric intake and energy expenditure at various ages.[91] Total daily energy expenditure declined each year by 12.4 kcal. The daily energy expenditure for physical activity fell more rapidly than the energy expenditure for basal needs (7.8 kcal compared to 5.2 kcal). Total daily caloric intake declined by about 450 kcal between the ages of 30 and 80 (2,604 to 2,163 kcal). A steep decline in daily caloric intake and expenditure occurred between the ages of 35 and 55, with little decline thereafter until age 70 and beyond. The total daily caloric intake calculated from food records and the daily energy expenditure calculated from measurements of basal metabolism plus daily activity records differed by 7% or less within particular age cohorts. Because these men were physically healthy and exercised regularly, they demonstrated a smaller decrease in total energy expenditure than men of similar ages in the general population.

Reports from NHANES II[93] indicate a decrease in daily caloric intake from 2,899 kcal in men ages 20 to 29 to 1,734 kcal in men ages 70 to 74. Caloric intake declined by about 350 kcal between the ages of 20 and 39 and by about 200 kcal per decade after age 40. In women caloric intake declined by about 400 kcal over this age range, from 1,675 kcal at ages 20 to 29 to 1,270 kcal at ages 70 to 74. Decreases in caloric intake in women were approximately 70 to 80 kcal per decade. The low caloric intakes observed in the oldest age groups, particularly among women, raise serious issues regarding the adequacy of protein, vitamin, and mineral intakes, and the importance of menu items high in nutrient density.

Recommended caloric intakes. In past years the recommended dietary allowances (RDAs) for energy divided people over age 50 into two categories; those ages 51 to 75, and those ages 76 and over.[28] The recommended intake of kilocalories for the latter group was adjusted downward to accommodate the anticipated decrease in energy expenditure, particularly for physical activity, in the oldest age group. The 1989 RDAs[29] grouped all individuals over the age of 50 with the recommendation that a further decrease in energy expenditure is neither inevitable nor desirable (Table 3-3).

The estimated REE for people over age 60 is calculated using the following prediction equations published by the World Health Organization and based on weight and age.

- Men over age 60   REE (kcal/day) = $(13.5 \times \text{wt in kg}) + 487$
- Women over age 60   REE (kcal/day) = $(10.5 \times \text{wt in kg}) + 596$

Prediction equations do not provide a precise estimate for each individual but do provide a guide for planning food intake. The 1980 RDAs[28] were based on the desirable weight for

height for each age group. The 1989 recommended caloric allowances[29] are based on the median heights and weights for each age and sex group as reported in NHANES II. Thus the body weights used in these calculations are higher and represent actual rather than desirable weights. Recommended caloric intakes are also higher compared to the 1980 recommendations.

The thermic effect of food, although rather small in relation to total energy expenditure, could have a significant long-term effect on energy balance. In developing the RDA, this thermic effect was considered to represent about 5% to 10% of the energy value of the food eaten and to contribute rather little to the energy requirement.

The recommended caloric intakes developed for those over age 50 are based on light to moderate activity levels and represent 1.5 times the basal requirement. Such an activity level might include 8 hours of rest, 13 hours of very light physical activity (activities involving sitting or standing), and 3 hours of light activity (activities involving walking on a level surface at 3 mph). A recent study[46] suggests that older women, even those over age 80, have more hours of light activity involving walking than do older men (Table 3-4). Older women may continue their usual routine of household tasks, or this increased activity may indicate a better health status among older women who may be caring for older husbands. Physical activity does drop in both sexes after age 80. The light-to-moderate activity level represented in the current RDAs may not be sufficient to achieve optimum cardiovascular fitness.[29]

Issues in Defining the Energy Requirement

Critical issues relating to the energy requirement of older people are (1) the caloric intake required for optimum rather than maintenance levels, and (2) the alteration of caloric intake or energy expenditure required for weight loss. In a metabolic evaluation of six healthy men over age 63,[13] the daily energy requirement for basal needs was 1,622 kcal; the caloric intake required to maintain body weight was 2,554 kcal

TABLE 3-3   *Recommended Energy Intake for Adults Over Age 50*

	Men	Women
Body weight (kg)	77	65
REE (kcal/day)	1,530	1,280
Total energy allowance (kcal/day)	2,300	1,900
Range to allow for individual differences (±20%)	1,840-2,760	1,520-2,280

Adapted from Food and Nutrition Board: *Recommended dietary allowances,* ed 10, Washington, DC, 1989, National Academy Press.

TABLE 3-4   Time Allocation (in Hours) of Older Men and Women*

Age (years)	Men		Women	
	60-69	80+	60-69	80+
Sleeping/resting	9.4	11.3	9.4	11.4
Sitting	7.7	8.4	7.2	8.4
Standing	3.6	2.0	2.0	1.0
Walking/moving about	3.2	2.4	5.3	3.1

*Based on a 24-hour period.
Adapted from James WPT, Ralph A, Ferro-Luzzi A: Energy needs of the elderly: a new approach. In Munro HN, Danford DE, editors: *Nutrition, aging, and the elderly,* New York, 1989, Plenum Press.

or about 1.6 times the basal energy requirement. (The RDA for energy for adults over age 50 is based on 1.5 times the basal requirement.) With the exception of 30 minutes of cycling on a stationary bicycle, these men were sedentary; in fact, most reported having higher levels of physical activity when at home than when in the metabolic unit. On this basis their caloric intake during the study was believed to represent their minimum requirement for maintenance.

Calloway and Zanni[13] considered the maintenance energy requirement for ambulatory but inactive older people to be about 1.5 times the basal requirement, in agreement with the RDA, but from their perspective this is a minimum rather than an optimum intake, and active older adults would require more than this level. The older men in that study, however, were in good physical health, which influenced both their level of muscle mass and physical activity. On the other hand, healthy older men are often reported to consume less than the RDA of 2,300 kcal,[93] and a consistent level of physical activity usually is required to avoid weight gain on intakes above this level.

This issue is further clouded by studies of long-term energy balance that suggest that individuals possess a regulatory mechanism that acts to ensure energy homeostasis.[84] Seldom do caloric intake and energy expenditure balance on a week-to-week basis; small shifts in metabolic rate conserve energy when fewer kilocalories are ingested and may dissipate unneeded kilocalories through thermogenesis when intake exceeds expenditure. This implies that decreasing caloric intake will result in energy conservation with no real benefit to the older individual. Changes in metabolic efficiency of more or less than 10% in response to increased or decreased caloric intake are considered to fall outside normal limits.[45] Decreases in resting energy metabolism have been reported in individuals adopting low-calorie weight reduction diets.[97]

Although these mechanisms require further study in older individuals, they raise questions about the efficacy of drastically reducing kilocalories in an effort to achieve weight reduction in older people in whom a metabolic pattern has developed over a lifetime. Although decreasing caloric intake may be necessary to prevent weight gain among individuals who are extremely limited in movement and cannot increase their physical activity, even severe restriction may not accomplish weight loss. Inappropriately low-calorie intakes, resulting in weakness and poor nutritional status, will further limit activity and decrease energy expenditure, setting in motion a vicious cycle. For those who are severely arthritic and chair-bound, arm exercises may help to increase energy expenditure. A serious health problem such as diabetes would mandate strict control of caloric intake.

Older overweight individuals should be encouraged to (1) avoid foods high in fat or sugar and low in nutrient density, (2) limit the number of servings of nutrient-dense foods that are high in kilocalories and fat, and (3) increase physical activity to increase energy expenditure. An attempt to reverse a lifelong weight pattern that does not include an exercise component will probably have only limited success.[20] Exercise using 150 to 200 kcal per day will help in weight control.

Summary

Evaluation of body composition in older people is difficult, because standards and methods developed for younger adults are not always appropriate for older adults. Whole body counting, body density measurements, and neutron activation and dilution techniques provide reasonable estimates of body fat and lean tissue but require expensive equipment, highly trained personnel, and in some cases extensive cooperation on the part of the client. Skinfold measurements can be unreliable for estimation of body fat in older people because of changes in skinfold compressibility and the age-related movement of body fat from the extremities to the trunk. Circumference measurements hold promise for estimation of fatness in older people, although standard values need to be developed.

Advancing age is accompanied by an increase in body fat and a loss of lean body mass, particularly muscle mass. Since this pattern is not evident among aging individuals with limited caloric intakes and continuing physical exercise, life-style and overconsumption of kilocalories rather than normal aging are likely causes. Loss of lean body mass with a consequent drop in resting energy metabolism and decreasing physical activity lead to a decline in the total energy expenditure of the older individual. At the same time protein, vitamin, and mineral requirements remain unchanged. Nutrition counseling should stress the selection of nutrient-dense foods and development of a physical activity program.

REVIEW QUESTIONS

1. How does aging influence body composition, specifically fat-free mass, total body water, body fat, and body weight?
2. What are the beneficial effects of physical exercise on body composition in aging adults? What types of exercise are best suited to older people, and what factors influence adherence to an exercise plan?
3. What factors contribute to the resting energy expenditure (REE) in older people? What is the best method for determining REE in older people? What method is the most practical to the clinician working with older adults?
4. What are the implications for meal planning for older adults, based on the fact that total energy expenditure changes as people age?
5. What nutritional suggestions can be made to the older person who is overweight? Will exercise help weight reduction in the older person? If so, how much exercise is recommended?

SUGGESTED LEARNING ACTIVITIES

1. Visit a nutrition assessment laboratory, and view a demonstration of body composition analyses. Research the pros and cons of estimating body fat by use of skinfold calipers, bioelectrical impedance, dual photon absorption, and neutron analysis.
2. Determine body mass index (BMI) for 10 older adults, using Quetelet's formula and a nomogram. Compare the differences.
3. Write a lesson plan for a 20-minute class to be presented at a senior citizens center on the advantages of strength training for older adults.
4. Plan the energy requirements for (1) a 64-year-old man who competes in masters' swimming events; (2) an 89-year-old woman who lives in her own home and gardens for 1 hour each day; and (3) a 74-year-old woman who is institutionalized.

Key Terms

Provided here for review is a list of the major terms in this chapter. The definitions can be found in the Glossary, which begins on p. 336. To help you understand how these terms are applied, the page number is given for the first mention of each term in the chapter.

aerobic capacity, 68
anthropometric measurements, 50
basal metabolism, 64
bioelectrical impedance, 53
body cell mass (BCM), 49
body mass index (BMI), 54
computed tomography, 50
dual photon absorption, 50
envelope measurements, 55

REFERENCES

1. Albrink MJ, Meigs JW: Serum lipids, skinfold thickness, body bulk, and body weight of native Cape Verdeans, New England Cape Verdeans, and United States factory workers, *Am J Clin Nutr* 24:344, 1971.

2. Aloia JF and others: Relationship of menopause to skeletal and muscle mass, *Am J Clin Nutr* 53:1378, 1991.

3. Anonymous: Walk, don't run—or saunter if you wish, *Tufts University Diet and Nutrition Letter,* vol 9, no 12, February 1992.

4. Barlett HL and others: Fat-free mass in relation to stature: ratios of fat-free mass to height in children, adults, and elderly subjects, *Am J Clin Nutr* 53:1112, 1991.

5. Baumgartner RN and others: Body composition in elderly people: effect of criterion estimates on predictive equations, *Am J Clin Nutr* 53:1345, 1991.

6. Berdanier CD: Weight loss–weight regain: a vicious cycle, *Nutr Today* 26(5):6, 1991.

7. Blanchard J and others: Comparison of methods for estimating body composition in young and elderly women, *J Gerontol* 45:B119, 1990.

8. Bloesch D and others: Thermogenic response to an oral glucose load in man: comparison between young and elderly subjects, *J Am Coll Nutr* 7:471, 1988.

9. Bogardus C and others: Familial dependence of the resting metabolic rate, *N Engl J Med* 315:96, 1986.

10. Bouchard C and others: Inheritance of the amount and distribution of human body fat, *Int J Obes* 12:205, 1987.

11. Bouchard C and others: Genetic effect in resting and exercise metabolic rates, *Metabolism* 38:364, 1989.

12. Bray GA: Obesity. In Brown ML, editor: *Present knowledge in nutrition,* ed 6, Washington, DC, 1990, International Life Sciences Institute–Nutrition Foundation.

13. Calloway DH, Zanni E: Energy requirements and energy expenditure of elderly men, *Am J Clin Nutr* 33:2088, 1980.

14. Chumlea WC, Baumgartner RN: Status of anthropometry and body composition data in elderly subjects, *Am J Clin Nutr* 50:1158, 1989.

15. Chumlea WC, Roche AF, Steinbaugh ML: Anthropometric approaches to the nutritional assessment of the elderly. In Munro HN, Danford DE, editors: *Nutrition, aging, and the elderly,* New York, 1989, Plenum Press.

16. Chumlea WC, and others: Distributions of serial changes in stature and weight in a healthy elderly population, *Hum Biol* 60:917, 1988.

17. Clarys JP and others: The skinfold: myth and reality, *J Sports Sci* 5:3, 1987.

18. Cohn SH and others: Compartmental body composition based on total body nitrogen, potassium, and calcium, *Am J Physiol* 239:E523, 1980.

19. Cohn SH and others: Improved models for determination of body fat by in vivo neutron activation, *Am J Clin Nutr* 40:255, 1984.

20. Council on Scientific Affairs: Treatment of obesity in adults, *JAMA* 260:2547, 1988.

21. Deurenberg P, Weststrate JA, van der Kooy K: Is an adaptation of Siri's formula for the calculation of body fat percentage from body density in the elderly necessary? *Eur J Clin Nutr* 43:559, 1989.

22. Deurenberg P and others: Body mass index as a measure of body fatness in the elderly, *Eur J Clin Nutr* 43:231, 1989.

23. Deurenberg P and others: Assessment of body composition by bioelectrical impedance in a population aged over 60 years, *Am J Clin Nutr* 51:3, 1990.

24. Evans WJ: Exercise and muscle metabolism in the elderly. In Hutchinson ML, Munro HN, editors: *Nutrition and aging,* New York, 1986, Academic Press.

25. Evans WJ, Meredith CN: Exercise and nutrition in the elderly. In Munro HN, Danford DE, editors: *Nutrition, aging and the elderly,* New York, 1989, Plenum Press.

26. Fiatarone MA and others: High-intensity strength training in nonagenarians: effects on skeletal muscle, *JAMA* 263:3029, 1990.

27. Flynn MA and others: Total body potassium in aging humans: a longitudinal study, *Am J Clin Nutr* 50:713, 1989.

28. Food and Nutrition Board: *Recommended dietary allowances,* ed 9, Washington, DC, 1980, National Academy Press.

29. Food and Nutrition Board: *Recommended dietary allowances,* ed 10, Washington, DC, 1989, National Academy Press.

30. Forbes GB: *Human body composition: growth, aging, nutrition, and activity,* New York, 1987, Springer-Verlag.

31. Forbes GB: Body composition. In Brown ML, editor: *Present knowledge in nutrition,* ed 6, Washington, DC, 1990, International Life Sciences Institute–Nutrition Foundation.

32. Forbes GB, Brown MR, Griffiths HJL: Arm muscle plus bone area: anthropometry and CAT scan compared, *Am J Clin Nutr* 47:929, 1988.

33. Fredrix EWHM and others: Estimation of body composition by bioelectrical impedance in cancer patients, *Eur J Clin Nutr* 44:749, 1989.

34. Fredrix EWHM and others: Resting and sleeping energy expenditure in the elderly, *Eur J Clin Nutr* 44:741, 1990.

35. Fukagawa NK and others: Protein-induced changes in energy expenditure in young and old individuals, *Am J Physiol* 260:E345, 1991.

36. Garrow JS: New approaches to body composition, *Am J Clin Nutr* 35:1152, 1982.

37. Gregerman RI, Gaffney GW, Shock NW: Thyroxine turnover in euthyroid man with special reference to changes with age, *J Clin Invest* 41:2065, 1962.

38. Harris SS and others: Physical activity counseling for healthy adults as a primary preventive intervention in the clinical setting, *JAMA* 261:3590, 1989.

39. Heymsfield SB, Waki M: Body composition in humans: advances in the development of multicompartment chemical models, *Nutr Rev* 49(4):97, 1991.

40. Heymsfield SB and others: Dual-photon absorptiometry: comparison of bone mineral and soft tissue mass measurements in vivo with established methods, *Am J Clin Nutr* 49:1283, 1989.

41. Hoeldtke RD, Cilmi KM: Effects of aging on catecholamine metabolism, *J Clin Endocrinol Metab* 60:479, 1985.

42. Hofstetter A and others: Increased 24-hour energy expenditure in cigarette smokers, *N Engl J Med* 314:79, 1986.

43. Hopkins DR and others: Effect of low-impact aerobic dance on the functional fitness of elderly women, *J Am Geriatr Soc* 30:189, 1990.

44. James WPT: Energy. In Horwitz A and others, editors: *Nutrition in the elderly,* New York, 1989, Oxford University Press.

45. James WPT, McNeill G, Ralph A: Metabolism and nutritional adaptation to altered intakes of energy substrates, *Am J Clin Nutr* 51:264, 1990.

46. James WPT, Ralph A, Ferro-Luzzi A: Energy needs of the elderly: a new approach. In Munro HN, Danford DE, editors: *Nutrition, aging, and the elderly,* New York, 1989, Plenum Press.

47. Kern PA and others: The effects of weight loss on the activity and expression of adipose tissue lipoprotein lipase in very obese humans, *N Engl J Med* 322:1053, 1990.

48. Kuczmarski RJ: Need for body composition information in elderly subjects, *Am J Clin Nutr* 50:1150, 1989.

49. Lukaski HC: Methods for the assessment of human body composition: traditional and new, *Am J Clin Nutr* 46:537, 1987.

50. Lukaski HC and others: Assessment of fat-free mass using bioelectrical impedance measurements of the human body, *Am J Clin Nutr* 41:810, 1985.

51. Marshall WA and others: Anthropometric measurements of the Tristan da Cunha islanders, 1962-68, *Hum Biol* 43:112, 1971.

52. Meredith CN and others: Peripheral effects of endurance training in young and old subjects, *J Appl Physiol* 66:2844, 1989.

53. Micozzi MS and others: Correlations of body mass indices with weight, stature, and body composition in men and women in NHANES I and II, *Am J Clin Nutr* 44:725, 1986.

54. Moore FD and others: *The body cell mass and its supporting environment,* Philadelphia, 1963, WB Saunders.

55. Morey MC and others: Two-year trends in physical performance following supervised exercise among community-dwelling older veterans, *J Am Geriatr Soc* 39:549, 1991.

56. Must A, Dallal GE, Dietz WH: Reference data for obesity: 85th and 95th percentiles of body

mass index (wt/ht²) and triceps skinfold thickness, *Am J Clin Nutr* 53:839, 1991.

57. Nelson ME and others: Hormone and bone mineral status in endurance-trained and sedentary postmenopausal women, *J Clin Endocrinol Metab* 66:927, 1988.

58. Nichols JF and others: Effect of age and aerobic capacity on resting metabolic rate and the thermic effect of food in healthy men, *Nutr Res* 10:1161, 1990.

59. Noppa H and others: Body composition in middle-aged women with special reference to the correlation between body fat mass and anthropometric data, *Am J Clin Nutr* 32:1388, 1979.

60. Ohlson MA and others: Anthropometry and nutritional status of adult women, *Hum Biol* 28:189, 1956.

61. Poehlman ET, Horton ES: Regulation of energy expenditure in aging humans, *Annu Rev Nutr* 10:255, 1990.

62. Poehlman ET, Melby CL, Badylak SF: Resting metabolic rate and postprandial thermogenesis in highly trained and untrained males, *Am J Clin Nutr* 47:793, 2988.

63. Ravussin E, Bogardus C: Relationship of genetics, age, and physical fitness to daily energy expenditure and fuel utilization, *Am J Clin Nutr* 49:968, 1989.

64. Ravussin E and others: Determinants of 24-hour energy expenditure in man: methods and results using a respiratory chamber, *J Clin Invest* 78:1568, 1986.

65. Rodin J and others: Weight cycling and fat distribution, *Int J Obes* 14:303, 1989.

66. Rosenthal MJ and others: Thyroid failure in the elderly, *JAMA* 358:209, 1987.

67. Rudman D: Nutrition and fitness in elderly people, *Am J Clin Nutr* 49:1090, 1989.

68. Rudman D and others: Effects of human growth hormone in men over 60 years old, *N Engl J Med* 323:1, 1990.

69. Schlenker ED: Nutritional status of older women, doctoral dissertation, East Lansing, Mich, 1976, Michigan State University.

70. Schutz Y and others: Postprandial thermogenesis at rest and during exercise in elderly men ingesting two levels of protein, *J Am Coll Nutr* 6:497, 1987.

71. Schwartz RS: Effects of exercise training on high-density lipoproteins and apolipoprotein A-1 in old and young men, *Metabolism* 37:1128, 1988.

72. Schwartz RS, Jaeger LF, Veith RC: The thermic effect of feeding in older men: the importance of

the sympathetic nervous system, *Metabolism* 39:733, 1990.

73. Schwartz RS and others: Body fat distribution in healthy young and older men, *J Gerontol* 45:M181, 1990.

74. Schwartz RS and others: The effect of intensive endurance exercise training on body fat distribution in young and older men, *Metabolism* 40:545, 1991.

75. Segal KR and others: Estimation of human body composition by electrical impedance methods: a comparative study, *J Appl Physiol* 58:1565, 1985.

76. Seltzer CC and others: Reliability of relative body weight as a criterion of obesity, *Am J Epidemiol* 92:339, 1970.

77. Sidney KH, Shephard RJ, Harrison JE: Endurance training and body composition of the elderly, *Am J Clin Nutr* 30:326, 1977.

78. Skerji B and others: Subcutaneous fat and age changes in body build and form in women, *Am J Phys Anthropol* 11:577, 1953.

79. Society of Actuaries: Build study 1979, Chicago, 1980, The Society.

80. Solomon DH: The normal and diseased thyroid gland. In Abrams WB, and Berkow R, editors: *Merck manual of geriatrics,* Rahway, NJ, 1990, Merck, Sharp & Dohme.

81. Steen B: Body composition and aging, *Nutr Rev* 46:45, 1988.

82. Steen B: Body composition. In Horwitz A and others, editors: *Nutrition in the elderly,* New York, 1989, Oxford University Press.

83. Streat SJ, Beddoe AH, Hill GL: Measurement of body fat and hydration of the fat-free body in health and disease, *Metabolism* 34:509, 1985.

84. Sukhatme PV, Margen S: Autoregulatory homeostatic nature of energy balance, *Am J Clin Nutr* 35:355, 1982.

85. Sullivan DH and others: An approach to assessing the reliability of anthropometrics in elderly patients, *J Am Geriatr Soc* 37:607, 1989.

86. Svendsen OL and others: Measurement of body fat in elderly subjects by dual-energy x-ray absorptiometry, bioelectrical impedance, and anthropometry, *Am J Clin Nutr* 53:1117, 1991.

87. Tibaldi JM and others: Thyrotoxicosis in the very old, *Am J Med* 81:619, 1986.

88. Tremblay A and others: Impact of dietary fat content and fat oxidation on energy intake in humans, *Am J Clin Nutr* 49 799, 1989.

89. Trotter M, and Gleser G: The effect of aging on stature, *Am J Phys Anthropol* 9:311, 1951.

90. US Department of Health and Human Services:

Anthropometric data and prevalence of overweight for Hispanics: 1982-84, DHHS Pub No (PHS) 86-1689, Washington, DC, 1986, US Government Printing Office.

91. US Department of Health and Human Services: Normal human aging: the Baltimore Longitudinal Study of Aging, NIH Pub No 84-2450, Washington, DC, 1984, US Government Printing Office.

92. US Department of Health and Human Services: Anthropometric reference data and prevalence of overweight: United States, 1976-80, DHHS Pub No (PHS) 87-1688, Washington, DC, 1987, US Government Printing Office.

93. US Department of Health and Human Services, US Department of Agriculture: Nutrition monitoring in the United States: an update report on nutrition and monitoring, DHHS Pub No (PHS) 89-1255, Washington, DC, 1989, US Government Printing Office.

94. Van Itallie TB, Lew EA: Health implications of overweight in the elderly. In Prinsley D, Sandstead HH, editors: *Nutrition and aging,* New York, 1990, Alan R Liss.

95. Vance ML: Growth hormone for the elderly, *N Engl J Med* 323:52, 1990.

96. Vaughan L, Zurlo F, Ravussin E: Aging and energy expenditure, *Am J Clin Nutr* 53:821, 1991.

97. Wadden TA and others: Long-term effects of dieting on resting metabolic rate in obese outpatients, *JAMA* 264:707, 1990.

98. Young CM and others: Predicting specific gravity and body fatness in older women, *J Am Diet Assoc* 45:333, 1964.

4 Nutrient Digestion and Absorption

Objectives

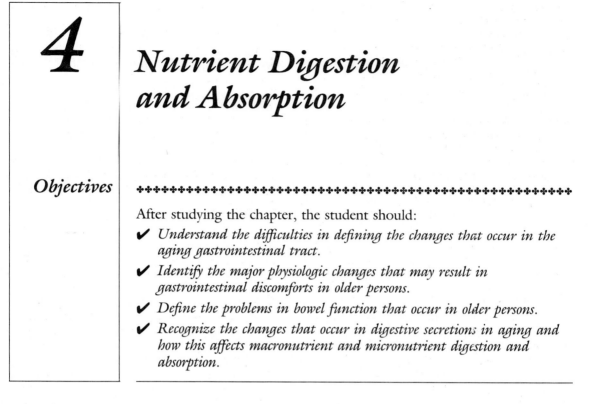

++

After studying the chapter, the student should:

✔ *Understand the difficulties in defining the changes that occur in the aging gastrointestinal tract.*

✔ *Identify the major physiologic changes that may result in gastrointestinal discomforts in older persons.*

✔ *Define the problems in bowel function that occur in older persons.*

✔ *Recognize the changes that occur in digestive secretions in aging and how this affects macronutrient and micronutrient digestion and absorption.*

Introduction

The changes in the gastrointestinal tract that occur with normal aging are not well understood; yet such changes could have important implications for the nutritional status of older adults. Incomplete digestion and consequent reduced absorption of nutrients would result in nutrient deficiencies, regardless of the adequacy of nutrient intake. Also, if changes in the functional capacity of the gastrointestinal tract cause physical discomfort, the older person may eat less, thereby increasing the likelihood of nutrient deficiency. For these reasons complaints from older individuals about gastrointestinal upset require careful evaluation. At the same time, healthy older adults may experience no change in gastrointestinal function even beyond age 80.

AGING AND GASTROINTESTINAL FUNCTION
Level of Function

Function in the gastrointestinal tract is generally well preserved into advanced age. The large reserve capacity of the many organs that make up the gastrointestinal system is mostly responsible for the preservation of generally adequate function. No change in the dietary requirement of any particular nutrient is justified, according to available clinical evidence on changes in the gastrointestinal tract.[8] Nevertheless, it is commonly believed that gastrointestinal function declines significantly with increasing age.

Of all organ systems, the gastrointestinal tract is the most common source of chronic discomfort in older people, and some gastrointestinal disorders, including diverticulosis and atrophic gastritis, are more common among older than younger adults. Holt[29] pointed out that gastrointestinal disease can be more difficult to diagnose in older patients with several concomitant disorders that can distort the usual features of the primary disorder. Clinical signs may be atypical because of age-related differences in gastrointestinal motility or the localized perception of pain induced by medications or changes in the central nervous system.

Gastrointestinal distress does not necessarily indicate **malabsorption**; individuals with no symptoms may absorb nutrients poorly, whereas others with constant gastrointestinal discomfort may absorb nutrients normally. Because of the potential impact of gastrointestinal problems on nutritional status and the fact that such symptoms often signal organic disease, all complaints should be investigated carefully.

Prevalence of Problems

As with most chronic conditions, chronic digestive disorders increase with age. Among 42,000 adults participating in the National Health Interview Survey,[38] the age gradient was especially steep for ulcers, diverticulitis, and gallbladder problems. About 10% of those over age 64 reported having diverticulitis, compared to 3% of younger adults. Between two age groups (ages 45 to 64, and 65 and older), the proportion of adults who had ever had gallbladder problems increased from 6% to 12% among men and from 14% to 23% among women. However, these reports were based on general interviews and did not include physical examination.

Although women are more likely to have gallbladder problems in later years, men are more likely to have ulcers. About 14% of middle-aged men reported ever having ulcers; this increased to 20% in the oldest age group. General digestive disorders and bowel complaints are especially characteristic of older women. Smaller numbers of black and Hispanic elderly report ever having had digestive disorders. The lower reporting of these disorders may relate to fewer physician visits for diagnosis of these conditions rather than reduced incidence.

Eating problems and symptoms of digestive distress do increase with age in older people. Nevertheless, data collected in the **Georgia Centenarian Study**[9] suggest that most older people living in the community are relatively free of gastrointestinal distress (Table 4-1). Although chewing, biting, and bowel problems (**constipation** or diarrhea) were more frequent in the centenarians compared to those ages 60 to 89, food intolerance was less common (5% versus 48%). This would suggest that gastrointestinal dysfunction is more closely related to chronic diseases than aging per se, although both factors probably are involved.

Basis of Problems

Unfortunately, digestive symptoms are often nonspecific, and it is not always possible to determine a specific organic cause or disease. This was the case among a group of outpatients over age 65 seeking help for digestive problems: 56% had no demonstrable disease; 20% had an ulcer, gallbladder disease, or **diverticulosis;** 10% had cancer; and 14% had other disorders.[59]

A wide variety of commonly used prescription and over-the-counter drugs, including digitalis, anticonvulsants, diuretics, and aspirin, can cause gastrointestinal distress. The gastrointestinal tract is sensitive to mental and emotional stress, which can lead to gastric upset or a change in bowel habits. The interplay of age-related changes in the structure, motility, and secretions of the gastrointestinal tract, as influenced by psychologic or physical stress, can cause digestive disorders or exacerbate existing organic disease.[54]

Xerostomia

Xerostomia, or dry mouth, is a common problem among older people, and it can arise from several causes.[46,47] A decrease in the secretion of saliva may be related to changes in sensory receptors or in functioning of the central nervous system. Drugs, including antidepressants, antihypertensive agents, and bronchodilators, can decrease secretion of saliva. **Autoimmune diseases** and both radiation and chemotherapy cancer treatments can cause xerostomia. Difficulty lubricating, masticating, tasting, and

TABLE 4-1   *Percentage of Older People With Particular Nutrition Risk Factors**

	Ages 60-69 (n = 46)	Ages 80-89 (n = 44)	Ages 100+ (n = 19)
Any illness that interferes with eating?	13	14	26
Any trouble biting or chewing certain foods?	17	16	37
Any foods not eaten because they disagree with you?	48	48	5
Any abdominal pain or discomfort in the last month?	4	9	5
Any trouble swallowing in the last month?	2	2	5
Any vomiting in the last month?	2	5	0
Any problems with your bowels (diarrhea or constipation)?	17	25	37
On a special diet?	9	16	16

*People answering yes to the questions in the table; preliminary data from the Georgia Centenarian Study.
Modified from Bowman BA, Rosenberg IH, and Johnson MA: Gastrointestinal function in the elderly. In Munro H, Schlierf G, editors: *Nutrition of the elderly,* Nestle Nutrition Workshop Series, vol 29, New York, 1992, Raven Press.

swallowing food is a critical effect of this condition. Saliva also plays an important role in lubricating and maintaining the teeth and oral mucosa, destroying harmful microorganisms and neutralizing potentially toxic substances taken into the mouth. Infections, ulcers in the oral cavity, and increases in tooth decay are other consequences of dry mouth. Dry mouth can have nutritional consequences as well in older adults.

Rhodus and Brown[47] compared the nutrient intakes of independently living and institutionalized adults being treated for xerostomia and control subjects of similar age. Mean age was 68 to 69 years in all three groups. The institutionalized individuals with xerostomia had lower intakes of all nutrients than their counterparts living in the community. Caloric intake was only 1,190 kcal in the institutionalized patients, compared to 1,739 kcal in those living in the community. Older people of similar age with normal salivary secretion were consuming 2,164 kcal each day. None of the control subjects had less than the recommended dietary allowance (RDA) for energy, protein, vitamins A and C, thiamin, and riboflavin, and only 5% were low in calcium and iron. In contrast, 25%

to 90% of those with xerostomia fell below the RDA for these nutrients. Diets were most inadequate for vitamin B_6, calcium, potassium, and zinc. Body mass index (BMI) was significantly lower, and the number of individuals with inadequate serum albumin was higher among those with xerostomia. General health was similar across all groups.

Xerostomia is an important risk factor for inadequate nutrient intake. Using artificial salivas or hard, sugarless candy may help relieve discomfort. When possible, therapeutic drugs with no known effect on salivary gland functioning might be substituted for those that induce or exacerbate xerostomia. Trying a softer diet and experimenting with textures and seasonings may help the older individual with xerostomia to eat more.

Dysphagia

Dysphagia is characterized by difficulty in swallowing and passing food from the oral cavity to the stomach. As described in Fig. 4-1, swallowing is a complex process involving three phases[41,64]:

- In the oral phase, food is masticated, mixed with salivary secretions, and prepared for

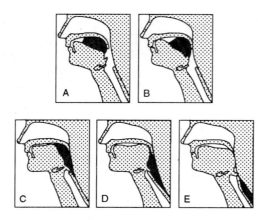

FIG. 4-1 Sequence of events in swallowing. **A,** Food is moved to rear of mouth. **B,** Soft palate rises and obstructs nasal passage. **C,** Epiglottis closes to obstruct trachea. **D,** Bolus passes through upper esophageal sphincter. **E,** Bolus moves down esophagus.

(Adapted from Davenport HW: *Physiology of the digestive tract,* Chicago, 1982, Year Book Medical Publishers.)

swallowing; the liquid or food bolus is then moved to the rear of the mouth
- In the pharyngeal phase, the food is forced into the throat; for the moment respiration ceases, the soft palate rises to prevent food from entering the nasal passages, the epiglottis closes to prevent food from entering the trachea, and the upper esophageal sphincter relaxes
- In the esophageal phase, the food bolus or liquid enters the esophagus and moves down the passage; the lower esophageal sphincter relaxes, and the food enters the stomach; the soft palate and epiglottis return to their normal positions, and breathing resumes

Dysphagia in older people usually is caused by changes in the central nervous system and deterioration of neuromuscular control. A **cerebrovascular accident** or stroke, **Parkinson's disease,** or **organic brain syndrome** can influence neural control of the muscles involved in swallowing and tongue movement. **Diabetic neuropathy** also can lead to swallowing disorders.[42]

Once food enters the esophagus, a peristaltic wave initiated by the swallowing reflex moves food along the passageway. As the peristaltic wave nears the stomach, it is preceded by a wave of relaxation that acts on the lower esophageal sphincter, causing it to open and allow food to enter the stomach. In some older individuals, normal peristaltic waves do not occur or their amplitude is decreased, resulting in delayed esophageal emptying.[13] Consequently, the esophagus becomes dilated as food accumulates. This results in muscle contractions that can be both painful and ineffective in propelling the food bolus. Liquids, particularly thin liquids such as water, may be even more difficult to handle than solid foods.[42]

The incidence of dysphagia increases with age. It is estimated that 30% to 40% of institutionalized older people have swallowing disorders.[64] In a survey of 136 community residents over age 87,[6] 16% reported bouts of coughing and choking when eating and drinking, or having to swallow more than once to remove the same bite of food from the mouth. For six of the 21 people the swallowing problem was severe. Four reported daily choking, and two had restricted their diet to thick soups because of their dysphagia. It is noteworthy that none of the six had discussed these symptoms with their physician, believing this problem to be an inevitable consequence of advancing age.

Dysphagia has implications for both nutritional and physical health. This condition can limit the type and quantity of food and liquids consumed, contributing to malnutrition or dehydration. A more immediate danger is choking or the aspiration of food into the lung and development of pneumonia.[58] Thus care in feeding and selecting appropriately prepared foods is paramount. Evaluation and a treatment plan require a team approach that includes a speech pathologist and a nutritionist.

Matthews[41] recommends the following guidelines for working with dysphagic adults:

Positioning: The individual should be sitting up at a 90-degree angle, both when eating and for about 30 minutes before and after eating to take advantage of gravity flow and to properly align the esophagus for swallowing.

Food of appropriate consistency: Thick liquids, pureed meats in sauce or gravy, and foods that easily form a bolus in the mouth are preferred; sticky foods, foods with stringy fibers such as celery, foods with small seeds or pits, and foods with two consistencies (e.g., soups containing small pieces of meat or vegetables) increase the risk of choking and aspiration.

Environment: A relaxed, unhurried atmosphere is important, so that the individual can take small amounts of food at a time and eat at a pace he or she finds comfortable.*

Food Intolerance

Perceived discomfort in the gastrointestinal tract after eating a particular food influences whether a person will eat that food and foods considered similar in form or content. Older adults report a higher frequency of **food intolerance** than younger adults, although severe symptoms of intolerance, including nausea, vomiting, or diarrhea, are relatively infrequent.[65,71] Ten percent of 477 community living Swedish elderly singled out dietary fat as a food component causing distress, although the severity of the symptoms was not discussed.[71]

Vegetables are sometimes singled out as foods causing gastrointestinal distress because of their fiber content or undigestible carbohydrates, such as raffinose, that lead to gas production. Zimmerman and Krondl[74] studied food intolerance in older people receiving home-delivered meals in Toronto. Forty percent of the recipients had one or more perceived food intolerances, and 60% had none. Vegetables were the most frequently cited food group causing symptoms. The vegetables most poorly tolerated were cauliflower, cabbage, brussels sprouts, onions, and corn. Carrots, peas, and broccoli, although poorly tolerated raw, were well tolerated cooked. Celery and lettuce were the only raw vegetables well tolerated by those with food intolerance. Burping was the most common symptom reported, followed by flatulence, **heartburn,** and abdominal pain. Zimmerman and Krondl emphasized that many

well-tolerated vegetables, including raw vegetables, were not being included in home-delivered meals because planners believed them to cause intolerance. It is important to note that broccoli, spinach, carrots, and yams, good sources of folacin and the carotenoids, were well tolerated in both groups when cooked.

Dyspepsia

Abdominal discomfort after eating can have many causes. Drugs such as digitalis, levodopa, or aspirin may be at fault. Overconsumption of food or alcohol can cause gastrointestinal distress. Discomfort from burning sensations caused by irritation of the stomach mucosa or from distention often leads to constant swallowing in an effort to relieve the distress.[11] However, swallowing air can exacerbate the problem and lead to more discomfort. Psychologic stress and tension can cause gastric distress. Reporting of frequent indigestion does increase with age. In a national survey,[66] 19% of young adults (compared to 44% of adults over age 64) had this problem. Fewer blacks report frequent indigestion, regardless of age.

Although chronic indigestion can signal the presence of ulcers or other organic disorder, some individuals have **chronic dyspepsia** with no identifiable cause.[25] Those with **nonulcer dyspepsia** have a similar rate of gastric emptying, and their levels of gastric acid and intestinal gas are no higher than those without symptoms. Efforts to identify particular personality types that are more likely to have nonulcer dyspepsia have been unsuccessful.[62]

Recent work suggests that people with this condition are more sensitive to gastric events than other people.[25] Messages of peristaltic contractions usually do not reach the nerve centers of the brain, where physical sensations are processed, and thus are not perceived. It appears, however, that some individuals have a lower threshold for recognition of these signals. These people felt pain when their stomach wall was stretched with an inflatable bag to the same size that produced no discomfort in control subjects. Although we have no cure for this condition, symptoms can be reduced by avoiding alcohol, aspirin, and other known stomach irritants. Severe gastric distress can be treated

---

*Further suggestions and additional readings are listed in Tripp F, Cordero O: Dysphagia and nutrition in the acute care geriatric patient, *Top Clin Nutr* 6:60, 1991.

with H_2-blockers, drugs that reduce the secretion of gastric acid.[11] Chronic dyspepsia in an older person must be evaluated carefully for possible organic disease. Indigestion and gastrointestinal dysfunction are not normal consequences of advancing age.

Diverticulosis

Diverticulosis is a common disorder among older people in Western societies; the prevalence increases rapidly after age 40, and by age 80 over half of the population has diverticula in the colon.[56] Diverticulosis is characterized by pouchlike projections along the inner wall of the colon, particularly where the colon joins the rectum. This condition should be distinguished from diverticulitis, or infection and inflammation of the diverticula that can result in bleeding or obstruction of the bowel. In most people diverticulosis is asymptomatic; symptoms that do occur as a result of uncomplicated diverticulosis include abdominal discomfort and erratic bowel habits (diarrhea or constipation). It has been theorized that diverticula are caused by increases in intraluminal pressure caused by low-fiber diets and low bulk, particularly as the tissue becomes less elastic with increasing age. Although this idea is popular, intraluminal studies have not demonstrated increased luminal pressure in older people with or without diverticula of the colon.[56] Cashman[11] recommends that the dietary modifications used to treat chronic constipation also be used with diverticulosis, recognizing that certain individuals may not be able to tolerate increased levels of dietary or supplemental fiber.

Problems in Bowel Function

Prevalence of constipation. Constipation is the most common gastrointestinal problem in the United States, and it is estimated that more than $400 million is spent on laxatives each year.[23] Evaluation is difficult, because we lack a standard definition of this condition.[52] Constipation is a chronic condition involving decreased frequency of bowel movements, difficult passage of stools, passage of hard stools, or a sensation of incomplete emptying of the bowel. Normal bowel habits range from three bowel movements a week to two bowel move-

ments a day. A common definition of constipation is fewer than three bowel movements a week.[12]

Unfortunately, many individuals who by this definition have normal bowel function consider themselves to be constipated. Among the 15,000 individuals between the ages of 12 and 74 who were evaluated in the first National Health and Nutrition Examination Survey (NHANES I),[52] 31% of those with four to six bowel movements a week reported constipation. Both age and race are related to this problem (Fig. 4-2). Fewer than 13% of those under age 45 (compared to 64% to 75% of those over age 65) considered constipation a problem.[66] Blacks are more likely to report this condition than whites. In a random sample of 209 older Baltimore adults ranging in age from 65 to 93,

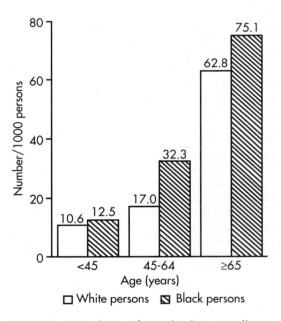

FIG. 4-2   Prevalence of constipation according to age and race. Black adults over age 44 and white adults over age 64 are the most likely to report constipation.

(Data from US Department of Health and Human Services: Health of black and white Americans: 1985-87, DHHS Pub No (PHS) 90-1599, Hyattsville, Md, 1990, US Government Printing Office.)

30% reported being constipated at least once a month.[72] At the same time, only 3% reported a stool frequency of fewer than three a week. Among these older people, having to strain to pass stools was regarded as a primary symptom of constipation.

Causes of constipation. Constipation can have many causes.[12,23] Normal bowel habits may be interrupted by a change in the diet or activity level or after a bout with diarrhea resulting from a viral infection or other gastrointestinal upset. **Irritable bowel syndrome** or **spastic colon,** generally associated with stress, often results in alternating patterns of diarrhea and constipation.

Certain metabolic conditions lead to constipation.[12] Hypothyroidism or hyperthyroidism, abnormal serum calcium or potassium levels, reduced or excessive secretion of the adrenocorticoid hormones, or dehydration can cause constipation. Degenerative neurologic disorders, including Parkinson's disease, or neural damage resulting from a stroke can contribute to constipation. Sluggish bowel movements can be a sign of depression in both younger and older adults. Many medications are potential causes of constipation. Various antihypertensive, anticholinergic, and antidepressant drugs, as well as narcotics used to control pain, can alter normal bowel habits. Calcium and iron supplements and antacids that contain aluminum contribute to the problem.

Individuals who have used laxatives for a long period and have become dependent on these drugs may not be able to establish normal bowel function. Chronic use of irritant laxatives containing **phenolphthalein** or **senna extract** appears to result in neural changes in the wall of the colon, with loss of motility and contraction of the colonic muscle. A less common but serious cause of constipation is obstruction of the lower bowel as a complication of cancer or some other disorder. Constipation accompanied by blood in the stool; severe cramps; a tender, distended abdomen; or markedly narrowed stools requires immediate medical evaluation.[12,15,23]

Some older people have constipation over a period of years or even decades.[16] Studies using markers that are visible on x-ray suggest that intestinal transit time does not increase with age in older individuals with normal bowel function.[11] In contrast, older people who chronically use laxatives have a prolonged transit time and physiologic changes in colonic and rectal function. If a person has a long-term history of using laxatives, dietary intervention may not be successful. Effective treatment of chronic constipation requires careful evaluation of underlying and complicating factors.

Constipation often can be alleviated and usually can be prevented by (1) increasing dietary fiber, (2) increasing fluid intake (daily fluid intake should equal at least 2,000 ml), and (3) getting more exercise.[12,24]

Even persistent constipation may respond to relatively simple measures. Laxatives should be used only after other measures have failed.

Dietary fiber and bowel habits. Dietary treatment of constipation usually involves increasing the individual's fiber intake, either with fiber-rich foods or fiber supplements. Eating 10 to 20 g of wheat bran daily (4 to 8 g dietary fiber) was shown to alleviate constipation in up to 60% of the older institutionalized individuals treated.[11] Transit time was also reduced by this treatment. It must be recognized, however, increasing dietary fiber to this extent initially will result in flatulence, abdominal distress, and in some cases even more irregular bowel habits than when the person was dependent on laxatives.[68] Institutionalized older people usually require about 2 weeks to adapt to a high-fiber diet. Before initiating dietary treatment of irregular bowel habits, it is imperative that organic causes of constipation (e.g., bowel obstruction or fecal impaction) be eliminated as possible factors.

All increases in dietary fiber should be accompanied by a generous intake of fluids. Bran supplements or preparations containing psyllium can obstruct the esophagus and are not appropriate for older people with dysphagia or esophageal problems. Stool bulking agents are not appropriate for severely debilitated older patients. Using bran supplements in institutional settings has been reported to be successful in reducing the need for laxatives, adding to the general comfort of many older patients, and resulting in significant cost savings.[11] **Lactitol,** a nondigestible disaccharide that draws water into the gastrointestinal tract and thereby softens and increases stool mass, is also being evaluated as a treatment for constipation in elderly, institutionalized individuals.[68]

Encouraging an individual to eat lots of foods high in fiber is a desirable alternative to fiber supplements for older people who can eat reasonable amounts of food. Such foods not only contribute dietary fiber but also important vitamins and minerals. Unfortunately, daily fiber intake often is less than optimal in institutionalized older people and those living in their own homes. The mean dietary fiber intake in 209 independently living Baltimore elderly was 8.3 g.[72] Current recommendations of the Committee on Diet and Health suggest a fiber intake of 25 to 35 g per day, to be achieved by eating five or more servings of vegetables and fruits and six or more servings of breads, cereals, and legumes.[63]

Findings from NHANES I[52] indicated that people who reported problems with constipation ate fewer servings of dried peas and beans, fruits, and vegetables. Twenty-one percent of those who never ate legumes were constipated, compared to 9% of those who ate legumes about once a day. In this survey the number of servings of breads and cereals was not related to incidence of constipation; however, data analysis did not differentiate between whole-grain products high in fiber and refined products from which most of the fiber has been removed. It is interesting to note that constipated individuals consumed fewer kilocalories and less food overall than those with normal bowel habits.

Older individuals with chewing or swallowing problems may not eat much high-fiber food. Matthews[40] pointed out that green peas, baked beans, and lentils can be cooked to a soft consistency or made into soup so they can be eaten fairly easily by those who are edentulous or have some degree of dysphagia. Whole-grain muffins, cookies, and hot breads may be attractive to older people who may not be receptive to whole-grain breads or cereals. Wheat bran becomes more palatable when incorporated into baked products, soups, casseroles, or meat loaf.

The mechanism by which dietary fiber improves bowel function is still a matter of debate.[60] **Soluble fibers** (e.g., pectin found in fruits or psyllium seeds) trap water during their passage through the gastrointestinal tract and thereby soften the stools and increase stool weight. Soluble fibers are also digested by bacteria found in the colon, which increases stool weight. **Insoluble fibers,** found in wheat bran and legumes, are not digested by the colonic microflora. The action of these fibers on stool mass may be in part related to their bulk and ability to hold water.[60] However, other physical or chemical properties also may be involved. Coarse bran, for example, acts as a laxative, but finely ground bran does not. Moreover, plastic flakes of the same diameter as coarse bran brought about the same softening effect and increase in stool weight as bran itself.[11] Thus Cashman[11] concluded that mechanical stimulation of the inner lining of the colon leads to the effect observed with both materials. In any case the increase in stool weight, about double the amount of the indigestible material, is an important component of the beneficial effect observed.

The effect of bran supplements on the absorption of important minerals must be considered in nutrition recommendations. Among seven healthy volunteers who ranged in age from 59 to 76 years, calcium absorption decreased from 22% to 9% of total intake as the level of dietary fiber increased.[3] Dietary fiber averaged 9 g per day on the self-selected diets and increased to 21 g per day when wheat bran was added as a dietary supplement. The effect of the wheat bran on calcium absorption was gradual and did not become evident until the third week of the study. This effect should be evaluated carefully, particularly in older women for whom calcium balance is already precarious.

AGING AND PHYSIOLOGIC CHANGES IN THE GASTROINTESTINAL TRACT

Our understanding of the normal physiology of the gastrointestinal tract is limited in both younger and older adults. Functional and noninvasive tests to define normal function and changes in healthy older adults are generally lacking. Nevertheless, it is likely that physiologic changes associated with the aging process influence gastrointestinal function in some older people. Disorders in gastrointestinal function could arise from changes in muscle innervation or the muscle fibers or brain and hormonal control. Most older people have normal gastrointestinal function under average conditions but are less able to compensate for changes in the type or amount of food eaten or for the effects of pathogens or chronic disease.[61]

Physiologic Changes in the Mouth

A major age-related change in the mouth is loss of teeth, which can influence food intake. Ill-fitting dentures irritate the tongue and mucosal tissues, resulting in pain when masticating food. Although loss of teeth is common in current cohorts of older people, improved dental care and attention to oral health suggest that tooth loss will be less extensive in future cohorts.[9] Changes in the tongue and the number and function of the taste buds can diminish taste perception and recognition (see Chapter 12).

Physiologic Changes in the Esophagus

The esophagus is responsible for transporting food from the mouth to the stomach. Normal motor activity in the esophagus consists of orderly peristaltic waves that move from the upper esophageal sphincter through the smooth muscle in the esophageal wall to the lower esophageal sphincter, leading into the stomach. The peristaltic wave terminates with the closing of the lower sphincter, thus preventing backflow from the stomach into the esophagus. In older people without diabetes or neural disability, the nerve pathways remain intact, although the esophageal smooth muscle may thicken and weaken.[21]

"Presbyesophagus" is the term used for the changes in esophageal motility described in older individuals. Disordered esophageal contractions are observed more frequently in people over age 70, although most of these individuals can swallow normally[50] (swallowing problems are discussed in detail later in this chapter).

A problem in some older people is **gastroesophageal reflux,** or the backflow of stomach contents into the esophagus. This comes from weakening of the lower esophageal sphincter. Because the gastric contents are very acidic, they can damage the esophageal mucosa, and the older person may have heartburn. Antacids may help alleviate this condition, although they interfere with the absorption of particular nutrients, including iron and vitamin B_{12}. Fat and alcohol tend to decrease the pressure of the lower esophageal sphincter, and large meals delay gastric emptying, thereby contributing to this problem.[11] These factors might be considered when counseling individuals with heartburn.

Physiologic Changes in the Stomach

Bowman and coworkers[9] suggest that the most prominent effect of aging on gastrointestinal function involves the stomach. Changes in the gastric mucosa have important implications for secretion of **hydrochloric acid,** which is essential for absorption of various nutrients and control of bacterial microflora. The gastric mucosa also secretes **intrinsic factor,** which is necessary for the absorption of vitamin B_{12}.

Gastric mucosa. The populations of cells that make up the gastric mucosa renew at varying rates. In adults the loss of cells from the mucosal surface usually is balanced by the proliferation of new cells.[21] Decreased rates of cell division or increased rates of cell loss alter the integrity of the gastric mucosa, resulting in atrophy or ulceration and diminished functional capacity.

Atrophic gastritis is a chronic inflammation of the stomach accompanied by deterioration of the mucosa.[32] Among 359 older people in Boston (257 lived in the community and 102 were institutionalized), the prevalence of atrophic gastritis increased with age.[35] Twenty-four percent of those ages 60 to 69 and 37% those ages 80 to 99 had this condition.

Various explanations, including alterations in cell division, changes in immune function, and particular drugs have been offered for the increase in atrophic gastritis in older adults.[31]

One logical consideration is a possible decrease in cell proliferation. It has been reported[33] that the blood supply to the gastric mucosa is diminished in older age, and energy metabolism and the production of high-energy intermediates is slowed in human mucosal cells. These changes in the delivery and use of nutrients by this tissue could influence the rate of cell proliferation.

One type of atrophic gastritis that occurs in older people is associated with altered immune response. This includes a decrease in the immunoglobulins known to protect the mucosal surface and an increase in the immune factors responsible for autoimmune damage to mucosal tissues.[53] *Helicobacter pylori,* a microorganism associated with both gastritis and the development of peptic ulcers, is also being studied as a possible cause of atrophic gastritis in older people.[11]

The increasing use of **nonsteroidal antiinflammatory drugs** in the treatment of arthritis and other chronic pain is receiving attention in regard to the incidence of gastritis, loss of blood from the gastrointestinal tract, and peptic ulcers in older people. People over age 60 who regularly take aspirin or similar drugs are three times as likely to have severe gastrointestinal disease requiring hospitalization than those under age 60 with similar drug usage.[20] These drugs may exacerbate the age-related physiologic changes described above.

Gastric motility. The control of gastrointestinal motility is not well understood. The sequential contractions of the smooth muscle, responsible for moving the gastrointestinal contents along the tract, are controlled partly by the inherent innervation of the smooth muscle and partly by the autonomic nervous system.[45] The gastrointestinal hormones secretin and **cholecystokinin** also help to regulate gastrointestinal motility.[1]

Gastric motility usually is evaluated on the basis of gastric emptying time in individuals fed a test meal or liquid. Available studies comparing **gastric emptying time** in younger and older adults present conflicting results. When older subjects with no gastrointestinal disease were fed a high-carbohydrate test meal, gastric emptying time was somewhat slowed.[70] Another report[1] indicated that gastric emptying time was two and one half times longer in older adults than in younger adults. However, most of those older subjects had neurologic disorders or organic diseases, such as hypothyroidism, that influence gastrointestinal motility. Other workers[37] suggested that older individuals emptied liquids from the stomach more rapidly than younger people in response to the sensation of gastric fullness. Delayed gastric emptying, when it exists, is a factor in the absorption of drugs and delayed onset of pharmacologic action.

Physiologic Changes in the Small Intestine

Intestinal mucosa. Relatively little work is available describing age-related changes in the intestinal mucosa of humans. General health and nutritional status appear to be more important than age in determining cell morphology and function in the small intestine.[51] There appeared to be very little difference in cell structure between older well-nourished adults and young controls, although the villi were somewhat shorter in the older group.[51] There are no differences in the number of villi per unit area as a function of age.[50] Differences might exist in the level of enzyme activity in the mucosal cells, because in animal studies the time required for cell maturation was extended; however, this has not been confirmed in humans.[11]

A significant change that does occur in the small intestine of older individuals with atrophic gastritis is the colonization of bacteria, primarily **lactobacilli** and **streptococci**.[32] When normal levels of hydrochloric acid are secreted by the gastric mucosa, only limited numbers of bacteria are found in the proximal small intestine. When secretion of hydrochloric acid is absent or extremely limited, bacterial overgrowth of the small bowel ensues. **Bacterial overgrowth** has important implications for nutritional status. These bacteria can compete for the available B vitamins and may induce vitamin deficiencies. Particular bacteria interfere with the absorption of fat and other macronutrients. The significant impact that bacterial overgrowth can have on nutritional status was demonstrated in a study of institutionalized, underweight older people whose diets were monitored.[28] After treatment with antibiotics, 13 of the 16 began to gain weight on intakes equal in kilocalories to those consumed previously. Only two of the 16 had been consuming less than 1,600 kcal per day. Bacterial overgrowth should be considered as a possible cause of malnutrition in older people with demonstrated weight loss or poor weight gain and generally adequate nutrient intakes.

Intestinal motility. There appears to be no change of clinical importance in **intestinal motility** of the upper bowel in healthy older people. When individuals free of gastrointestinal disease and young controls were given a test meal consisting of whole-wheat bread, scrambled eggs, and orange juice, transit time from the mouth to the entrance to the colon did not differ.[70] Decreasing transit time in the small intestine may not be beneficial, for if the digested food passes too rapidly through the small intestine, important nutrients may not be absorbed.

Physiologic Changes in the Colon

The most important functions of the colon are to complete the absorption of water, electrolytes, and bile acids and to act as a reservoir for fecal matter until it is excreted.[11] Information is limited on age-related morphologic changes in the colon. There is some degree of mucosal atrophy and change in the mucus-secreting cells. The inner smooth muscle layer of the colon wall weakens as a result of a loss of collagen and an increase in connective tissue. The major structural change in the aging colon is diverticulosis; the major functional change is constipation[56] (both conditions are discussed in detail elsewhere in this chapter).

Physiologic Changes in the Pancreas

It is likely that advancing age leads to morphologic and functional changes in the pancreas. The pancreas is smaller and weighs less in people over age 70; however, this finding may relate to the larger body size of younger people.[21] In any case, the functional reserve of this organ is so great that 90% of its secretory capacity can be lost before clinical consequences become apparent.[11] When pancreatic function is no longer sufficient to support normal digestion and absorption, it usually is because of pancreatic disease or chronic pancreatitis. **Pan-** **creatic insufficiency** is associated with steatorrhea, diabetes, and weight loss.[11]

Physiologic Changes in the Liver and Gallbladder

Liver function. The liver is one of the largest organs in the body, comprising about 2.5% of body weight in a young adult.[21] Based on a study of more than 400 livers obtained at autopsy, liver weight as a function of body weight increases up to the age of 50 and then declines, parallel to the observed decrease in lean body mass. In those over age 90, the liver is disproportionately small.[11] This change in liver weight reflects the loss of liver parenchymal cells that carry on general liver function. Although blood flow to the liver declines in advancing age, older people who are free of liver disease show no change in liver secretions. Of greater importance may be possible changes in drug metabolism and clearance, although current knowledge of these functions in elderly people is limited.

The influence of chronic diseases on liver function has received little attention. Chronic alcohol use, protein malnutrition, obesity, diabetes mellitus, and hypothyroidism can alter the flux of fatty acids delivered to the liver or the balance in fatty-acid oxidation, storage, and excretion by liver cells.[11] In general, fat accumulation in the liver produces only an enlargement of this organ and not a change in function.[21]

Gallbladder function. Diseases in the gallbladder and bile ducts account for about one third of the abdominal surgery performed in people over age 70.[36] The development of **gallstones**, or **calculi**, in the gallbladder is extremely common in older people. Gallstones usually consist of condensed cholesterol, bile pigments, and calcium salts. The prevalence of gallstone disease is higher in women than in men, and in whites than in blacks. Prevalence rates in white women increase from 15% among those ages 40 to 49 to 30% among those ages 60 to 69.[36] Most of the time gallstone disease is asymptomatic and unrecognized. **Biliary colic** or intense, unexpected pain lasting one or several hours is the only symptom of uncomplicated gallstones. Biliary complications such as obstruction of the bile duct are rather infrequent. Treatments that dissolve gallstones now offer alternatives to surgery for the older individual with a recurring or acute problem.

Various investigators[22] have evaluated dietary habits as related to the development of gallstones. Although current intakes of protein, fat, or fiber were not significantly related to the incidence of gallstones in older adults, it does appear that dietary habits earlier in life may influence the development of gallstones in later life. Populations who as children and young adults consumed relatively low levels of fat and protein and relatively high levels of fiber appear to have a reduced incidence of gallstone disease in middle age and beyond.

AGING AND DIGESTIVE SECRETIONS
Problems in Evaluation

Studies evaluating digestive secretion in older people have been limited and the results inconsistent. In some cases findings were probably influenced by the selection of institutionalized or hospitalized older people as subjects. Previous diet influences the levels of digestive enzymes. The influence of age may differ if the level of secretion is measured under basal rather than stimulated conditions.

Although the volume of several digestive secretions appears to decrease in older adults (Table 4-2), the functional significance of these changes is not understood. Digestive secretions normally are produced in amounts substantially above what is required, allowing a margin of safety. The degree of malabsorption caused by changes in digestive secretions is also influenced by individual dietary habits. Eating one or two very large meals rather than several smaller meals is more likely to result in some degree of malabsorption if enzyme levels are significantly reduced. The form in which a nutrient is consumed (e.g., heme versus inorganic iron) influences the digestive secretions required. Chronic use of antacids may raise the pH in the stomach and alter digestive function. Thus older people must be evaluated individually.

Digestive Secretions in the Mouth

Salivary gland function generally is well preserved into advanced age in healthy adults.[4,67,69] **Parotid** salivary flow, under both basal and stimulated conditions, was similar in young (39 or younger), middle age (40 to 59), and old (60 or older) men in the Baltimore Longitudinal Study of Aging (BLSA).[4] Salivary flow does not decrease significantly despite the fact that the salivary glands in people over age 75 have about one third fewer fluid-secreting cells. Baum[4] pointed out that either the fluid-secreting cells remaining in older people become more efficient and increase their output, or the salivary glands have a significant **reserve capacity** that is used in later life.

A recent study[69] evaluated the **amylase** concentration in the saliva of older adults from a retirement community. The enzyme concentration was actually higher in the older adults than in the younger controls. It is possible that the proportion of water in the salivary fluid is reduced in older groups, thereby increasing the concentration of enzyme. As noted earlier, a quantitative reduction in salivary fluid results in xerostomia and degenerative changes in the mouth. There has been no research describing the effects of salivary amylase and **lingual lipase** on the digestion of dietary fat and carbohydrate in older people.

Digestive Secretions in the Stomach

Hydrochloric acid. The major components of gastric juice are hydrochloric acid, pepsinogen, **intrinsic factor,** and mucus.[21] The reduction in acid secretion in some older people parallels the decrease in the number of parietal cells in the gastric mucosa. **Hypochlorhydria,** caused by the loss of a variable number of cells, can range from mild to severe.[32] When all parietal cells have been lost, no hydrochloric acid is secreted (**achlorhydria**), even with chemical stimulation. Although the prevalence of atrophic gastritis increases with age, many healthy older people have gastric acid secretion levels similar to younger people, and in some older people acid secretion is actually higher. Among 41 healthy men ranging in age from 44 to 71 years, acid secretion under basal, meal-

TABLE 4-2 *Age-Related Changes in Digestive Hormones and Secretions*

	Digestive Function	Level of Secretion
Hormones		
Gastrin	Stimulates flow of gastric enzymes and hydrochloric acid	No change; may increase in some individuals
Secretin	Stimulates secretion of pancreatic juice rich in bicarbonate and promotes production of bile by the liver	No change observed
Cholecystokinin (CCK)	Stimulates secretion of pancreatic juice rich in enzymes and bicarbonate and causes ejection of bile, from the gallbladder to the duodenum	Increased
Secretions		
Saliva	Moistens food and aids in mastication and swallowing	Generally no change; decreased in some individuals
Salivary amylase	Breaks down starch to dextrins and some maltose	No change; may increase in some individuals
Hydrochloric acid	Activates pepsinogen to pepsin for protein digestion; causes some breakdown of sucrose to glucose and fructose	Decreased to some extent in many individuals
Pepsin	Breaks down complete proteins to peptides and peptones	May decrease in volume
Pancreatic juice	Contains pancreatic amylase, pancreatic lipase and trypsin for digestion of carbohydrates, lipids, and proteins, respectively; contains bicarbonate, which neutralizes the acidity of chyme	May decrease in volume
Pancreatic amylase	Breaks down starch and glycogen to maltose	May decrease in volume
Trypsin	Splits peptide bonds to form small polypeptides and amino acids	No change observed
Pancreatic lipase	Hydrolyzes triglycerides to monoglycerides, fatty acids and glycerol	May decrease in volume
Bile	Emulsifies lipids to smaller fat particles for digestion; combines with lipids and fatty acids to form micelles	No change
Disaccharidases	Breaks down disaccharides to monosaccharides	Lactase—decreased Maltase—unchanged Sucrase—unchanged

stimulated, and gastrin-stimulated conditions was significantly higher in the older men than in the younger men ages 23 to 42 years.[26] Serum gastrin levels were similar in both groups. This unexplained increase in acid secretion in some older men may contribute to the rising incidence of peptic ulcer observed in older people. It should be noted, however, that the mean age of the older men described above was 57 years, suggesting that a reasonable number were of middle age or among the young-old (see Chapter 1). Several reviewers[31] have emphasized that relatively few elderly people have a totally normal gastric mucosa; however, more studies of healthy older people are needed.

When evaluating the sources of hydrogen ions in the gastrointestinal tract, it is important to remember that eating acid foods will provide hydrogen ions. Also, complete digestion of 30 g of triglyceride will produce 100 mEq of fatty acids.[31] Decreases in gastric acid secretion do not appear to influence gastric motility,[7] although this issue remains controversial. A significant rise in pH does allow bacterial growth and the survival of pathogens entering the gastrointestinal tract.

Pepsin and intrinsic factor. The pepsin activity in the gastric juice was reported to be reduced by 25% in people over age 60, compared to young controls.[18,50] This could relate to a reduced synthesis of the enzyme precursor **pepsinogen** by the chief cells in the gastric mucosa. The conversion of pepsinogen to pepsin requires hydrogen ions, which may be reduced in the older individual. The effect of decreased pepsin activity on protein digestion is unknown. Reduced secretion of intrinsic factor could limit absorption of vitamin B_{12}. Based on the stomach's extensive reserve capacity for secreting intrinsic factor, only in the most severe cases of gastric atrophy does malabsorption of vitamin B_{12} become a problem.[51] According to Russell,[51] a more important limitation to vitamin B_{12} absorption is the increase in stomach pH, which reduces the bioavailability of this vitamin. (The absorption of vitamin B_{12} is discussed further in Chapter 6.)

Digestive Secretions in the Small Intestine

Digestive secretions that act on food in the small intestine include disaccharidases synthesized in the brush border of the mucosa, amylase, **lipase, proteases,** and **bicarbonate** secreted by the pancreas, and bile secreted by the liver and stored and released by the gallbladder. A well-recognized change in disaccharidase secretion is the decrease in the enzyme lactase in older adults.[11,49,55] This results in a decreased tolerance for milk and other dairy products high in lactose. At the same time, it appears that brush border concentrations of sucrase and maltase are unchanged.[11]

Pancreatic secretions appear to decrease in older people, although digestive function does not seem to be impaired. Under stimulated conditions the pancreatic secretion of bicarbonate, lipase, and amylase was 40% lower in older adults compared to younger adults. Nevertheless, none of the older adults reported any abdominal discomfort after meals nor showed signs of malabsorption.[21] Gullo and coworkers[27] evaluated pancreatic function using a water-soluble ester that is hydrolyzed by pancreatic enzymes. When compared on the basis of age, pancreatic function did not differ between those ages 66 to 79 and those ages 80 to 88.

Bile salts are secreted in normal amounts in healthy older people. The response time and rate of emptying of the gallbladder after a fat meal are similar in young and aged adults (60 to 82 years).[34] The aging gallbladder does become less sensitive to cholecystokinin, so that increased levels are required to bring about contraction. In response to this situation, the duodenal mucosa appears to secrete greater amounts of cholecystokinin; consequently, the actual sequence of gallbladder emptying is similar in adults of all ages.

The ability of the gastrointestinal mucosa to adapt to certain nutrition conditions such as an abrupt change in nutrient intake is being evaluated through animal models.[30] This has important implications for older individuals who have an acute illness or are undergoing surgery. The disaccharidases found in the brush border of the small intestine decrease at similar rates in both young and old animals when food is withheld. Upon refeeding, however, older animals demonstrated an exaggerated response, producing excessive levels of enzymes and leading to increased protein turnover. This observation requires further evaluation in terms of its relevance to aging humans.

AGING AND NUTRIENT ABSORPTION
Factors Influencing Nutrient Absorption

Nutrient absorption depends on many factors, including the completeness of digestion, the integrity of the intestinal mucosa, the presence of competing or inhibiting substances, and the blood supply to the absorptive surface. In healthy older people, digestion is reasonably complete, and nutrients are presented in the molecular or ionic form necessary for absorption. Structural changes in the cell membrane cause a decline in the transport capacity of aging cells in other organs, and this may be true for mucosal intestinal cells as well.[11]

Decreased blood perfusion to the small intestine can influence the rate or degree of nutrient absorption. Reduced blood flow lowers the concentration gradient between the mucosal cell and the portal vein, thus slowing absorption. Evidence for this concept comes from work evaluating drug absorption.[48] The compounds affected most by the level of blood flow were those with the highest absorption rates. When uptake occurred by passive diffusion, the degree of absorption did not change when blood flow fell to 10% of normal. The rate of uptake of lipid-soluble compounds decreased by one half when blood flow fell by 35%. In light of the fact that **splanchnic blood perfusion** to the intestinal region drops by about one half in older age groups, the influence of blood flow rate on the absorption of specific nutrients should be examined. Current evidence suggests that the absorption of carbohydrate, fat, and protein generally is unaffected in healthy older people at normal intake levels.

Absorption of Carbohydrate

Glucose absorption. Carbohydrate absorption in older people has been studied using D-xylose excretion levels and hydrogen levels in expired air after a high-carbohydrate meal. D-xylose is absorbed by active transport similar to the mechanism for glucose and galactose. Since D-xylose is not metabolized, the rate and completeness of absorption of a test dose can be measured by renal excretion.[51] Serum levels of D-xylose at either 1 or 2 hours after ingestion of the test dose did not differ in older adults ages 56 to 86 compared to young controls. Urinary excretion of D-xylose was slowed in direct proportion to increasing age.[2,51] It has since been determined, however, that in all but the oldest subjects (those over age 80) the decline in D-xylose excretion was caused by the decline in renal function common in older people, not by a change in carbohydrate absorption.

To avoid the influence of renal function on test results, other workers have measured **breath hydrogen** after ingestion of a test carbohydrate meal. An increase in breath hydrogen over baseline level results from bacterial action on unabsorbed carbohydrate in the distal small intestine or the colon. This test is commonly used to evaluate lactose digestion and absorption but can be used to evaluate these processes in other disaccharides and polysaccharides.

Test meals containing 25 to 200 g of carbohydrate were given to 21 older people who had no gastrointestinal complaints and who ranged in age from 65 to 89 years.[17] Only 31% had no increase in hydrogen expiration after the test meals containing 200 g of carbohydrate. Conversely, 69% were unable to completely digest and absorb that level of carbohydrate when given at one time. Feibusch and Holt[17] concluded that the mean absorptive capacity for carbohydrate was approximately 125 g in people ages 65 to 75 and possibly lower in those over age 85. No differences in anthropometric measurements existed between those with positive breath tests, indicating some degree of malabsorption, and those with negative tests. Older people, who tend to have low caloric intakes (see Chapter 3), would be unlikely to consume even 100 g of carbohydrate at one meal; therefore this finding may be of limited practical importance. It is also unclear whether the elevated hydrogen expiration observed in these older people was the result of bacterial overgrowth of the small intestine, arising from reduced gastric acid production, or actual malabsorption of ingested carbohydrate.

Lactose absorption. Reduced levels of **lactase** in the small intestine and consequent lactose intolerance have been implicated in the relatively low consumption of milk by some older people. In some individuals lactase activity in adulthood remains very similar to that in infancy, whereas in others it drops to low levels. Lactose intolerance is more prevalent among blacks than among whites. In one urban study,[55] 70% of black adults (compared to 6% to 12% of white adults) were intolerant to the level of lactose equivalent to 1 quart of milk.

The relationship between demonstrated lactase deficiency based on administration of a large dose of lactose dissolved in water and the ability to consume milk or milk products with a meal without developing symptoms is a source of controversy. Evaluation of milk-drinking habits at a Title III-C congregate meal program[39] did reveal differences among racial and ethnic groups (Table 4-3). Although a higher percentage of Mexican Americans refused milk, other groups also indicated either a dislike for milk or the incidence of symptoms suggesting lactose intolerance. The type of milk available may be a critical factor, since a higher proportion of black participants chose buttermilk, whereas relatively few of the Mexican Americans chose that milk. Since buttermilk contains only about 0.5% less lactose than whole milk, it is questionable whether the lactose content alone would significantly influence acceptability. Marrs[39] suggests that the cultural acceptance of milk may be as important as the ability to digest lactose in older adults.

An evaluation of 87 healthy older adults in Boston (mean age = 77 years)[49] confirmed that factors other than physiologic responses to lactose may be important in the appearance of symptoms after ingestion of a milk product. On subsequent days, each subject in a double-blind design was given 240 ml of a chocolate drink that was either lactose free or contained 11 g of lactose (4.5% lactose by weight). Twenty-six percent of those tested malabsorbed lactose on the basis of the hydrogen breath test. The incidence of malabsorption was 70% to 75% among black, Jewish, and Italian subgroups, compared to 12% among Northern European groups. Malabsorption was not related to digestive symptoms. About equal numbers (28% and 30% of absorbers and malabsorbers, respectively) reported digestive symptoms after drinking chocolate drink with lactose. About one fifth of the malabsorbers experienced gastrointestinal distress after both the lactose-containing and the lactose-free chocolate drink, suggesting that a component other than lactose was causing the problem. More than half of the malabsorbers reported drinking more than one glass of milk a day.

Lactose malabsorption may not in itself restrict milk consumption in most older people, particularly at the moderate intake usually recorded in this age group. Expectation of discomfort, whether based on known lactose intolerance or distress after drinking milk, regardless of the cause, could be an important consideration in the consumption of dairy products by older adults. Enzyme preparations that can be added to milk products to break down the lactose are commercially available.[43]

Absorption of Fat

Currently there is no evidence to suggest that fat digestion or absorption is altered in healthy

TABLE 4-3   *Percentage of Title III-C Congregate Meal Participants Who Do Not Drink Milk*

	Digestive Symptoms	General Dislike	Total
Mexican American elderly	6	9	15
Black elderly	1	5	6
White elderly	3	3	6

Modified from Marrs DC: Milk drinking by the elderly of three races, *J Am Diet Assoc* 72:495, 1978.

older people.[2,14,51] When fat absorption is impaired in older adults, two different factors may be involved.[2,5,71] First, the older individual could have decreased secretion of pancreatic lipase or bile salts as a result of altered pancreatic, hepatic, or gallbladder function. Second, an overgrowth in the small intestine of bacteria with the ability to split bile salts effectively reduces the concentration of bile salts to form micelles necessary for fat absorption. Among 114 adults ranging in age from 19 to 91 who were given 100 g of fat a day, fat malabsorption was not evident.[2,51] In those ages 20 to 60, **fecal fat** was 3.3 g per day; in those ages 60 to 70, it was 2.5 g; and in the oldest group, ages 70 to 91, it was 2.9 g. Fat absorption in all age groups was above the normal value of 95%. These subjects were also given a labeled dose of bile salts, and over the next 6 hours, the expiration of labeled carbon dioxide was monitored to test for the action of intestinal bacteria on bile salts. There was no evidence of an age-associated increase in the splitting of bile salts by intestinal bacteria.

Even debilitated older people continue to absorb a high percentage of their dietary fat. This suggests that high-fat formulas can be effective in supplying kilocalories to severely undernourished patients. Older individuals with a mean age of 64 who were fed 350 g of fat per day by nasogastric tube absorbed 93% of the fat delivered.[57] Although fecal fat reached a level of 23 g per day, fat excretion still represented less than 10% of the fat fed. Over the 22-day test period, these patients gained an average of 5 kg, and nitrogen retention reached 4.9 g per day. Simko and Michael[57] concluded that a high intestinal absorptive reserve is maintained into old age, even with complicating disease. Although the amount of fat fed to these patients would not be appropriate over an extended period, it provided an available and usable source of energy for short-term rehabilitation.

The ability of these patients to absorb a high percentage of the fat delivered to the gastrointestinal tract may relate to its being given in small amounts over a 24-hour period. The amount of fat fed at one meal influenced the degree of both digestion and absorption in older Swedish men ages 67 to 72 years.[71] When fed 115 g of fat at one meal, their fecal fat ranged from 5 to 16 g, compared to 3 to 9 g in young control subjects. The fat excreted was predominantly neutral fat. In a subsequent evaluation, the same level of fat (115 g) was distributed across three meals and snacks; 10 to 40 g of fat were fed at one time. Fecal fat dropped to 5 to 7 g in the older subjects, indicating absorption of 93% to 95% of the amount fed. This level of dietary fat is considerably higher than that usually consumed by older adults. In NHANES II,[67] the mean fat intake in men ages 60 to 69 was 82 g; this fell to 72 g in men ages 70 to 74. Fat intakes of women of comparable ages were 53 and 48 g, respectively.

In general older people are able to tolerate and digest normal amounts of dietary fat when it is distributed over several meals. Fat appearing in the stool usually is in the form of neutral fat or triglyceride, indicating that the amount of pancreatic lipase needed to digest the fat is the limiting factor.[71] Normally, neutral fat constitutes only a minor portion of fecal fat, with fatty acids the predominant form.

Absorption of Protein

Despite the importance of protein to general health, evaluation of the effectiveness of protein digestion and absorption in older people has been limited. Based on available evidence, however, the completeness of digestion and degree of absorption do not differ in older and younger adults at normal levels of intake. On protein intakes of 1 g per kilogram of body weight, fecal nitrogen in older adults does not exceed 2 g (1 to 2 g per 24 hours is considered within the normal range).[73] Healthy older men and women with a mean age of 77 who were consuming self-selected diets supplying 0.97 g of protein per kilogram of body weight absorbed 85% of their protein intake.[10] Absorption fell to 81% in housebound older adults of similar age with a high level of chronic disease.[10] The digestibility factor for protein generally is considered to be 92%.[19]

In older debilitated patients receiving a liquid diet containing protein derived from casein and soybeans, protein absorption was 88% of total intake.[57] This group received 81 g of protein per day delivered by nasogastric tube over a 24-hour period, thus presenting the gastrointestinal tract with small amounts of protein at a time.

The amount of protein consumed may be a factor in overall digestion and absorption in older people. At protein levels of 1.5 g per kilogram of body weight or above, the amount of nitrogen in the feces of older subjects exceeded that in younger subjects.[71] In the older subjects fecal nitrogen ranged from 1.9 to 4.4 g, compared to 1.9 to 2.2 g in the younger subjects. Rosenberg and coworkers[50] concluded that older adults may tolerate high-protein diets less well than younger adults, but they noted that very few individuals have been studied. There is no evidence to suggest that healthy elderly people, as well as those with superimposed chronic disease, cannot effectively digest and absorb available protein and amino acids.

Absorption of Vitamins and Minerals

Age-related changes in the absorption of vitamins and minerals are beginning to receive more attention. For the most part these nutrients are being studied in a clinical context considering age-related changes in nutrient metabolism, nutritional status, and incidence of deficiency. For this reason the absorption of specific vitamins and minerals is discussed in Chapters 6 and 7.

Issues in Malabsorption

When malabsorption of the macronutrients occurs in older people, several factors usually are involved. Among 70 patients over age 65 who were referred with unexplained chronic gastrointestinal disorders, weight loss, anemia, or general malnutrition, the problem was seldom related to only one cause.[44] Pancreatic insufficiency, diverticulosis in the small intestine, complications following partial **gastrectomy, celiac disease,** atrophic gastritis, and bacterial overgrowth were identified in these patients. Fifteen of the 70 had an anatomically normal small intestine but still experienced malabsorption. Only four of the 14 with pancreatic disease had abdominal pain.

General malabsorption in older people usually involves several structural or functional changes in the gastrointestinal tract. Chewing problems limit food mastication and reduce the surface area exposed to the action of digestive secretions. Laxatives that produce inappropriately rapid transit of the food bolus through the gastrointestinal tract reduce the relative amount of nutrients absorbed. The presentation of smaller amounts of food and nutrients at one time may maximize function. Spreading food intake over three meals and snacks may be advantageous, rather than eating one or two very large meals. These considerations should be shared with older people in nutrition counseling.

Summary

Disturbances of the gastrointestinal tract, including dysphagia, xerostomia, and constipation, increase in number and severity with age as a result of changes in muscle or neural control, dietary habits, or the use of drugs. Digestive secretions are reduced in some older individuals, although the functional significance of this finding is unknown. It is believed that digestion can proceed normally despite a significant reduction in digestive enzymes because of the vast reserve capacity of the pancreas and other secretory organs. The most common change in digestive secretions occurs in the stomach as a result of atrophic gastritis, with loss of the parietal cells and a decline in the secretion of hydrochloric acid. The subsequent rise in pH has implications for the absorption of various nutrients, including vitamin B_{12}, and bacterial overgrowth.

Digestion and absorption of carbohydrates appear to be complete in older individuals, except for lactose. Fat and protein absorption patterns are unchanged at normal intake amounts or when high amounts are spread over several meals throughout the day. The presence of neutral fat in the feces suggests that pancreatic lipase is limiting in some older individuals. Lactose intolerance, whether real or perceived, requires further evaluation in older people. Newly developed, noninvasive tests offer the potential for further study of digestion and absorption in healthy and physiologically compromised older adults.

REVIEW QUESTIONS

1. Why is it a common belief that gastrointestinal function drastically declines with advancing age? What functional changes occur in the gastrointestinal tract with aging? Are there any gender differences in the changes?
2. Define *xerostomia* and *dysphagia*. How common are these two problems in older persons? What dietary alterations might be necessary when they occur?
3. What are some of the most common causes of dyspepsia in the older person? What is the difference between chronic indigestion and nonulcer dyspepsia?
4. How common are complaints of constipation in the older population? How is constipation defined, and what dietary measures are recommended to alleviate the problem?
5. What are the major changes in the mouth, the esophagus, the stomach, and the intestinal tract in older persons? How do these changes affect the digestion and absorption of carbohydrate, protein, fat, vitamins, and minerals?

SUGGESTED LEARNING ACTIVITIES

1. Select one of the following medications and present a 15-minute oral drug report, emphasizing the nutrient/drug interactions.
   - metoclopramide HCl
   - phenolphthalein
   - famotidine
   - docusate sodium
   - cimetidine
   - ranitidine
2. Plan a 2-day menu for a 77-year-old man who is experiencing dysphagia following a cerebrovascular accident.
3. Make a list of the vegetables that Zimmerman and Krondl cited as difficult to tolerate by older people. Survey 20 clients receiving home-delivered meals in a program nearby and discover if any of these vegetables are also cited by older persons in your community.
4. Prepare a 1-page nutrition education tool on the benefits of a high-fiber diet, including examples of high-fiber foods and easy ways to incorporate them into the meal plan of older persons.

Key Terms

Provided here for review is a list of the major terms in this chapter. The definitions can be found in the Glossary, which begins on p. 336. To help you understand how these terms are applied, the page number is given for the first mention of each term in the chapter.

REFERENCES

1. Anuras S, Loening-Baucke V: Gastrointestinal motility in the elderly, *J Am Geriatr Soc* 32:386, 1984.
2. Arora S and others: Effect of age on tests of intestinal and hepatic function in healthy humans, *Gastroenterology* 96:1560, 1989.
3. Balasubramanian R, Johnson EJ, Marlett JA: Effect of wheat bran on bowel function and fecal calcium in older adults, *J Am Coll Nutr* 6:199, 1987.
4. Baum BJ: Salivary gland fluid secretion during aging, *J Am Geriatr Soc* 37:453, 1989.
5. Becker GH, Meyer J, Necheles H: Fat absorption in young and old age, *Gastroenterology* 14:80, 1950.
6. Bloem BR and others: Prevalence of subjective dysphagia in community residents aged over 87, *Br Med J* 300:722, 1989.
7. Bortolotti M and others: Influence of gastric acid secretion on interdigestive gastric motor activity and serum motilin in the elderly, *Digestion* 38:226, 1987.
8. Bowman BB, Rosenberg IH: Digestive function and aging, *Hum Nutr Clin Nutr* 37C:75, 1983.
9. Bowman BA, Rosenberg IH, Johnson MA: Gastrointestinal function in the elderly. In Munro H, Schlierf G, editors: *Nutrition of the elderly*, Nestle Nutrition Workshop Series, vol 29, New York, 1992, Raven Press.
10. Bunker VW and others: Nitrogen balance studies in apparently healthy elderly people and those who are housebound, *Br J Nutr* 57:211, 1987.
11. Cashman MD: The aging gut. In Chernoff R, editor: *Geriatric nutrition: the health professional's handbook,* Gaithersburg, Md, 1991, Aspen Publications.
12. Castle SC: Constipation: endemic in the elderly, *Med Clin N Am* 73:1497, 1989.
13. Clouse RE, Abramson BK, Todorczuk JR: Achalasia in the elderly: effects of aging on clinical presentation and outcome, *Dig Dis Sci* 36:225, 1991.
14. Cohn JS and others: Postprandial plasma lipoprotein changes in human subjects of different ages, *J Lipid Res* 29:469, 1988.
15. Donatelle E: Constipation: pathophysiology and treatment, *Am Fam Physician* 42:1335, 1990.
16. Everhart JE and others: A longitudinal survey of self-reported bowel habits in the United States, *Dig Dis Sci* 34:1153, 1989.
17. Feibusch JM, Holt PR: Impaired absorptive capacity for carbohydrate in the aging human, *Dig Dis Sci* 27:1095, 1982.
18. Fikry ME: Gastric secretory functions in the aged, *Gerontol Clin* 1:216, 1965.
19. Food and Nutrition Board: *Recommended dietary allowances,* ed 10, Washington, DC, 1989, National Academy of Sciences.
20. Fries JF and others: Toward an epidemiology of gastropathy associated with nonsteroidal antiinflammatory drug use, *Gastroenterology* 96:647, 1989.
21. Geokas MC and others: The aging gastrointestinal tract, liver, and pancreas, *Clin Geriatr Med* 1:177, 1985.
22. Gilat T and others: Gallstones and diet in Tel Aviv and Gaza, *Am J Clin Nutr* 41:336, 1985.
23. Goldfinger SE: Constipation. I. The hard facts, *Harvard Health Letter* 16:1, 1991.
24. Goldfinger SE: Constipation. II. Remedies, *Harvard Health Letter* 16:5, 1991.
25. Goldfinger SE: Sensitive stomachs, *Harvard Health Letter* 17:4, 1992.
26. Goldschmiedt M and others: Effect of age on gastric acid secretion and serum gastrin concentrations in healthy men and women, *Gastroenterology* 101:977, 1991.
27. Gullo L and others: Aging and exocrine pancreatic function, *J Am Geriatr Soc* 34:790, 1986.
28. Haboubi NY, Cowley PA, Lee GS: Small bowel bacterial overgrowth: a cause of malnutrition in the elderly, *Eur J Clin Nutr* 42:999, 1988.
29. Holt PR: General perspectives on the aged gut, *Clin Geriatr Med* 7:185, 1991.
30. Holt PR, Kotler DP: Adaptive changes of intestinal enzymes to nutritional intake in the aging rat, *Gastroenterology* 93:295, 1987.
31. Holt PR, Rosenberg IH, Russell RM: Causes

and consequences of hypochlorhydria in the elderly, *Dig Dis Sci* 34:933, 1989.

32. Kassarjian Z, Russell RM: Hypochlorhydria: a factor in nutrition, *Annu Rev Nutr* 9:271, 1989.

33. Kawano S and others: Age-related change in human gastric mucosal energy metabolism, *Scand J Gastroenterol* 26:701, 1991.

34. Khalil T, Poston GJ, Thompson JC: Effects of aging on gastrointestinal hormones. In Prinsley DM, Sandstead HH, editors: *Nutrition and aging,* New York, 1990, Alan R Liss.

35. Krasinski SD and others: Fundic atrophic gastritis in an elderly population: effect on hemoglobin and several serum nutritional indicators, *J Am Geriatr Soc* 34:800, 1986.

36. Krasman ML, Gracie WA, Strasius SR: Biliary tract disease in the aged, *Clin Geriatr Med* 7:347, 1991.

37. Kupfer RM and others: Gastric emptying and small-bowel transit rate in the elderly, *J Am Geriatr Soc* 33:340, 1985.

38. LeClere FB and others: Prevalence of major digestive disorders and bowel symptoms, 1989, advance data from Vital and Health Statistics, No 212, Hyattsville, Md, 1991, National Center for Health Statistics.

39. Marrs DC: Milk drinking by the elderly of three races, *J Am Diet Assoc* 72:495, 1978.

40. Matthews LE: Using high-fiber foods to meet resident needs, *J Nutr Elderly* 7:47, 1988.

41. Matthews LE: Techniques for feeding the person with dysphagia, *J Nutr Elderly* 8:59, 1988.

42. Mendez L, Friedman LS, Castell DO: Swallowing disorders in the elderly, *Clin Geriatr Med* 7:215, 1991.

43. Miller RW, Lecos C: Sweet milk and sour stomachs, *FDA Consumer* 18(2):23, 1984.

44. Montgomery RD and others: Causes of malabsorption in the elderly, *Age Ageing* 15:235, 1986.

45. Piccione PR and others: Intestinal dysmotility syndromes in the elderly: measurement of orocecal transit time, *Am J Gastroenterol* 85:161, 1990.

46. Rhodus NL: Nutritional intake in both free-living and institutionalized older adults with xerostomia, *J Nutr Elderly* 10(1):1, 1990.

47. Rhodus NL, Brown J: The association of xerostomia and inadequate intake in older adults, *J Am Diet Assoc* 90:1688, 1990.

48. Richey DP: Effects of human aging on drug absorption and metabolism. In Goldman R, Rockstein M, editors: *Physiology and pathology of human aging,* New York, 1975, Academic Press.

49. Rorick MH, Scrimshaw NS: Comparative tolerance of elderly from differing ethnic backgrounds to lactose-containing and lactose-free dairy drinks: a doubleblind study, *J Gerontol* 24:191, 1979.

50. Rosenberg IH, Russell RM, Bowman BB: Aging and the digestive system. In Munro HN, Danford DE, editors: *Nutrition, aging, and the elderly,* New York, 1989, Plenum Press.

51. Russell RM: Gastrointestinal function and aging. In Morley JE, Glick Z, Rubenstein L, editors: *Geriatric nutrition: a comprehensive review,* New York, 1990, Raven Press.

52. Sandler RS and others: Demographic and dietary determinants of constipation in the US population, *Am J Public Health* 80:185, 1990.

53. Schmucker DL, Daniels CK: Aging, gastrointestinal infections, and mucosal immunity, *J Am Geriatr Soc* 34:377, 1986.

54. Schuster MM: Influence of aging on gastrointestinal disorders. In Abrams WB, Berkow R, editors: *Merck manual of geriatrics,* Rahway, NJ, 1990, Merck Sharp & Dohme Research Laboratories.

55. Scrimshaw N, Murray EB: Introduction: the acceptability of milk and milk products in populations with a high prevalence of lactose intolerance, *Am J Clin Nutr* 48:1083-5, 1988.

56. Shamburek RD, Farrar JT: Disorders of the digestive system in the elderly, *N Engl J Med* 322:438, 1990.

57. Simko V, Michael S: Absorptive capacity for dietary fat in elderly patients with debilitating disorders, *Arch Intern Med* 149:557, 1989.

58. Sitzmann JV: Nutritional support of the dysphagic patient: methods, risks, and complications of therapy, *J Parent Enteral Nutr* 14:60, 1990.

59. Sklar M: The gastrointestinal system. In Chinn AB, editor: *Working with older people, vol 4, Clinical aspects of aging,* Rockville, Md, 1971, US Government Printing Office.

60. Slavin JL: Dietary fiber: mechanisms or magic on disease prevention? *Nutr Today* 25:6, 1990.

61. Szurszewski JH, Holt PR, Schuster M: Proceedings of a workshop, "Neuromuscular Function and Dysfunction of the Gastrointestinal Tract in Aging," *Dig Dis Sci* 34:1135, 1989.

62. Talley NJ and others: Relation among personality and symptoms in nonulcer dyspepsia and the irritable bowel syndrome, *Gastroenterology* 99:327, 1990.

63. Thomas PR, editor: *Improving America's diet and health: from recommendations to action,* Washington, DC, 1991, National Academy Press.

64. Tripp F, Cordero O: Dysphagia and nutrition in the acute care geriatric patient, *Top Clin Nutr* 6:60, 1991.

65. US Department of Health and Human Services: Normal human aging: the Baltimore Longitudinal Study of Aging, NIH Pub No 84-2450, Washington, DC, 1984, US Government Printing Office.

66. US Department of Health and Human Services: Health of black and white Americans, 1985-87, DHHS Pub No (PHS) 90-1599, Hyattsville, Md, 1990, US Government Printing Office.

67. US Department of Health and Human Services, US Department of Agriculture: Nutrition monitoring in the United States: an update report on nutrition monitoring, DHHS Pub No (PHS) 89-1255, Washington, DC, 1989, US Government Printing Office.

68. Vanderdonckt J and others: Study of the laxative effect of lactitol (Importal) in an elderly institutionalized but not bedridden population suffering from chronic constipation, *J Clin Exp Gerontol* 12:171, 1990.

69. Wand C-H, Woolfolk CA: Salivary amylase activity of the aged, *Gerontology* 36:193, 1990.

70. Wegener M and others: Effect of aging on the gastrointestinal transit of a lactulose-supplemented mixed solid-liquid meal in humans, *Digestion* 39:40, 1988.

71. Werner I, Hambraeus L: The digestive capacity of elderly people. In Carlson LA, editor: *Nutrition in old age,* Symposia Swedish Nutrition Foundation X, Stockholm, 1972, Almqvist & Wiksell.

72. Whitehead WE and others: Constipation in the elderly living at home, *J Am Geriatr Soc* 37:423, 1989.

73. Zanni E, Callaway DH, Zezulka AY: Protein requirements of elderly men, *J Nutr* 109:513, 1979.

74. Zimmerman SA, Krondl MM: Perceived intolerance of vegetables among the elderly, *J Am Diet Assoc* 86:1047, 1986.

5 Nutrient Requirements and Metabolism

Objectives

✦✦

After studying this chapter, the student should be able to:

✔ *Understand how the recommended dietary allowances (RDAs) for older adults were developed, and why the recommendations are controversial*

✔ *Recognize the need for an adequate energy intake in older people and understand how energy intake influences protein status*

✔ *Identify appropriate food sources of carbohydrate, protein, and fat for the older person*

✔ *List the methods of protein evaluation useful in determining the protein status of older adults*

✔ *Recognize the causes of protein-energy malnutrition (PEM) in older people and understand the impact PEM has on quality of life.*

Introduction

The **recommended dietary allowances (RDAs),** as applied to older adults, continue to be a source of controversy. Because research defining the specific requirements of older people is lacking, current recommendations for older adults have been extrapolated from those developed for younger adults. The influence of the aging process on the requirements for and the metabolism of the macronutrients is poorly understood. It is known that an inappropriately high intake of fat can accelerate degenerative changes and promote usual rather than successful aging. Both dietary fat and serum lipoprotein are receiving increasing attention because of their relationship to the development of cardiovascular disease. New methodology allowing estimation of protein turnover in various body compartments has contributed to the current understanding of protein needs in both health and disease. Determining protein requirements may be particularly important for older individuals with compromised renal function or for those whose intake of quality protein is limited because of cost. Foods high in complex carbohydrates usually are good sources of important vitamins and minerals as well as fiber and should represent a major portion of the caloric intake. In this chapter we will consider the appropriate amounts of carbohydrate, fat, and protein for the older adult and the metabolic basis for these recommendations.

RECOMMENDED DIETARY ALLOWANCES

Recommendations for Younger versus Older Adults

The RDAs have been developed as an estimate of the nutrient needs of all healthy people.[16] For younger age groups research studies are available on which to base these recommendations. Because similar research studies with older adults have been few in number, the RDAs for people over age 50 have been extrapolated from those developed for younger adults. For many nutrients, including protein and most vitamins and minerals, the recommended intakes are the same for younger adults ages 25 to 50 and older adults ages 51 and over (see Appendix A). Exceptions include the iron allowance for women and the thiamin, riboflavin, and niacin allowances for men and women. The RDA for iron decreases from 15 to 10 mg daily for women over age 50 because of the cessation of menstruation and associated iron loss. The requirements for thiamin, riboflavin, and niacin decline in response to the lower caloric intake of people over age 50. Before 1989 the Food and Nutrition Board suggested a further adjustment in energy intake for those age 76 or older, based on the reduced physical activity of people in this age group. However, as noted in Chapter 3, a low level of physical activity should not be viewed as normal in older adults, and downward adjustments in caloric intake should be handled on an individual basis.

Limitations of the Recommended Dietary Allowances

The RDAs have many limitations when applied to older people. Factors that contribute to these problems include (1) the **heterogeneity** among aging people, (2) the physiologic changes associated with the aging process, (3) the degenerative changes related to chronic dis-

ease, and (4) the heavy use of prescription and over-the-counter drugs by this age group.[50]

People continue to change in body composition, physiologic function, and degree of metabolic adaptation as they age. Aging changes are complicated further by chronic disease and drug treatment. Munro[40] considers it unrealistic to assume that all individuals over age 50 have similar nutrient requirements. The energy needs of an active man in his seventies who exercises regularly differ markedly from those of a frail 90-year-old who is confined to his home and spends most of his time sitting in a chair.

Changes in digestion or absorption brought about by a decrease in the secretion of **hydrochloric acid** or **intrinsic factor** will increase the need for particular nutrients. Estrogen withdrawal after menopause alters calcium absorption and metabolism and thereby influences the calcium requirement. At the same time, reduced kidney function in older adults indicates that excessive amounts of protein should be avoided.

Another concern about the RDAs for older adults is the interrelation between particular nutrients and degenerative diseases. Chronic disease influences nutrient requirements, both as a result of the disease process itself and in relation to the therapeutic drugs prescribed to manage the condition. Impaired gallbladder function that results in less efficient absorption of fat can increase the requirements for the fat-soluble vitamins. Diuretics prescribed in the management of hypertension can deplete body stores of potassium, magnesium, zinc, pyridoxine, or folic acid, depending on the particular drug (see Chapter 9). For the older individual receiving continuous drug therapy, the RDAs may not provide a realistic estimate of nutrient needs.

Approaches to Dietary Recommendations

There are many differences of opinion as to the feasibility of or the need for specific RDAs for older age groups. A major issue in this controversy is the extreme heterogeneicity among the elderly, especially as influenced by medical problems and chronic disease. On this basis Munro[39] suggested the development of two sets of recommendations, one for healthy elderly and one for those with chronic disease. Another possible approach is the establishment of a range of suggested intakes: (1) the minimum level required to prevent the development of deficiency diseases; (2) a desirable level to be used in diet planning; and (3) an upper level of safe intake to prevent adverse or toxic effects.[17]

In contrast to these proposals, others view the available research information as too limited to allow specific recommendations for the elderly and see no reason to suggest that healthy older people should consume a diet different from that recommended for younger people.[28] Also, the extreme individual differences among physically impaired older people indicate that one set of standards would not be applicable to all. Hegsted[28] points to the need to develop standards that will help individuals with diet planning. In his opinion, the RDAs tend to encourage the use of supplements, since individuals are unprepared to select diets that will provide the levels of nutrients assumed to be required.

A reasonable approach suggested by Harper[25] stresses the importance of evaluating older people as individuals, considering their general health, level of physical activity, and degree of chronic disease. Appropriate goals are (1) to prevent nutrient depletion and (2) to avoid providing excessive amounts of nutrients, which cannot be used and must be excreted. Either situation is undesirable for optimum health and well-being. At the same time, there is a continuing need for detailed study of the nutrient requirements of older people. A special area for emphasis might be nutrient requirements after age 75, when physiologic limitations increase and nutrient needs are most influenced by long-term drug use. An important group for study is the healthy elderly, from whom we might learn what levels of nutrient intake promote successful aging.

DIETARY CARBOHYDRATE AND METABOLISM
Carbohydrate Intake

Foods high in complex carbohydrates include fruits, vegetables, and whole-grain breads and cereals. These foods contribute energy, fiber, iron and other trace minerals, and important vitamins to the diet. An unfortunate trend among all age groups is the addition of high-sucrose carbohydrate foods to the diet in place of complex carbohydrate foods containing fiber and other nutrients. A recent survey of older vegetarian and nonvegetarian California women[30,42] whose mean age was 72 indicated that sugar provided about 20% of their caloric intake. Average caloric intakes ranged from 1,360 to 1,450 kcal per day.

The proportion of total kilocalories supplied by carbohydrate foods differed in the vegetarian and nonvegetarian women.[30,42] The vegetarian women obtained 60% of their total energy from carbohydrate and 32% from fat. The nonvegetarian women had lower intakes of carbohydrate, which supplied only 50% of total kilocalories, and higher intakes of fat, which supplied 36% of total kilocalories. The vegetarian women also had significantly higher intakes of vitamins A and E, thiamin, copper, and manganese.

Data from the second National Health and Nutrition Examination Survey (NHANES II)[64] indicate that older women obtain more of their kilocalories from carbohydrate than do older men. The percentage of energy coming from carbohydrate was 43% in men and 47% in women ages 60 to 69. Carbohydrate intake increased with age, since men between ages 70 and 74 obtained 46% of their total kilocalories from carbohydrate and women of that age range obtained 50% from that source. Bread and cereal products tend to be comparatively low in cost and are popular among older people who may have chewing problems. Complex carbohydrate foods rather than carbohydrate foods high in sucrose should predominate in low-calorie diets.

The current guidelines of the Food and Nutrition Board[16] suggest that at least half of all kilocalories be supplied by carbohydrate. The Committee on Diet and Health of the National Academy of Sciences[13] has recommended that Americans obtain more than 55% of their total caloric intake from carbohydrate. Eating generous amounts of complex carbohydrate foods increases dietary levels of important vitamins, minerals, and fiber and decreases the amount of dietary fat.[57]

The Body's Need for Carbohydrate

Glucose is a major energy source for many body tissues, including the brain and nervous system. Because other dietary components can be converted to glucose, there is no absolute dietary requirement for carbohydrate under most circumstances.[16] Other simple sugars, including fructose and galactose, can be converted to glucose, as can many amino acids and the glycerol component arising from the breakdown of triglycerides. When dietary carbohydrate is absent or very limited, stored triglycerides are broken down at a rapid rate, the oxidation of fatty acids is enhanced, and ketone bodies begin to accumulate. A carbohydrate-free diet can lead to a breakdown of body proteins and losses of potassium, sodium, and fluid. Normal metabolic function is maintained on a daily intake of 50 to 100 g of carbohydrate.

Very-low-carbohydrate diets advocated for weight loss that substitute protein for carbohydrate are inappropriate and can be dangerous for older individuals. An excessive intake of protein, with subsequent increases in nitrogenous waste, put additional stress on the renal system of an older person, who may already be in a state of **hyperfiltration** and **hyperperfusion.** Fluid and electrolyte balance, already precarious in older people with advanced cardiac or renal disease, can be further distorted by very-low-carbohydrate diets. Older people who want to lose weight should be advised to avoid such regimens.

Dietary Fiber

Individuals of all ages are being encouraged to eat generous amounts of plant foods high in fiber. Foods high in dietary fiber are associated with appropriate serum lipoprotein patterns and decreased incidence of cardiovascular disease, diabetes, and colon cancer. The Food and Nutrition Board's Committee on Diet and Health[13] suggests that people eat five or more servings of a combination of fruits and vegetables and six or more servings of a combination of legumes and breads and cereals. Breads and cereals appear frequently in the diets of older people, although whole-grain items are less commonly used and should be encouraged. Appropriate intakes of fiber obtained from the foods mentioned above also contribute to normal bowel function. Fiber supplements are unnecessary, and in excessive amounts they contribute to bowel dysfunction and interfere with the absorption of important minerals.

LIPID REQUIREMENTS AND METABOLISM

Fat Intake

Recent national surveys[64] indicate that older people are consuming dietary levels of total fat and saturated fat above those recommended for adults of all ages (Table 5-1). Older men are consuming higher levels of fat than older women, and fat intakes decrease with age to a

TABLE 5-1 Fat Consumption by Older People (percentage of total kilocalories)

Age (years)	Men		Women		Recommended Level
	60-69	70-74	60-69	70-74	
Total fat	38	37	36	34	≤30
Saturated fat	13	13	12	12	<10
Monounsaturated fat	14	14	13	12	10-15
Polyunsaturated fat	5	5	5	4	≤10

Adapted from Food and Nutrition Board: *Recommended dietary allowances,* ed 10, Washington, DC, 1989, National Academy of Sciences; US Department of Health and Human Services, US Department of Agriculture: Nutrition monitoring in the United States: an update report on nutrition monitoring, DHHS Pub No (PHS) 89-1255, Washington, DC, 1989, US Government Printing Office.

greater extent in older women. Intakes of poly-unsaturated fatty acids are rather low (4% to 5% of total kilocalories) and may indicate less-than-optimum intakes of the essential fatty acids and the **omega-3 fatty acids** found in fish. Omega-3 fatty acids are believed to offer some protection against the development of coronary heart disease.[52] Nutrition education for older people should address the reduction of total dietary fat and offer suggestions for substituting foods higher in polyunsaturated fatty acids for those high in saturated fatty acids. Appropriate changes in dietary fat can be achieved by (1) switching to dairy foods lower in total fat, (2) eating more fish, poultry, and vegetable proteins, and (3) cutting back on meats that are high in total and saturated fat.

Essential Fatty Acids

Role of essential fatty acids. Dietary fat is a source of both energy and **linoleic acid,** which is necessary to maintain health. Linoleic acid, the essential fatty acid, can be converted to **arachidonic acid,** which does not need to be supplied by the diet when linoleic acid is available.[16] Linoleic and **arachidonic acids,** which are found in phospholipids, form an important component of cellular membranes. **Linolenic acid,** an omega-3 fatty acid, has also been classified as an essential fatty acid, although until recently its specific role in human nutrition was unclear. It is now recognized that linolenic acid is a substrate for the synthesis of eicosapentaenoic acid and docosahexaenoic acid, also found in fatty fish.[16] **Eicosapentaenoic** and **docosahexaenoic acids,** whether synthesized by the body from available linolenic acid or consumed in the diet, can influence blood platelet aggregation and other physiologic responses.

Essential fatty acid requirements. Essential fatty acid deficiency seldom occurs in adults, although it has been described in patients maintained on parenteral feedings that did not contain fat and in individuals with serious fat malabsorption problems. A linoleic acid intake equal to 1% to 2% of total caloric intake will prevent clinical or biochemical signs of deficiency.[16] One tablespoon of vegetable oil supplies about 6 g of linoleic acid, which would help meet the required amount. Because essential

fatty acid deficiency has not been observed in individuals with normal fat absorption, an RDA has not been assigned to either linoleic or arachidonic acids or the omega-3 polyunsaturated fatty acids. However, recent work[16,52] suggests that the ratio of dietary linoleic acid to dietary omega-3 fatty acids is related to physiologic function, **platelet aggregation,** the development of coronary heart disease, and the inflammatory responses involved in the development of rheumatoid arthritis. It would seem pertinent to consider the establishment of RDAs for these polyunsaturated fatty acids.

Essential fatty acids in older people. Dietary evaluations of both community-living and institutionalized older people suggest that linoleic acid status declines with age. In a group of 70 women ranging from 62 to 99 years, the intake of linoleic acid was lowest in those over age 85.[26] This group consumed only 5.8 g per day, compared to the 62- to 75-year-old group, who consumed 6.4 g per day. The older group also consumed less total fat. In that study the institutionalized women had a higher intake of linoleic acid (6.8 g) than the women of similar age living in the community (5.6 g).

Institutionalized older people can have a very low intake of linoleic acid despite a high intake of fat. In a French nursing home, linoleic acid intake was only 4 g per day, although total dietary fat provided more than 40% of total energy.[5] Younger people living in that region who ate similar types of food got 12 g of linoleic acid per day on a similar intake of total fat. The older institutionalized subjects had lower concentrations of both linoleic acid and arachidonic acid in their serum lipids, compared to the young subjects. According to Asciutti-Moura and coworkers,[5] the decreased levels of arachidonic acid in the serum lipids of the older adults could relate to a decreased ability to metabolize linoleic acid to arachidonic acid, its usual metabolic product. The enzyme needed for this conversion requires vitamin B_6 as a cofactor, and this enzyme activity level would be reduced if vitamin B_6 status was poor. Vitamin B_6 status was not evaluated in these older people.

Holman and coworkers,[29] who reviewed the linoleic acid content of serum lipids in more than 200 people from the general population, concluded that the reduced levels of linoleic acid in the older subjects were not as low as in essential fatty acid deficiency but suggested declining status. The classic symptoms of linoleic acid deficiency are skin changes and atrophy of the **sebaceous glands** that lubricate the hair follicle and surrounding skin. A Michigan survey[49] reported that older women who ate less than 6 g of linoleic acid a day were more likely to have skin problems and **hyperkeratosis** of the elbows and knees. Poor linoleic acid status also increases the older person's risk of cardiovascular disease.[65]

Lipid Metabolism and Serum Cholesterol

The major focus of research in lipid metabolism in older people has been on the factors influencing serum cholesterol and lipoprotein levels. Serum cholesterol levels are related to both age and sex. Findings from NHANES II and the Hispanic HANES indicate that total serum cholesterol increases with age, peaking in men between the ages of 45 and 54 and in women between the ages of 55 and 64.[64] At ages 55 and beyond, total serum cholesterol was higher in women. Mean serum cholesterol levels do not differ on the basis of race or ethnic background; values were similar in black, white, and Hispanic populations. At the same time, older women are more likely than men to have a serum cholesterol of 240 mg/dl or higher, placing them at high risk for coronary heart disease. Men may be more likely to receive intervention treatment to reduce elevated serum cholesterol, or men at high risk may have died before age 60. (The proportion of older people with inappropriate levels of serum cholesterol is discussed in Chapter 10.)

Little information is available about changes in serum cholesterol after age 60. In the Baltimore Longitudinal Study of Aging (BLSA), serum cholesterol declined from 232 to 213 mg/dl between the ages of 65 and 102.[63] Among 70 institutionalized women,[26] serum cholesterol values were 238 mg/dl between ages 62 and 75, 226 mg/dl between ages 76 and 85, and 217 mg/dl between ages 86 and 99.

Dietary Influences on Serum Cholesterol

The influence of diet on lipoprotein patterns in older people continues to be a matter of interest. Omega-3 polyunsaturated fatty acids, found in the oil of fatty fish, lower serum triglyceride and total serum cholesterol.[52] These fatty acids appear to interfere with the synthesis of very-low-density lipoproteins and have a beneficial effect on the composition of low-density lipoprotein (LDL) cholesterol by changing the cholesterol/protein ratio.[2] In general, increased amounts of dietary fiber decrease serum triglyceride and LDL cholesterol concentrations, but this could relate partly to the decrease in dietary fat that usually accompanies this change in food sources. **Soluble fiber,** found in legumes, oats, and fruit pectins, is more effective in lowering serum lipid than is insoluble fiber, found in wheat bran. Carbohydrate consumed in the form of simple sugars will aggravate an existing **hyperinsulinemia** and lower the level of high-density lipoprotein (HDL) cholesterol. When consumed in small amounts, alcohol seems to raise serum HDL cholesterol, particularly the **apo-1-lipoprotein,** which facilitates the transport and excretion of cholesterol from the body.[2]

Recent evidence suggests that oxidation of LDL cholesterol is critical to its destructive effect on the arterial wall and the formation of fatty streaks.[18] If so, natural antioxidants obtained from food containing vitamins C and E and beta-carotene may prevent the progression of coronary heart disease.

Dietary Intervention in Aged Adults

Albrink[2] suggests that both age and risk factors be considered when planning a diet for an older adult. The length of time required for an individual to benefit from a dietary change should be a factor when considering aggressive dietary intervention. Cholesterol-lowering regimens have demonstrated a positive effect in preventing heart disease within 7 years. From that standpoint, it seems inappropriate to attempt radical dietary changes in someone age 80 or older for whom the burden of change or the loss of favorite foods might outweigh any possible benefit. For the young-old, who are looking forward to 25 or more years of life, gradual changes that still preserve the individual food pattern can lead to long-term benefits. A family history of heart disease may be helpful in deciding for whom dietary changes are most critical.

A diet that conforms to the recommendations of the Food and Nutrition Board's Committee on Diet and Health[13] (fat 30% or less of total kilocalories) is appropriate for people of all ages. At the same time, it is important to recognize that any change that brings the daily food pattern closer to that goal should be commended. Decreasing dietary fat to any degree, even if total intake is still above 30%, contributes to physical well-being.

An overriding issue for the aged adult is weight control. For a person of average weight or one who is overweight, continued weight gain can adversely affect risk factors for heart disease and mobility. Regular physical exercise to prevent weight gain can also increase HDL cholesterol and decrease LDL cholesterol.[13] Factors influencing HDL cholesterol levels are primary areas for intervention; for example, a recent analysis of major epidemiologic studies concluded that an increase of 1 mg/dl in HDL cholesterol led to a 2% decrease in the risk of coronary heart disease in men and a 3% decrease of the risk in women.[24]

EVALUATION OF PROTEIN REQUIREMENTS
Uncertainties in Protein Requirements

Evaluating protein requirements is an intensive process requiring substantial resources on the part of the researchers and a high degree of commitment on the part of the individuals being studied. Consequently, there have been few studies evaluating the protein requirements of older people, and little information is available describing the changes, if any, that occur in protein metabolism over adult life. Because protein requirements are related to protein synthesis and breakdown in skeletal muscle and body organs, changes in body composition can influence protein needs. Emotional stress, infection, and chronic diseases, which are known to

increase protein requirements, are common in older people. Also, a relatively low-calorie diet can influence the utilization of ingested protein. These factors make the older individual vulnerable to marginal or poor protein status and protein loss.

The Body's Need for Protein

Protein needs of adults. Protein metabolism continues as a dynamic process throughout adult life. Although physical growth has ceased, sufficient protein must be consumed to replace body nitrogen losses, which include (1) **desquamated cells** from the gastrointestinal tract and skin, (2) body secretions, including perspiration or digestive enzymes lost through the gastrointestinal tract, and (3) end products of body metabolism excreted in the urine. Proteins oversee the maintenance of cell and organ function in their roles as enzymes, hormones, and mediators of immune responses. Thus age-related changes in protein availability and synthesis could have important consequences for physical well-being.[54]

In the older individual, **positive nitrogen balance** can relate to the repletion of body protein stores after illness, malnutrition, or stress. Strength training leading to an increased muscle mass is associated with nitrogen retention and a positive nitrogen balance. When nitrogen excretion exceeds nitrogen intake, as occurs in infection, after surgery, in debilitating illness, or with glucocorticoid therapy, protein depletion ensues.[70] Nitrogen balance measurements reflect the sum total of nitrogen gain or loss; however, they do not provide answers as to the relative gain or loss of individual tissues. Hegsted[27] pointed out that an adult is seldom in nitrogen equilibrium with a net gain or loss of zero, but rather has fluctuating periods of nitrogen accretion and loss that on the average produce a net balance.

Loss of body protein. Even well-nourished adults appear to lose body protein as a function of age. As described in Chapter 3, both longitudinal and cross-sectional studies have demonstrated a progressive decline in body potassium throughout adult life. Potassium is more highly concentrated in the muscle than in the nonmuscle portion of the fat-free body. This has led

Cohn and coworkers[12] to the conclusion that the nonmuscle protein mass (made up of the brain, lungs, and organs in the abdominal cavity) generally is unaffected by age-related protein losses. In contrast, skeletal muscle decreases by 46% between the ages of 20 and 80. This estimate of the age-related decline in skeletal muscle is in agreement with other workers, who reported that skeletal muscle made up 25% of body weight at birth, increased to 45% of body weight in the young adult, and declined to 27% of body weight after age 70.[68] This loss in muscle tissue is believed to contribute to the decrease in maximum oxygen consumption observed in older as compared to younger men (see Chapter 1).

The changes in body muscle and protein content have led to different interpretations of the protein requirements of older people.[40] First, the observed decrease in active metabolic tissue could reduce the need for protein and amino acids. An opposing point of view is that an inadequate intake of protein and amino acids contributes to protein loss, and increased amounts of protein are required to maintain appropriate body functions and reestablish protein reserves. Evaluations of protein metabolism and requirements in older individuals have not completely resolved this issue.

Age-Related Changes in Protein Metabolism

Estimating protein turnover. Protein synthesis and breakdown, referred to as **protein turnover,** has been estimated in particular organs and tissues as well as in the total body. Using labeled glycine, it is possible to estimate total protein turnover as related to body weight, creatinine excretion, or some other measure of body composition. The amino acid **3-methylhistidine,** a breakdown product of the major muscle proteins, is quantitatively excreted in the urine in proportion to total muscle protein turnover. The measurement of total body protein turnover obtained with labeled glycine combined with the measurement of total muscle protein turnover obtained with 3-methylhistidine excretion allows us to evaluate the relative contribution of muscle and nonmuscle compartments to total body protein turnover: total body protein turnover minus total muscle protein turnover equals the nonmuscle protein turnover.[68]

Rate of protein turnover. Whole-body protein synthesis and breakdown does not differ between older and younger men when based on body weight. However, when differences in body composition are taken into consideration, the rates of whole-body protein turnover are significantly different. Whole-body protein synthesis and breakdown expressed on the basis of creatinine excretion or body cell mass are higher in older than in younger adults.[68]

Although whole-body protein turnover is higher in older adults, the contribution of the muscle compartment to total protein turnover is strikingly lower. This is because older adults have less muscle mass, not because of changes in protein synthesis and breakdown in remaining muscle. Young and coworkers[67] propose that muscle protein turnover accounts for only 20% of whole-body protein turnover in older men, compared to 30% in younger men. Conversely, the contribution of the nonmuscle mass or the **visceral organs** to total protein metabolism is higher in older people. The greater contribution of the visceral organs to total protein turnover is responsible for the higher rate of whole-body protein turnover in older people. The visceral organs (the liver, kidneys, and heart) have a higher rate of protein metabolism than does skeletal muscle. As was pointed out in Chapter 3, the higher rate of metabolism in the visceral organs needs to be considered when evaluating the nutritional needs of the debilitated older person in whom muscle mass is severely compromised and body weight is very low.

The nutritional significance of the age-related reduction in muscle mass and its relative contribution to total body protein metabolism is unclear. It is known that skeletal muscle serves as a protein reserve and plays an important role in metabolic adaptation in situations of stress such as infection, surgery, or reduced food intake. A reduced muscle reserve would appear to increase the vulnerability of the older person to unfavorable nutritional consequences under conditions of physical stress or interrupted food intake.[69]

PROTEIN REQUIREMENTS IN OLDER PEOPLE
Methods for Evaluating Protein Requirements

Protein requirements can be evaluated through two different approaches. The **factorial method** evaluates all possible routes of nitrogen loss and establishes a level of protein intake that will be expected to replace those losses. Body nitrogen is lost through the skin, urine, and feces in the form of desquamated cells, secretions, and metabolic waste products, even when no protein is provided in the diet. These losses, referred to as **obligatory nitrogen losses,** represent the minimum amount of nitrogen that must be replaced each day. According to this method, the protein requirement is the amount of protein that is equivalent to these losses plus an adjustment of 30% for individual variability and an adjustment of 30% for efficiency of protein utilization. Protein is used less efficiently as protein intake increases. This value is then adjusted to reflect the biologic availability of the proteins ingested in a typical Western diet.[40]

The second approach for determining protein requirements is the **balance method.** In a balance study, individuals are fed graded amounts of protein to determine the minimum level of protein that will maintain the individual in nitrogen equilibrium or zero nitrogen balance. This level of protein is then increased by 30% to allow for individual variability.[40]

Using the Factorial Method in Older People

A major issue when using the factorial method to determine the protein requirements of older people is the ability of older adults to adapt to a protein-free diet and reduce their urinary nitrogen excretion to a minimum level. In a comparison of young men, older men, and older women, neither the number of days required for urinary nitrogen to reach minimum

levels nor the rate of decrease in urinary nitrogen differed among groups.[51]

Obligatory nitrogen losses are influenced by both body composition and the age-related change in the relative contributions of the muscle and nonmuscle compartments to total protein turnover.[61] Differences in nitrogen losses per kilogram of body weight, as seen in men as compared with women, are related to the higher proportion of muscle tissue and lower proportion of body fat in men. Obligatory nitrogen losses were found to be 52 mg/kg body weight in older men and 39 mg/kg body weight in older women. Differences in obligatory nitrogen losses calculated per gram of creatinine excretion are somewhat higher in older than in younger adults because of the higher contribution of the visceral organs to total body protein turnover in older adults. It is interesting to note that Zanni and coworkers[71] found no age-related differences in obligatory nitrogen losses calculated on the basis of creatinine excretion in older men in whom muscle mass was well preserved.

Although data are limited, it appears that total obligatory nitrogen losses do not differ appreciably on the basis of age. Protein requirements, however, may still differ between older and younger people with similar nitrogen losses if older people use dietary protein less efficiently to replace proteins that are lost. For this reason it has been concluded that protein recommendations for adults should be based on balance studies.[16,40]

Nitrogen Balance Studies in Older People

Limitations of balance studies. Although nitrogen balance studies are the method of choice for evaluating protein requirements, they have several limitations of particular concern with older people. First, the prior nutritional status of the individual can influence the level of protein at which nitrogen equilibrium is achieved. An older person who has been on a low-protein diet and has poor protein stores is more likely to retain protein and reach equilibrium on a lower protein intake than an older person whose protein status is optimum.[23] Secondly, caloric intake influences protein utilization.[23] Protein is used more efficiently when caloric intakes are high than when caloric intakes are low or barely adequate. On low-calorie intakes, protein may be used for energy rather than for protein replacement. Finally, balance studies usually are conducted in controlled environments and are likely to include test diets that differ markedly from the usual food pattern. This requires both a psychologic and a metabolic adjustment to the study situation. Because of the cost and intense commitment required of participants, the time period allowed for adjustment may be relatively short. Whether older people require a longer period of time to adapt to a new dietary pattern or level of nutrient intake is unclear.

Nitrogen balance studies with test diets. The protein requirements of older people have been evaluated using various levels of protein and energy. Nitrogen balance on graded levels of egg protein was evaluated in seven men and seven women ranging in age from 68 to 84 years.[60] After 1 week of standardization, the subjects were rotated on three different protein levels for a period of 10 days each. As described in Fig. 5-1, both the men and the women were losing nitrogen on protein intakes below 0.7 g/kg body weight. Women appeared to be even more likely to lose nitrogen on low-protein diets than men, since they were not retaining nitrogen on intakes of 0.8 g/kg body weight. At an intake of 0.85 g/kg body weight, the men were retaining nitrogen and appeared to be replacing the body protein lost when the protein intake was low. Uauy and coworkers[60] concluded that the inability of many older individuals to maintain a consistent pattern of nitrogen balance precluded the determination of a minimum protein requirement.

For older people with chronic disease who are taking prescription drugs, even the current RDA for protein, 0.8 g/kg body weight, may not be adequate to establish nitrogen equilibrium. The adequacy of the current RDA for protein was evaluated over a 30-day period in older men with a mean age of 75 and older women with a mean age of 78.[23] Although free of diabetes or other endocrine disorders, these

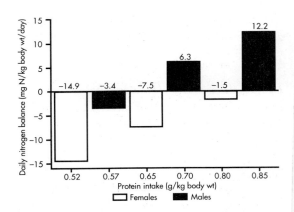

FIG. 5-1 Loss and retention of nitrogen in older people given increasing amounts of egg protein. Most older women were still losing nitrogen when given the recommended level of protein, 0.8 g per kg of body weight.

(Data from Uauy R, Scrimshaw NS, Young VR: Human protein requirements: nitrogen balance response to graded levels of egg protein in elderly men and women, *Am J Clin Nutr* 31:779, 1978.)

older people had heart disease, hypertension, and gastrointestinal problems, including peptic ulcer and diverticulosis, and were representative of the older population with chronic diseases. After 30 days, four of the eight women and three of the seven men were still in negative nitrogen balance. Nitrogen balance did improve over the 30-day period in the men, although in the women improvement was slight. At the end of the first 10 days, all of the men and six of eight women were losing nitrogen. In the women hemoglobin levels declined from 13.7 to 13 g/dl over the study period. Older women appear to be more vulnerable to protein loss, as suggested by the observed decrease in hemoglobin. This probably is a result of their reduced muscle mass and, consequently, diminished reserve of protein and amino acids.

There are reports in the literature suggesting that older men can maintain nitrogen balance on protein intakes well below the RDA.[10,71] Zanni and coworkers[71] reported that the older men in their study achieved nitrogen equilibrium on a protein intake of 0.59 g/kg body weight. The discrepancy between their findings and the study described above, which suggests that a protein level of 0.8 g/kg body weight may be inadequate in some cases, could relate to both the individuals being studied and the experimental protocol. Those given the lower protein diet (0.59 g/kg body weight) consumed a protein-free diet immediately before the test diet, and the resulting protein depletion could have led to increased nitrogen retention when protein was restored. In addition, the men achieving nitrogen equilibrium on the low-protein diet were younger; five of six were below age 70. Of the men fed 0.8 g/kg body weight, six of seven were over age 71. Moreover, the latter group of men, who were living in the community, had various chronic problems that may have influenced protein absorption and utilization.

Nitrogen balance studies on self-selected diets. The nitrogen balance studies described heretofore were conducted in metabolic units, and the subjects consumed defined formula diets. These conditions could be stressful and could influence the quantity of protein required to achieve nitrogen equilibrium. These influences were avoided in an evaluation of 44 British men and women, ranging in age from 70 to 85 years, who were studied in their homes on self-selected diets.[6] The 24 healthy older people had no apparent disease and did their own food shopping and meal preparation. The 20 housebound individuals could not leave their homes unaccompanied and had various chronic disorders, including lung disease, osteoarthritis, and heart disease. Their food was bought by family members, friends, homemaker aides, or the older people themselves if someone took them shopping. Nitrogen balance was determined over a 5-day period.

As described in Table 5-2, the healthy men and women had higher intakes of total protein and higher intakes of protein per kilogram of body weight. The healthy group was in nitrogen equilibrium, with a mean nitrogen balance of $+0.04$ to -0.06 g per day. Their self-selected diets were about 15% protein. The housebound men and women were similar in age to the healthy men and women but had lower intakes of both protein and energy, although protein supplied 12% to 14% of total energy. These individuals were losing 1.1 to 1.7 g of nitrogen a day.

Both protein intake and health status influenced nitrogen balance. Mean daily nitrogen losses among the housebound elderly were similar in those who consumed 0.8 g of protein per kilogram of body weight and those who consumed less. Caloric intakes did not influence nitrogen retention in either the healthy or housebound older people. The healthy group did absorb protein more efficiently; the level of absorption was 85% in the healthy versus 81% in the homebound elderly.

The levels of protein intake and nitrogen loss in this homebound population have important implications for providers of home care. Of the

TABLE 5-2 *Nitrogen Balance in Healthy and Housebound Older People*

	Healthy		Housebound	
	Men	Women	Men	Women
Age (years)	78	76	79	79
Energy intake (kcal)	2,071	1,571	1,500	1,143
Total protein intake (g)	69	60	46	39
Energy intake (kcal/kg body wt)	30	25	22	19
Protein intake (g/kg body wt)	1.00	0.94	0.69	0.65
Nitrogen (g lost or gained per day)	−0.06	+0.04	−1.74	−1.11

Data from Bunker VW and others: Nitrogen balance studies in apparently healthy elderly people and those who are housebound, *Br J Nutr* 57:211, 1987.

20 homebound older people in this study, only seven received one home-delivered meal each day, whereas the others were dependent on food delivered or prepared by relatives, friends, or homemaker aides who visited once or twice a week. The fact that the protein intake of the homebound older people was only two thirds that of the mobile, healthy older group demonstrates the importance of adequate food delivery. When the homebound subjects were approached 6 to 12 months later about another study, their health had deteriorated to the point that none were able to participate. Bunker and coworkers[6] raised the question whether this deterioration could have been prevented with additional food.

Energy Intake and Nitrogen Balance

The classic studies in protein metabolism described the protein-sparing action of carbohydrate and emphasized the need for sufficient kilocalories to promote the utilization of protein and amino acids. In both younger and older people, the level of protein required to achieve nitrogen balance (as g/kg body weight) is inversely related to the level of kilocalories being consumed. The older men studied by Zanni and coworkers,[71] for whom protein intakes of 0.59 g/kg body weight appeared adequate, had caloric intakes of 45 kcal/kg body weight. The older people who had negative nitrogen balances on intakes providing the recommended level of protein (0.8 g/kg body weight) had caloric intakes of only 29 to 32 kcal/kg body weight.[23]

The caloric intake currently recommended by the Food and Nutrition Board for men and women over age 50 is 30 kcal/kg body weight.[16] This represents a substantial decrease from the levels recommended for younger adults, which are 36 kcal/kg for women and 37 kcal/kg for men. Increasing energy expenditure to allow additional energy intake can improve protein status whether or not the food added contains protein. Adding 400 kcal to the diet in the form of carbohydrates increased nitrogen retention in older men to the same extent as adding 5 to 10 g of protein.[31] Older Michigan women required daily caloric intakes of 1,500 kcal or more to maintain nitrogen equilibrium

on daily protein intakes of 50 to 60 g.[43] In the United States most older women consume less than 1,500 kcal each day. In NHANES II,[64] the mean reported intake among women ages 60 to 69 was 1,340 kcal; intake declined to 1,270 kcal in those ages 70 to 74.

The additional nitrogen retained when caloric intake is increased is handled differently from that retained when protein intake is increased.[21] Serum albumin and **transferrin** and other labile protein stores increase when protein is added to a marginal diet. In contrast, the additional nitrogen retained when kilocalories are increased is not as easily lost even when caloric intake is reduced to former levels. Encouraging physical activity to allow greater flexibility in caloric intake should be a priority in all nutritional counseling.

Recommended Dietary Intake for Protein

The current RDA for protein for adults of all ages is 0.8 g/kg body weight.[16] Because older adults are likely to have less lean body tissue per kilogram of body weight than younger people, this protein allowance actually is higher per unit of lean body mass and should allow for any age changes in protein utilization or metabolism.[40] Because older individuals have lower caloric intakes than younger individuals, it is recommended that protein provide 12% to 14% of the total energy intake.[16]

Factors Influencing Protein Requirements and Utilization

Previous protein intake. The metabolic response to a particular type or level of protein can be influenced more by the protein intake of the previous months than by the current intake.[27] As long as 3 months may be required to adapt to a low-protein intake when the previous intake was liberal. An individual with marginal protein status and limited protein reserves will respond with a strongly positive nitrogen balance when placed on a high-protein diet as protein stores are being repleted.[23] Alternatively, a well-nourished individual may not demonstrate protein retention regardless of the level and quality of protein fed.

Over a lifetime individuals may adapt to a diet actually considered inadequate by general standards. DaCosta and Moorhouse[14] described two older people, a man of 76 and a woman of 81, who usually consumed about 30 g of protein a day. Despite protein intakes that were only 50% to 60% of the RDA, their serum albumin levels were 4.8 and 4.1 g/dl, respectively, and both were in good health. An older individual who has adapted to a particular type and level of protein appears to retain that accommodation throughout life, if reasonable health is maintained. Previous diet should be considered when developing a therapeutic regimen for an older person.

Individual variability. Protein requirements vary both among individuals of a particular age and sex as well as within the same individual from one time to another. Healthy, active, normal-weight older women with moderate but consistent patterns of protein intake (0.6 to 0.8 g/kg body weight) appeared to have less need for protein than overweight, inactive women with numerous health complaints and irregular meal patterns.[44] Physiologic stress, such as inflammation and infection, increases protein requirements and often results in substantial nitrogen losses, mediated in part by the stress response of the glucocorticoid hormones.[70]

Emotional stress can be equally detrimental to nitrogen balance, and even liberal protein intakes may not be sufficient to prevent nitrogen loss when emotional upset is severe. Swanson[56] described an older woman living alone who went from negative to positive nitrogen balance on an equivalent level of protein when a grandson came to live with her and her psychologic outlook improved. Many older people endure constant emotional stress from declining health and possible loss of independence, financial problems, or loneliness after the death of a spouse. The long-term impact of such psychologic distress on nitrogen balance has not been evaluated.[66]

Amino Acid Requirements

The protein requirement includes the need for the nine essential amino acids that cannot be synthesized by the body. There have been few balance studies evaluating amino acid requirements in older people, but the results of these studies have suggested that some older people may be consuming less-than-optimum intakes of lysine and methionine.[40] Munro[40] described studies evaluating tryptophan and threonine requirements in older people by using the **plasma amino acid response curve.** This technique involves increasing the intake of one essential amino acid at a time and monitoring the plasma level. For most essential amino acids, the plasma level rises sharply when intake exceeds the requirement. The level of intake at which this occurs is considered the requirement for that essential amino acid.

Comparisons of the amino acid requirements of younger and older adults using the plasma response curve have suggested that the need for some essential amino acids may change with age.[67] The minimum daily requirement for tryptophan was found to be 2 mg/kg body weight in older healthy adults, and 3 mg/kg body weight in younger adults. On the other hand, the daily requirement for threonine appears to be the same in all adults when expressed per unit of body weight. Since older people do have a lower proportion of lean body mass per unit of body weight than younger people, the requirements for certain essential amino acids may actually be somewhat higher per unit of active metabolic tissue in the elderly adult.

Young and coworkers[67] consider the requirements for essential amino acids to be similar in healthy older people and healthy younger people. However, they have raised questions about the adequacy of current recommendations for essential amino acid intakes in adults.[69] The World Health Organization recommends that essential amino acids constitute 11% of the total protein requirement of young adults. Based on recent work using labelled amino acids, Young and coworkers consider the essential amino acid requirement of adults to be about 33% of total protein; however, this proposal remains controversial. In light of the fact that animal protein makes up 65% of the total protein in the average American diet, all essential amino acids are likely to be provided in adequate amounts.[16]

Plasma Amino Acid Levels

The fasting plasma amino acid profile can provide useful information about an individual's nutritional status.[47] An intake deficient in protein or any single essential amino acid will be reflected in changes in plasma amino acid levels. Protein-energy malnutrition (PEM) results in a lower ratio of essential amino acids to nonessential amino acids in the plasma. Studies of healthy older people consuming adequate amounts of protein suggest that plasma amino acid levels are not influenced by age.[7]

Plasma levels of essential amino acids were similar in healthy younger men and healthy older men consuming more than 1 g of protein per kilogram of body weight.[7] Another report[47] indicated that apparently healthy older men living in the community had lower plasma levels of methionine, threonine, phenylalanine and the branched-chain essential amino acids (leucine, isoleucine, and valine). Although none of the older men with lower plasma amino acid levels had a serum albumin below 3.5 g/dl, protein nutrition may still have been marginal, as suggested by their lower ratio of essential to nonessential amino acids.

The plasma amino acid profile of older institutionalized men is influenced by their overall level of nutrition, their health status, and their intake of prescription drugs.[47] Older men with neurologic disorders who were orally fed had reduced ratios of essential to nonessential amino acids. About one third of these men also had clinical evidence of protein and energy deficiency. The drugs prescribed for older neurologic patients may complicate their clinical condition. Levodopa, used to treat Parkinson's disease, competes with the branched-chain amino acids for transport across the blood-brain barrier. Low levels of the branched-chain amino acids will indirectly promote the uptake of levodopa by the brain. This effect on the uptake of levodopa may be partly responsible for the variability in individual responsiveness to this drug.

Debilitated older patients given one to one and a half times the RDA for protein and at least the recommended levels of the essential amino acids may still have low plasma levels of methionine and the branched-chain amino acids

compared to healthy young men.[47] Whether the anorexia and weight loss sometimes observed in older people in poor health are caused or exacerbated by altered amino acid plasma levels or metabolism requires further evaluation. In light of the apparent abnormalities in plasma amino acid patterns in older people with marginal protein status and high intakes of neuroactive drugs, further research in amino acid metabolism is justified.

Hormonal Control of Amino Acid Metabolism

Insulin and amino acid metabolism. The major hormone controlling the utilization and retention of amino acids is insulin. The rise in plasma levels of both glucose and amino acids after the ingestion of a meal containing carbohydrate and protein stimulates the secretion of insulin from the beta cells of the pancreas. Insulin promotes the movement of plasma amino acids into the skeletal muscle for protein synthesis and inhibits the breakdown of existing muscle proteins and subsequent flow of amino acids into the peripheral circulation. The branched-chain amino acids (leucine, isoleucine, and valine) play a particular role in the control of protein metabolism.[69] The branched-chain amino acids carry amino groups into the skeletal muscle and regulate protein synthesis and breakdown. When the branched-chain amino acids are in short supply, the breakdown of protein is curtailed in an effort to conserve body protein. When the amino acid pool increases, protein synthesis is stimulated. Insulin plays an important role in promoting the movement of the branched-chain amino acids from the plasma into the skeletal muscle.[20,36,53]

The aging process is associated with reduced sensitivity of skeletal muscle and adipose cells to the action of insulin and transport of glucose. This resistance of peripheral tissues to the action of insulin contributes to the deterioration in glucose tolerance observed in many older people.[20] Recent work[20,36] has attempted to determine whether the influence of insulin on amino acid metabolism is similarly changed. In contrast to the age-related decline in the effect of insulin on glucose metabolism, plasma amino acid levels and protein metabolism appear to remain sensitive to insulin action into advanced age. Among men age 50 and older, plasma levels of the branched-chain amino acids decreased significantly after ingestion of 75 g of glucose.[36] However, the overall decrease in plasma amino acids was less among those over age 80. It has been reported that plasma amino acid levels are higher in individuals with higher proportions of body fat. The increased plasma amino acid levels in the oldest men could relate to their increased level of body fat and reduced number of muscle cells.

The ability of insulin to regulate the movement of particular amino acids into the cell could have important implications for neural function in older people.[19] The ratio of the plasma concentrations of particular amino acids appears to influence the rate of synthesis of **serotonin** and other neurotransmitters in the central nervous system. It is believed that the synthesis of serotonin from its precursor, tryptophan, is controlled by the level of tryptophan in neural tissues and, in turn, by the level of uptake of tryptophan from the plasma.[19] Tryptophan competes with the branched-chain amino acids, phenylalanine, and tyrosine for transport across the cell membrane into the brain. Insulin could bring about an increase in the synthesis of neural transmitters by lowering the plasma levels of the competing amino acids and thereby increasing the uptake of tryptophan. After an infusion of insulin, the plasma levels of the competing amino acids decreased to the same degree in both younger and older men.[20] Nevertheless, the plasma ratio of tryptophan to these competing amino acids was still somewhat lower in the older adults. Whether this decrease in the tryptophan ratio results in a decrease in the uptake of tryptophan and subsequent production of neurotransmitters is not known.

Nutritional Implications of Changes in Protein Metabolism

The reduced muscle mass and changes in total body protein synthesis associated with aging may have important implications for nutritional health. Skeletal muscle serves as a source of amino acids during adaptation to physiologic stress or reduced intake of protein and energy. Under those conditions, amino acids mobilized from the breakdown of muscle proteins maintain protein synthesis in vital organs and the immune system.[53,70] **Glutamine** is considered important in maintaining the cells of the immune system.[53] When muscle protein and nitrogen are decreased as a consequence of aging, glutamine reserves may also be reduced. This could have serious consequences for the older adult who has a serious infection or is recovering from surgery. Reduced numbers of **T cells** and **neutrophils** have been observed in older people with an inadequate protein intake or protein-energy malnutrition.[9,32] Providing sufficient amounts of protein and energy and encouraging regular exercise to maintain body muscle mass are important considerations in the nutritional support of both healthy and physiologically compromised older people.

Practical Aspects of Protein Intake

High-quality protein foods generally are among the more expensive items in the food budget. Less expensive plant or incomplete proteins such as nuts, cereals, bread, pasta, and legumes contribute toward meeting the protein requirement, although complete proteins of animal origin including meat, fish, poultry, eggs, and dairy products should also be consumed in reasonable amounts. Animal-plant protein combinations such as cereal and milk or macaroni and cheese enhance protein quality at a reasonable cost and should be encouraged in nutrition education for older people. Plant proteins can be complementary and when used in combination provide an amino acid pattern similar to animal proteins. Plant-plant combinations that provide high-quality protein include beans and rice or beans and bread, peanut butter and bread, or split pea soup and bread. A further advantage to consuming more plant proteins is that these foods tend to be lower in fat than particular meat, poultry, or dairy foods.[4]

Animal protein foods are good sources of iron, calcium, and zinc and provide these minerals in forms that are well absorbed. Prepared or convenience items, popular because they require little or no effort in preparation, tend to be expensive sources of protein (Table 5-3). Certain frankfurters and luncheon meats, less desirable choices because of their fat and sodium content, also cost more per 20 g of protein than many other sources of high-quality protein. Milk, one of the less expensive sources of quality protein, contributes calcium, riboflavin, and vitamins A and D to the diet and can be low in fat. Two 8-ounce glasses of milk each day will provide one fourth and one third of the daily protein needs of the older man and woman, respectively. Dairy products; ground meat; well-cooked, skinless chicken and fish; or eggs provide high-quality protein for older people with chewing problems.

PROTEIN STATUS
Factors Influencing Protein Intake

The protein intake of most older people is adequate, although race, sex, and age influence

TABLE 5-3 *Comparative Cost of 20 g of Protein**

Food	Amount to Be Eaten	Total Cost (cents)
Chicken leg	3 ounces	15
Eggs	3	17
Milk, dried skim (reconstituted)	2 cups	22
Beef liver	3 ounces	22
Peanut butter	5 tablespoons	27
Tuna, canned	3 ounces	27
Milk, fluid	2 cups	31
Hamburger	3 ounces	34
Cheddar cheese	3 ounces	40
Baked beans (preprepared)	1⅔ cups	43
Beef, stew meat	3 ounces	49
American cheese	3 ounces	55
Flounder, frozen	3 ounces	56
Cottage cheese	¾ cup	58
Frankfurters	3	62
Split pea soup (preprepared)	2 cups	89
Bologna (beef)	6 1-ounce slices	120

*Based on prices in Blacksburg, Va, Spring, 1992.

protein intake.[34,41,62,64] Men have higher protein intakes compared to women, whites have higher protein intakes compared to blacks and people age 75 or younger have higher protein intakes than those over age 75.

Living arrangements, income, and state of health influence protein intake. Older urban men and women interviewed at family practice medical centers[58] had protein intakes of 69 and 56 g, respectively, compared to older rural men and women whose intakes were 53 and 42 g, respectively. The mean ages of the four groups were similar, ranging from 72 to 75 years. The urban residents with higher incomes were consuming over 100% of the RDA, whereas the rural residents were consuming only 84% to 88% of the recommended level.

Daily protein intake was significantly lower in Boston men ages 76 and over compared to those ages 60 to 75 (74 and 83 g, respectively).[41] In contrast, daily protein intake did not change in women over this age span who had intakes of 64 to 65 g. In that study protein intake calculated on the basis of body weight ranged from 1.02 to 1.06 g/kg, suggesting that the lower protein intakes among the women and the men over age 75 were related to their lower body weights. Level of income is negatively associated with protein intake. In a national survey,[62] 10% of all men and women ages 65 to 74 had less than two thirds the RDA for protein, but 18% of low-income older adults had less than this amount.

Institutionalized older people in relatively good health do not always have lower protein intakes than older adults living in the community. The protein intakes of institutionalized older people in Boston with no apparent wasting diseases were similar to those of elderly individuals of equivalent age residing in their own homes.[48] Food intake records obtained by observation of the food actually consumed indicated that none of the 158 institutionalized women and only one of the 102 institutionalized men consumed less than 67% of the RDA for protein.

Energy Intake and Protein Status

The greatest deterrent to optimum protein status in older people may be their relatively low caloric intakes. As described in Table 5-4,

TABLE 5-4   *Mean Energy Protein Intake According to the RDA**

	Protein (% RDA)	Energy (% RDA)
Men		
50-59 yr	140	96
60-69 yr	125	85
70-74 yr	109	75
Women		
50-59 yr	112	75
60-69 yr	108	70
70-74 yr	98	67

*Based on 1989 Recommended Dietary Allowances.
Data from US Department of Health and Human Services, US Department of Agriculture: Nutrition monitoring in the United States: an update report on nutrition monitoring, DHHS Pub No (PHS) 89-1255, Washington, DC, 1989, US Government Printing Office.

the mean caloric intakes of many men and women in older age categories are 75% or less of that recommended.[64] At greatest risk are those who regularly consume inadequate amounts of both protein and energy. An evaluation of 3-day food records collected from 75 frail elderly attending an adult day care center[34] confirmed that nutrient intakes falling below the RDA are rather common among older people who are dependent on others for their food. Seventy-two percent of that group had less than the recommended level of kilocalories and 35% had less than the recommended level of protein (based on the 1980 RDAs). Of even greater concern was the number consuming less than three fourths of the RDA (41% fell below this level for energy and 14% fell below this level for protein). Because diets low in kilocalories are also likely to be low in protein, many of those consuming less than 75% of the RDA for protein probably were also deficient in kilocalories. These older people may be using important amino acids as sources of energy, adding further to a deteriorating protein status.

Even well-nourished older people with no clinical or biochemical evidence of poor protein status may have caloric intakes that fall below 30 kcal/kg body weight, the level recommended for men and women ages 51 and over.[16] In an older Boston population[34] with high protein intakes, caloric intake was only 25 kcal/kg body weight among the men and 24 kcal/kg body weight among the women. Among hospitalized elderly people[45] and the housebound British women[6] described earlier, caloric intakes fell to 19 kcal/kg body weight. Attention to providing adequate kilocalories is critical when planning a diet for an older person.

Serum Albumin Levels in Older People

Serum albumin levels and chronic disease. Albumin, which is synthesized in the liver, has many functions, including transporting hormones and enzymes, binding drugs, and maintaining osmotic pressure and appropriate fluid distribution in body compartments.[8] The effect of aging on serum albumin levels is not understood. Although decreases in serum albumin have been reported in older people, these evaluations generally did not control for protein status or health conditions that influence serum albumin levels.[8] Albumin synthesis is reduced in liver disease, and albumin losses are accelerated in renal disease and gastrointestinal disorders. Serum albumin levels are decreased in conditions that lead to expanded fluid volume, as occurs in congestive heart failure and renal disease.[38] Moreover, low plasma albumin levels can exacerbate fluid retention in cardiac failure, hypertension, and sodium imbalance.[3] Some workers have suggested that postural changes associated with extended bed rest can bring about a decline in serum albumin levels.[37]

The chronic conditions described above will contribute to changes in serum albumin levels despite optimum intakes of protein and calories. In 260 older adults residing in long-term care facilities[48] who had protein and calorie intakes equivalent to the RDA, the median plasma albumin level was 3.7 to 3.8 g/dl. This level is significantly lower than the 4.2 g/dl observed in noninstitutionalized healthy elderly of similar age. About one fourth of the institutionalized population had plasma albumin levels below 3.5 g/dl. (Serum albumin levels below 3.5 g/dl indicate declining protein status.)

Serum albumin levels and age. Healthy

older people with adequate intakes of protein and calories appear to maintain normal serum albumin levels into advanced age. An ongoing longitudinal study of about 1,100 men[8] between the ages of 39 and 90 reported only a slight decrease in serum albumin levels over this age range (Fig. 5-2). Only one man between the ages of 70 and 79 had a serum albumin level below 3.5 g/dl. Multiple regression analysis indicated that less than 5% of the variation in serum albumin levels among these men could be explained on the basis of age. The rate of decline in serum albumin levels in these men was 0.05 g/dl per decade.

Further study is needed to explore the effects of both age and protein intake on albumin synthesis and catabolism. An evaluation of albumin metabolism in healthy younger and older men suggested that the set point for albumin synthesis is lower in older people and is less responsive to changes in protein intake.[22] When protein intakes are low, the rates of albumin synthesis and catabolism are similar in older and younger people. However, when protein intake is optimum, younger individuals increase their rate of albumin synthesis, whereas older people do not.

Plasma albumin levels generally are used as a measure of visceral protein status.[37] A disadvantage of this measurement is the relatively long **half-life** of albumin (about 14 to 20 days). This means that albumin levels are somewhat slow to respond to nutritional therapy, and 2

weeks or more may be required before an improvement in protein status becomes evident.[37] Serum transferrin, **prealbumin,** and **retinol-binding protein** need further evaluation as possible indicators of protein status in older people. (The influence of iron status on plasma transferrin levels is discussed in Chapter 7.)

Protein Energy Malnutrition

Incidence of protein-energy malnutrition. A primary physiologic effect of malnutrition, whether undernutrition or overnutrition, is a change in body composition. **Protein-energy malnutrition (PEM)** is characterized by a loss of lean body mass and adipose tissue. As the condition progresses, serum albumin levels decline, accompanied by changes in immunologic and **hematopoietic function.**[33]

PEM in older people is caused by inadequate nutrient intake, increased nutritional requirements, or a combination of these.[46] PEM resulting from inadequate intake occurs in both institutionalized older people and those living at home. Physical disability, low income, or poor appetite can lower nutrient intake in older individuals living at home. An institutionalized adult may be served a nutritionally adequate meal but because of difficulty swallowing, inability to self-feed, or dislike of the food provided, the meal is not consumed.

PEM has been defined as the metabolic response to stress associated with increased requirements for kilocalories and protein.[33] Lipschitz[33] suggested that older people are more susceptible to PEM than younger people and develop this disorder more rapidly and under conditions of less stress. Trauma, surgery, infection, and inflammatory conditions such as rheumatoid arthritis can result in PEM. Among British men and women over age 70 who were living at home, PEM was associated with chronic bronchitis, emphysema, and gastrectomy.[40]

The initial responses to metabolic stress play a positive role in enabling the individual to make an optimum physiologic response to the infection or trauma that initiated the stress.[33] One characteristic response is an enhanced rate of catabolism of muscle protein. This breakdown of muscle protein yields a supply of amino acids for the synthesis of new proteins

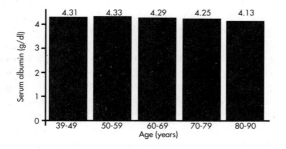

FIG. 5-2 Mean serum albumin levels according to age. Serum albumin levels did not change with age in healthy men.

(Data from Campion EW, deLabry LO, Glynn RJ: The effect of age on serum albumin in healthy males: report from the normative aging study, *J Gerontol* 43:M18, 1988.)

essential for an immune response or to serve as a source of energy while nutrient intake is reduced. Younger people who have a greater muscle mass and protein reserve can have a reduced nutrient intake for up to 10 days with no apparent change in nutritional status and disease outcome.[33] After that, inadequate intakes of protein and energy result in a significant lowering of serum albumin levels and impaired immunologic, hematologic, and hepatic function, which can adversely affect recovery. In contrast to younger people, older people experience the negative effects of reduced protein and caloric intakes within 2 to 3 days, with increased morbidity and mortality. A serum albumin level below 3.5 g/dl was the best single predictor of mortality among 80 consecutive patients between the ages of 85 and 100 admitted to a major medical center.[1] This held true regardless of age or disease diagnosis. In those patients a low serum albumin level was associated with infection and reduced immunologic capability.

PEM also carries increased risk of death for older adults living at home. Involuntary weight loss that was not related to a terminal disease or an increased level of exercise was associated with increased mortality among older men discharged from a geriatric rehabilitation unit.[55] Involuntary weight loss often is an indicator of severe PEM. Following an extensive review of the literature, Rudman and Feller[46] estimated that 3% of older people living at home and 15% to 60% of those in institutions showed evidence of PEM. Among older underweight patients in an extended-care facility in Great Britain, body build was related to caloric and protein intake before rather than after admission.[35] The poorly nourished patients had problems with mobility as a result of rheumatoid arthritis or bone fractures and had some degree of disability before entering the extended-care facility. A segment of the older population about whom little information is available is the homebound. Many homebound elderly are dependent on meal delivery programs, which provide fewer than three meals a day and deliver only 5 days a week. Thus the risk of PEM in this group remains high.

Hematologic changes in protein-energy malnutrition. One physiologic consequence of PEM is anemia and reduced hematopoietic function in the bone marrow.[38] Unfortunately, it is difficult to separate changes that result from normal aging complicated by disease from changes that result from PEM, since they are remarkably similar. In fact Lipschitz[32] has suggested that protein deficiency may contribute to the changes in hemopoietic function usually ascribed to aging. The anemia associated with PEM is identical to the anemia of chronic disorders that is related to infection and inflammation. Hemoglobin levels range from 10 to 12 g/dl, and serum iron and transferrin are low. Although hemoglobin and serum iron levels are similar to those seen in iron-deficiency anemia, iron stores are normal or may actually be elevated in the anemia associated with PEM.[11]

Increased intakes of protein and kilocalories bring about a rise in serum iron and transferrin within 48 hours, suggesting a nutritional role in the hematopoietic impairment that occurs in PEM.[32] Hemoglobin levels rise after nutritional supplementation, presumably because iron stores are being diverted to the formation of red blood cells. It is difficult to establish, however, whether the improved hematopoietic function observed in older patients who are given supplements is the result of their improved protein-energy status or a general improvement in their overall medical condition.

Immunologic changes in protein-energy malnutrition. Immunologic function declines with age and the effects of age, and PEM may be additive as PEM leads to more severe immunologic changes in older adults.[33] Older patients with PEM have reduced levels of neutrophils, the white blood cells that act as phagocytes and engulf bacteria and foreign substances. Examination of the bone marrow in these individuals reveals reductions in the number of stem cells and other cell precursors important in immunologic function.[32] Poor protein status results in not only reduced numbers of white blood cells but also changes in their function. Neutrophils, **B cells**, and **T cells** appear to have decreased **antigenic** and **bacteriocidal** activities when nutrition is inadequate.[9]

Older adults are ill more often than young adults. One survey[47] suggested that 15% to 20% of nursing home patients have active infections involving the urinary tract, respiratory tract, skin, or eye. Protein supplementation does result in a significant increase in the bone marrow of precursors of cells necessary for normal immunologic function, although levels do not reach those of healthy elderly persons.[32]

Protein-energy supplementation. Nutrition support providing adequate protein and kilocalories will prevent the development of PEM or ameliorate the problem when it does occur. The best approach with older people at risk for PEM is to promote their consumption of a nutritionally dense, well-balanced diet. Individuals should be encouraged to eat as much as they can, keeping in mind their dental status, functional status, and medical condition.[11] For frail elderly, those with long-standing PEM, or the critically ill, eating sufficient food to overcome existing nutritional deficiencies may not be possible, and dietary or liquid supplements or enteral feeding may be required. One care team noted that only 10% of their older patients with PEM could eat sufficient food at meal time to correct their nutritional deficiencies.[11]

Between-meal or bedtime snacks of nutrient-dense foods such as cheese and crackers, peanut butter and crackers, hard-cooked eggs, milkshakes or frappes, or a half sandwich will supply protein and energy as well as vitamins and minerals. Commercial liquid supplements can provide added nutrients when food intake is low. In a study of older British women[15] admitted to the hospital following a hip fracture, a liquid supplement given at bedtime reduced both the length of the hospital stay and the incidence of complications. Six months after these women were discharged from the hospital, complication rates were still significantly lower in the group that received the supplement (40%) than in the group that did not (74%).

Increasing energy and protein intakes of hospitalized older people may be difficult if their usual intake is only about 1,000 kcal per day and they are unable to consume additional food or liquids. Carbohydrate and protein powders that do not change the flavor, color, or texture of foods can be added to soup, cereal, juice, milk, or other soft foods to increase nutrient density. Items such as a milkshake, hot chocolate, or orange juice can be doubled in caloric content. In one report, daily caloric intake was increased by about 1,200 kcal, and weight loss was halted.[59] Mean serum albumin levels increased by 0.8 g/dl, indicating an improvement in protein status. The degree of improvement, however, varied widely among individual patients, since increases in serum albumin ranged from 0.2 to 1.8 g/dl.

The biochemical and physiologic parameters of PEM do not always respond to protein-energy supplementation. Among malnourished, homebound older people, commercial liquid supplements effectively raised serum albumin levels and led to increases in body weight.[32] Yet despite these indicators of improved nutritional status, immune function remained abnormal and hemoglobin levels did not increase. Lipschitz[32] concluded that poor nutritional status can aggravate existing abnormalities in immune and hematopoietic function in older people. Although nutrient repletion of those who are severely malnourished will lead to some improvement in immune response, it will not restore function to normal levels. Changes in immunologic and hematopoietic function observed in healthy or mildly malnourished elderly people are not related to nor responsive to changes in protein or calorie status.

Summary

Because little is known about the nutrient requirements of older people, the RDAs for those over age 50 have been extrapolated from those developed for younger people. Caloric requirements decrease with advancing age, and iron requirements are lower in women after menopause. Although there is no established recommendation for carbohydrate, older people are encouraged to get more than half of their kilocalories from carbohydrate foods, with emphasis on complex carbohydrates rich in fiber. A daily source of linoleic acid is encouraged, although a quantitative recommendation has not been developed.

Protein requirements in advanced age are influenced by changes in body compartments, caloric intake, previous protein intake, emotional stress, and chronic disease. Protein metabolism tends to shift from the muscle compartment to the visceral organs as skeletal muscle is lost. Healthy older people can conserve nitrogen when protein intake is low, although obligatory nitrogen loss, calculated per kilogram of body cell mass, is higher in older people as a result of the shift in protein metabolism from the skeletal muscle to the visceral organs. Obligatory nitrogen loss per kilogram of body weight is higher in men, who have a greater proportion of lean body mass and a lower proportion of body fat compared to women.

Nitrogen balance studies indicate that many older people lose nitrogen on intakes below 0.8 g of protein per kilogram of body weight, and for some even this level is not sufficient. Caloric intakes below recommended levels prevent efficient utilization of the protein consumed. Protein metabolism does remain sensitive to insulin action into advanced age. Insulin acts to promote protein synthesis by moving amino acids from the plasma into the skeletal muscle and prevents the breakdown of existing proteins within the cell. Serum albumin levels in healthy older people are similar to those of younger people.

Nutrition surveys suggest that some older people are at risk for PEM because their intakes of both protein and kilocalories are below recommended levels. The relative cost of quality protein sources may contribute to the problem. PEM has been identified in both community-living and institutionalized older people who have reduced nutrient intakes or increased nutrient requirements as a result of infection, trauma, or inflammation. PEM leads to hematopoietic and immunologic changes that further increase the risk of illness or death. Increasing the intake of food or commercial nutritional supplements can reverse some but not all of these changes. Encouraging the intake of appropriate amounts and types of food can prevent the development of PEM in older individuals.

REVIEW QUESTIONS

1. How were the recommended dietary allowances (RDAs) for older adults developed? What are the limitations of the current RDAs? What is the feasibility of specific RDAs for older people?
2. How much carbohydrate should be consumed by older adults? What type of carbohydrates should be eaten? Are fiber supplements a useful way to increase dietary fiber? Are diets that are very low in carbohydrates recommended for older adults?
3. What is the role of the essential fatty acids in the diets of older persons? Is it reasonable to assume a beneficial risk reduction of cardiovascular disease by lowering blood lipids in older adults?
4. What methods are used to measure protein status in older adults? How does aging affect protein status? What level of dietary protein is recommended for older persons? What factors might influence the recommendation for dietary protein?
5. What biochemical markers can be used to assess protein-energy malnutrition in the older person? What are the causes of PEM in older adults? What effects does PEM have on immunological and hematological function? What dietary recommendations can be made to crrect PEM?

SUGGESTED LEARNING ACTIVITIES

1. Compare and contrast the RDAs of a 21-year-old college student with a 79-year-old retired college professor. Plan a 3-day diet, using a computer nutrient analysis program, to meet the RDAs of each. Each diet should contain 55% to 60% carbohydrate, 15% protein, and 25% to 30% fat.
2. Illustrate the end products of metabolism of linoleic and linolenic acids. Identify the roles of each in immune function, platelet aggregation, and blood lipid reduction.
3. Prepare answers to the following questions, which were asked by older adults attending a lecture on diet and heart disease at a senior center:
   - Is it beneficial for a 75-year-old woman to try to reduce a total blood cholesterol level of 253 mg/dl?
   - Should a 65-year-old man be advised to change his high-fat diet and high waist-to-hip ratio following angioplasty?
   - Give five tips for reducing saturated fat content of a typical American diet.
4. Contact the director of a local senior center and ask if you can conduct a taste test on 10 different liquid nutritional supplements. Develop an instrument for rating each supplement by taste, smell, texture, and overall desirability.
5. Plan a 3-day diet for a 90-year-old woman who is housebound, edentulous, and has protein-energy malnutrition.

Key Terms

Provided here for review is a list of the major terms in this chapter. The definitions can be found in the Glossary, which begins on p. 336.

To help you understand how these terms are applied, the page number is given for the first mention of each term in the chapter.

REFERENCES

1. Agarwal N and others: Predictive ability of various nutritional variables for mortality in elderly people, *Am J Clin Nutr* 48:1173, 1988.
2. Albrink MJ: Advisability (or lack of it) of lipid-lowering diets for the elderly. In Prinsley DM, Sandstead HH, editors: *Nutrition and aging,* New York, 1990, Alan R Liss.
3. Anderson WF and others: Clinical and subclinical malnutrition in old age. In Carlson LA, editor: *Nutrition in old age,* Symposia Swedish Nutrition Foundation X, Stockholm, 1972, Almqvist & Wiksell.
4. Anonymous: Things nobody ever told Rocky Balboa about protein, *Tufts University Diet and Nutrition Letter,* 8(12):3, 1991.
5. Asciutti-Moura LS and others: Fatty acid composition of serum lipids and its relation to diet in an elderly institutionalized population, *Am J Clin Nutr* 48:980, 1988.
6. Bunker VW and others: Nitrogen balance studies in apparently healthy elderly people and those who are housebound, *Br J Nutr* 57:211, 1987.
7. Caballero B, Gleason RE, Wurtman RJ: Plasma amino acid concentrations in healthy elderly men and women, *Am J Clin Nutr* 53:1249, 1991.
8. Campion EW, deLabry LO, Glynn RJ: The effect of age on serum albumin in healthy males: report from the normative aging study, *J Gerontol* 43:M18, 1988.
9. Chandra RK: Nutritional regulation of immunocompetence and risk of disease. In Horwitz A and others, editors: *Nutrition in the elderly,* New York, 1989, Oxford University Press.
10. Cheng AHR and others: Comparative nitrogen balance study between young and aged adults using three levels of protein intake from a combination wheat-soy-milk mixture, *Am J Clin Nutr* 31:12, 1978.
11. Chernoff R: Nutritional support in the elderly. In Chernoff R, editor: *Geriatric nutrition: the health professional's handbook,* Gaithersburg, Md, 1991, Aspen Publishers.
12. Cohn SH and others: Improved models for determination of body fat by in vivo neutron activation, *Am J Clin Nutr* 40:255, 1984.

13. Committee on Diet and Health, Food and Nutrition Board: *Diet and health: implications for reducing chronic disease risk,* Washington, DC, 1989, National Academy Press.
14. DaCosta F, Moorhouse JA: Protein nutrition in aged individuals on self-selected diets, *Am J Clin Nutr* 22:1618, 1969.
15. Delmi M and others: Dietary supplementation in elderly patients with fractured neck of the femur, *Lancet* 335:1013, 1990.
16. Food and Nutrition Board: *Recommended dietary allowances,* ed 10, Washington, DC, 1989, National Academy of Sciences.
17. Freeland-Graves JH, Bales CW: Dietary recommendations of minerals for the elderly. In Bales CW, editor: *Mineral homeostasis in the elderly,* New York, 1989, Alan R Liss.
18. Frei BB: Battling the bad fat, *Harvard Health Letter* 17:6, 1992.
19. Fukagawa NK and others: Plasma tryptophan and total neutral amino acid levels in men: influence of hyperinsulinemia and age, *Metabolism* 36(7):683, 1987.
20. Fukagawa NK and others: Glucose and amino acid metabolism in aging man: differential effects of insulin, *Metabolism* 37(4):371, 1988.
21. Garza C, Scrimshaw NS, Young VR: Human protein requirements: the effect of variations in energy intake within the maintenance range, *Am J Clin Nutr* 29:280, 1976.
22. Gersovitz M and others: Albumin synthesis in young and elderly subjects using a new stable isotope methodology: response to level of protein intake, *Metabolism* 29:1075, 1980.
23. Gersovitz M and others: Human protein requirements: assessment of the adequacy of the current Recommended Dietary Allowance for dietary protein in elderly men and women, *Am J Clin Nutr* 35:6, 1982.
24. Gordon DJ and others: High-density lipoprotein cholesterol and cardiovascular disease, *Circulation* 79:8, 1989.
25. Harper AE: Recommended dietary allowances for the elderly, *Geriatrics* 33:73, 1978.
26. Harrill I, Jansen C, Barthrop J: Serum cholesterol and triglycerides and hyperlipoproteinemia in elderly women, *J Gerontol* 33:347, 1978.
27. Hegsted DM: Proteins. In Beaton GH, McHenry EW, editors: *Nutrition. A comprehensive treatise: macronutrients and nutrient elements,* vol 1, New York, 1964, Academic Press.
28. Hegsted DM: Recommended dietary intakes of elderly subjects, *Am J Clin Nutr* 50:1190, 1989.
29. Holman RT, Smythe L, Johnson S: Effect of sex and age on fatty acid composition of human serum lipids, *Am J Clin Nutr* 32:2390, 1979.
30. Hunt IF, Murphy NJ, Henderson C: Food and nutrient intake of Seventh-day Adventist women, *Am J Clin Nutr* 48:850, 1988.
31. Kountz WB, Ackermann PG, Kheim T: The effect of added carbohydrate and fat on nitrogen balance in the elderly, *J Am Geriatr Soc* 3:691, 1955.
32. Lipschitz DA: Nutrition and the aging hematopoietic system. In Hutchinson ML, Munro HM, editors: *Nutrition and aging,* New York, 1986, Academic Press.
33. Lipschitz DA: Impact of nutrition on the age-related decline in hematopoiesis. In Chernoff R, editor: *Geriatric nutrition: the health professional's handbook,* Gaithersburg, Md, 1991, Aspen Publishers.
34. Ludman EK, Newman JM: Frail elderly: assessment of nutrition needs, *J Gerontol* 26:198, 1986.
35. MacLennan WJ, Martin P, Mason BJ: Energy intake, disability disease, and skinfold thickness in a long-stay hospital, *Gerontol Clin* 17:173, 1975.
36. Marchesini G and others: Insulin resistance in aged man: relationship between impaired glucose tolerance and decreased insulin activity on branched-chain amino acids, *Metabolism* 36:1096, 1987.
37. Mitchell CO, Chernoff R: Nutritional assessment of the elderly. In Chernoff R, editor: *Geriatric nutrition: the health professional's handbook,* Gaithersburg, Md, 1991, Aspen Publishers.
38. Mitchell CO, Lipschitz DA: Detection of protein-calorie malnutrition in the elderly, *Am J Clin Nutr* 35:398, 1982.
39. Munro HN: Major gaps in nutrient allowances: the status of the elderly, *J Am Diet Assoc* 76:137, 1980.
40. Munro HN: Protein nutriture and requirements of the elderly. In Munro HN, Danford DE, editors: *Nutrition, aging, and the elderly,* New York, 1989, Plenum Press.
41. Munro HN and others: Protein nutriture of a group of free-living elderly, *Am J Clin Nutr* 46:586, 1987.
42. Nieman DC and others: Dietary status of Seventh-day Adventist vegetarian and nonvegetarian elderly women, *J Am Diet Assoc* 89:1763, 1989.
43. Ohlson MA and others: Intakes and retentions of nitrogen, calcium, and phosphorus by 136 women between 30 and 85 years of age, *Fed Proc* 11:775, 1952.

44. Ohlson MA and others: Utilization of an improved diet by older women, *J Am Diet Assoc* 28:1138, 1952.

45. Rammohan M, Juan D, Jung D: Hypophagia among hospitalized elderly, *J Am Diet Assoc* 89:1774, 1989.

46. Rudman D, Feller AG: Protein-calorie undernutrition in the nursing home, *J Am Geriatr Soc* 37:173, 1989.

47. Rudman D and others: Fasting plasma amino acids in elderly men, *Am J Clin Nutr* 49:559, 1989.

48. Sahyoun NR and others: Dietary intakes and biochemical indicators of nutritional status in an elderly, institutionalized population, *Am J Clin Nutr* 47:524, 1988.

49. Schlenker ED: Nutritional status of older women, doctoral dissertation, East Lansing, Mich, 1976, Michigan State University.

50. Schneider EL and others: Recommended dietary allowances and the health of the elderly, *N Engl J Med* 314:157, 1986.

51. Scrimshaw NS, Perera WDA, Young VR: Protein requirements of man: obligatory urinary and fecal nitrogen losses in elderly women, *J Nutr* 106:665, 1976.

52. Simopoulos AP: Omega-3 fatty acids in health and disease. In Prinsley DM, Sandstead HH, editors: *Nutrition and aging,* New York, 1990, Alan R Liss.

53. Skeie B and others: Branch-chain amino acids: their metabolism and clinical utility, *Crit Care Med* 18:549, 1990.

54. Stadtman ER: Protein modification in aging, *J Gerontol* 43:B112, 1988.

55. Sullivan DH, Walls RC, Lipschitz DA: Protein-energy undernutrition and the risk of mortality within 1 year of hospital discharge in a select population of geriatric rehabilitation patients, *Am J Clin Nutr* 53:599, 1991.

56. Swanson P: Adequacy in old age. I. Role of nutrition, *J Home Econ* 56:651, 1964.

57. Thomas PR: *Improving America's diet and health: from recommendations to action,* Washington, DC, 1991, National Academy Press.

58. Thompson MP and others: Comparison of dietary intake of urban and rural elderly patients in family practice centers, *South Med J* 80:1216, 1987.

59. Tomaiolo PP, Enman S, Draus V: Preventing and treating malnutrition in the elderly, *J Parent Enteral Nutr* 5:46, 1981.

60. Uauy R, Scrimshaw NS, and Young VR: Human protein requirements: nitrogen balance response to graded levels of egg protein in elderly men and women, *Am J Clin Nutr* 31:779, 1978.

61. Uauy R and others: Human protein requirements: obligatory urinary and fecal nitrogen losses and the factorial estimation of protein needs in elderly males, *J Nutr* 108:97, 1978.

62. US Department of Health and Human Services: Dietary intake source data: United States, 1976-80, DHHS Pub No (PHS) 89-1681, Washington, DC, 1983, US Government Printing Office.

63. US Department of Health and Human Services: Normal human aging: the Baltimore Longitudinal Study of Aging, NIH Pub No 84-2450, Washington, DC, 1984, US Government Printing Office.

64. US Department of Health and Human Services, US Department of Agriculture: Nutrition monitoring in the United States: an update report on nutrition monitoring, DHHS Pub No (PHS) 89-1255, Washington, DC, 1989, US Government Printing Office.

65. Wahle KWJ and others: Concentrations of linoleic acid in adipose tissue differ with age in women but not men, *Eur J Clin Nutr* 45:195, 1990.

66. Watkin DM: The assessment of protein nutrition in aged man, *Ann NY Acad Sci* 69:902, 1958.

67. Young VR: Amino acids and proteins in relation to the nutrition of elderly people, *Age Ageing* 19:S10, 1990.

68. Young VR: Protein and amino acid metabolism with reference to aging and the elderly. In Prinsley DM, Sandstead HH, editors: *Nutrition and aging,* New York, 1990, Alan R Liss.

69. Young VR, Bier DM: Amino acid requirements in the adult human: how well do we know them? *J Nutr* 117:1484, 1987.

70. Young VR, Munro HN, Fukagawa N: Protein and functional consequences of deficiency. In Horwitz A and others, editors: *Nutrition in the elderly,* New York, 1989, Oxford University Press.

71. Zanni E, Callaway DH, Zezulka AY: Protein requirements of elderly men, *J Nutr* 109:513, 1979.

6

Vitamins in the Aged

✶✶✶

After studying the chapter, the student should:

✔ *Identify the digestive alterations that influence absorption of vitamins in the older person.*

✔ *Outline the requirements of the fat-soluble and water-soluble vitamins in the elderly.*

✔ *Understand the role of vitamins in health maintenance of the older person.*

✔ *Recognize disease states that are common in the elderly and how they can affect vitamin status.*

✔ *Recognize the influence that vitamins may play in the prevention of chronic diseases.*

Introduction

Vitamin requirements and metabolism are receiving increasing attention as epidemiologic findings suggest that intakes of particular vitamins are related to the incidence of chronic diseases. Vitamins that act as antioxidants appear to have a role in preventing coronary artery disease and cancer. Current work is focusing on the actions of vitamins as related to immune function, the formation of cataracts, and the development of osteoporosis, all problems associated with aging. Physiologic processes, including neural function, formation of red blood cells, and tissue repair, require specific vitamins. The potential for vitamin toxicity may be increased in older people with compromised kidney function who ingest inappropriate types or amounts of vitamin supplements. Research exploring these relationships is continuing, although much remains to be learned. The current recommended intake of all the vitamins can be found in Appendix A.

FAT-SOLUBLE VITAMINS
Factors Influencing Absorption

Digestive secretions. Dietary fat, essential for the absorption of the **fat-soluble vitamins,** usually is consumed in the form of triglycerides, which must be broken down into monoglycerides or free fatty acids for absorption to take place. The fat-soluble vitamins (A, D, E, and K) become associated with lipid globules in the stomach and then join with **bile salts** in the intestinal lumen to form **micelles.** The micelles carry both fatty acids and the fat-soluble vitamins to the mucosal surface, where absorption takes place. **Pancreatic lipase,** required for the digestion of dietary fat, usually is present in sufficient amounts in older adults to allow this process to proceed normally. Bile salts secreted by the liver and stored in the gallbladder are necessary for the formation of micelles. Older people with pancreatic or liver disease can have problems absorbing both fat and the fat-soluble vitamins. For those unable to absorb sufficient lipid, fat-soluble vitamins can be administered in **water-miscible emulsions** either orally or intramuscularly.

Dietary constituents. Dietary fat has two important functions in the absorption of fat-soluble vitamins. First, lipids serve as a transport mechanism to move the vitamins from the stomach into the small intestine; second, lipids delay gastric emptying and ensure the delivery of only small amounts of fat at a time, thereby promoting formation of micelles. At least 5 g of dietary fat a day are required to support absorption of the fat-soluble vitamins.[70] Polyunsaturated fatty acids, compared to saturated fatty acids, lower absorption of the fat-soluble vitamins. Although the mechanism by which this occurs is not known, the absorption of vitamin A is depressed by the presence of peroxidized fat.[70,102] Peroxidized fatty acids arising from the oxidation of polyunsaturated fatty acids may be detrimental to other fat-soluble vitamins as well.

Vitamin A appears to compete with vitamins E and K for binding sites, and high levels of vitamin A supplements will depress absorption of those two vitamins.[102] Conversely, large amounts of **alpha-tocopherol** (vitamin E) inhibit the absorption of **beta-carotene.** Highly concentrated supplements of fat-soluble vitamins appear to have potential for creating nutrient imbalances as well as toxicity.

Vitamin A and Carotenoids

Vitamin A is supplied to the body as **preformed vitamin A** found only in animal foods, and as vitamin A precursor **carotenoids** found in vegetables and fruits. Vitamin A is important for visual function and the maintenance of epithelial tissues and resistance to infection.

Absorption of vitamin A. Preformed vitamin A is present in animal foods and vitamin supplements in the form of **retinyl esters.** Retinyl esters are hydrolyzed through digestion to yield **retinol,** the form of vitamin A that enters the mucosal cell.[70] In the mucosal cells of the small intestine, retinol is reesterified into retinyl esters and incorporated into the core of triglyceride-rich chylomicrons, which enter the lymph and then the general circulation.

Recent work has confirmed that the removal of vitamin A esters from the plasma after absorption is slowed in older adults.[3] Krasinski and coworkers[50] administered 3,000 retinol equivalents (RE) in the form of retinyl esters to healthy older adults (mean age = 65) and younger adults (mean age = 32) in Boston. Plasma retinyl esters were measured in both groups for 8 hours. The increase in plasma retinyl esters above fasting levels was similar in both groups for the first 4 hours after ingestion of the vitamin A, but the older group had significantly higher levels for hours 5 through 8 (Fig. 6-1). When vitamin A was consumed along with a high-fat meal, it became apparent that the postprandial rise in plasma retinyl esters occurred in parallel to the rise in the plasma triglyceride-rich chylomicron fraction. The slowed removal of retinyl esters from the plasma appears to be related to delayed removal of this lipid fraction in older adults. The slowed removal of chylomicrons from the plasma could relate to decreased levels of **lipoprotein lipase** enzyme. This enzyme, located on the endothelial surface of the capillary, hydrolyzes the triglyceride in the chylomicron and allows the fatty acids to move into the cell. When the triglyceride has been removed, the **chylomicron remnant** containing the retinyl esters is removed from the plasma by the liver. Plasma retinyl esters are the major postprandial metabolites of vitamin A.

When older and younger adults were given a test dose of beta-carotene, results were similar; plasma clearance of beta-carotene occurred at a faster rate in younger subjects.[57] Another important observation in that study was the in-

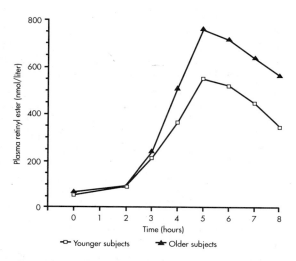

FIG. 6-1 Effect of age on postprandial plasma retinyl ester (vitamin A) level. Mean plasma retinyl ester levels in older people, age 50 and over (▲), and younger people, under age 50 (□), given 3,000 retinol equivalents of vitamin A. Mean levels at 4 hours and beyond are significantly different.

(With permission from Krasinski SD and others: Postprandial plasma retinyl ester response is greater in older subjects compared with younger subjecst, *J Clin Invest* 85:883, 1990.)

crease in plasma retinyl esters in the older subjects after the test dose of beta-carotene. This indicated that beta-carotene was not only effectively absorbed but also converted to retinol in the intestinal mucosa and reesterified for incorporation in the chylomicrons. Maiani and colleagues[57] believed that the elevated plasma retinyl ester level in the older subjects indicated more efficient absorption and conversion of beta-carotene in older age groups. Conversely, a reduced rate of uptake of retinyl esters by the liver would also contribute to the elevated plasma levels.

Metabolism of vitamin A. An evaluation of vitamin A status in 562 healthy Boston adults between 60 and 98 years of age has confirmed the high bioavailability of retinyl esters contained in vitamin supplements.[49] Plasma retinol levels did not differ between those who took vitamin A supplements and those who did not,

but plasma retinyl ester levels were more than doubled in those taking daily supplements containing 5,000 to 10,000 IU and nearly tripled in those taking daily supplements containing more than 10,000 IU. In these older people the fraction of total plasma vitamin A (retinol plus retinyl esters) circulating as retinyl esters was 13%. In **hypervitaminosis A,** the proportion of plasma vitamin A in the form of retinyl esters is 30%. Nevertheless, the older people who had been taking vitamin A supplements containing at least 5,000 IU for longer than 5 years did have plasma retinyl ester levels associated with elevated serum levels of **aspartate aminotransferase,** which indicates liver damage. Whether this liver damage was the direct result of vitamin A overload could not be confirmed.

Many older people take concentrated supplements of both vitamin A and vitamin E. It has been shown in animals that vitamin E decreases the activity of **hepatic retinyl ester hydrolase,** the enzyme required to mobilize retinyl esters stored in the liver.[50] This relationship has not been demonstrated in older human subjects; nevertheless, it suggests that vitamin E supplements could exacerbate the risk associated with prolonged use of vitamin A supplements in excess of the recommended dietary allowance (RDA).

Vitamin A requirements. Total vitamin A intake includes both preformed vitamin A found in animal products and the vitamin A precursor carotenoids found in fruits and vegetables. Unfortunately, analytical methods that can ascertain the specific carotenoids present in a particular food item have only recently been perfected. Consequently, food composition tables based on international units (IU) still include carotenoids since found to have little or no vitamin A activity.[76] Beta-carotene is the carotenoid with the highest vitamin A activity, and it is used as a standard. The Food and Nutrition Board[27] recommends the use of retinol equivalents based on established conversion factors for expressing vitamin A activity. The 1989 RDAs expressed in retinol equivalents are 1,000 RE for men and 800 RE for women over age 50. The 1980 RDAs were expressed in IU.[26] The recommended levels for adults over age 50 were 5,000 IU for men and 4,000 IU for women.

Vitamin A intake and biochemical status. Mean intake of vitamin A tends to exceed the RDA and increase with age. In the second National Health and Nutrition Examination Survey (NHANES II),[93] mean intake equalled 6,163 IU in men ages 60 to 69 and 6,731 IU in those ages 70 to 74. Mean intake was lower among women, 5,400 IU in the 60- to 69-year-old group and 5,469 IU in the 70- to 74-year-old group. Mean intake of vitamin A tended to skew to the right as a result of the exceedingly high intake among those consuming foods exceptionally rich in vitamin A (liver) or carotenoids (e.g., carrots, broccoli) or vitamin supplements. For example, intakes expressed as a percentage of the RDA ranged from 1% to 775% in 268 elderly South Carolina residents.[80]

Despite the fact that mean vitamin A intake equals or exceeds the RDA in most older populations, there are older individuals with poor intakes. In healthy Boston older people, 15% to 19% of the men and 7% to 11% of the women consumed less than the RDA for vitamin A based on food intake.[49] Frail older people or those with physical problems are more likely to have low intakes of vitamin A. Half of older xerostomia patients consumed less than the recommended level.[74] Thirty percent of a frail elderly group attending an adult day care center consumed *less than half* of the RDA for vitamin A over a 3-day period.[56]

Plasma or serum vitamin A levels tend to increase until about age 40 in men and age 60 in women and then plateau. A 4-year study of 200 healthy white elderly people in New Mexico[30] reported no changes over that period; mean plasma retinol levels were 57 μg/dl in the men and 59 μg/dl in the women. Only two individuals, one man and one woman, consumed less than half of the RDA for vitamin A; 44% consumed, on the average, 2,000 RE of vitamin A a day (two to two and a half times the RDA). The older men using a supplement had significantly higher plasma retinol levels than nonusers.

Older whites tend to have higher serum vitamin A levels than older blacks.[91] Among older Hispanic adults, men have higher serum retinol levels than women; those of Mexican American background have lower serum levels than those of Cuban background.[54] Environmental and ethnic differences in food choices very likely contribute to these differences.

Although they are fairly simple to determine, plasma vitamin A levels do not always identify older individuals at risk of deficiency. Among 30 institutionalized older people over age 80, dietary intakes met or exceeded recommended levels for all but four subjects, and plasma retinol levels were above 30 μg/dl for all but two subjects.[4] However, response to a 450 RE test dose of retinyl esters indicated that seven of the 30 had depleted liver stores.

Chronic disease, infection, and weight loss are associated with depletion of liver vitamin stores. Liver content of retinyl esters measured at autopsy was more than twice as high in older people who died suddenly of a heart attack or stroke compared to those of similar age who had long-term illnesses or wasting diseases.[11] In several of the latter group, liver stores were near the critical level of less than 10 μg/g of liver tissue—the point at which plasma retinol levels can no longer be maintained and functional impairment becomes obvious. Liver vitamin A stores do not decline as a function of age, per se.

There is a need for functional tests that will detect declining vitamin A status before deficiency becomes overt. Visual abnormalities can be detected when serum levels range from 20 to 40 μg/dl. One third of 18 adults with serum levels between 30 and 39 μg/dl[17] had impaired dark adaptation, which became normal after vitamin A supplementation and an increase in serum levels to 40 μg/dl or above. This raises serious questions about the appropriateness of the standard of 20 μg/dl often used to define risk. Rasmussen and colleagues[73] also emphasize the importance of fasting blood samples when evaluating vitamin A status in the elderly in light of the elevated postprandial rise in plasma vitamin A levels in this group.

Roles of the carotenoids. At one time the major function of the carotenoids was thought to be that of precursor of vitamin A. Recent research has pointed to the carotenoids as **antioxidants** in cancer prevention, a role independent of vitamin A activity.[76] The ability of these compounds to prevent oxidative damage to tissues also has been related to prevention of cataracts. Among middle-aged and older people, those with plasma carotenoid levels in the upper quintiles had less than one fourth the risk of cataracts as those whose plasma level was in the lowest quintile.[42] Supplementation with beta-carotene also brings about changes in the immune system in older people.[99] This stimulatory effect tended to reverse changes in the types and characteristics of immune cells usually associated with the aging process. The level necessary to achieve this response, however, was 30 mg or more of beta-carotene a day. This is the equivalent of the beta-carotene found in more than 1 pound of carrots.[76]

Beta-carotene is considered safe at intakes ranging from 15 to 50 mg a day.[10] It does appear, however, that older people both absorb beta-carotene and convert a portion of the amount absorbed to retinol. As described earlier, older people given a test dose of beta-carotene had increased serum levels of both beta-carotene and retinyl esters.[57] In light of the evidence of liver damage among the Boston elderly people who were ingesting concentrated vitamin A supplements over several years,[49] this age group may have a higher susceptibility to vitamin A overload. Older people should be discouraged from consuming supplemental doses of beta-carotene or vitamin A that exceed recommended levels.[88]

Vitamin E

Vitamin E functions as an important antioxidant[27] in trapping **free radicals** and preventing tissue damage. Vitamin E has long received attention as a possible means of delaying the onset and severity of age changes or chronic disease. It is only recently that research has been initiated to provide experimental evidence to support or dispel these claims.

Absorption of vitamin E. Currently there is no evidence to suggest that absorption of vitamin E (alpha-tocopherol) is influenced by age. Vitamin E deficiency, when it has been identified, was associated with serious fat malabsorption. Alpha-tocopherol is absorbed and utilized more efficiently than **gamma- or beta-tocopherol** by both younger and older people.[32]

Vitamin E requirements. The vitamin E requirement in **tocopherol equivalents** (TE) is influenced by the level of intake of polyunsaturated fatty acids (PUFA). The RDA is designed to maintain the suggested ratio of 0.4 mg TE per gram of PUFA on the customary American diet.[27] In general, foods high in PUFA, such as vegetable oils, are also high in vitamin E; thus as intakes of PUFA rise, so should intakes of vitamin E. However, this is not always the case. Chicken, a food recommended as a substitute for protein foods higher in saturated fat, has a relatively high content of PUFAs but a low content of vitamin E and a ratio of only 0.2.[64] Data from NHANES II[64] suggest that both men and women over age 65 are consuming less than the RDA for vitamin E (10 mg TE for men; 8 mg TE for women). Mean intakes were 8.3 mg TE and 6.6 mg TE in men and women, respectively. Median intakes were 60% of the RDA in men and 49% of the RDA in women, suggesting that more than half of this age group have intakes that are seriously low.

A recent study evaluating vitamin E status and **lipid peroxidation** in individuals receiving fish oil supplements[62] emphasizes the importance of the relationship between vitamin E and PUFA intakes. In both younger and older women daily receiving 2 g of fish oil high in **omega-3 fatty acids,** the positive changes in plasma lipid patterns—a decrease in triglycerides and an increase in the ratio of polyunsaturated to saturated fatty acids—were accompanied by a significant increase in the degree of peroxidation of serum lipids. Plasma vitamin E levels did not change over the 3-month period of supplementation, although the ratio of plasma vitamin E to plasma omega-3 fatty acids declined significantly. The fish oil capsules being consumed contained 3 IU of vitamin E per gram of lipid.

As we continue to stress the need to reduce intake of items high in saturated fatty acids and suggest substitutions that are high in PUFAs or that provide omega-3 fatty acids, it is important to encourage increased intakes of fruits and vegetables that will increase total vitamin E intake without additional fat.

Vitamin E intake and biochemical status. Surveys of community-living and institutionalized older adults have not revealed significant numbers at risk of vitamin E deficiency (a plasma level below 0.5 mg/dl). In a Boston study,[49] healthy older subjects had higher plasma tocopherol levels than young controls, and supplement users had higher levels than nonusers regardless of age. Vitamin E intakes from food were not reported, but mean supplemental intakes of vitamin E were 178 mg a day in men and 140 mg a day in women. Researchers from Belgium evaluated vitamin E status in 95 healthy volunteers ranging in age from 20 to 94 years[95]; 23 of these individuals were age 80 or older. Only one volunteer, who was 94 years of age, had a plasma vitamin E level indicative of deficiency. Plasma vitamin E levels were significantly related to plasma cholesterol and triglyceride levels and age. Both plasma vitamin E and lipid levels were highest in those ages 40 to 59 and lowest in those over age 80. Barnes and Chen[9] evaluated 84 independent-living and 22 institutionalized older adults between 60 and 90 years of age and found no significant serum vitamin E differences on the basis of age, sex, or living situation.

Role of vitamin E in immune function. The aging process is associated with a decline in **cell-mediated immune response** despite the absence of serious disease. The major change is a decrease in the number of **T cells,** which are important for the body's defense against virus and tumor cells and certain bacteria. A double-blind study with 32 healthy older people[60] tested the effect of vitamin E supplementation on immune response. Along with a controlled diet, the subjects were given a tablet containing either 800 mg of alpha-tocopherol acetate or a placebo. By the end of the 30-day period, the individuals receiving the vitamin E had significantly increased plasma vitamin E levels and improved responses to tests evaluating immune function, including cell-mediated immunity. Not all of the subjects receiving supplements demonstrated an improvement in immune response, but those who did improved in all measurements. Meydani

and colleagues[60] emphasized that long-term studies using lower levels of vitamin E are required before recommendations can be developed. Nevertheless, this observation supports the need to maintain vitamin E intakes that meet the current RDA.

Among 209 older people living in the community,[19] vitamin E status based on plasma alpha-tocopherol levels was negatively related to the number of infections reported during the previous 3 years. It has been suggested that vitamin E prevents the peroxidation of the polyunsaturated fatty acids in the membranes that control the recognition of foreign bodies and the active response of immune cells.

Vitamin D

Although vitamin D traditionally has been considered a vitamin, recent evidence indicates that it is actually a hormone. A hormone is a chemical substance produced in one organ of the body that regulates an activity in another organ of the body. Major functions of vitamin D are the regulation of blood calcium levels, the absorption of calcium in the intestine, and the mobilization of calcium from the bone.[100]

Sources of vitamin D. Vitamin D can be supplied to the body through food or supplements, or it can be synthesized in the skin. The form of vitamin D commonly used in food fortification and also produced in the skin is **vitamin D_3, cholecalciferol.** Vitamin D_3 is synthesized in the skin by the irradiation of **7-dehydrocholesterol,** a sterol naturally found in skin cells. The concentration of 7-dehydrocholesterol and the quantity and quality of ultraviolet radiation are major factors in the control of vitamin D_3 synthesis.[100]

Aging influences vitamin D_3 synthesis in several ways. First, older people have a lower concentration of 7-dehydrocholesterol in their skin compared to younger people. Under similar lighting conditions, individuals age 80 synthesized less than half the amount of vitamin D_3 as individuals age 20.[100] Second, older people with some degree of physical disability spend most of their time indoors and thus have limited exposure to ultraviolet light. Dietary vitamin D is found in a limited number of foods with milk, fortified to the level of 400 IU per quart,[27] the most common source. Unfortunately, many older people drink a limited amount of milk.

Absorption of vitamin D. Aging, per se, does not adversely affect vitamin D absorption.[100] After administration of an oral dose of 50,000 IU of vitamin D, peak serum concentrations in healthy elderly people were similar to those in young people, although serum levels returned to basal levels more rapidly in the younger individuals.[20] Vitamin D is not well absorbed by those with general malabsorption problems. Absorption of an orally administered dose of vitamin D was less than 4% when the flow of bile into the small intestine was interrupted.[21] Skin synthesis is an important source of vitamin D in people of all ages.

Metabolism of vitamin D. Vitamin D obtained from food, supplements, or endogenous synthesis undergoes two biochemical reactions in the conversion to its biologically active form[100]: (1) in the liver, vitamin D is hydroxylated to **25-hydroxyvitamin D (25[OH]D),** and (2) in the kidneys, 25(OH)D is hydroxylated to **1,25-dihydroxyvitamin D (1,25[OH]$_2$D).** It is 1,25(OH)$_2$D that is responsible for the metabolic effects attributed to vitamin D.

Serum levels of vitamin D metabolites are influenced by age, vitamin D availability, **parathyroid hormone (PTH),** and kidney function. In general, serum levels of 25(OH)D are similar in younger and older adults if vitamin D intakes are adequate; they are also remarkably similar in older individuals from different geographic areas.

Studies with healthy older people indicate that serum 25(OH)D levels tend to decrease with advancing age, whereas serum levels of the active metabolite, 1,25(OH)$_2$D, tend to increase up to age 65 and then plateau.[24] Eastell and coworkers[24] consider this increase in 1,25(OH)$_2$D to represent an increased production of this metabolite in response to an intestinal resistance to the action of vitamin D. When calcium absorption declines because of intestinal resistance, serum calcium levels also decline, triggering the secretion of increased amounts of PTH. PTH attempts to restore serum calcium levels to normal by increasing the production of

1,25(OH)$_2$D, thereby raising calcium absorption to its normal level.

At times institutionalized older people given supplements of vitamin D demonstrate increased serum levels of 25(OH)D but no increase in serum levels of 1,25(OH)$_2$D.[1,18,35] This has been attributed to a deficiency of 1-α-hydroxylase, the enzyme present in the kidneys that is necessary for the conversion of 25(OH)D to the active dihydroxy metabolite.[35] The activity of 1-α-hydroxylase decreases with age, and the magnitude of the decrease is proportional to the age-related decrease in renal function. The glomerular filtration rate at which the reduced enzyme level becomes critical is believed to be 50 ml/min/1.73 m^2.[35] The glomerular filtration rate reported in healthy older men ages 75 to 84 in the Baltimore Longitudinal Study of Aging (BLSA) was 97 ml/min/1.73 m^2.[92] Thus it would seem that renal function must be greatly impaired before the loss of 1-α-hydroxylase becomes clinically important. Nevertheless, Rudman and colleagues[78] observed that bone fractures in institutionalized elderly men were more common among those with low blood levels of 1,25(OH)$_2$D and high blood urea nitrogen levels. It is likely that changes in renal function, as well as alterations in PTH secretion, account for the wide variability in serum vitamin D metabolite levels observed in older people.

Intake, sun exposure, and vitamin D requirements. Dietary intakes of vitamin D seldom equal the RDA of 5 μg (200 IU). Among 304 healthy older people in New Mexico,[72] the median dietary intake of vitamin D was 88 IU, although 26% were taking a vitamin D supplement. Those taking a supplement had higher plasma levels of 25(OH)D, although overall, mean plasma levels were only half those observed in young controls. In a Canadian population of 137 women and 49 men who were low income and lived alone,[23] mean intakes were 2 μg in the women and 1.9 μg in the men, approximately 40% of the RDA. Intakes of vitamin D were closely related to intakes of calcium in 426 older middle-class subjects in southern California.[36] Women consuming at least 440 mg of calcium each day were most likely to consume the recommended level of vitamin D, suggesting that milk products fortified with vitamin D contributed significantly to the intakes of both nutrients.

Because of the importance of sunlight and skin synthesis to vitamin D status, serum concentrations of 25(OH)D vary seasonally in those with some sun exposure.[100] Krall and coworkers[47] evaluated dietary vitamin D, serum 25(OH)D levels, and PTH concentrations in 333 healthy white postmenopausal women in Boston with a mean age of 58 years. These women had low mean intakes of calcium (408 mg per day) and vitamin D (112 IU per day). Each of these intakes is about 50% of the RDA. Vitamin D intake was higher, 427 IU, among users of supplements. The inverse relationship between serum PTH and 25(OH)D levels was dependent upon vitamin D intake (Table 6-1). When vitamin D intake was greater than 220 IU per day, serum PTH and 25(OH)D levels did not vary with the season. When intakes fell below 220 IU, serum 25(OH)D levels were highest between August and October, when sun exposure could be expected to be relatively high, and lowest between March and May, after the cold winter months. Serum 25(OH)D levels dropped by more than one third between the summer and winter examination periods, and serum PTH levels rose over that period.

When vitamin D intake or synthesis is not sufficient to maintain serum 25(OH)D and calcium absorption as needed to provide sufficient calcium to maintain normal blood calcium levels, PTH levels rise and bone calcium is mobilized to restore blood calcium levels to normal. Thus a major goal in the maintenance of bone health in older women is to prevent a rise in serum PTH levels and the subsequent loss of bone mineral. Knoll and others[47] concluded that a daily dietary intake of more than 220 IU of vitamin D a day would prevent a seasonal increase in PTH levels and the potential mobilization of skeletal calcium.

Webb and coworkers[101] evaluated the contribution of sunlight exposure to vitamin D status in men and women with mean ages of 81 to 83 years. They concluded that a daily total of 10 μg or 400 IU of vitamin D was necessary to maintain optimum 25(OH)D levels in those with minimal exposure to sunlight. Based on the large proportion of their elderly people who had elevated PTH despite 25(OH)D levels in the normal range, these authors suggest that older people may require higher 25(OH)D levels to maintain adequate synthesis of 1,25(OH)$_2$D. Low levels of 25(OH)D and low sunshine scores have been associated with hip fractures in elderly individuals.[53] A daily supplement containing 10 μg of vitamin D was sufficient to maintain normal 25(OH)D levels in these institutionalized people despite limited

TABLE 6-1   *Seasonal Variations in Serum Parameters in Older Women With Low Intakes of Vitamin D*

	March-May	November-February	August-October
Age (years)	60	59	58
Calcium intake (mg/day)	381	412	440
Serum total calcium (mmol/L)	2.29	2.30	2.34
Serum parathyroid hormone (ng/L)	37	34	30*
Serum 25(OH)D (nmol/L)	63	75	93*

*The August-October levels are significantly different from the March-May levels.
Modified from Krall EA and others: Effect of vitamin D intake on seasonal variations in parathyroid hormone secretion in postmenopausal women, *N Engl J Med* 321:1777, 1989.

sunlight exposure. At the same time, it is ill-advised for older individuals to consume supplements containing more than 10 μg of vitamin D in light of its known toxic effects.[27]

Vitamin K

Vitamin K intake and serum levels. Relatively few studies exist that describe the usual dietary intakes and normal blood levels of vitamin K in adults of all ages. This is related to the fact that analytical methods that can ascertain the **phylloquinone** (vitamin K) content of food, blood, and tissues are only now being developed. It has been estimated that current dietary intakes of vitamin K are in the range of 300 to 500 μg a day, levels five to 10 times the estimated requirement. Since major dietary sources of phylloquinone are green vegetables, intakes may be less than adequate in older people who eat few vegetables because of cost, chewing problems, or personal preference. In younger adults (mean age = 36) serum phylloquinone levels were not related to age, sex, or number of servings of green vegetables eaten per week.[63]

A comparison of younger and older adults revealed that serum phylloquinone levels were positively related to plasma triglyceride levels.[81] Although the older individuals had higher plasma levels of phylloquinone, they had decreased vitamin levels when expressed per millimole of plasma triglyceride. There does appear to be a seasonal variation in plasma vitamin K levels, with higher values recorded in September and October. This may relate to a seasonal variation in the consumption of green vegetables or the fourfold increase in the vitamin K content of milk and dairy products in the summer months. Low plasma phylloquinone levels are being evaluated as possible prognostic indicators of **hypoprothrombinemia** in older patients taking antibiotics.

WATER-SOLUBLE VITAMINS

Thiamin

Absorption of thiamin. Little is known about age-related changes, if any, in the requirements and metabolism of thiamin. Thiamin absorption is not impaired in older people unless associated with use of alcohol. At physi-

ologic concentrations, thiamin is absorbed by an energy-requiring, carrier-mediated process. Folic acid is required for the synthesis of these carrier proteins and is therefore considered essential for thiamin absorption. Among older women in Ireland,[83] however, thiamin status was not influenced by folate status either before or after supplementation with folic acid. **Polyphenols** found in tea and coffee have been described as having **antivitamin** activity. Thiamin status in the older Irish women was unrelated to polyphenol intake despite high daily intakes of tea (1,170 g) and coffee (60 g).

Thiamin requirements. The minimum requirement for thiamin is 0.3 mg/1,000 kcal, although the recommended level is 0.5 mg/1,000 kcal. Daily intake should not fall below 1 mg even if total energy intake is less than 2,000 kcal. The 1989 RDA suggests 1.2 mg for men and 1 mg for women over age 50.[27] Thiamin plays an important role in the metabolism of neurotransmitters and the control of nerve transmission and fatty acid metabolism, and it is necessary regardless of caloric intake. An early study comparing thiamin metabolism in younger (mean age = 34) and older (mean age = 70) men[38] found no differences in (1) the rate of decrease in thiamin excretion when placed on a deficient diet, (2) the appearance of clinical signs of deficiency during 3 months of vitamin depletion, and (3) the rate of increase in urinary excretion after vitamin supplementation. Thiamin requirements and utilization in alcoholism are discussed in Chapter 9.

Thiamin intake and biochemical status. Thiamin intake decreases with age, although this more likely results from the observed decrease in caloric intake rather than a change in the type of food consumed. In a comparison of healthy elderly, institutionalized elderly, and healthy young adults,[69] daily thiamin intake was significantly lower in the older groups who consumed 1.09 and 0.73 mg, respectively, versus 1.44 mg in the younger group. In contrast, thiamin intake per 1,000 kcal was the same among the three groups, 0.67 to 0.71 mg. In a survey of older Canadian women,[14] thiamin intake per 1,000 kcal was 0.8 mg in those ages 55 to 64 and 0.9 mg in those ages 65 to 74 and 75 and over. Among healthy, independently living older adults in Boston,[59] low intakes of thiamin were associated with caloric intakes below 22 kcal/kg body weight.

The most appropriate test for the evaluation of thiamin status is the **erythrocyte transketolase assay,** which measures enzyme activity before and after the addition of thiamin pyrophosphate. The percentage of increase in enzyme activity after the addition of thiamin pyrophosphate indicates the degree of deficiency. The erythrocyte transketolase test is highly sensitive; enzyme activity remains normal on an intake of 0.5 mg of thiamin daily.[15] Estimates of the prevalence of thiamin deficiency have ranged from 1% in older people in New York,[15] to 37% in older Japanese adults,[39] to 48% in older Irish women.[83] O'Rourke and coworkers[69] measured erythrocyte thiamin levels and found that 13% of community-living older people were at risk of thiamin deficiency, compared to 46% of institutionalized elderly people.

In most cases thiamin deficiency can be reversed by increasing thiamin intake. In a double-blind study of older Irish women living in their own homes, erythrocyte transketolase activity was restored to normal in those receiving 10 mg of thiamin a day, whereas enzyme activity remained low in those given a placebo[84] (Table 6-2). Also, the symptoms of thiamin deficiency (fatigue and poor appetite) decreased and caloric intake increased in those

women given the vitamin but not in those given the placebo. Daily intakes of 2.5 mg of thiamin (two times the RDA) will not maintain appropriate biochemical status in older men who drink alcoholic beverages regularly and are deficient in folic acid.[96] Good sources of dietary thiamin such as whole-grain or enriched breads and cereals, lean pork, legumes, and nuts should be emphasized to older clients.

Riboflavin

Absorption and metabolism of riboflavin. The absorption of riboflavin, essential for energy metabolism in the cell, does not appear to differ in older and younger adults. Alexander and coworkers[2] evaluated riboflavin nutriture in 24 ambulatory, institutionalized older women whose mean intake from food was 1.8 mg a day. (The RDA is 1.2 mg for women and 1.4 mg for men.) On this level of intake, **erythrocyte glutathione reductase enzyme activity** (which requires riboflavin as a cofactor) was normal, and urinary riboflavin equalled 1.64 µg/mg creatinine. When dietary intake was nearly doubled by the addition of a riboflavin supplement of 1.7 mg, urinary excretion also about doubled to 3.41 µg/mg creatinine.

Riboflavin intake and biochemical status. Riboflavin status may actually improve with advancing age in both people who take supplements and those who don't, with the most striking change occurring after age 50. This

TABLE 6-2   *Influence of Thiamin Supplementation on Energy Intake and Well-Being in Older Irish Women*

	Placebo Group (n = 40)		Thiamin-Supplemented Group (n = 40)	
	Before	After	Before	After
Number thiamin deficient	19	18	19	0
Energy intake (kcal)	1,648	1,662	1,679	1,970
Appetite score	5.9	6.1	6.0	9.5*
Fatigue score	5.0	4.9	5.4	1.2*
General well-being score	4.8	4.8	5.2	8.8*

*The women rated each physical parameter on a scale from 0 (I never have this condition) to 10 (I have this condition all of the time); a high score is appropriate for appetite and general well-being; a low score is appropriate for fatigue.
Modified from Smidt LJ and others: Influence of thiamin supplementation on the health and general well-being of an elderly Irish population with marginal thiamin deficiency, *J Gerontol* 46:M16, 1991.

suggestion comes from a screening of 667 people ranging from 20 to 87 years of age at a state fair.[28] In that group, 6% of those over age 50 who were not taking supplements had less-than-acceptable enzyme activity levels compared to 11% of those ages 20 to 49. The relationship between total riboflavin intake and enzyme activity is more closely defined at lower levels of intake; little change in enzyme activity occurs when intake reaches 3 to 4 mg daily and the enzyme system is saturated with riboflavin.

Riboflavin intake generally is adequate among healthy older people with average caloric intakes; however, particular food groups influence riboflavin intake. Among 19 older lacto-ovo-vegetarian women,[66] none consumed less than the RDA for riboflavin, whereas three of 14 nonvegetarian women of similar age consumed less than the standard. The lacto-ovo-vegetarian women appeared to consume more milk and fortified cereal products. In contrast, frail elderly subjects with a mean age of 76[56] who had caloric intakes well below the RDA and low consumption of milk and dairy products were consuming less than three fourths of the recommended level of riboflavin. Some reports[90] indicate lower intakes of riboflavin in elderly blacks, which could relate to their lower consumption of dairy products.

One benefit of obtaining riboflavin from dairy products is the contribution these foods make toward meeting the calcium requirement. Based on the food intake patterns of 24 healthy older women,[2] when 40% or more of the RDA for riboflavin is provided by milk and dairy products, the individual is likely to meet at least 80% of the RDA for calcium.

Niacin

Niacin intake and status. Niacin requirements and metabolism in aging people have received little attention recently. An older study of niacin status in elderly people did reveal little evidence of biochemical deficiency. Among 116 institutionalized and independent-living older people,[33] only three had urinary excretions of niacin metabolites below the acceptable level. However, in a national survey,[90] more than one third of low-income older people consumed less than 67% of the RDA for niacin. In a Tennessee study,[97] older men living in the community had mean intakes of niacin that were below the RDA; they were consuming 13.1 mg, compared to the RDA of 15 mg or equivalent. The women in that study had a mean intake of 14 mg, compared to their RDA of 13 mg or equivalent. The Food and Nutrition Board[27] notes that some foods such as milk and eggs that are not high in preformed niacin do contain high levels of tryptophan, which can be used to synthesize niacin (60 mg tryptophan = 1 mg niacin). The relative efficiency of niacin synthesis from tryptophan in older people has not been evaluated.

Ascorbic Acid

Absorption of ascorbic acid. The association of ascorbic acid with antioxidant functions that may help prevent the development of atherosclerotic plaques and cataracts, physiologic problems of great importance to older people, has brought renewed attention to this vitamin. In general ascorbic acid is highly absorbed; at levels of intake usually supplied in food (20 to 120 mg a day), absorption is 90% or higher.[71] There is no current evidence to suggest that ascorbic acid absorption in healthy older adults differs from that in young adults with similar ascorbic acid status.[12,13] Ascorbic acid was reported to be poorly absorbed by hospitalized elderly women (mean age = 83), but the medical condition and ascorbic acid status of these women were not described.[22]

Metabolism of ascorbic acid. Controlled studies evaluating ascorbic acid absorption, tissue uptake, and excretion in young and elderly men and women indicate that ascorbic acid status rather than age is the major influence on these processes.[12,13] All subjects consumed a vitamin C–restricted diet supplying less than 10 mg of ascorbic acid daily for several weeks until plasma ascorbic acid levels fell to 0.4 mg/dl; then, all were given a 500 mg supplement daily for 3 weeks. Vitamin C metabolism was evaluated in the depleted and supplemented states.

Depleted subjects, regardless of age, had lower plasma levels of ascorbic acid after administration of a 500 mg test dose than supplemented subjects and excreted a smaller amount of ascorbic acid in the urine. This was expected, since absorbed ascorbic acid would be taken up more rapidly by the tissues in depleted individuals. In depleted subjects 96% of the test dose entered tissue storage sites, compared to about 48% in the supplemented individuals. Conversely, supplemented subjects excreted about 40% of the test dose, although excretion was somewhat slowed in the older group. Vitamin C urinary excretion is controlled by glomerular filtration and active tubular reabsorption. At plasma concentrations up to 1.4 mg/dl, about 97% of the ascorbic acid in the glomerular filtrate is reabsorbed. Above this threshold ascorbic acid spills over into the urine.

Ascorbic acid requirements. Ascorbic acid metabolism does differ between men and women regardless of age, and this probably relates to the gender differences in fat-free mass. In older men and women on controlled intakes ranging from 30 to 280 mg a day, plasma levels were significantly lower in men at all levels of intake[94] (Table 6-3). All were nonsmokers. Women reached a plasma level of about 1 mg/dl on an intake of about 90 mg a day; in contrast, older men required an intake of 150 mg a day (the RDA for both sexes is 60 mg). On intakes of 60 mg, the current recommended daily allowance, the older men had marginal plasma ascorbic acid levels (0.5 mg/dl), suggesting risk of vitamin C deficiency. In men plasma levels do not exceed about 1 mg/dl regardless of intake.

The total body pool of ascorbic acid is believed to reach a maximum at 20 mg/kg body weight with a steady-state plasma level of 1 mg/dl.[71] These values are based on young adult men, and currently no such data are available for women or older people of either sex. It does appear that older men require more than two times the current RDA to maintain this steady state. The RDA for ascorbic acid requires further evaluation in aging adults. Older men and smokers are at particular risk.

Ascorbic acid intake and biochemical status. In older people socioeconomic status, gender, and ascorbic acid status are related. Median ascorbic acid intakes of women ages 65 to 74 were 71 and 92 mg, respectively, in those with incomes below and above the poverty line.[25] Equivalent intakes for men were only 45 and 85 mg. In a national survey,[91] 7% of low-income white women, 14% of low-income white men, and more than half of low-income black men had serum ascorbic acid levels indicative of deficiency. In contrast, among 677 older economically advantaged people in Boston,[40] only one had a plasma level indicative of deficiency (less than 0.2 ml/dl); 6% of the men and 3% of the women had marginal status (0.2 to 0.4 mg/dl). There was no relationship between plasma ascorbic acid level and age (ages ranged from 60 to 98), although women had higher levels and smokers somewhat lower levels. One fourth of this community-living population consumed at least 300 mg of ascorbic acid daily; 42% reported using supplements.

Assessment of 260 institutionalized older people in Boston[82] revealed that nine were consuming less than 67% of the RDA for vitamin C; median plasma values for men and women were 1 to 1.14 mg/dl. When ascorbic acid deficiency is observed in chronically ill older patients, it usually is related to prior intake and can be corrected with supplementation of 100 mg a day.[65] Ascorbic acid is lost if cooked vegetables are held at serving temperature for several hours, as sometimes happens in home-delivered meal programs (see Chapter 13). Citrus fruits are a better source of ascorbic acid under such circumstances.

TABLE 6-3 *Ascorbic Acid Intake and Resulting Plasma Levels in Older Men and Women*

Total Ascorbic Acid Intake (mg/day)*	Plasma Ascorbic Acid Level (mg/dl)	
	Men	Women
45	0.28	0.50
60	0.50	0.90
90	0.79	1.09
150	1.05	1.27
280	1.09	1.43

*RDA, 60 mg.
Modified from VanderJagt DJ, Garry PJ, Bhagavan HN: Ascorbic acid intake and plasma levels in healthy elderly people, *Am J Clin Nutr* 46:290, 1987.

Current research with ascorbic acid. The role of ascorbic acid as an antioxidant is being evaluated in regard to several problems of aging, including cataracts and atherosclerosis. The incidence of **senile cataracts** in the United States is 4% (ages 52 to 64), 18% (ages 65 to 74), and 46% (ages 75 to 85).[87] Senile cataracts are caused by chemical changes in the proteins in the lens of the eye that result in protein aggregates, a loss of transparency, and obscured vision. These chemical changes involve oxidation reactions, and current work is evaluating the relationship between an individual's antioxidant status and the development of cataracts. Ascorbic acid concentration in the lens of the eye is more than 30 times the concentration in the plasma and thus may play a role in preventing oxidation reactions.[87]

Ascorbic acid also appears to inhibit the oxidation of low-density lipoprotein (LDL).[98] Oxidized LDL attaches to the intima of the arterial wall and promotes the development of atherosclerotic lesions. When added to cell cultures at physiologic levels, ascorbic acid was more effective in preventing the oxidation of LDL than was alpha-tocopherol.[44]

Plasma ascorbic acid levels were related to high-density lipoprotein (HDL) cholesterol levels in a group of 672 Boston elderly.[41] Average HDL cholesterol levels ranged from 43 mg/dl in those whose plasma ascorbic acid levels were less than 1 mg/dl to 50 mg/dl in those whose plasma ascorbic acid levels were at least 1.5 mg/dl. This remained true after adjustment for sex, age, race, skinfold thickness, exercise, and dietary intakes of related nutrients. Placebo-controlled trials of long duration are needed to examine and confirm the relationship between ascorbic acid and plasma cholesterol fractions.

Vitamin B_6 (Pyridoxine)

Vitamin B_6 is an important coenzyme in the metabolism of protein and amino acids and has been studied in relation to the level of protein in the diet. Vitamin B_6 has a role in immune function and the synthesis of neurotransmitters, issues of great importance to the health and well-being of aging adults. A major concern, however, is appropriate measures of vitamin B_6 status, as it appears that biochemical parameters used in younger people may not be valid in older people.

Vitamin B_6 absorption and metabolism. Many studies have reported decreased levels of **plasma pyridoxal phosphate (PLP)** in older people; however, decreased vitamin intakes or metabolic changes, rather than impaired absorption, seem to be the cause. In men ages 25 to 35, 45 to 55, and 65 to 75 given 2.9 mg of vitamin B_6, neither the maximum rise in plasma pyridoxine levels nor the time required to reach the maximum level differed among age groups.[45] After pyridoxine is absorbed, it goes to the liver, where it is phosphorylated. The rise in plasma PLP as a proportion of total plasma vitamin B_6 was also similar in all age groups, indicating that the activity of liver phosphorylation enzymes was unchanged in older adults. Nevertheless, basal levels of both plasma PLP and total plasma vitamin B_6 in the two older age groups were about 60% of those in the youngest age group. Basal plasma PLP levels were 76 mmol/L in those ages 25 to 35, compared to 48 and 42 mmol/L in those ages 45 to 55 and 65 to 75, respectively. Plasma PLP is bound to albumin, which protects it from hydrolysis; therefore a decrease in circulating albumin could bring about a decrease in plasma PLP; however, albumin levels were unchanged in the older age groups. Since PLP is stored in skeletal muscle, Lee and Leklem[52] suggested that differences in vitamin B_6 metabolism between younger and older adults may relate to decreased muscle mass in older age groups.

Vitamin B_6 requirement. Recent work at the Human Nutrition Research Center on Aging in Boston indicates that the vitamin B_6 requirements of healthy elderly men and women are about 1.96 and 1.90 mg a day, respectively.[75] These values are based on the amount of vitamin B_6 required to bring about normal excretion levels of **xanthurenic acid** after administration of a tryptophan load. Vitamin B_6 is a cofactor for several enzyme reactions in the conversion of tryptophan to niacin. When vitamin B_6 is not available in required amounts, tryptophan metabolism cannot proceed normally and xanthurenic acid, an intermediary metabolite, begins to accumulate and is excreted in the urine. In the Boston study, the older subjects were depleted of vitamin B_6 and then fed gradually increasing amounts of the vitamin at two different levels of dietary protein (0.8 and 1.2 g/kg body weight). In contrast to younger individuals, in whom protein intakes significantly influence vitamin B_6 requirements, the vitamin B_6 requirements in these older individuals did not vary according to protein intake. Older women developed biochemical signs of vitamin B_6 deficiency faster than older men. This could relate to the smaller skeletal mass and vitamin B_6 stores of older women compared to older men.

This study[75] raised serious questions about the sensitivity of biochemical measures of vitamin B_6 status as applied to older people. The **tryptophan load test** was the most sensitive to vitamin B_6 nutriture. Increases in urinary xanthurenic acid excretion became evident within 5 days after the institution of a vitamin B_6-deficient diet, and excretion returned to baseline levels when vitamin B_6 intake became adequate. In contrast, **erythrocyte aspartate transaminase enzyme activity** (commonly used to evaluate vitamin B_6 status in all age groups) did not respond to small changes in vitamin B_6 intake after vitamin depletion. Dutch workers[55] have also expressed concern about the sensitivity of this measurement to marginal vitamin B_6 status. They suggested that lower levels of erythrocyte PLP lead to reduced synthesis of the aspartate transaminase apoenzyme, thereby introducing a second variable in addition to availability of the vitamin B_6 coenzyme.

This work also points to a discrepancy between the current RDA[27] for vitamin B_6 for people over age 50 and the apparent requirement; this is especially pertinent for women. The *apparent requirement* of older men was found to be 1.96 mg, whereas the RDA designed to provide a measure of safety is 2 mg. In women the *apparent requirement* of 1.90 mg is above the current RDA of 1.6 mg. Moreover, the form of vitamin B_6 fed in the Boston study is highly bioavailable; the vitamin found in dietary sources may be bound and in part unavailable. Thus a goal for older people should be daily consumption of at least the current RDA. Further work is needed to confirm

this apparent age-related increase in vitamin B_6 requirements.

One important consequence of vitamin B_6 deficiency in older people is impaired cell-mediated immunity. Vitamin B_6 depletion resulted in a decreased number of lymphocytes and depressed mitogenic responses in older men and women.[61] These indices were restored to normal after vitamin repletion. Vitamin B_6 deficiency may in fact contribute to the age-related decline in immune function in some older people.

Vitamin B_6 intake and biochemical status. Age, sex, health, and use of supplements influence vitamin B_6 status. Plasma PLP levels in 617 healthy men from the BLSA are described in Fig. 6-2.[92] Among those not taking supplements, plasma levels decreased by 0.9 ng/ml per decade. Plasma levels were higher in supple-

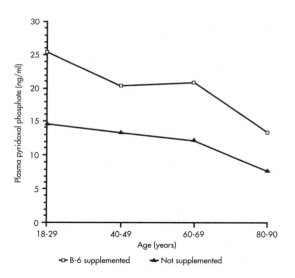

FIG. 6-2 Effect of age and supplementation on plasma pyridoxal phosphate (vitamin B_6) level. Healthy older men have lower plasma pyridoxal phosphate levels than healthy younger men regardless of supplementation. These men were participants in the Baltimore Longitudinal Study of Aging.

(Data from US Department of Health and Human Services: Normal human aging: the Baltimore Longitudinal Study of Aging, NIH Pub No 84-2450, Washington, DC, 1984, US Government Printing Office.)

ment users at all ages and were not significantly different in older versus younger people. In those not using supplements, the number of plasma values indicating marginal status increased from 3% in the group ages 40 to 49 to 12% in the group age 80 and over.

Less-than-optimum vitamin B_6 status is common in older people based on dietary intake or biochemical measurements. Erythrocyte enzyme activity levels identified vitamin B_6 deficiency in 70% of a group of institutionalized older people[31]; 48% of the men and 55% of the women were consuming less than 1 mg of vitamin B_6 a day. A survey by the U.S. Department of Agriculture (U.S.D.A.)[89] of 394 low-income people age 75 and over reported that mean intakes of vitamin B_6 were about half that recommended.

Vitamin B_6 status appears to be influenced by health status as well as by total intake. Manore and coworkers[58] studied vitamin B_6 status in 198 low-income older people in Arizona using 3-day dietary records and plasma PLP levels. Thirty-two percent of this population had plasma levels indicative of deficiency, and only 5% of those were using supplements. In contrast, 95% of those with the highest plasma PLP levels were using supplements. Mean intakes from food were 1.5 and 1.8 mg a day, respectively, in the groups with low and high plasma levels.

Several individuals with the lowest plasma PLP levels were consuming appropriate levels of vitamin B_6 (2.5 mg a day); however, they also reported two or more serious health problems (e.g., heart disease, kidney disorders, diabetes). Such problems were less common among those with higher plasma vitamin levels. This raises questions about the vitamin B_6 status of elderly people with significant chronic disease, in spite of appropriate dietary intakes. It is also prudent to avoid vitamin B_6 supplements above the RDA in light of reported toxicity and neural dysfunction in those consuming inappropriately high amounts (see Chapter 9).

Good dietary sources of vitamin B_6 should be emphasized in diet planning with older people. In the NHANES II study,[46] dietary vitamin B_6 was supplied in about equal amounts by animal and vegetable foods. Meat and milk are good sources and also contain high amounts of protein. Fruits, potatoes, and other vegetables and ready-to-eat cereals add to the vitamin B_6 intake without adding protein, thus increasing the vitamin B_6-to-protein ratio. Vitamin B_6 intakes in the NHANES II study were significantly lower in elderly blacks compared to elderly whites. Median dietary intakes were 1.36 and 0.98 mg in the white men and women over age 65 and 0.98 and 0.81 mg in the black men and women over age 65. The cost of foods high in vitamin B_6, as well as differences in the use of milk products, may contribute to this difference.

Folate

Absorption of folate. Folate, or **folacin,** is a general term referring to the family of compounds that have a structure and biologic action similar to folic acid (**pteroylglutamic acid**). About three fourths of the folates occurring naturally in foods are present as polyglutamates,[7] containing more than one glutamic acid residue per molecule; however, only monoglutamates are absorbed in the small intestine. **Folylpolyglutamate hydrolase enzyme,** secreted by the intestinal mucosa, cleaves the polyglutamate molecule to a monoglutamate molecule that is absorbed. It had been suggested that older people lacked sufficient hydrolase to release and absorb naturally occurring folates in food.[8] That report was disproven by Bailey and coworkers,[7] who administered labeled **folylpolyglutamate** and **folylmonoglutamate** to a group of younger and older individuals. They recovered similar amounts of labeled metabolites in the urine from both age groups. Also, mucosal biopsy samples revealed a similar activity level of hydrolase enzyme in younger and older subjects. Although age per se does not decrease folate absorption, gastrointestinal problems associated with chronic disease or the use of particular drugs can lead to reduced folate uptake.

Poor folate status resulting from low dietary intake or other causes can itself impair folate absorption. Folate deficiency leads to both structural and functional changes in the upper jejunum, the primary site of folate absorption.

If mucosal damage is severe, even monoglutamate absorption is limited. Intestinal changes related to folate deficiency can be reversed with folate supplementation.

Atrophic gastritis (see Chapter 4) and the rise in pH in the proximal small intestine from 6.7 (normal) to 7.1 (atrophic gastritis) can impair folate absorption, which requires the acid environment. Absorption of a test dose of folic acid was 51% in healthy elderly people (mean age = 70 years) but only 31% in those with atrophic gastritis (mean age = 72 years).[79] When the folic acid was administered with acid, absorption rose to 54% in those with atrophic gastritis but remained unchanged in those with normal acid secretion. Surprisingly, older people with atrophic gastritis have been found at times to have higher serum levels of folate than normal elderly subjects (9.6 versus 7.9 ng/ml).[48] It appears that the reduced level of acid in the upper small intestine allows the growth of large numbers of folate-synthesizing bacteria, which provide a compensatory source of folate.

Liver folate content is believed to provide a direct measure of body folate stores. Liver folate stores determined in 560 liver specimens obtained at autopsy tended to be lower in people who had died after age 60.[37] Vitamin levels were also lower among individuals who had long-term illnesses than among those who died accidentally. Only two subjects had liver folate levels below 3 μg/g, a level indicative of severe deficiency. Although severe deficiency was not a general problem in that population, older people with long-standing chronic disease would appear to be at greater risk.

Folate requirement. The folate requirement of older people has been surrounded by controversy. Questions relating to the older person's ability to absorb folate led some to suggest an elevated requirement. Alternatively, surveys of adults of various ages led the Food and Nutrition Board[27] to reduce the recommended intake for folate from 400 μg a day in all adults to 200 μg a day for men and 180 μg a day for women.

According to Herbert,[34] serum folate levels are a sensitive measure of early negative folate balance. If folate intake or absorption is severely reduced, folate serum levels will fall below 3 ng/ml within a few weeks. If the situation persists, the individual eventually will reduce tissue and liver stores. **Red cell folate** levels are a good measure of liver folate stores. When red cell folate levels drop below 160 ng/ml, tissue stores are depleted and liver stores are below 1.6 μg/g (normal liver stores are 5 to 17 μg/g).

Older people have been reported to maintain appropriate biochemical folate levels on intakes even lower than the current RDA. Jagerstad and Westesson[43] studied a group of 35 healthy Swedish pensioners who maintained appropriate whole blood folate levels over a period of 6 years on daily intakes of 145 to 175 μg of folate. Among 270 healthy older adults in New Mexico,[29] about 40% consumed less than 200 μg a day of folate; however, only 8% had low serum folate levels and only 3% had low red blood cell folate levels. These data suggest that the recommended level of folate is sufficient to maintain appropriate storage levels in generally healthy people. Low serum folate levels are twice as likely to occur in hospitalized or institutionalized older people than in those residing in their own homes.[77] The greater prevalence of folic acid deficiency in chronically ill older people could be the result of drugs that interfere with folic acid absorption and metabolism and thereby elevate the requirement.

Folate intake and biochemical status. Income and folate status are related. In a Florida dietary survey,[5,77] 65% of low-income elderly had less than 200 μg of folic acid daily, compared to only 37% of those with higher incomes. Moreover, more than one third of the low-income group had intakes below 100 μg, or 50% of the RDA; this was true for only 3% of the upper income group. Most of the low-income people were at risk of folate deficiency according to their red cell folate concentrations (Fig. 6-3). Food records revealed that intakes of folate-rich foods were low; only 17% regularly used fresh vegetables, and only 30% regularly used citrus fruits. It was customary to boil vegetables for long periods of time; such cooking methods destroy folate. Irregular shopping trips can limit use of fruits and dark green vegetables and lower folate intakes. Low-cost sources of folate, with emphasis on preparation methods that enhance nutrient retention,

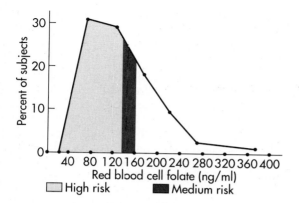

FIG. 6-3 Red blood cell folate level and risk of deficiency in low-income elderly blacks. Many low-income older blacks are at high risk of folate deficiency based on their red blood cell folate levels.

From Baily LB and others: Folacin and iron status and hematological findings in predominantly black elderly persons from urban low-income households, *Am J Clin Nutr* 32:2346, 1979. © American Society for Clinical Nutrition.)

should be stressed in nutrition education programs.

Vitamin B_{12}

Absorption of vitamin B_{12}. Vitamin B_{12} is required for the normal metabolism of neural tissue, and a deficiency results in degenerative changes in the **myelin sheath** and irreversible neurologic damage. Vitamin B_{12} is also required for the replication and metabolism of DNA and the maturation of the red blood cells. Intrinsic factor secreted by the chief cells of the gastric mucosa is required for the absorption of vitamin B_{12}. Lack of intrinsic factor leads to vitamin B_{12} deficiency and **pernicious anemia** (see Chapter 8).

Vitamin B_{12} absorption studies performed on 76-year-olds from the Goteborg, Sweden longitudinal study (n=38) who had normal serum vitamin B_{12} levels revealed urinary excretions of the labeled test dose ranging from 8.6% to 45.2%.[57] This compared favorably to the reference interval of 10% to 38% established with young people in that laboratory. When elderly subjects from the same study with low vitamin B_{12} concentrations (below 130

pmol/L) were tested, 13 of the 20 had normal absorption levels.

Suter and Russell[86] suggest that many older patients with poor vitamin B_{12} absorption have a problem other than a failure to secrete intrinsic factor. Atrophy of the gastric mucosa, with decreased production of acid, is a major cause of vitamin B_{12} malabsorption, even when intrinsic factor is available. Decreased secretion of hydrochloric acid results in decreased hydrolysis of proteins and decreased conversion of pepsinogen to pepsin, which further breaks down protein and releases protein-bound vitamin B_{12}. Many older people with apparently normal vitamin B_{12} absorption, based on tests performed with free cobalamin (vitamin B_{12}) are unable to absorb the food-bound vitamin.[16] Even in the presence of intrinsic factor, an acid environment enhances the binding of vitamin B_{12} to carrier proteins that facilitate its transfer to intrinsic factor. A rise in gastric pH permits bacterial overgrowth that can reduce vitamin B_{12} availability. Bacteria may bind the vitamin, thereby inhibiting its absorption, or metabolize or alter its structure. Individuals with gastrointestinal atrophy may require more dietary vitamin B_{12} than is currently recommended.[86] When all ability to absorb vitamin B_{12} is lost, **cobalamin** may have to be provided by injection.

Vitamin B_{12} intake and biochemical status. Information is limited on dietary intakes of vitamin B_{12} in older populations. This is particularly pertinent for low-income or vegetarian older people, since this vitamin is found only in animal foods, which tend to be expensive or consumed in lower amounts by vegetarians. In a U.S.D.A. survey[89] of low-income aged, however, dietary vitamin B_{12} was not a problem; mean intake for both sexes, including those age 75 and over, equaled the current RDA. Older vegetarian women in California[66] had vitamin B_{12} intakes much like nonvegetarian women of similar age. In a survey of institutionalized elderly people in Boston,[82] only 8% consumed less than two thirds of the RDA for vitamin B_{12}. A continuing problem is the limited information available on the true vitamin content of both fresh and processed foods.

Most healthy older people appear to have appropriate blood levels of vitamin B_{12}. In older people living in the community in New Mexico,[29] only 3% had deficient blood levels; among the Goteborg, Sweden, population,[68] 5% of the 70-year-olds (n = 293) and 6% of the 75-year-olds (n = 486) were at risk. An evaluation of low-income urban black and Hispanic older people[6] found no one at risk for vitamin B_{12} deficiency based on serum levels. There is always the possibility, however, that serum levels were being maintained at the expense of liver stores.

Many older people routinely receive injections of **cyanocobalamin** for treatment of a variety of symptoms, including fatigue and weakness. In a rural clinic 10% of older patients received injections of vitamin B_{12}.[51] This practice may contribute to the relatively low proportion of older people with blood levels indicative of deficiency.

Pantothenic Acid

Pantothenic acid is widely distributed in foods, and deficiency is unlikely in individuals consuming a varied diet. An evaluation of pantothenic acid intakes and biochemical levels in an elderly population[85] revealed no differences between those living in the community and those who were institutionalized with a higher incidence of chronic diseases. Average dietary intake was 5.9 mg per day, well within the estimated safe and adequate intake of 4 to 7 mg per day.[27] Blood pantothenic acid levels were similar in both groups, although vitamin excretion levels were higher in those consuming supplements. At this time there is no evidence to suggest that pantothenic acid status is a problem in older adults.

Biotin

Currently, information about biotin intake or status in older people is practically nonexistent. The safe and adequate daily intake is suggested to be 30 to 100 μg per day.[27] Biotin deficiency has been reported in alcoholics and in those consuming raw egg whites, which contain avidin. This binds biotin and inhibits its absorption. It has been suggested that a decrease in stomach acid may impair the release of food-bound biotin, thus making it unavailable for absorption.[86]

Summary

The roles of vitamins and the specific vitamin requirements of the aging adult are receiving increasing attention. The action of vitamin D acting as a hormone in controlling calcium metabolism and bone health and suggestions that vitamin E and ascorbic acid may participate in preventing atherosclerotic lesions have critical implications for health and well-being and the prevention of chronic disease. Both vitamin E and vitamin B_6 influence immune responses in older people, and ascorbic acid in its role as an antioxidant may retard development of cataracts. Despite our growing knowledge of vitamin actions, the particular vitamin requirements of older people remain uncertain. In healthy older people, vitamin absorption appears normal, but both prescription and over-the-counter drugs and changes in the gastrointestinal tract may interfere with vitamin absorption in older adults with chronic medical problems. Decreases in the gastric acid, which is normally required to release vitamin B_{12} from food and make it available for absorption, can result in a vitamin B_{12} deficiency even when intrinsic factor is present. The ascorbic acid requirement of healthy older men may be higher than indicated by the current RDA; also, the current RDA for vitamin B_6 may not offer any margin of safety for older adults and in the case of women may be lower than the actual requirement. Folic acid status is a problem in elderly people who consume low levels of citrus fruits and dark green vegetables. Older adults need to be cautioned about the inappropriate use of vitamin supplements, especially fat-soluble vitamin supplements; long-term use at levels above two times the RDA can result in toxicity.

REVIEW QUESTIONS

1. Are the RDAs adequate for most older persons? What evidence exists to suggest a decreased or an increased need for some vitamins as we age? Which vitamins are included in this group?

2. How do changes in the aging gastrointestinal tract influence digestion and absorption of vitamins? Are fat-soluble or water-soluble vitamins more affected by gastrointestinal changes in older persons? How can dietary constituents influence digestion and absorption of vitamins?
3. Why is vitamin D considered to be a hormone? How is vitamin D supplied to the body, and what factors influence absorption and use of the vitamin? Are any groups of older persons more likely than are others to suffer from poor vitamin D status?
4. What is known about the age-related changes in the requirements of the water-soluble vitamins? Do elderly persons consume adequate amounts of the water-soluble vitamins? For which water-soluble vitamins is there evidence that the RDA may be inadequate?
5. How can vitamins affect the immune system of the older person? Which vitamins play a role in enhancing immune status? Which vitamins may play a role in atherosclerosis and heart disease prevention?

SUGGESTED LEARNING ACTIVITIES

1. Go to the drug store and find two vitamin supplements that are marketed for the older consumer. Compare the levels of vitamins in each supplement to the RDA for older people and to a common multivitamin. How do they compare? Based on your investigation, would you recommend the vitamin supplement to an older person?
2. Go to the library and find an article on the Shute brothers (Evan and Wilfrid Shute) and their claims for vitamin E supplementation. Compare their claims to the current scientific evidence on vitamin E as an antioxidant.
3. Write a lesson plan for a three-part nutrition education program for an audience of older persons attending programs at an elder hostel. The title of the lesson plan is, "Vitamize your breakfast, lunch, and dinner—how to incorporate more vitamin-rich foods in all of your meals."
4. Diagram the differences between cell-mediated and humoral immunity. Show where vitamins are known to play a role in immune function.
5. Prepare a nutrition education handout on preserving vitamins when cooking vegetables. Include tips on purchasing, storing, and preparing the vegetables and show where nutrient losses commonly occur.

Key Terms

Provided here for review is a list of the major terms in this chapter. The definitions can be found in the Glossary, which begins on p. 336. To help you understand how these terms are applied, the page number is given for the first mention of each term in the chapter.

alpha tocopherol, 124
antioxidant, 127
antivitamin activity, 131
aspartate aminotransferase, 125
avidin, 140
beta carotene, 124
beta tocopherol, 127
bile salt, 123
carotenoid, 124
cell-mediated immune response, 128
chylomicron remnant, 124
cobalamin, 138
cyanocobalamin, 140
erythrocyte aspartate transaminase enzyme activity, 136
erythrocyte glutathione reductase enzyme activity, 132
erythrocyte transketolase assay, 132
fat soluble vitamin, 123
folacin, 137
folylmonoglutamate, 137
folylpolyglutamate, 137
folylpolyglutamate hydrolase enzyme, 137
free radical, 127
gamma tocopherol, 127
hepatic retinyl ester hydrolase, 125
hypervitaminosis A, 125
hypoprothrombinemia, 131
lipid peroxidation, 127
lipoprotein lipase, 124
micelle, 124
myelin sheath, 139
omega-3 fatty acids, 127
pancreatic lipase, 124
parathyroid hormone (PTH), 129

REFERENCES

1. Aksnes L and others: Serum levels of vitamin D metabolites in the elderly, *Acta Endocrinol* (Copenh) 121:27, 1989.
2. Alexander M and others: Relation of riboflavin nutriture in healthy elderly to intake of calcium and vitamin supplements: evidence against riboflavin supplementation, *Am J Clin Nutr* 39:540, 1984.
3. Anonymous: Processing of dietary retinoids is slowed in the elderly, *Nutr Rev* 49:116, 1991.
4. Asciutti-Moura LS and others: Vitamin A intake and vitamin A status in an elderly, institutionalized population, *Nutr Rep Int* 39:1107, 1989.
5. Bailey LB and others: Folacin and iron status and hematological findings in predominately black elderly persons from urban low-income households, *Am J Clin Nutr* 32:2346, 1979.
6. Bailey LB and others: Vitamin B_{12} status of elderly persons from urban low-income households, *J Am Geriatr Soc* 28:276, 1980.
7. Bailey LB and others: Effect of age on poly- and monoglutamyl folacin absorption in human subjects, *J Nutr* 114:1770, 1984.
8. Baker H, Jaslow SP, Frank O: Severe impairment of dietary folate utilization in the elderly, *J Am Geriatr Soc* 26:218, 1978.
9. Barnes KJ, Chen LH: Vitamin E status of the elderly in central Kentucky, *J Nutr Elderly* 1(3-4):41, 1981.
10. Bendich A: The safety of β-carotene, *Nutr Cancer,* 11:207, 1988.
11. Black DA, Heduan E, and Mitchell D: Hepatic stores of retinol and retinyl esters in elderly people, *Age Ageing* 17:337, 1988.
12. Blanchard J, Conrad KA, Garry PJ: Effects of age and intake on vitamin C disposition in females, *Eur J Clin Nutr* 44:447, 1990.
13. Blanchard J and others: Vitamin C disposition in young and elderly men, *Am J Clin Nutr* 51:837, 1990.
14. Bourn DM and others: Selected nutrient intakes of a cohort of Canadian postmenopausal women estimated from 3-day dietary records: sources of variance in nutrient intakes and probability estimates of their adequacy, *Nutr Res* 10:391, 1990.
15. Brin M and others: Some preliminary findings on the nutritional status of the aged in Onondaga County, New York, *Am J Clin Nutr* 17:240, 1965.
16. Carmel R and others: Food cobalamin malabsorption occurs frequently in patients with unexplained low serum cobalamin levels, *Arch Intern Med* 148:1715, 1988.
17. Carney EA, Russell RM: Correlation of dark adaptation test results with serum vitamin A levels in diseased adults, *J Nutr* 110:552, 1980.
18. Chapuy M-C, Chapuy P, Meunier PJ: Calcium and vitamin D supplements: effects on calcium metabolism in elderly people, *Am J Clin Nutr* 46:324, 1987.
19. Chavance M and others: Vitamin status, immunity and infections in an elderly population, *Eur J Clin Nutr* 43:827, 1989.
20. Clemens TL and others: Serum vitamin D_2 and vitamin D_3 metabolite concentrations and absorption of vitamin D_2 in elderly subjects, *J Clin Endocrinol Metab* 63:656, 1986.
21. Clements MR, Chalmers TM, Fraser DR: Enterohepatic circulation of vitamin D: a reappraisal of the hypothesis, *Lancet* 1:1376, 1984.
22. Davies HEF and others: Studies on the absorption of 1-xyloascorbic acid (vitamin C) in young and elderly subjects, *Hum Nutr Clin Nutr* 38C:463, 1984.
23. Delvin EE, Imbach A, Copti M: Vitamin D nutritional status and related biochemical indices in an autonomous elderly population, *Am J Clin Nutr* 48:373, 1988.

24. Eastell R and others: Interrelationship among vitamin D metabolism, true calcium absorption, parathyroid function, and age in women: evidence of an age-related intestinal resistance to 1,25-dihydroxyvitamin D action, *J Bone Miner Res* 6:125, 1991.
25. Fanelli MT, Woteki CE: Nutrient intakes and health status of older Americans: data from the NHANES II, *Ann NY Acad Sci* 561:94, 1989.
26. Food and Nutrition Board: *Recommended dietary allowances,* ed 9, Washington, DC, 1980, National Academy of Sciences.
27. Food and Nutrition Board: *Recommended dietary allowances,* ed 10, Washington, DC, 1989, National Academy of Sciences.
28. Garry PJ, Goodwin JS, Hunt WC: Nutritional status in a healthy elderly population: riboflavin, *Am J Clin Nutr* 36:902, 1982.
29. Garry PJ, Goodwin J, Hunt WC: Folate and vitamin B$_{12}$ status in a healthy elderly population, *J Am Geriatr Soc* 32:719, 1984.
30. Garry PJ and others: Vitamin A intake and plasma retinol levels in healthy elderly men and women, *Am J Clin Nutr* 46:989, 1987.
31. Guilland JC and others: Evaluation of pyridoxine intake and pyridoxine status among aged institutionalised people, *Int J Vitam Nutr Res* 54:185, 1984.
32. Handelman GJ and others: Oral α-tocopherol supplements decrease plasma γ-tocopherol levels in humans, *J Nutr* 115:807, 1985.
33. Harrill I, Cervone N: Vitamin status of older women, *Am J Clin Nutr* 30:431, 1977.
34. Herbert V: Nutritional anemias in the elderly. In Prinsley DM, Sandstead HH, editors: *Nutrition and aging,* New York, 1990, Alan R Liss.
35. Himmelstein S and others: Vitamin D supplementation in elderly nursing home residents increases 25(OH)D but not 1,25(OH)$_2$D, *Am J Clin Nutr* 52:701, 1990.
36. Holbrook TL, Barrett-Connor E: Calcium intake: covariates and confounders, *Am J Clin Nutr* 53:741, 1991.
37. Hoppner K, Lampi B: Folate levels in human liver from autopsies in Canada, *Am J Clin Nutr* 33:862, 1980.
38. Horwitt MK: Dietary requirements of the aged, *J Am Diet Assoc* 29:443, 1953.
39. Itoh R and others: Biochemical assessment of vitamin status in "healthy" elderly Japanese: relationships between intakes and biochemical measures of thiamine, riboflavin and ascorbic acid, *Nutr Rept Int* 39:509, 1989.
40. Jacob RA and others: Vitamin C status and nutrient interactions in a healthy elderly population, *Am J Clin Nutr* 48:1436, 1988.
41. Jacques PF and others: Ascorbic acid, HDL, and total plasma cholesterol in the elderly, *J Am Coll Nutr* 6:169, 1987.
42. Jacques PF and others: Nutritional status in persons with and without senile cataract: blood vitamin and mineral levels, *Am J Clin Nutr* 48:152, 1988.
43. Jagerstad M, Westesson A-K: Folate, *Scand J Gastroenterol* 14(suppl 52):196, 1979.
44. Jialal I, Vega GL, Grundy SM: Physiologic levels of ascorbate inhibit the oxidative modification of low-density lipoprotein, *Atherosclerosis* 82:185, 1990.
45. Kant AK, Moser-Veillon PB, Reynolds RD: Effect of age on changes in plasma, erythrocyte, and urinary B$_6$ vitamers after an oral vitamin B$_6$ load, *Am J Clin Nutr* 48:1284, 1988.
46. Kant AK, Block G: Dietary vitamin B$_6$ intake and food sources in the US population: NHANES II, 1976-1980, *Am J Clin Nutr* 52:707, 1990.
47. Krall EA and others: Effect of vitamin D intake on seasonal variations in parathyroid hormone secretion in postmenopausal women, *N Engl J Med* 321:1777, 1989.
48. Krasinski SD and others: Fundic atrophic gastritis in an elderly population: effect on hemoglobin and several serum nutritional indicators, *J Am Geriatr Soc* 34:800, 1986.
49. Krasinski SD and others: Relationship of vitamin A and vitamin E intake to fasting plasma retinol, retinol-binding protein, retinyl esters, carotene, α-tocopherol, and cholesterol among elderly people and young adults: increased plasma retinyl esters among vitamin A–supplement users, *Am J Clin Nutr* 49:112, 1989.
50. Krasinski SD and others: Postprandial plasma retinyl ester response is greater in older subjects compared with younger subjects, *J Clin Invest* 85:883, 1990.
51. Lawhorne L, Ringdahl D: Cyanocobalamin injections for patients without documented deficiency: reasons for administration and patient responses to proposed discontinuation, *JAMA* 261:1920, 1989.
52. Lee CM, and Leklem JE: Differences in vitamin B$_6$ status indicator responses between young and middle-aged women fed constant diets with two levels of vitamin B$_6$, *Am J Clin Nutr* 42:226, 1985.
53. Lips P and others: Determinants of vitamin D status in patients with hip fracture and in el-

derly control subjects, *Am J Clin Nutr* 46:1005, 1987.

54. Looker AC, Johnson CL, Underwood BA: Serum retinol levels of persons aged 4 to 74 years from three Hispanic groups, *Am J Clin Nutr* 48:1490, 1988.

55. Löwik MRH and others: Dose-response relationships regarding vitamin B_6 in elderly people: a nationwide nutritional survey (Dutch Nutritional Surveillance System), *Am J Clin Nutr* 50:391, 1989.

56. Ludman EK, Newman JM: Frail elderly: assessment of nutrition needs, *Gerontologist* 26:198, 1986.

57. Maiani G and others: Beta-carotene serum response in young and elderly females, *Eur J Clin Nutr* 43:749, 1989.

58. Manore MM and others: Plasma pyridoxal 5′-phosphate concentration and dietary vitamin B_6 intake in free-living, low-income elderly people, *Am J Clin Nutr* 50:339, 1989.

59. McGandy RB and others: Nutritional status survey of healthy, noninstitutionalized elderly: energy and nutrient intakes from 3-day diet records and nutrient supplements, *Nutr Res* 6:785, 1986.

60. Meydani SN and others: Vitamin E supplementation enhances cell-mediated immunity in healthy elderly subjects, *Am J Clin Nutr* 52:557, 1990.

61. Meydani SN and others: Vitamin B_6 deficiency impairs interleukin-2 production and lymphocyte proliferation in elderly adults, *Am J Clin Nutr* 53:1275, 1991.

62. Meydani M and others: Effect of long-term fish oil supplementation on vitamin E status and lipid peroxidation in women, *J Nutr* 121:484, 1991.

63. Mummah-Schendel LL, Suttie JW: Serum phylloquinone concentrations in a normal adult population, *Am J Clin Nutr* 44:686, 1986.

64. Murphy SP, Subar AF, Block G: Vitamin E intakes and sources in the United States, *Am J Clin Nutr* 52:361, 1990.

65. Newton HMV and others: The cause and correction of low blood vitamin C concentrations in the elderly, *Am J Clin Nutr* 42:656, 1985.

66. Nieman D and others: Dietary status of Seventh-day Adventist vegetarian and nonvegetarian elderly women, *J Am Diet Assoc* 89:1763, 1989.

67. Nilsson-Ehle H: Cyanocobalamin absorption in the elderly: results for healthy subjects and for subjects with low sodium cobalamin concentration, *Clin Chem* 32:1368, 1986.

68. Nilsson-Ehle H and others: Low serum cobalamin levels in a population study of 70- and 75-year-old subjects, *Dig Dis Sci* 34:716, 1989.

69. O'Rourke NP and others: Thiamine status of healthy and institutionalized elderly subjects: analysis of dietary intake and biochemical indices, *Age Ageing* 19:325, 1990.

70. Olson JA: Recommended dietary intakes (RDI) of vitamin A in humans, *Am J Clin Nutr* 45:704, 1987.

71. Olson JA, Hodges RE: Recommended dietary intakes (RDI) of vitamin C in humans, *Am J Clin Nutr* 45:693, 1987.

72. Omdahl JL and others: Nutritional status in a healthy elderly population: vitamin D, *Am J Clin Nutr* 36:1125, 1982.

73. Rasmussen HM and others: Serum concentrations of retinol and retinyl esters in adults in response to mixed vitamin A and carotenoid containing meals, *J Am Coll Nutr* 10:460, 1991.

74. Rhodus NL, Brown J: The association of xerostomia and inadequate intake in older adults, *J Am Diet Assoc* 90:1688, 1990.

75. Ribaya-Mercado JD and others: Vitamin B_6 requirements of elderly men and women, *J Nutr* 121:1062, 1991.

76. Ritenbaugh C: Carotenoids and cancer, *Nutr Today* 22:14, 1987.

77. Rosenberg IH and others: Folate nutrition in the elderly, *Am J Clin Nutr* 36(suppl):1060, 1982.

78. Rudman D and others: Fractures in the men of a Veterans Administration nursing home: relation to 1,25-dihydroxyvitamin D, *J Am Coll Nutr* 8:324, 1989.

79. Russell RM and others: Folic acid malabsorption in atrophic gastritis: possible compensation by bacterial folate synthesis, *Gastroenterology* 91:1476, 1986.

80. Ryan VC, Bower ME: Relationship of socioeconomic status and living arrangements to nutritional intake of the older person, *J Am Diet Assoc* 89:1805, 1989.

81. Sadowski JA and others: Phylloquinone in plasma from elderly and young adults; factors influencing its concentration, *Am J Clin Nutr* 50:100, 1989.

82. Sahyoun NR and others: Dietary intakes and biochemical indicators of nutritional status in an elderly, institutionalized population, *Am J Clin Nutr* 47:524, 1988.

83. Smidt LJ and others: Influence of folate status and polyphenol intake on thiamin status of Irish women, *Am J Clin Nutr* 52:1077, 1990.

84. Smidt LJ and others: Influence of thiamin sup-

plementation on the health and general well-being of an elderly Irish population with marginal thiamin deficiency, *J Gerontol* 46:M16, 1991.

85. Srinivasan V and others: Pantothenic acid nutritional status in the elderly—institutionalized and noninstitutionalized, *Am J Clin Nutr* 34:1736, 1981.

86. Suter PM, Russell RM: Vitamin requirements of the elderly, *Am J Clin Nutr* 45:501, 1987.

87. Taylor A: Associations between nutrition and cataract, *Nutr Rev* 47:225, 1989.

88. Thomas RR: *Improving America's diet and health: from recommendations to action*, Washington, DC, 1991, National Academy Press.

89. US Department of Agriculture: Food and nutrient intakes of individuals in 1 day: low-income households. November 1979-March 1980, National Food Consumption Survey 1977-78, Preliminary Report No 13, Washington, DC, 1982, US Government Printing Office.

90. US Department of Health and Human Services: Dietary intake source data: United States, 1976-1980, DHHS Pub No (PHS) 83-1681, Washington, DC, 1983, US Government Printing Office.

91. US Department of Health and Human Services: Hematological and nutritional biochemistry reference data for persons 6 months to 74 years of age: United States, 1976-1980, DHHS Pub No (PHS) 83-1682, Hyattsville, Md, 1982, US Government Printing Office.

92. US Department of Health and Human Services: Normal human aging: the Baltimore Longitudinal Study of Aging, NIH Pub No 84-2450, Washington, DC, 1984, US Government Printing Office.

93. US Department of Health and Human Services, US Department of Agriculture: Nutrition monitoring in the United States: an update report on nutrition monitoring, DHHS Pub No (PHS)89-1255, Washington, DC, 1989, US Government Printing Office.

94. VanderJagt DJ, Garry PJ, and Bhagavan HN: Ascorbic acid intake and plasma levels in healthy elderly people, *Am J Clin Nutr* 46:290, 1987.

95. Vandewoude MF, Vandewoude MG: Vitamin E status in a normal population: the influence of age, *J Am Coll Nutr* 6:307, 1987.

96. Vir SC, Love AH: Nutritional status of institutionalized and noninstitutionalized aged in Belfast, Northern Ireland, *Am J Clin Nutr* 32:1934, 1979.

97. Walker D, Beauchene R: The relationship of loneliness, social isolation, and physical health to dietary adequacy of independently living elderly, *J Am Diet Assoc* 91:300, 1991.

98. Wartanowicz M and others: The effect of α-tocopherol and ascorbic acid on the serum lipid peroxide level in elderly people, *Ann Nutr Metab* 28:186, 1984.

99. Watson RR and others: Effect of β-carotene on lymphocyte subpopulations in elderly humans: evidence for a dose-response relationship, *Am J Clin Nutr* 53:90, 1991.

100. Webb AR, Holick MF: The role of sunlight in the cutaneous production of vitamin D_3, *Ann Rev Nutr* 8:375, 1988.

101. Webb AR and others: An evaluation of the relative contributions of exposure to sunlight and of diet to the circulating concentrations of 25-hydroxyvitamin D in an elderly nursing home population in Boston, *Am J Clin Nutr* 51:1075, 1990.

102. Webb F: Absorption mechanisms for fat-soluble vitamins and the effect of other food constituents. In *Nutrition in health and disease and international development, Symposia from the XII International Congress of Nutrition*, New York, 1981, Alan R Liss.

7

Minerals in the Aged

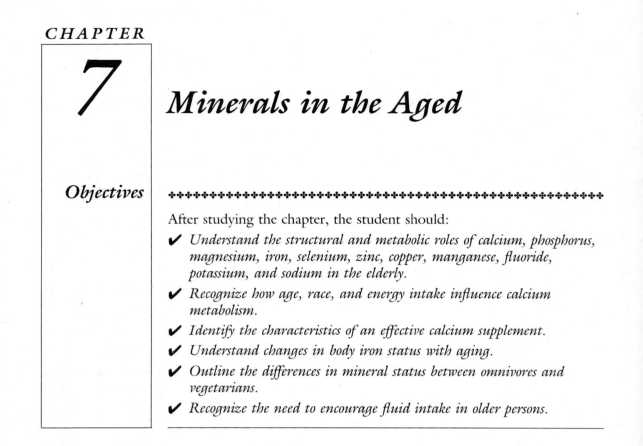

Objectives

❖❖❖

After studying the chapter, the student should:

✔ *Understand the structural and metabolic roles of calcium, phosphorus, magnesium, iron, selenium, zinc, copper, manganese, fluoride, potassium, and sodium in the elderly.*

✔ *Recognize how age, race, and energy intake influence calcium metabolism.*

✔ *Identify the characteristics of an effective calcium supplement.*

✔ *Understand changes in body iron status with aging.*

✔ *Outline the differences in mineral status between omnivores and vegetarians.*

✔ *Recognize the need to encourage fluid intake in older persons.*

Introduction

Balance techniques traditionally used to ascertain mineral requirements are both costly and tedious, and they demand extraordinary cooperation on the part of the subjects. The development of new methods using **labeled trace minerals** or **isotopes** has made it possible to measure minute amounts of minerals in tissues and fluids and has sparked renewed interest in both the structural and metabolic roles of these nutrients. This is especially true for older people because of age-related degenerative changes that involve particular minerals. Bone metabolism, glucose tolerance, and immune function undergo changes with advancing age and are closely related to mineral requirements and metabolism. The association of **selenium, calcium,** **potassium,** and **sodium** with the development of hypertension and cardiovascular disease has encouraged research evaluating these relationships. This chapter focuses on current knowledge about mineral requirements in the later years.

MACROMINERALS
Calcium

Of the **macrominerals,** a healthy adult has approximately 1,200 g of body calcium, about 99% of which is contained in the skeleton.[21] The remaining 1%, found in cell membranes and extracellular fluids, plays an important role in nerve transmission, muscle contraction, and membrane function. Calcium metabolism has important implications for both nutritional and physical health. Aging is accompanied by a gradual loss of bone mineral which, if accelerated, leads to increased risk of bone fracture.

Control of calcium metabolism. Serum calcium must be maintained within very narrow limits (4.5 to 5.5 mmol/L)[1] to ensure normal functioning of the heart and nervous system. Serum calcium levels and overall calcium metabolism are controlled by the interaction of several hormones, including **parathyroid hormone (PTH), estrogen** or **testosterone, calcitonin,** and the active metabolite of vitamin D $(1,25[OH]_2D)$. If calcium intake or absorption is inadequate, serum calcium concentrations are maintained at the expense of bone mineral. A slight decrease in serum calcium increases PTH secretion and decreases calcitonin secretion. PTH restores the serum calcium concentration to its former level by (1) stimulating the conversion of $25(OH)D$ to $1,25(OH)_2D$ in the kidneys to promote increased absorption of calcium in the intestine; (2) decreasing renal excretion of calcium by enhancing calcium reabsorption in the renal tubule; and (3) increasing bone **resorption** and mobilization of bone calcium.[1]

As a consequence of these actions, serum calcium concentration rises slightly above its usual level, resulting in a decrease in secretion of PTH and an increase in secretion of calcitonin. By opposite actions, calcitonin decreases production of $1,25(OH)_2D$ and calcium absorption, increases renal calcium excretion, and decreases bone resorption, thereby effecting a decrease in serum calcium. The repetition of these events effectively maintains serum calcium concentration within narrow limits (see Chapter 6 for a discussion of vitamin D and PTH).

Estrogen modulates the effects of PTH and calcitonin by stimulating the synthesis of **renal 1-α-hydroxylase,** the enzyme necessary to convert $25(OH)D$ to $1,25(OH)_2D$. Estrogen and probably testosterone suppress the action of PTH on bone resorption. After estrogen withdrawal, bone becomes increasingly sensitive to PTH, and calcium mobilization is accelerated.[1] The influence of the sex steroid hormones on bone metabolism is more pronounced in women, who experience a cessation of estrogen secretion, compared to men, who experience a gradual decline in testosterone secretion.

Calcium absorption

Mechanisms of calcium absorption. Calcium is absorbed in the small intestine by both active transport and passive diffusion. Active calcium transport is controlled by **1,25-dihydroxyvitamin D,** which stimulates the synthesis of carrier proteins and **calcium-dependent ATPase.** At high concentrations, calcium absorption also occurs by passive diffusion. Calcium absorption by passive diffusion is significant when intakes are high. When a person drinks a glass of milk, about 20% of the calcium absorption that occurs is by passive diffusion.[15]

It has been recognized for many years that calcium absorption decreases with age. In an early study, younger women absorbed 67% of a calcium dose; women ages 80 and over absorbed only 26%.[15] Although the rather high percentage of absorption among the younger women would suggest they had a low calcium intake before the study, it is generally recognized that calcium absorption drops by 30% to 50% over adulthood in both sexes, with major changes occurring after age 60.

Young adults also have the ability to adapt the rate of calcium absorption to the level of intake. The percentage of calcium absorbed increases as intake decreases. Older individuals are less able to respond to low intake. On a high-calcium diet containing 2,000 mg of calcium, young adults absorbed more than one third more calcium than did older adults. When allowed to adapt to a low-calcium diet providing 300 mg of calcium, the young adults absorbed 45% more of the calcium provided than the older adults. Elderly people with **osteoporotic bone disease** absorb calcium even less well than nonosteoporotic elderly of similar age. For some older people, a deficiency of $1,25(OH)_2D$, related to inadequate levels of renal 1-α-hydroxylase, contributes to decreased calcium absorption. In those with normal vitamin D metabolite levels, changes in the intestine may hinder absorption.[15]

Source of dietary calcium. In general, calcium absorption is enhanced when the calcium is in a solubilized form, such as in milk, or in a highly soluble form, such as in the **calcium-citrate-malate compound** now added to citrus juices.[15] Calcium is less available from relatively insoluble salts such as **calcium carbonate.** However, environmental factors in the gastrointestinal tract also influence absorption.[76] Young women absorbed only 25% of a dose of 250 mg of calcium consumed as calcium carbonate on an empty stomach but increased their absorption to 33% when the test dose was administered with a meal.[29] Although it has been suggested that lactose facilitates calcium absorption, this has not been observed in humans,[35] and the carbohydrate included in this test meal was a starch (bread). Heaney and coworkers[29] suggest that the presence of food stimulates more gastric acid secretion than does the supplement alone, which enhances the breakdown of insoluble salts. Ingestion of a meal slows gastric emptying and delivers the calcium to the duodenum in smaller amounts, which may enhance absorption from milk or other food products.

The role of gastric acid in calcium absorption becomes important for older people with **achlorhydria.** Calcium absorption from calcium carbonate (250 mg) was more than tenfold higher in older people with normal gastric secretion than in those with achlorhydria.[68] When the test dose was administered without food, the normal subjects absorbed about 45%, and the achlorhydric subjects only 4%. However, when the test dose was given with a breakfast of eggs, toast, juice, and coffee, absorption in the achlorhydric group increased to 21%, a value within the normal range for individuals on similar daily calcium intakes. Although gastric acid may be necessary to solubilize a calcium salt in the fasting state, calcium-food complexes may assist absorption in the fed state. Gastric acid has no effect on the diminished absorption of calcium from a high-fiber meal.[41] The presence of **phytates** or **oxalates** or both lowers the bioavailability of calcium. Absorption of calcium from spinach, a vegetable high in oxalates, was found to be about 5%.[28]

Calcium intake

Influence of age. The recommended calcium intake for men and women ages 25 and over is 800 mg.[21] Calcium intakes in women tend to fall below two thirds of the recommended dietary allowance (RDA). In the **second National Health and Nutrition Survey Examination (NHANES II)**, the calcium intake of men exceeded that of women in all age groups (Fig. 7-1). Decreases in calcium intake over adulthood are also more striking among men. Calcium intake averaged 1,096 mg in men ages 20 to 29 but fell to 664 mg by age 70. Young women ages 20 to 29 consumed only 662 mg of calcium, and those over age 69 consumed only 546 mg. Income level does not appear to influence calcium intake in people age 65 or over.[18] Median calcium intake in men ages 65 to 74 was 595 mg in those below the poverty level and 597 mg in those at or above the poverty level. In women the median calcium intakes were 477 and 473 mg. The intakes of the women were only about 60% of the RDA.[18]

Influence of race. Race can influence calcium intake.[80] Older black men and women in Alabama[80] were consuming 668 to 687 mg of calcium, but less than the white men and women

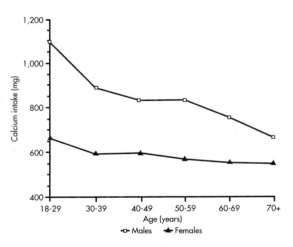

FIG. 7-1 Calcium intake of adults by sex and age. Calcium intake decreases with age in both men and women; women of all ages consume less calcium than men.

(Data from US Department of Health and Human Services, US Department of Agriculture: Nutrition monitoring in the United States: an update report on nutrition monitoring, DHHS Pub No [PHS] 89-1255, Washington, DC, 1989, US Government Printing Office.)

of similar age, who had mean intakes of 710 and 735 mg, respectively. Twenty-nine percent of all subjects were consuming less than 67% of the RDA. Lactose intolerance is thought to be more prevalent among blacks; nevertheless, the mean calcium intakes of these elderly blacks were 85% of the RDA. These individuals may have been consuming some dairy products or possibly large amounts of dark green vegetables high in calcium. It was noted that use of vitamin and mineral supplements was higher in the elderly blacks, which may have added to the calculated calcium intakes.

The media attention being given to the need for calcium has increased the use of calcium supplements in older age groups. A recent report[79] indicated that 12% of women ages 55 to 74 and 9% of women ages 75 or older were using calcium supplements. Use of supplements is higher among women than men, and higher in the white and Hispanic populations than in the black population. Milk-based products appear to be popular foods among institutionalized older people; only 4% to 5% of 270 institutionalized elderly in Boston consumed less than 67% of the RDA.[74]

Influence of caloric intake. The association of calcium and caloric intakes in older people has not been consistent. In 291 independent-living Boston elderly,[53] those with diets lowest in kilocalories were the most likely to be consuming less than two thirds the recommended level of calcium. Sixty percent of the women with caloric intakes below 20 kcal/kg were deficient in calcium, compared to only 4% of those consuming at least 26 kcal/kg. In the men, these differences were 39% versus 4%. In contrast, Holbrook and Barrett-Connor[33] evaluated 24-hour recall records of 426 men and 531 women between the ages of 50 and 79 and found no relationship between calcium intake and total energy intake. They did observe higher levels of protein, saturated fatty acids, vitamin D, magnesium, and phosphorus among those consuming more than 440 mg of calcium a day. This was true for both sexes. It would be prudent to emphasize lower fat dairy products when counseling older adults.

The higher vitamin D intake among those consuming more calcium-rich foods points to the value of milk and other vitamin D–fortified

dairy products as sources of calcium. In a California population,[33] dairy products, dark green leafy vegetables, and beans also contributed magnesium to the diet, so that those with the highest calcium intakes also had high magnesium intakes (90% of the RDA). However, only about one third of both men and women were consuming at least 440 mg of calcium a day (approximately 55% of the RDA). The tertile with the lowest calcium intakes (less than 284 mg) was consuming only 36% of the recommended level.

Consistency of intake. Current findings regarding bone health point to the importance of longitudinal evaluations of calcium intake. Heaney and coworkers[30] reviewed food records collected from 164 women from a religious order who were studied intensively every 5 years over a 22-year period as part of a study in bone metabolism. Current calcium intake did not provide a reliable estimate of past intake. The range of uncertainty for estimating an earlier intake was ± 568 mg. Thus a woman with a current intake of 800 mg could have had an earlier intake as low as 232 mg or as high as 1,368 mg. One factor contributing to this variability is the calcium content of over-the-counter and prescription medications. In many cases individuals are unaware of the calcium in these products, and label information can be incomplete. Although the contribution of medications may be insignificant in those with a high intake from food, it can more than double the apparent intake of women who do not consume dairy products regularly.[30]

Calcium requirement. The requirement for calcium in middle and advanced age is among the more controversial of all the requirements. Nordin and coworkers[58] have pointed out that calcium differs from other minerals in that plasma levels provide no indication of nutritional status. Bone density could provide some measure of calcium status, but the wide interindividual variation in bone loss precludes the establishment of an endpoint for evaluation, and the slow turnover of bone tissue necessitates long-term review to discern changes in total bone mass.

Calcium is lost from the body through the urine, feces, and, to a smaller extent, the skin. Dermal and digestive secretion losses amount to about 150 mg a day.[21] Urinary losses are controlled by PTH but can vary according to age, race, or bone problems. Blacks have lower and osteoporotic patients higher levels of urinary calcium.[26] Combined obligatory calcium losses from all routes are estimated to be 200 to 250 mg a day.[21] Based on an estimated absorption rate of 30% to 40%, the Food and Nutrition Board has established a recommended intake of 800 mg.[21]

Based on calcium balance studies in 85 normal subjects, Nordin and Heaney[57] propose that an intake of 1,100 mg of calcium is required to ensure absorption of about 200 mg of calcium. It is their contention that when active transport mechanisms are saturated, increased absorption occurs only by diffusion. Consequently, at higher levels of intake, the percent absorption of added calcium may be only 6% to 10%. After estrogen withdrawal at menopause, absorption by active transport declines, renal conservation is reduced, and calcium losses escalate.

Early work suggested that calcium balance could be improved in older women by increasing calcium intake.[27] Although the rate of absorption may be low, the net amount of calcium absorbed from a larger, compared to a smaller, intake will be greater. After studying the calcium balance in 168 healthy women, Heaney and coworkers[27] concluded that estrogen-deprived women could achieve calcium balance on a daily intake of 1,500 mg of calcium. **Premenopausal** or estrogen-repleted postmenopausal women required 990 mg of calcium a day to avoid calcium losses.

Calcium supplementation. In recent years research has focused on the level of calcium intake required to prevent **negative calcium balance** as measured by bone mineral losses in middle age and beyond; but clinical trials have yielded conflicting results. Factors contributing to these differences have included the length of the study period, the form in which the calcium was consumed, and the menopausal status of the women evaluated.[16]

Source of calcium. In clinical trials calcium has been supplied in the form of dairy products, calcium carbonate, calcium-citrate-malate complex, and combinations of calcium salts.[17,57,65,71] Polley and coworkers[65] followed 210 postmenopausal women supplemented daily with 1,000 mg of calcium supplied by a combination of calcium salts or 800 mg of calcium in dairy products. Total calcium intake from the usual diet plus the supplemental calcium equalled 1,586 mg in the group receiving dairy products and 1,658 mg in those receiving the tablets. Both groups had a reduced rate of bone loss from the forearm, compared to untreated controls, but differed in their urinary response to supplementation. Those given the calcium tablets significantly increased their urinary calcium excretion, whereas those given the dairy products did not.

Dawson-Hughes and coworkers[17] provided postmenopausal women with 500 mg calcium supplements in the form of calcium carbonate or calcium-citrate-malate, which is used to fortify citrus juices. The calcium-citrate-malate appeared to be more effective in preventing bone loss than the calcium carbonate. However, those workers recommended milk and dairy foods as the best calcium sources on the basis of the protein, riboflavin, and vitamin D also provided.

Period after menopause. The rate at which calcium is lost from the skeleton is accelerated during the **early postmenopausal period** (first 5 years after menopause) compared to the later postmenopausal period.[26,57] The rate of bone loss has been estimated to be 2% to 3% a year during the early period, compared to about 1% a year during the later period. The rapid loss of bone immediately after menopause is believed to represent a lowering of the set point regulating bone mass, and calcium is released until the lower set point is reached.[16,26] During this period there is little or no dependence on external calcium sources, and calcium supplementation has no effect. When the new set point has been established, the regulatory hormones once again become sensitive to dietary calcium levels.

The relative efficacy of calcium supplementation in late as compared to early menopause may account for the differing results of clinical trials evaluating the benefits of high-calcium intake in preventing bone loss.[16] For example, over a 2-year period, Riis and coworkers[71] evaluated the effect on bone mineral loss of estrogen replacement, a calcium supplement of 2,000 mg daily, or a placebo in 43 early postmenopausal women. Bone mineral loss was prevented in the estrogen-treated group but reached significant levels in both the placebo and calcium-treated groups. Those workers concluded that added calcium, even at this level, had only a minor effect on slowing total bone losses.

In a controlled study[17] Dawson-Hughes and coworkers evaluated bone loss in 301 healthy postmenopausal women. Half had a usual calcium intake of less than 400 mg a day, and the other half had usual daily intakes of 400 to 650 mg. Subjects received either a placebo or 500 mg of calcium daily in the form of calcium carbonate or calcium-citrate-malate for 2 years. Those in early menopause experienced a rapid loss of bone regardless of their calcium intake. However, findings among the women who had undergone menopause at least 6 years before indicated that postmenopausal women who consume less than 400 mg a day of calcium can significantly reduce their loss of bone by increasing their calcium intake to at least 800 mg. In those with the lowest dietary calcium intakes, the calcium-citrate-malate supplement prevented bone loss at the hip, spine, and forearm; the calcium carbonate supplement prevented loss in the hip and forearm bones but not the spine.

The women with higher calcium intakes to begin with who were consuming at least 400 to 650 mg of calcium a day from food received no significant benefit from the calcium supplement; both placebo and treatment groups with higher intakes from food maintained bone density in the hip and forearm but lost bone from the spine. This study provides evidence that supplements at a level of 500 mg that will raise total intake to about 800 mg a day can positively influence bone health.

Marcus[51] noted that increasing calcium intake to between 1,000 and 1,500 mg a day is a formidable undertaking and, according to the Food and Nutrition Board,[21] is not without risk. An extremely high calcium intake can induce constipation and in men with **hypercalciuria** can increase the risk of urinary stone formation.[21] A nutritional risk for both sexes may be the interference of high calcium intake with the absorption of iron, zinc, or other **divalent cations**. A provocative paper by Hallberg and others[25] reported that doses of 300 to 600 mg of calcium at a meal decreased the absorption of both **heme** and **nonheme iron** by 50% to 60%. This raises serious questions about the use of high-level calcium supplements at mealtime by those whose iron status is already precarious.

An important goal with adult men and women regardless of age should be raising calcium intake to the RDA of 800 mg. This can be done with three or more servings of calcium-rich foods each day, including milk and dairy products, canned salmon with bones, sardines, or calcium-fortified citrus juices. For individuals who cannot or will not increase their food sources of calcium, various factors should be considered in selecting a supplement:

- *Price:* The form and brand that provides the most elemental calcium for the lowest cost per tablet should be used.
- *Dosage:* Doses above 500 mg can lead to gastrointestinal discomfort by enhancing acid secretion or can lead to constipation.[51]
- *Bioavailability:* Calcium carbonate, calcium lactate, calcium gluconate, calcium citrate, and calcium-citrate-malate are all reasonably well absorbed.
- *Safety:* Calcium supplements such as bone meal or **dolomite** should be avoided because they can contain toxic contaminants; the dosage should be checked carefully on calcium supplements containing vitamin D to ensure that daily usage does not provide potentially toxic levels of this vitamin.

Calcium relationships with other nutrients. Protein and phosphorus have opposite effects on urinary calcium excretion.[21] An increase in protein intake reduces renal tubular reabsorption of calcium and increases urinary calcium loss. On the other hand, an increase in dietary phosphorus increases tubular reabsorption of calcium and thereby decreases urinary calcium loss. Careful evaluation of current diet patterns has revealed that protein and phosphorus intakes tend to rise simultaneously when use of milk, eggs, and meat is increased.[21] Thus there appears to be little effect on calcium balance when recommended levels of calcium are consumed.

Increased sodium intakes increase urinary calcium losses in postmenopausal women.[92] In a clinical trial of calcium supplementation,[65] restricting sodium intake to 1,800 mg a day increased the effectiveness of an 800 mg calcium supplement in reducing bone mineral loss. The influence of sodium intake on calcium excretion requires further evaluation.

Phosphorus

Phosphorus plays an important role in energy metabolism as a component of high-energy molecules such as **adenosine triphosphate.** About 85% of body phosphate is found in bone mineral in the ratio of 1 phosphorus to 2 calcium ions.[21] It is generally recommended that calcium and phosphorus be consumed in a ratio of 1:1, but in the presence of adequate calcium, the ratio is considered unimportant. The RDA for phosphorus is 800 mg.[21] In 1985 dairy products provided 36% of the phosphorus in the food supply; meat, poultry, and fish provided 29%, and grain products provided 13%.[87] Dairy products contain more calcium than phosphorus, whereas meat, poultry, and fish (without bones) contain 15 to 20 times more phosphorus than calcium.[21]

In the NHANES II study,[87] men ages 60 to 69 consumed 1,290 mg of phosphorus daily, and women, 894 mg. It has been suggested that phosphorus intakes are underestimated because of incomplete information relating to phosphate-containing food additives in processed food. Nevertheless, phosphorus intakes still exceed calcium intakes by a considerable margin. Calcium intakes were 755 mg and 552 mg, respectively, in these men and women. Phosphorus deficiency, characterized by weakness, pain, and bone mineral loss, has been identified in older individuals with prolonged use of antacids containing **aluminum hydroxide.**[1,21] Aluminum hydroxide binds to phosphorus, thus preventing absorption.

Magnesium

Magnesium participates in biochemical and physiologic processes involving energy metabolism and nerve transmission. About 60% of body magnesium is in the bone.[21] Although magnesium deficiency has not been reported in adults consuming natural diets, particular chronic problems experienced by older adults contribute to magnesium loss and magnesium toxicity.

Magnesium intake. No information currently exists on magnesium absorption in older people, although there is no reason to believe that absorption is seriously impaired. Data from the 1977-1978 National Food Consumption Survey[86] indicate that men age 65 or older consume approximately 80% of their RDA of 350 mg, and women of that age consume about 75% of their RDA of 280 mg. Blacks consume less magnesium than whites with a similar income.[87] This may relate to blacks' lower use of milk and dairy products, which supply about 16% of the magnesium in the U.S. food supply.[87] Good sources of magnesium are nuts, legumes, unmilled grains, bananas, and vegetables. Higher intakes of plant foods and dairy products may have contributed to the higher dietary magnesium levels observed among older vegetarian women compared to older nonvegetarian women.[56] A survey of low-income older people by the U.S. Department of Agriculture found that magnesium intake was 263 mg in men ages 65 to 74 and 216 mg in those 75 or older. Magnesium intake did not decline after age 65 in the women, who consumed about 200 mg a day.

Magnesium plasma levels and metabolism. Plasma magnesium levels in healthy individuals are remarkably constant; the site of regulation is the kidneys. About 70% of plasma magnesium is unbound and filtered by the kidneys. On the average 95% of the filtered magnesium is reabsorbed, although the kidneys can adjust this level in response to changes in the plasma magnesium concentration.[21] Magnesium stores in the bone also serve to protect against radical fluctuations in extracellular magnesium levels. Magnesium losses occur when **renal tubular reabsorption** is impaired as a result of **nephritis,** particular **diuretics,** or inappropriate hormone secretion.[44] Diuretics such as **furosemide** decrease magnesium reabsorption. **Digoxin** enhances magnesium excretion, and magnesium depletion increases sensitivity to digoxin toxicity. In **hyperparathyroidism,** high urinary calcium levels competitively inhibit the reabsorption of magnesium.

An evaluation of serum magnesium levels in 75 nursing home residents (mean age = 68 years) suggested that despite the existence of chronic diseases and related medications, the major risk factor for magnesium depletion was poor intake.[14] Only three residents had serum magnesium levels below normal, and all had poor eating habits. Sherwood and coworkers[77] found the range of serum magnesium levels among 177 older people admitted to a geriatric clinic to be similar to those of healthy young adults. Diuretics were not a factor, since four of 53 patients receiving diuretic therapy and four of 51 patients not using diuretics had inadequate plasma magnesium levels.

Erythrocyte magnesium concentration may be a more appropriate indicator of magnesium status than serum magnesium levels in older people. In one elderly population 20% were found to be at risk based on erythrocyte magnesium concentrations; only 10% of these were identified based on plasma magnesium levels.[83]

Magnesium deficiency and toxicity. Magnesium deficiency can result from laxative abuse and the loss of large amounts of secretions containing high levels of magnesium (5 to 7 mmol/L) from the lower gastrointestinal tract. Chronic alcoholism leads to diminished magnesium intake and absorption and enhances renal excretion. Older individuals with uncontrolled diabetes mellitus are at risk of magnesium deficiency, since excretion is enhanced by the **osmotic diuresis** induced by high urinary glucose and ketone levels.[3]

Hypermagnesemia is a risk for older people who have impaired kidney function and excessive magnesium intakes. Common magnesium-containing antacids may provide 100 to 200 mg a dose, and magnesium-containing laxatives can provide as much as 500 mg a dose.[3] Drowsiness, lethargy, loss of coordination and reflexes, and changes in mental function are beginning signs of magnesium toxicity, and with increasing severity **cardiac arrhythmias** and cardiac arrest can occur. Overuse of magnesium-containing antacids and supplements also can lead to chronic, unexplained diarrhea with accompanying nutrient depletion.

TRACE ELEMENTS
Iron

Among the **trace elements** is iron, the status of which is influenced by both age and sex. For many nutrients general status may deteriorate with age as a result of poor intake or chronic disease, but iron status actually improves in women after middle age with the cessation of menstruation and monthly blood loss. At older ages women are actually at lower risk of iron deficiency than men.[32] After age 50, the RDA for iron is 10 mg for both sexes.[21]

Iron absorption. Iron absorption is a complicated and inefficient process in people of all ages. Because there is no established route for the excretion of iron once it has been taken into the body, control is exerted at the point of entry.[21] Iron absorption is influenced by body need, body stores, gastric pH, and foods eaten.

Body need for iron. In a healthy older adult with appropriate iron stores, iron is required to replace obligatory iron losses. Under normal circumstances the major routes of iron loss are through the **desquamation** of cells from the skin and gastrointestinal tract. The iron contained in red blood cells is recycled when aged erythrocytes are broken down, and the usual loss of red blood cells in the urine and feces is negligible.[31] Using labeled iron, Finch[20] estimated daily iron loss to be 0.61 mg in older men (mean age = 70) and 0.64 mg in nonmenstruating older women (mean age = 66). Normal iron losses in the young adult have been estimated to be 1 and 1.5 mg daily in men and women, respectively.

Body stores. Iron stores in a healthy man between ages 20 and 50 average about 1,000 mg. In contrast, iron stores in women of similar age are only about 300 mg as a result of monthly blood loss. After age 50 body iron stores increase proportionately to a greater extent in women than in men. By the age of 70 or 80, men have body iron stores of about 1,200 mg, whereas nonmenstruating women have more than doubled their iron stores, to about 800 mg.[32] As a result, iron deficiency is unlikely except in the case of blood loss or extremely low intake or absorption over an extended period of time. Under usual circumstances the percentage of iron absorbed increases as body stores decrease.

Gastric acidity. Decreased secretion of gastric juice by the gastric mucosa affects the absorption of iron in several ways. First, components within the gastric juice bind to iron and enhance its absorption; second, the hydrochloric acid in gastric juice maintains a low pH, which promotes the reduction of inorganic iron (found in enriched and fortified food products) from the **ferric** to the **ferrous** form required for absorption. Antacids that raise pH levels, and certain drugs (e.g., cholestyramine) that form complexes with both inorganic and organic iron decrease iron uptake.[31] At one time it was suggested that morphologic changes in the intestinal brush border modified the rate of absorption. However, recent workers[12] reported no change in villi height or density in mucosal sections between older and younger subjects.

In light of the importance of gastric acid to iron absorption, Krasinski and coworkers[42] evaluated blood parameters of iron status in normal older people and those with varying degrees of **atrophic gastritis.** Hemoglobin levels, serum iron levels, and serum ferritin levels did not differ among groups. An increased incidence of anemia was observed in those over age 75 compared to those ages 60 to 74. However, serum vitamin B_{12} levels were also lower in that age group, suggesting that the anemia was related to several factors and not merely iron status.

Food source. It has been recognized that heme iron (approximately 40% of the iron found in animal tissues) is more easily absorbed than nonheme iron (the remaining 60% of iron found in animal tissues and the iron found in plant foods).[21] Both heme iron and ascorbic acid have been found to facilitate the absorption of nonheme iron. Consuming at least 75 mg of ascorbic acid or 90 g (about 3 ounces) of meat, fish, liver, or poultry, or a combination of these will increase the level of nonheme iron absorbed from 3% to 8%. Absorption of heme iron is considered to be 23%.[31] Although the addition of ascorbic acid or animal tissues at the levels described are likely to increase the absorption of nonheme iron in people of all ages with a body need for iron, these values were derived in studies with women of childbearing age with body iron stores of about 500 mg. Also, the addition of heme iron or ascorbic acid cannot compensate for other substances that interfere with iron absorption such as phytates, bran, or the **polyphenols** found in tea. Iron absorption in the typical U.S. diet averages about 10%.[21]

Iron absorption and age. Metabolic studies using labeled iron in younger and older healthy adults indicate that age per se does not influence iron absorption.[84] Both groups absorbed about 8% of the labeled dose. Of interest, however, was the magnitude of difference in absorption among the older men studied. Percent absorption of iron could be expected to vary among older people with differing iron status; however, the older men in this study were judged to have adequate iron stores based on blood parameters and previous intake. Turnlund and colleagues[84] suggested that the previous iron intake of the men with increased absorption may have included iron that was largely biologically unavailable, and iron stores may have depleted. This points to the importance of suggesting food patterns that will improve iron bioavailability, particularly among older people whose primary iron sources are vegetables, legumes, and grain products.

Iron requirements and metabolism. A major physiologic role of iron is to transport oxygen as part of the **hemoglobin** molecule in the red blood cell and the **myoglobin** molecule in the muscle. The primary storage site for iron is the liver. When it is absorbed, iron enters the portal vein bound to the carrier protein **transferrin.** At that time it may be transported to the bone marrow for incorporation into an **erythrocyte** or to the liver, where it is stored in the **Kupffer cells.** In an adult with adequate iron status, about one third of the available transferrin is saturated with iron, and this parameter serves as an indicator of iron status. In an individual who is iron deficient, the synthesis of transferrin increases as a physiologic response to increase the amount of iron carried across the mucosal cell and into the body.[32]

Body iron stores can be estimated on the basis of the **plasma ferritin level.** Plasma ferritin iron is in direct equilibrium with storage iron and, according to Herbert,[32] the plasma ferritin level (in nanograms per milliliter) when multiplied by 10 will indicate the milligrams of iron stored. If plasma or serum ferritin falls to 20 ng/ml, it means that stores have declined to 200 mg. If iron depletion continues, a drop in **erythropoiesis** and anemia ensue. In a Spanish population experiencing accidental death,[31] only 3% of the older men and 8% of the older women had liver stores indicative of deficiency. Protein-energy malnutrition, infection, inflammation, defective erythropoiesis, or chronic blood loss can also result in iron-deficiency anemia and disordered iron metabolism (see Chapter 8). Based on average absorption levels, the current RDA of 10 mg will provide sufficient iron to replace normal losses.

Dietary iron and biochemical parameters. Iron intake and biochemical parameters of iron status are influenced by age, sex, income, and dietary pattern. Iron intake is closely related to caloric intake; thus older people with diets low in kilocalories are more likely to be low in iron; nevertheless, studies of healthy, community-living older people indicate a low prevalence of intakes below the RDA. Among 691 noninstitutionalized people in Boston who ranged in age from 60 to 98 years,[54] only 1% of the men and 2% to 5% of the women consumed less than two thirds of the RDA from food, although caloric intake was a factor. All of the women with low iron intakes were consuming less than 20 kcal/kg body weight (30 kcal/kg body weight is recommended).[53] Seventy percent of institutionalized xerostomia patients[70] whose mean energy intake was 1,190 kcal had less than the recommended level of iron. Over one third of the frail elderly[48] attending an adult day care program in New York City were consuming less than 75% of the RDA for iron.

Older people may compensate for a lowered caloric intake by deliberately choosing foods high in nutrient density, including iron. Although in general the American diet contains 6 mg of iron per 1,000 kcal,[31] **centenarians** studied in the state of Georgia had intakes of about 7 mg per 1,000 kcal,[38] and the diets of healthy Arizona women ages 75 and over[89] contained 8 mg per 1,000 kcal.

Income can be a significant factor in iron intake. This could be expected, since protein foods high in iron tend to be costly. In the NHANES II study, older people who were eligible for food stamps but were not participating in the program had a mean iron intake of only 6.8 mg.[45] A vegetarian diet pattern does not necessarily reduce total iron intake, although the bioavailability of the iron consumed

is likely to be decreased. Older vegetarian women in California[56] had higher iron intakes than their nonvegetarian counterparts; 4% of the vegetarian versus 7% of the nonvegetarian women consumed less than the RDA for iron.

Biochemical parameters of iron status differ on the basis of sex, level of iron intake, and age. Many older people continue to maintain appropriate iron status into advanced age. Among 69 independently living older adults in Arizona with a mean age of 80,[50] only two individuals had erythrocyte counts below 3.5 trillion/L, and only one woman and one man had hemoglobin concentrations indicative of deficiency (less than 12 g/dl for women and less than 14 g/dl for men). Ten of the subjects (14%) had low serum iron and transferrin saturation levels, but no one had a serum ferritin level below 20 ng/ml. The women had lower mean levels of all parameters with the exception of serum ferritin, which did not differ between the sexes. Only one person consumed less than 67% of the RDA, but 22% of the subjects took supplements.

Parameters of iron status do differ in well-nourished and poorly nourished older people. Elderly blacks tend to have lower dietary iron levels than elderly whites of the same sex. Among 186 black very low-income elderly adults in Washington, DC,[49] 48% of the men and 33% of the women had hemoglobin levels below established standards, and 23% of all participants had serum ferritin levels below 20 ng/ml. Forty-one percent of this group consumed less than the RDA for iron, and level of intake was directly related to biochemical status (Table 7-1). Those with lower intakes not only had lower erythrocyte counts and hemoglobin levels but also lower body iron stores, since serum ferritin equalled only 11 ng/ml. In addition to low iron intakes, these individuals may also have been consuming iron sources with low bioavailability. The low body weight of those with poor iron status suggests a low food intake overall.

A comparison by Löwik and coworkers[46,47] of older **omnivores** and older vegetarians in the Netherlands also raises the issue of iron bioavailability in elderly people. All subjects in this evaluation were at least age 65; the 44 vegetar-

TABLE 7-1   *Characteristics of Elderly Blacks With Adequate or Poor Iron Status*

	Poor Iron Status	Adequate Iron Status
Iron intake (mg)	8.6	11.2
Hemoglobin level (g/dl)	11.0	13.5
Red blood cell count (trillion/L)	4.2	4.5
Serum ferritin (ng/ml)	11	120
Relative weight for height	76	99

Adapted from Macarthy PO, Johnson AA, Walters CS: Iron nutritional status of selected elderly black persons in Washington, DC, *J Nutr Elderly* 6(2):3, 1986.

ians refrained from eating meat, fish, or poultry and had followed this practice for most of their adult lives. The vegetarians tended to have lower numbers of erythrocytes, decreased transferrin saturation, and significantly lower serum ferritin levels compared to the omnivores. The vegetarians also were older, which no doubt contributed to these findings; however, the low serum ferritin levels suggest that over time, iron absorption had been diminished.

Practical aspects of iron intake. Many older people, even those with low incomes, obtain a portion of their iron from animal tissues. In low-income elderly in Arizona,[89] 21% of their dietary iron was provided by flesh foods. Ready-to-eat cereals, however, are a popular food of older people at all income levels.[86] How well the iron salts added to enriched and fortified cereal products are absorbed by older people with some degree of **hypochlorhydria** requires further study.

There is the potential for **hemochromatosis** in older people with excessive iron intakes or absorption. Manore and coworkers[50] reported a median iron intake of 27 mg among their supplement users age 75 and over. Among Boston elderly people,[37] serum ferritin levels (and likely liver iron stores) were directly related to alcohol ingestion. Serum ferritin levels averaged 186 ng/ml among those consuming 15 g or more of

alcohol a day. Hemochromatosis should be suspected when serum iron levels reach 174 μg/dl and transferrin saturation exceeds 60%.[22]

Selenium

Selenium is a cofactor for **glutathione peroxidase,** an enzyme that, in concert with vitamin E, plays an important role in **antioxidant** function. Selenium deficiency in humans results in a degenerative disease of the **myocardium** identified in young people in areas of China where the soil is lacking in selenium. An RDA for selenium was established in 1989.[21]

Selenium intake and biochemical levels. Little is known about the usual daily intake of selenium in the aging population. Based on the selenium content of food composites typical of the American diet, the intake of the average adult is estimated to be 108 μg per day.[21] The RDA for selenium is 70 μg for adult men and 55 μg for adult women.[21] In older British men and women,[8] selenium intakes were 54 μg in those in good health who had a varied diet and 38 μg in those in poor health who were housebound and dependent on others for their food supply. It does appear that older people, including those in poor health, can absorb selenium whether consumed in food or in a selenium-containing yeast product. Apparent absorption was 57% of intake among the British elderly regardless of health status. In an institutionalized elderly population in Brussels,[61] plasma selenium levels increased almost twofold, from 0.84 to 1.66 μmol/L in those receiving 100 μg of selenium daily in the form of selenium-enriched yeast. Serum levels remained unchanged in those given a placebo.

Serum selenium levels decrease with age.[40] The major sources of dietary selenium are fish and grain products, although the selenium content of grains is related to the selenium content of the soil in which they were grown.[36] Because intake of grain products tends to be lower when kilocalories are reduced, the age-related decline in serum selenium levels observed in some populations could be in part the result of decreased use of grain products.

Requirement for selenium. Current research has pointed to a possible involvement of selenium in the development of cardiovascular disease and in immune function. The 5-year risk of death from all causes and from cardiovascular disease was higher in Finnish men between the ages of 55 and 74 years whose serum selenium levels were below 45 μg/L.[90] This relationship was particularly strong for stroke, since men with low serum levels had a risk of 3.7 compared to those with appropriate serum selenium status. A daily supplement of 100 μg of selenium given to older institutionalized people for 6 months increased their **lymphocyte** proliferation responses to the range observed in younger adults.[61] Further work is required to determine the long-term results of such supplementation. Feller and coworkers[19] emphasize the need for appropriate selenium levels in tube feedings. Their elderly patients required intakes of 100 μg of selenium per 1,600 kcal to maintain the serum selenium levels established in young controls.

Zinc

Zinc is required by enzymes involved in DNA and protein synthesis and is essential for cell growth and repair. Because we lack sensitive indicators of zinc status, the evaluation of zinc nutriture among older people, as well as the estimation of a daily requirement, is uncertain.[21]

Zinc absorption and metabolism. Controlled studies evaluating zinc absorption in older adults given either formula or natural food diets indicate an age-related decrease in absorption.[2,85] On a formula diet containing 15 mg of zinc (the RDA for adult men) the percent absorption was 31% and 17%, respectively, in younger and older men.[85] Absorption was somewhat higher on the natural food diet, 39% and 21%, respectively, in younger men and older men, and in women given their RDA of 12 mg of zinc; however, the trend of lower total absorption in the older adults continued.[2] Older adults are able to about double their percent absorption on restricted diets containing only 5 mg of zinc, but total absorption in elderly people is still less, even when the zinc content of the diet is low.[2]

Turnlund and coworkers[85] noted that endogenous losses of zinc are lower in older adults, and they suggest that the lower absorption is a response to a lower requirement for zinc. Conversely, decreased absorption could bring about a conservation of body zinc and the observed reduction in endogenous losses. In older individuals in poor health, chronic negative nitrogen balance contributed to endogenous zinc loss.[7]

Added calcium in a meal does not adversely affect zinc bioavailability. A recent study at the U.S. Department of Agriculture's Human Nutrition Research Center in Boston, involving postmenopausal women,[91] indicated that increased calcium (about 470 mg) whether consumed as 400 ml of fluid milk or as a calcium supplement, did not reduce zinc absorption or retention on a basal diet supplying 16 mg of zinc.

Zinc intake and biochemical parameters. Zinc intake falls below the RDA of 15 mg for men and 12 mg for women in many older people. The daily intake of people ages 65 or older, estimated from dietary records obtained in the 1977-1978 National Food Consumption Survey (NFCS) and the NHANES II study, ranged from 7 to 13 mg.[75] Age, sex, and income influence dietary zinc levels. Zinc intakes declined from 12.9 mg a day in the men ages 60 to 69 to 10.8 mg in those ages 80 and over in a population of economically advantaged Boston elderly.[54] Comparable intakes among the women in that study were 10.6 and 10.0 mg. In contrast, zinc intakes increased with age in an older low-income group in Arizona.[89] The men and women below age 75 consumed 10.1 and 8.2 mg, respectively, whereas those ages 75 and over consumed 10.7 and 8.9 mg. Independent-living **xerostomia** patients[70] had only 7.5 mg of dietary zinc a day, and **hypophagic** hospitalized aged[66] had intakes of zinc that were only 45% of the RDA.

Dietary zinc is influenced by total energy intake and increases proportionately as total kilocalories increase.[75] Older men with caloric intakes of 1,800 kcal consume about 10.6 mg of zinc. Older women consuming about 1,300 kcal take in about 7.2 mg of zinc (60% of the RDA). Those with low caloric intakes can compensate by selecting foods rich in zinc. In the average American diet, about 70% of the zinc is provided in animal products such as meat, seafood (especially oysters), eggs, and poultry, relatively expensive items in the food budget.[75] The most common food source is beef. Legumes and whole-grain products are rich in zinc, although it is in a less bioavailable form. A diet based on dairy products and highly processed breads and cereals will be limited in zinc. Older vegetarian women in California who avoided meat, fish, and poultry[56] had mean zinc intakes of only 6.2 mg.

Despite relatively low zinc intakes, zinc deficiency, defined on the basis of serum zinc or leukocyte zinc levels, is not widespread in the older population. In the NHANES II study,[64] only 3% of those ages 65 to 74 had serum levels indicative of deficiency, although serum zinc levels do decrease with age in men. Women at all ages have lower serum zinc levels and lower zinc intakes. Older Dutch vegetarians, however, had significantly lower serum zinc levels than omnivores similar in age (Fig. 7-2).[46,47] Older people who avoid flesh foods, regardless of reason, may be at greater risk of poor zinc status, based on the reduced bioavailability associated with other zinc sources.

Swanson and coworkers[81] evaluated zinc status in 53 healthy Swiss elderly and reported that all had normal zinc serum levels and urinary excretion levels despite a mean intake of only 9.2 mg per day. Sixty-five percent had intakes below two thirds of the recommended level. After supplementation for 4 weeks with 30 mg of zinc daily, serum levels increased by one fourth, and urinary excretion levels more than doubled; however, **leukocyte** and platelet zinc levels, potentially useful indices of zinc status, did not increase. Concentrations of the **visceral proteins** (e.g., serum albumin) and the **immunoglobulins** that were normal before supplementation remained unchanged when zinc intakes were increased.

Zinc status and metabolic function. Zinc plays a key role in several important functions of particular concern in aging. Wound healing, **taste acuity,** and immune function are altered in classic zinc deficiency. Alternatively, there is no convincing evidence that supplementation with zinc above recommended levels will reverse age-related changes in these functions.[75] Wound-healing is improved in malnourished elderly patients who are given physiologic levels of zinc;

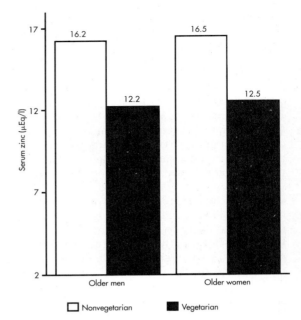

FIG. 7-2 Serum zinc levels in vegetarian and nonvegetarian older adults. Vegetarian men and women over age 64 have lower serum zinc levels than nonvegetarian men and women of similar age and geographic region.

(Data from Lowik MRH and others: Long-term effects of a vegetarian diet on the nutritional status of elderly people, [Dutch Nutrition Surveillance System], *J Am Coll Nutr* 9:18, 1990 and 9:600, 1990.)

wound-healing is not improved in older people with adequate zinc status before supplementation.

A more controversial area of research has been the effect of zinc supplementation on immune function. A well-controlled study[5] carried out with community-living older people between the ages of 60 and 89 indicated that zinc supplements of 100 mg a day exerted a transient improvement on natural killer cell function but depressed hypersensitivity immune function. Those receiving 15 mg of zinc a day showed some increase in delayed hypersensitivity immune function if their baseline measures had indicated marginal deficiency. Bogden and colleagues[5] thus concluded that older people should be cautioned against self-medication with high levels of zinc.

Further evidence that excessive intake of zinc adversely affects immune function comes from the report of Chandra,[10] who observed reduced **phagocytosis** and bacteriocidal action of leukocytes after supplementation with 300 mg daily. Even moderate levels of supplemental zinc (17 to 54 mg daily) blocked the rise in high-density lipoprotein (HDL) cholesterol levels associated with increased exercise.[24] It is pertinent that this effect on HDL cholesterol occurred in individuals age 65 and older who are vulnerable to advertising associating nutrient supplements and improved health.

Copper

Copper is a component of several important proteins and enzymes and is essential for erythropoiesis. The Food and Nutrition Board recommends 1.5 to 3 mg a day as a safe and adequate intake for adults. Current data suggest that average intakes fall below this amount, with men averaging 1.2 mg and women 0.9 mg a day.[21]

When it exists, poor copper status is more likely the result of low intake rather than poor absorption or retention. August and coworkers[2] studied young and elderly men and women given natural food diets containing about 3 mg of copper. Absorption levels were 60% in the younger subjects and 53% in the older ones. Moreover, the older individuals increased their rate of absorption to 67% when given a diet low in copper (about 0.5 mg). Healthy British elderly people[7] on self-selected diets were able to maintain copper balance on intakes of 1.28 mg.

It is of interest that older vegetarian women in California[56] had significantly higher copper intakes than older nonvegetarian women (1.42 versus 0.99 mg a day). Copper intakes of 100 older New Jersey men and women were 1.4 and 1.09 mg a day, respectively.[4] Organ meats, nuts, seeds, and legumes are good sources of copper. Elevated serum copper levels have been observed in patients with cardiovascular disease and are inversely related to serum HDL cholesterol levels. Because **ceruloplasmin,** the transport protein for copper, is elevated in many chronic diseases, including those associated with inflammation, increased serum copper levels may be a result and not a cause of cardiovascular risk.[34] These relationships between copper metabolism and chronic disease are worthy of further study.

Manganese

Manganese is a component of several mitochondrial **metalloenzymes** and is found in most edible plants; thus deficiency among people with access to plant foods is unknown. A safe and adequate daily intake for adults is 2 to 5 mg.[21] Gibson and coworkers[23] determined the manganese intakes of 90 noninstitutionalized Canadian women ranging in age from 58 to 89 years. Those workers chemically analyzed 24-hour duplicate diet composites collected by the subjects. Median manganese intake was 3.5 mg, although there were intakes as low as 1.6 mg and as high as 11 mg. In light of the limited information available describing the manganese content of common foods, it is surprising that the mean manganese intakes determined from the chemical analyses (3.8 mg) did not differ from the calculated intakes based on the food record for that day (3.9 mg).

The manganese intakes of these Canadian women[23] are about twofold higher than that of older vegetarian women and threefold higher than that of older nonvegetarian women studied in California.[56] Intakes in the California study[56] were calculated from 7-day food records. The vegetarian women had a mean intake of 2.18 mg, barely adequate under current standards, and the nonvegetarian women had a mean intake of 1.25 mg, considerably below the recommended level. Whole-grain bread and cereal products, the best sources of manganese, tend to be consumed in low amounts by women, although fruits and vegetables also contribute manganese to the diet. The higher intakes of the Canadian women[23] may have been due in part to their high consumption of tea; median intake was 1½ cups, or 360 ml a day. Tea is high in manganese, containing approximately 1.1 mg per 500 ml.

Chromium

Chromium is essential for maintaining normal glucose metabolism as it facilitates the interaction of insulin with the receptor site on the cell membrane. Glucose tolerance is impaired in chromium deficiency and returns to normal with chromium supplementation. Tissue chromium concentrations decline with increasing age and parallel the gradual deterioration in glucose tolerance that occurs in later adulthood. As a result, the chromium status of older people as related to impaired glucose tolerance and diabetes mellitus development has been a research topic of interest.

Chromium absorption. Chromium absorption is low in all age groups. In young adults, absorption is approximately 0.5% on intakes of at least 40 µg and increases to 2% on intakes below 40 µg.[21] In healthy older adults[60] fed 200 µg of trivalent chromium daily for 10 weeks, plasma chromium levels almost doubled, from 0.28 to 0.50 mg/ml. Plasma levels remained unchanged, however, in those receiving 5 µg of chromium per day in the form of brewer's yeast. In that population baseline plasma chromium levels were all within the range established in young adults.

In 22 apparently healthy older people on self-selected diets,[6] mean absorption appeared to be 2% to 3% of dietary intake. Mean intakes were 30 µg in men and 20 µg in women. Despite their low intakes, 20 of the 22 participants were in equilibrium (or had a positive balance); 2 had a slight negative balance; and 1 had a severe negative balance, losing about 24 µg of chromium per day. The individual losing significant amounts of chromium had a diet very high in fiber. It appears that older people are able to adjust to low intakes of chromium by increasing their level of absorption.

Chromium intake. Chromium is consumed at low levels in the United States. Chromium intakes of adults in Maryland (based on chemical analysis of self-selected diets) were 25 µg per day on an energy intake of 1600 kcal, and 33 µg per day on an energy intake of 2300 kcal. The current recommendation of the Food and Nutrition Board is 50 to 200 µg per day.[21] Mean chromium intake (based on food analysis) of 23 older adults living independently in New York[60] was 37 µg, with a range of 15 to 55 µg, well below the recommended level.

Older Canadian women[23] had chromium intakes ranging from 21 to 274 µg a day, with a mean of 96 µg. Mean caloric intake was 1,435 kcal. The Canadian women with the highest intakes of chromium consumed less protein than those with the lowest intakes, but there were no obvious differences in consumption of foods from particular food groups. On the day the food composite was collected for chemical analysis, 22% of the women consumed less than 50 µg of chromium, and 7% consumed more than 200 µg. The Canadian women were consuming high amounts of tea, reported to be a good source of chromium. Food sources of chromium include brewer's yeast, liver, potatoes, oysters, whole-grain bread and cereal products, cheese, and chicken. The milling of grain products results in the loss of almost 90% of the chromium.

Chromium status and glucose tolerance. Many factors related to physiologic aging, including changes in body composition and exercise patterns, contribute to impaired glucose tolerance (see Chapter 8). Chromium supplementation of older people with impaired glucose tolerance has met with varying degrees of success.[52,59,60] In general, improvement has been confined to individuals with marginal chromium status before supplementation. Among 85 older Canadian women supplemented with 200 µg of chromium,[52] decreased plasma glucose levels 2 hours after administration of 75 g of glucose was related to prior chromium intake. Median chromium intake was 56 µg a day among those exhibiting improved glucose tolerance, compared to 89 µg a day among those whose initial 2-hour glucose levels were in the normal range.

In double-blind, placebo controlled trials, Offenbacher and coworkers evaluated the effect of chromium supplementation on glucose tolerance in 24 institutionalized[59] and 23 free-living healthy older people[60] of similar age. Among the institutionalized individuals, supplementation with 10 µg of chromium in the form of brewer's yeast led to a slower increase and a more rapid decrease in serum glucose levels, although values after 2 hours were approximately the same. Plasma glucose, insulin, cholesterol, and triglyceride levels were unchanged in the healthy, free-living older people given either 5 µg of chromium in the form of brewer's yeast or 200 µg of chromium as chromium chloride ($CrCl_3$). Plasma chromium levels of all subjects were initially within the normal range. These workers concluded that even 5 μg of chromium, when supplied in the organically complexed form found in yeast, should have an effect in a marginally deficient individual; thus it would appear that alterations in glucose tolerance in this population were not related to chromium status. Chromium supplementation improves glucose tolerance by increasing the effectiveness, not the level, of available insulin.

Urberg and Zemel[88] have expanded the study of chromium status and glucose tolerance to include the possible role of **nicotinic acid** status. The chromium **glucose tolerance factor** contains two molecules of nicotinic acid along with chromium. When healthy elderly volunteers were given either 200 μg of chromium, 100 mg of nicotinic acid, or both for 4 weeks, neither chromium nor nicotinic acid alone had any effect. However, when chromium and nicotinic acid were given together, the area under the glucose curve decreased by 15%, indicating a more rapid decline in plasma glucose levels. These workers suggested that the lack of a consistent effect of chromium on glucose tolerance may relate to a limited availability of the nicotinic acid required for the synthesis of the glucose tolerance factor. Further work with both healthy and disease-impaired older people is required to validate this finding.

Fluoride

Fluoride currently is not classified as an essential element, although it does support optimum mineral crystallization in bones and teeth.[21] Epidemiologic comparisons of people living in areas with high or low levels of naturally occurring fluoride in the soil or drinking water point to a positive effect of fluoride in maintaining bone density and decreasing dental caries. Large bone crystals that develop in the presence of fluoride are less susceptible to resorption than smaller crystals. The potential toxicity of fluoride, however, has limited its use in treating bone disorders (see Chapter 8). The safe and adequate intake for fluoride is estimated to be 1.5 to 4 mg a day.[21] Fluoridation of public drinking water has been recommended when natural fluoride levels are low.

WATER AND ELECTROLYTES

Water and the principal **electrolytes (potassium, sodium,** and **chloride)** must be supplied to the body through the diet. Water balance and electrolyte concentrations can be altered in the older adult as a result of disordered control mechanisms or chronic disease.

Potassium

Potassium is the principal intracellular cation, and about 98% of body potassium is in the cell.[21] Plasma potassium levels are carefully controlled, since fluctuations affect the transmission of nerve impulses, the control of blood pressure, and the contraction of muscles, including the heart.

Potassium absorption and metabolism. Potassium is well absorbed (at a level of 90% or more), and there is no evidence to suggest less-than-adequate absorption at older ages.[21] The kidneys regulate potassium concentration in the extracellular fluid. The kidneys can both reabsorb and secrete potassium ions and are capable of reabsorbing up to 95% of the potassium in the **glomerular filtrate.** If this degree of potassium reabsorption was continuous, toxic and eventually lethal levels of potassium would accumulate.[21]

The reabsorption and secretion of potassium ions is controlled by two different feedback systems: (1) a rise in extracellular fluid potassium triggers an increase in tubular potassium secretion, and (2) an increase in **aldosterone** secretion indirectly increases potassium excretion, because the reabsorption of a sodium ion in the renal distal tubule results in the secretion of a potassium ion. Both low-sodium concentrations and high-potassium concentrations in the extracellular fluid stimulate the secretion of aldosterone by the adrenal cortex. Age-related changes in kidney function, as well as certain drugs, can alter potassium balance in older adults.[44]

Serum potassium levels are closely maintained between 3.8 and 5 mmol/L.[21] Replacing fecal and renal losses requires an intake of 1,600 to 2,000 mg (40 to 50 mmol). On low intakes of 800 mg (20 mmol), metabolic equilibrium is maintained at the expense of body stores, and potassium plasma levels may fall below 4 mmol/L.[21] Because increased levels of dietary potassium are believed to be beneficial in reducing hypertension, the Committee on Diet and Health[82] recommends five or more servings a day of vegetables and fruits, especially green and yellow vegetables and citrus fruits, which will provide about 3,500 mg (90 mmol) of potassium.

Potassium intake. Potassium intake varies widely, depending on an individual's food habits. The richest sources of dietary potassium are fruits and vegetables, and individuals who consume large amounts may have an intake of 8 to 11 g a day.[21] On the other hand, potassium intake among older people can be rather low. In the NHANES II study,[87] the potassium intakes of men and women ages 60 to 69 were 2,560 and 1,998 mg, respectively. Intakes decreased to 2,291 and 1,973 mg in those ages 70 to 74. Low-income elderly participating in the 1977-1978 National Food Consumption Survey[86] indicated that they consumed few citrus fruits and juices; only 17% of the men and 27% of the women had a citrus item on the day of record. Potatoes, which are rich in potassium, were consumed by 48% of the men ages 60 to 69 and 24% of the men ages 70 to 74. Among the women of comparable ages, 27% to 32% used potatoes. Older black men and women studied in Alabama[80] had potassium intakes of 1,723 and 1,607 mg, respectively.

The centenarians in good health participating in the Georgia study[38] had 16 servings of fruit a week and 23 servings of vegetables. Vegetables eaten included six servings of green and yellow vegetables, three servings of tomatoes, and one serving of carrots. Older people should be encouraged to have at least five servings a day from the fruit and vegetable group.

Potassium deficiency and toxicity

Hypokalemia. **Hypokalemia,** or a decreased level of potassium in the blood, can result from inadequate potassium intake, but the most common cause is the use of loop diuretics such as furosemide. Potassium depletion is also more likely to occur in older people with severely compromised kidney function, for whom minimum potassium losses may exceed 20 mmol (800 mg) a day.[39] Hypersecretion of aldosterone will lead to excessive potassium excretion. Potassium can be lost in large amounts through the chronic use of laxatives. Vomiting not only reduces food intake but also results in the loss of gastric acid. This loss of hydrogen ions can produce a metabolic **alkalosis** that causes potassium ions to move from the extracellular fluids into the cell, thus seriously reducing serum potassium levels.[44] Low potassium intake will exacerbate the potassium depletion associated with any of these conditions.

Serum potassium levels below 3.5 mmol/L are associated with impairment of several organ systems. Changes in the resting membrane potential and excitability of nerves and muscles can lead to disorientation and confusion, decreased motility of the gastrointestinal tract, inability of the kidneys to concentrate urine, cardiac arrhythmias, and deterioration in glucose tolerance.[44]

Susceptibility to digoxin intoxication increases in potassium deficiency.[39] Also, potassium appears to have a protective effect in reducing the hypertensive action of sodium. Unfortunately, hypokalemia can go unnoticed, since many of these clinical signs tend to be associated with aging and older patients in general.

The relative prevalence of hypokalemia and the advisability of potassium supplements is a matter of debate. In a double-blind study of older patients, Judge[39] reported that potassium chloride supplements improved both grip strength (muscle strength) and mental function; however, the dietary potassium intake of these elderly people was below recommended levels.

The major reason for using potassium supplements is to prevent losses in total body potassium. Lindeman[44] pointed out that follow-up studies of diuretic users over several years revealed no changes in total body potassium. Moreover, when potassium supplements were provided to patients who were losing body potassium, they had no effect. Up to 10% to 15% of intracellular potassium can be lost without a detrimental effect; tissue damage becomes apparent when losses reach 30%. In the opinion of that clinician,[44] foods rich in potassium can prevent a potassium deficiency even in people using thiazide or loop diuretics. When low serum potassium levels are accompanied by a metabolic alkalosis, potassium chloride is the appropriate supplement, since chloride is also required to correct the problem.

Hyperkalemia. **Hyperkalemia,** or an increased level of potassium in the blood, is most commonly associated with impaired kidney function, but inappropriate use of potassium supplements, metabolic or respiratory acidosis, **potassium-sparing diuretics** (e.g., triamterene), and adrenal insufficiency can also contribute to this condition.[39,44] Because of their compromised kidney function and reduced secretion of aldosterone, older people appear to be more susceptible to hyperkalemia when given potassium supplements than are younger people. In a drug surveillance program overseeing 16,000 patients, fewer than 1% of those under age 50 developed hyperkalemia, compared to 6% of those in advanced age.[44] Early symptoms of hyperkalemia are muscle weakness and apprehension; however, cardiac arrhythmias and cardiac arrest can occur suddenly with little prior warning. Older individuals taking potassium supplements or potassium-sparing diuretics require consistent monitoring of their serum potassium levels.

Sodium

Sodium intakes of all age groups are receiving increasing attention based on the fact that diets high in sodium are associated with elevated blood pressure.[21] Although sensitivity to **sodium-induced hypertension** is genetically related, we have no way to identify these individuals; thus some discretion in limiting sodium intake is appropriate for all adults, since it carries no risk for the general population.

Sodium homeostasis and requirement. Sodium is the principal cation in the extracellular fluid and is important in the regulation of extracellular fluid volume. Excessive sodium retention results in increased fluid retention with a possible rise in blood pressure and edema. Sodium excretion is controlled primarily by the **renin-angiotensin-aldosterone system.**[62,73] This system, which is activated in response to either decreased blood pressure or decreased sodium concentration in the filtrate in the renal tubule, stimulates the renal tubule to increase sodium reabsorption. The kidneys can reabsorb as much as 99% of the sodium in the glomerular filtrate.[21] When dietary sodium levels are high, aldosterone secretion is low and more sodium is excreted. When sodium intake is low, aldosterone secretion rises and sodium excretion can be reduced to almost zero.

Older individuals appear to be less able to adapt to changes in sodium intake and to conserve sodium when necessary.[73] Both circulating **renin** and aldosterone levels are decreased in older people, and this may influence both the time sequence and the degree of response to a change in sodium level.[62,73] Because secretion of aldosterone can be increased with administration of adrenal-stimulating hormones, the reduced secretion in response to a lower sodium intake likely relates to a defect in renin secretion or metabolism and not the adrenal gland.[73]

Another factor being evaluated in relation to sodium conservation and loss in older people is the role of **atrial natriuretic peptide.**[73] This hormone, secreted by the heart, acts to decrease water and sodium reabsorption in the kidneys, counteracting the action of the renin-angiotensin-aldosterone system. Levels of atrial natriuretic peptide are increased in older people. Based on their impaired ability to respond to altered sodium levels, it is judicious to avoid either extreme sodium restriction or administration of a sodium load.

Obligatory sodium losses have been estimated to be 5 mmol (115 mg) of sodium a day.[21] The safe minimum daily intake established by the Food and Nutrition Board is 500 mg.[21] The Committee on Diet and Health[82] recommends that all people limit their sodium intake to 2,400 mg, or 6,000 mg of salt. Sodium chloride, or table salt, is 40% sodium by weight, and 1 teaspoon of salt (5 g) contains 2,000 mg of sodium. Reducing sodium intake to 1,800 mg (4,500 mg of table salt) would probably benefit health even more.

Sodium intake. Estimates of sodium intake in the general population range from 4 to 5.8 g (10 to 14.5 g of sodium chloride).[21] In the United States a major source of sodium is sodium chloride, or table salt. A British study[82] concluded that only 10% of dietary sodium was naturally present in food, and only 15% came from salt added at home either in cooking or at the table; 75% was believed to come from salt or other sodium-containing additives used in food processing and manufacturing. This finding has important implications for elderly people who because of physical disability or living situation are dependent on preprepared food items. Also, food types fairly popular among older age groups; grain products, including white bread, rolls, and crackers; and processed meats such as hot dogs and luncheon meats were the two highest contributors of dietary sodium in the general population evaluated in the NHANES II study.[82]

Because individuals find it difficult to estimate the amount of salt they add in cooking and at the table, most surveys report sodium intake based on food composition tables, the amount of table salt in standard recipes for mixed dishes, and information on sodium content of processed foods provided by food manufacturers. Sodium intakes do decrease with age, which may relate to dietary advice given to older people being treated for cardiovascular disease, hypertension, or diabetes mellitus. In the NHANES II study,[87] reported sodium intakes were 3,916 mg in men ages 20 to 29 and only 2,975 and 2,804 mg at ages 60 to 69 and 70 to 74, respectively. Women appear to consume less sodium at all ages, with intakes of 2,404 mg at ages 20 to 29, and 2,108 and 1,903 mg at ages 60 to 69 and 70 to 74. A recent survey of California women[56] with a mean age of 71 years found their sodium intake to be 1,936 mg, very similar to the level reported in the national survey (1,903 mg).

Older black adults may consume lower levels of sodium than older white adults. In an Alabama study,[80] sodium intakes were 3,152 and 2,842 mg among the older white and black men, and 3,593 and 2,371 mg in older white and black women, respectively. The mean ages of these groups were 75 to 76 years, and the sodium intakes for the women in particular were higher than those reported in the NHANES II study for people of similar age. In all of these populations, it is likely that true sodium intake, which includes salt added at the table, sodium in drinking water, and sodium in various medications, is actually higher. In general women appear more likely than men to fall within the recommended level of 2,400 mg.

Sodium depletion and retention

Hyponatremia. **Hyponatremia,** or a below-normal concentration of sodium in the blood, is more likely to occur in older people than in younger people. For the most part older kidneys retain the ability to conserve sodium and maintain serum sodium concentrations in the normal range. Excessive amounts of diuretics, however, can lead to depleted volumes of both sodium and water.[44,62] Depleted fluid volume stimulates secretion of **antidiuretic hormone (ADH)** and subsequent reabsorption of water in the renal tubule. If sodium loss continues as water is being replaced, hyponatremia ensues.[44] Older adults also appear to become increasingly sensitive to **serum osmolality** and may secrete increased and inappropriate levels of ADH, leading to water retention and dilution of the sodium concentration in extracellular fluid.[62] Chronically ill older people who are taking a number of prescription drugs have a higher prevalence of hyponatremia. Vomiting and chronic diarrhea cause abnormal sodium loss. Mental impairment, confusion, and seizures resulting from fluid shifts in the brain are the major symptoms of this problem.[44]

Hypernatremia. An increase in serum sodium concentration is more likely related to insufficient intake of fluids than excessive water loss.[44] **Hypernatremia** is most common in frail, chronically ill older people who are unable to drink without help. An increase in serum sodium concentration is a powerful stimulator of the thirst mechanism; thus older people with access to water are less likely to develop serious hypernatremia, although a derangement in central nervous system function can blunt the thirst mechanism.[63] Continued vomiting or diarrhea causes significant loss of body water, as does an extremely elevated body temperature. Among hospitalized elderly people,[78] hypernatremia was associated with pneumonia and febrile illness, highly concentrated nutritional supplements following surgery, and **glycosuria** in poorly controlled diabetes. Hypernatremia is characterized by thirst and confusion in the early stages, progressing to delirium and coma.

Fluid Balance in the Older Adult

Water is the most abundant constituent in the human body. It accounts for about 60% of body weight in young adults and decreases to about 50% in older adults (see Chapter 3). Because the body cannot store water, fluid must be replaced daily. Normal daily body water turnover is estimated to be 4% of body weight.[69] This may be especially pertinent for the older adult in whom total available body water is reduced. It has been generalized that the loss of body water over adult life is related to the loss of body muscle, which is high in water content; however, a longitudinal study of healthy adults from ages 70 to 81[69] found the body water lost over that period to be from the extracellular fluid compartment. Reiff[69] suggests that the decline in body water may involve not only the loss of cells but also some decline in water content in existing cells as a result of changes in cell proteins and osmotic relationships.

Fluid intake. Fluid is supplied to the body in the form of water and other liquids, in foods, and as water of oxidation. In younger people the thirst mechanism tends to ensure an adequate fluid intake, but a diminished sensitivity to dehydration reduces fluid intake in older adults. The physically impaired or seriously ill individual who cannot drink without help is particularly vulnerable to low fluid intake. Those subject to **incontinence** may consciously restrict fluid intake to avoid embarrassment.

Among older adults in the National Food Consumption Survey,[86] intakes of liquids differed according to age and sex. Nonalcoholic liquid intake, which included coffee, tea, soda, fluid milk, juices, and fruit drinks, totalled 4.2 cups and 2.9 cups in the men and women ages 65 to 74, respectively. Liquid intake fell dramatically to 2.4 cups in the men ages 75 and over but remained about the same in the women of that age, who had a mean intake of 3 cups. It must be recognized, however, that these values do not include the plain water consumed by these older people. Other foods and the water derived from the complete oxidation of carbohydrates, fats, and proteins also contribute to fluid intake. Fruits and vegetables, for example, are 85% to 95% water by weight.[21]

The water of oxidation supplied by a 2,000 kcal diet is about 250 ml.

Water requirement. The water requirement of an adult is influenced by many factors. About half of the fluid to be replaced each day is that lost through the lungs and skin (**insensible water loss**).[21] These losses are increased in environments with high ambient temperatures or dry air, in physical exercise or exertion, or when body temperature is increased, as in febrile illness. Loss of fluid in the feces is rather limited under normal conditions but escalates dramatically in diarrhea. The water required to handle the solute load excreted through the kidneys varies according to diet composition. The breakdown products of protein metabolism, primarily urea but also sulfates and phosphates, are a major factor in the amount of water required for urine formation.

The Food and Nutrition Board[21] recommends 1 ml of water per kilocalorie as a general guideline for water consumption; others[9] suggest a minimum intake of 1,500 ml a day. Because water intoxication is unlikely in most individuals, the specified requirement often is increased to 1.5 ml/kcal[21] to allow for individual variations in activity level, insensible water loss, and urinary solute load. Because older adults are more vulnerable to dehydration as a result of less efficient kidney function, drugs that increase water loss, and reduced thirst sensation, they should be encouraged to raise their fluid intake to about 2,000 ml daily[9] unless this is contraindicated by particular cardiac or renal conditions necessitating fluid restriction.[13]

Regulation of water balance. Water and sodium homeostasis are interrelated and require a balance between intake and output. Intake is controlled by the thirst mechanism and the appetite for sodium. The excretion of both water and sodium is handled by the kidneys. Current work indicates that both the thirst mechanism and the kidneys' ability to conserve water are less efficient in healthy older adults, predisposing this age group to altered fluid balance.[63,72,73]

Excretion of water by the kidneys is controlled by ADH (**vasopressin**) secreted by the posterior lobe of the pituitary gland. ADH is secreted in response to (1) increased osmolality of the extracellular fluid acting on **osmoreceptors** in the hypothalamus, and (2) decreased blood volume and blood pressure acting on receptors in the major arteries. Osmoreceptor sensitivity appears to be enhanced in older people, and as noted earlier, ADH secretion is increased above the levels in younger adults.[62,73] An immediate action of ADH is to conserve water by increasing reabsorption in the renal tubule. Under normal circumstances this leads to an increase in urine solute concentration and a decrease in urine flow. However, aging kidneys cannot concentrate solute and conserve water to the extent possible at younger ages. Consequently, an older person requires a larger amount of water than a younger person to excrete the same solute load.[62]

Impairment of the thirst mechanism. A physiologic change of major significance to fluid homeostasis in older people is the alteration of the thirst mechanism. Medical textbooks over the years have pointed out that older patients do not ask for fluids.[72] Recent work[72,73] with healthy older men (ages 67 to 75) and healthy young controls (ages 20 to 31) has confirmed a blunting of the thirst mechanism. After 24 hours of water deprivation, resulting in about a 2% loss in body weight in both groups, the older subjects still experienced little thirst or unpleasant taste in the mouth, whereas the younger subjects were extremely thirsty and reported a high degree of taste unpleasantness.

Of great concern was the response of the older men when unlimited amounts of water were made available. The older individuals consumed only 3.4 ml/kg body weight, whereas the younger subjects consumed 8.5 ml/kg body weight (Fig. 7-3).[72] In other words, the younger men consumed the amount of fluid required to raise their plasma volume to predeprivation levels. The older subjects did not replace the water they had lost in spite of a significant increase in plasma sodium concentration, which normally stimulates thirst.[63] The younger men, on the other hand, had very little increase in plasma sodium levels yet experienced strong thirst. Older people seem to have a diminished ability to measure serum osmolality and appropriate fluid replacement levels.

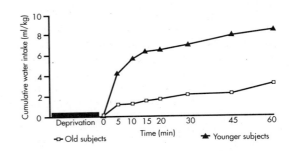

FIG. 7-3 Cumulative water intake of younger and older men following water deprivation. Because of an impaired thirst mechanism, older men do not consume a sufficient amount of water to replace body losses following water deprivation.

(With permission from Phillips PA and others: Reduced thirst following water deprivation in healthy elderly men, *N Engl J Med* 311:753, 1984.)

The **disordered thirst response** has serious implications for temperature regulation and response to heat stress. When placed in a heated chamber, older men had an increased body temperature and an increased hemoconcentration compared to younger men, yet had a reduced sensation of thirst.[55] Sweating, a usual means of lowering body temperature, is less effective in older people.

Several physiologic and hormonal systems may contribute to these changes in thirst and fluid regulation.[63,73] First, the osmoreceptors that respond to dehydration within the cell, and the **baroreceptors** that respond to changes in plasma volume may be less sensitive. It was pointed out that renin-angiotensin-aldosterone activity decreases with age, and angiotensin II is thought to be a strong stimulant of thirst. The increased levels of atrial natriuretic peptide observed in older people probably contribute to diminished thirst, since this peptide not only inhibits renin but also directly inhibits thirst.

Dehydration in the older adult. The older person's inability to recognize the need for fluid, coupled with limited access to water in some situations, increases the risk of dehydration, with significant consequences.[69] Body water is a diluent for medication, and a dehydrated individual is more vulnerable to drug toxicity. Temperature regulation is less efficient with a decreased level of body water to act as a **thermal buffer**.[41] As a result, older people living in hot, humid conditions are more susceptible to heat exhaustion or heat stroke.

Physical signs of dehydration include dry tongue, flushing, reduced turgor of the skin, and confusion or delirium as the condition increases in severity.[62] Serum sodium and blood urea nitrogen usually are elevated. Among 339 nursing home residents, 103 were determined to be dehydrated based on elevated serum sodium and an elevated blood urea nitrogen to creatinine ratio.[43] Dehydrated patients were most likely to be women, over age 85, and bedridden with several chronic conditions and several medications. Use of laxatives was a risk factor for severe dehydration. Those requiring assistance with feeding or drinking were 11 times more likely to be dehydrated than those able to feed themselves. This suggests a need for a dietary prescription for fluids among those needing constant care, whether institutionalized or at home.

Dehydration has been reported in older individuals receiving tube feedings high in protein (1 g/kg body weight). Chernoff[11] recommends a fluid intake of 30 ml/kg body weight or a fluid level 125% of the volume of the formula when patients are given this level of protein. When dehydration has been reported in patients receiving tube feedings, total fluid intake was about 2 L per day, and the onset of dehydration was gradual.[78]

The prevalence of dehydration among older people at home is unknown; however, the finding that laxatives predispose chronically ill older people to dehydration emphasizes the need to educate healthy older people about appropriate amounts of fluid. Reduced fluid intake exacerbates a constipation problem and puts a greater burden on the kidneys, particularly among those with high intakes of protein and electrolytes. Individuals who have problems with mobility may consciously restrict their fluid intake to avoid frequent trips to the bathroom, particularly if they must ask for help or climb stairs. Food records and diet histories obtained for nutrition counseling should include water intake as well as intake of other fluids.

Summary

Minerals are beginning to receive increasing scrutiny in relation to the health and well-being of older people. The absorption and metabolism of most minerals are unchanged as a consequence of increasing age, although zinc and calcium are absorbed less well in older adults. For calcium this change is likely related to hormonal influences and estrogen withdrawal at menopause. For calcium and many of the trace minerals, including chromium, copper, manganese, and zinc, intakes fall below even two thirds of the RDA in many older groups. Encouraging the use of milk and dairy foods, whole-grain breads and cereals, and fruits and vegetables will contribute to improved intakes of these nutrients. For the most part the mineral requirements of older people have been assumed to approximate those of younger people, and further work is needed. Calcium requirements are controversial, and some workers advocate that recommended levels be raised to 1,000 to 1,500 mg daily, whereas other evidence suggests that intakes meeting the current RDA will improve bone health if consumed on a consistent basis. Similarly, chromium supplements, while improving glucose tolerance in the poorly nourished, have little effect on those whose chromium status is adequate. Zinc requirements may be lower in older adults, since impaired function is not evident in people consuming less than recommended amounts.

Water and electrolyte balance in aged individuals who are ill or in good health requires continual attention. Impaired thirst and the kidneys' decreased ability to conserve water increases the risk of dehydration and potentially dangerous alterations in electrolyte levels. Although the institutionalized older person who cannot drink without help is especially vulnerable to low fluid intake, older people who live in areas with high ambient temperatures, who exercise regularly, who use laxatives, or who consume large amounts of protein also need to be advised about appropriate fluid intakes.

REVIEW QUESTIONS

1. Why is there a renewed interest in the role of minerals in elderly persons? What is the difference

between a macromineral and a trace mineral? Which minerals are associated with immune status, hypertension, bone metabolism, glucose tolerance, and cardiovascular disease?

2. What hormones are involved in the control of calcium balance? What role does each hormone play in maintaining normal serum calcium levels? Are serum calcium levels an accurate reflection of bone density?

3. What is the RDA for calcium for premenopausal and postmenopausal women? Is there any controversy over the calcium RDA? If so, explain. When is a calcium supplement useful? What are the characteristics of an effective calcium supplement?

4. How can laxative intake, alcohol intake, and prescription medications for hypertension and congestive heart failure influence mineral status? If kidney function is impaired, which minerals are more likely to rise to higher levels? How do vegetarian diets influence mineral status?

5. What factors contribute to lowered total body water in elderly persons? Why is this a dangerous situation for the older person? What is the water requirement for the elderly? What situations predispose the older person to dehydration?

SUGGESTED LEARNING ACTIVITIES

1. Divide the class into three teams with the goal of developing a brochure entitled, "Boning Up On Calcium." The first team will collect data on the calcium supplements available in the major drug store chains in your community, and the data collection will include name of supplement, form of calcium, other minerals or vitamins contained in the supplement, and the price per tablet. The second team will identify calcium-rich food sources and easy-to-fix calcium-rich recipes. The third team will work with a media specialist to come up with ideas for a brochure design and a marketing plan to distribute the brochure.

2. Prepare short answers to the following questions that you have received from elderly persons through the local "Dial-A-Dietitian" service in your community:
   A. "I read that zinc supplements will strengthen my immune system and make my food taste better. Should I start taking a supplement of zinc?"
   B. "Will drinking tea with my meals cause poor absorption of the minerals in my foods?"
   C. "I just started going through menopause. Should I start taking a calcium supplement to protect my bones?"

3. Prepare a 1-page handout to be used at a senior

center on choosing convenience foods for the older person who has hypertension and is concerned about sodium intake.

4. Go to the library and look up the following article: Salonen JT and others: High stored iron levels are associated with excess risk of myocardial infarction in eastern Finnish men, *Circulation* 89:803-811, 1992. Write a 2-page essay on risk factors for heart disease in the elderly, and include this newest hypothesis on iron and heart disease in your paper.

Key Terms

Provided here for review is a list of the major terms in this chapter. The definitions can be found in the Glossary, which begins on p. 336. To help you understand how these terms are applied, the page number is given for the first mention of each term in the chapter.

achlorhydria, 148
adenosine triphosphate, 152
aldosterone, 161
alkalosis, 162
aluminum hydroxide, 152
antidiuretic hormone (ADH), 164
antioxidant, 156
atrial natriuretic peptide, 163
atrophic gastritis, 154
baroreceptor, 166
calcitonin, 147
calcium, 146
calcium carbonate, 148
calcium-citrate-malate compound, 148
calcium-dependent ATPase, 147
cardiac arrhythmia, 153
centenarian, 155
ceruloplasmin, 159
chromium, 159
desquamation, 153
digoxin, 152
disordered thirst response, 166
diuretic, 152
divalent cation, 151
dolomite, 151
early postmenopausal period, 150
electrolyte, 161

REFERENCES

1. Arnaud CD, Sanchez SD: Calcium and phosphorus. In Brown ML, editor: *Present knowledge in nutrition*, ed 6, Washington, DC, 1990, International Life Sciences Institute, Nutrition Foundation.
2. August D, Janghorbani M, Young VR: Determination of zinc and copper absorption at three dietary Zn-Cu ratios by using stable isotope

methods in young adult and elderly subjects, *Am J Clin Nutr* 50:1457, 1989.

3. Berkelhammer C, Bear RA: A clinical approach to common electrolyte problems. IV. Hypomagnesemia, *Can Med Assoc J* 132:360, 1985.

4. Bogden JD and others: Zinc and immunocompetence in the elderly: baseline data on zinc nutriture and immunity in unsupplemented subjects, *Am J Clin Nutr* 46:101, 1987.

5. Bogden JD and others: Effects of 1-year supplementation with zinc and other micronutrients on cellular immunity in the elderly, *J Am Coll Nutr* 9:214, 1990.

6. Bunker VW and others: The uptake and excretion of chromium by the elderly, *Am J Clin Nutr* 39:797, 1984.

7. Bunker VW and others: Metabolic balance studies for zinc and copper in housebound elderly people and the relationship between zinc balance and leukocyte zinc concentrations, *Am J Clin Nutr* 46:353, 1987.

8. Bunker VW and others: Selenium balance studies in apparently healthy and housebound elderly people eating self-selected diets, *Br J Nutr* 59:171, 1988.

9. Carter WJ: Macronutrient requirements for elderly persons. In Chernoff R, editor: *Geriatric nutrition: the health professional's handbook,* Gaithersburg, Md, 1991, Aspen Publishers.

10. Chandra RK: Excessive intake of zinc impairs immune responses, *JAMA* 252:1443, 1984.

11. Chernoff R: Nutritional support in the elderly. In Chernoff R, editor: *Geriatric nutrition: the health professional's handbook,* Gaithersburg, Md, 1991, Aspen Publishers.

12. Corazza GR and others: Ageing and small-bowel mucosa: a morphometric study, *Gerontology* 32:60, 1986.

13. Crowe MJ and others: Altered water excretion in healthy elderly men, *Age Ageing* 16:285, 1987.

14. Dave DM, Katz PR, Gutman S: Serum magnesium levels in nursing home patients, *Nutr Res* 7:981, 1987.

15. Dawson-Hughes B: Osteoporosis and aging; gastrointestinal aspects, *J Am Coll Nutr* 5:393, 1986.

16. Dawson-Hughes B: Calcium supplementation and bone loss: a review of controlled clinical trials, *Am J Clin Nutr* 54:274S, 1991.

17. Dawson-Hughes B and others: A controlled trial of the effect of calcium supplementation on bone density in postmenopausal women, *N Engl J Med* 323:878, 1990.

18. Fanelli MT, Wotecki CE: Nutrient intakes and health status of older Americans: data from the NHANES II, *Ann NY Acad Sci* 561:94, 1989.

19. Feller AGF and others: Subnormal concentrations of serum selenium and plasma carnitine in chronically tube-fed patients, *Am J Clin Nutr* 45:476, 1987.

20. Finch CA: Body iron exchange in man, *J Clin Invest* 38:392, 1959.

21. Food and Nutrition Board: *Recommended dietary allowances,* ed 10, Washington, DC, 1989, National Academy of Sciences.

22. Gable CB: Hemochromatosis and dietary iron supplementation: implications from US mortality, morbidity, and health survey data, *J Am Diet Assoc* 92:208, 1992.

23. Gibson RS, Macdonald AC, Martinez OB: Dietary chromium and manganese intakes of a selected sample of Canadian elderly women, *Hum Nutr Appl Nutr* 39A:43, 1985.

24. Goodwin JS and others: Relationships between zinc intake, physical activity, and blood levels of high-density lipoprotein cholesterol in a healthy elderly population, *Metabolism* 34:519, 1985.

25. Hallberg L and others: Calcium: effect of different amounts on nonheme- and heme-iron absorption in humans, *Am J Clin Nutr* 53:112, 1991.

26. Heaney RP: Effect of calcium on skeletal development, bone loss, and risk of fractures, *Am J Med* 91:(suppl 5B), 1991.

27. Heaney RP and others: Calcium nutrition and bone health in the elderly, *Am J Clin Nutr* 36(suppl.):986, 1982.

28. Heaney RP and others: Calcium absorbability from spinach, *Am J Clin Nutr* 47:707, 1988.

29. Heaney RP and others: Meal effects on calcium absorption, *Am J Clin Nutr* 49:372, 1989.

30. Heaney RP and others: Long-term consistency of nutrient intakes in humans, *J Nutr* 120:869, 1990.

31. Herbert V: Recommended dietary intakes (RDI) of iron in humans, *Am J Clin Nutr* 45:679, 1987.

32. Herbert V: Nutritional anemias in the elderly. In Prinsley DM, Sandstead HH, editors: *Nutrition and aging,* New York, 1990, Alan R Liss.

33. Holbrook TL, Barrett-Conner E: Calcium intake: covariates and confounders, *Am J Clin Nutr* 53:741, 1991.

34. Honkanen VE and others: Plasma zinc and copper concentrations in rheumatoid arthritis: influence of dietary factors and disease activity, *Am J Clin Nutr* 54:1082, 1991.

35. Horowitz M and others: Lactose and calcium absorption in postmenopausal osteoporosis, *Arch Intern Med* 147:534, 1987.
36. Imai H and others: Dietary habit and selenium concentrations in erythrocyte and serum in a group of middle-aged and elderly Japanese, *Nutr Res* 10:1205, 1990.
37. Jacques PF and others: Moderate alcohol intake and nutritional status in nonalcoholic elderly subjects, *Am J Clin Nutr* 50:875, 1989.
38. Johnson MA and others: Nutritional patterns of centenarians, *Int J Aging Hum Dev* 34:57, 1992.
39. Judge TG: Potassium and magnesium. In Exton-Smith AN, Caird FI, editors: *Metabolic and nutritional disorders in the elderly,* Bristol, England, 1980, John Wright & Sons.
40. Kivelä S-L and others: Vitamin A, vitamin E, and selenium status in an aged Finnish male population, *Int J Vitam Nutr Res* 59:373, 1989.
41. Knox TA and others: Calcium absorption in elderly subjects on high- and low-fiber diets: effect of gastric acidity, *Am J Clin Nutr* 53:1480, 1991.
42. Krasinski SD and others: Fundic atrophic gastritis in an elderly population: effect on hemoglobin and several serum nutritional indicators, *J Am Geriatr Soc* 34:800, 1986.
43. Lavizzo-Mourey R, Johnson J, Stolley P: Risk factors for dehydration among elderly nursing home residents. *J Am Geriatr Soc* 36:213, 1988.
44. Lindeman RD: Mineral metabolism, aging, and the aged. In Young ED, editor: *Nutrition, aging, and health,* New York, 1986, Alan R Liss.
45. Lopez LM, Habicht J-P: Food stamps and the iron status of the US elderly poor, *J Am Diet Assoc* 87:598, 1987.
46. Löwik MRH and others: Long-term effects of a vegetarian diet on the nutritional status of elderly people (Dutch Nutrition Surveillance System), *J Am Coll Nutr* 9:600, 1990.
47. Löwik MRH and others: Nutrition and aging: nutritional status of "apparently healthy" elderly (Dutch Nutrition Surveillance System), *J Am Coll Nutr* 9:18, 1990.
48. Ludman EK, Newman JM: Frail elderly: assessment of nutrition needs, *Gerontologist* 26:198, 1986.
49. Macarthy PO, Johnson AA, Walters CS: Iron nutritional status of selected elderly black persons in Washington, DC, *J Nutr Elderly* 6(2):3, 1986.
50. Manore MM, Vaughan LA, Carroll SS: Iron status in free-living, low-income very elderly, *Nutr Rep Int* 39:1, 1989.
51. Marcus R: Calcium intake and skeletal integrity: is there a critical relationship? *J Nutr* 117:631, 1987.
52. Martinez OB and others: Dietary chromium and effect of chromium supplementation on glucose tolerance of elderly Canadian women, *Nutr Res* 5:609, 1985.
53. McGandy RB: Nutrition and the aging cardiovascular system. In Hutchinson MC, Munro HN, editors: *Nutrition and aging,* New York, 1986, Academic Press.
54. McGandy RB and others: Nutritional status survey of healthy, noninstitutionalized elderly: energy and nutrient intakes from 3-day diet records and nutrient supplements, *Nutr Res* 6:785, 1986.
55. Miescher E, Fortney SM: Responses to dehydration and rehydration during heat exposure in young and older men, *Am J Physiol* 257:R1050, 1989.
56. Nieman DC and others: Dietary status of Seventh-day Adventist vegetarian and nonvegetarian elderly women, *J Am Diet Assoc* 89:1763, 1989.
57. Nordin BEC, Heaney RP: Calcium supplementation of the diet: justified by present evidence, *Br Med J* 300:1056, 1990.
58. Nordin BEC and others: The problem of calcium requirement, *Am J Clin Nutr* 54:1295, 1987.
59. Offenbacher EG, Pi-Sunyer FX: Beneficial effect of chromium-rich yeast on glucose tolerance and blood lipids in elderly subjects, *Diabetes* 29:919, 1980.
60. Offenbacher EG, Rinlo CJ, Pi-Sunyer FX: The effects of inorganic chromium and brewer's yeast on glucose tolerance, plasma lipids, and plasma chromium in elderly subjects, *Am J Clin Nutr* 42:454, 1985.
61. Peretz A and others: Lymphocyte response is enhanced by supplementation of elderly subjects with selenium-enriched yeast, *Am J Clin Nutr* 53:1323, 1991.
62. Pfeil LA, Katz PR, Davis PS: Water metabolism. In Morley JE, Glick Z, Rubenstein LZ, editors: *Geriatric nutrition: a comprehensive review,* New York, 1990, Raven Press.
63. Phillips PA and others: Reduced osmotic thirst in healthy elderly men, *Am J Physiol* 261:R166, 1991.
64. Pilch SM, Senti FR, editors: Assessment of the zinc nutritional status of the US population based on data collected in the second National Health and Nutrition Examination Survey,

1976-1980, Bethesda, Md, 1984, Federation of American Societies for Experimental Biology.

65. Polley KJ and others: Effect of calcium supplementation on forearm bone mineral content in postmenopausal women: a prospective, sequential controlled trial, *J Nutr* 117:1929, 1987.

66. Rammohan M, Juan D, Jung D: Hypophagia among hospitalized elderly, *J Am Diet Assoc* 89:1774, 1989.

67. Rea IM: Sex and age changes in serum zinc levels, *Nutr Res* 9:121, 1989.

68. Recker RR: Calcium absorption and achlorhydria, *N Engl J Med* 313:70, 1985.

69. Reiff TR: Body composition with special reference to water. In Horwitz A and others, editors: *Nutrition in the elderly,* New York, 1989, Oxford University Press.

70. Rhodus NL, Brown J: The association of xerostomia and inadequate intake in older adults, *J Am Diet Assoc* 90:1688, 1990.

71. Riis B and others: Does calcium supplementation prevent postmenopausal bone loss? *N Engl J Med* 316:173, 1987.

72. Rolls BJ: Regulation of food and fluid intake in the elderly, *Ann NY Acad Sci* 561:217, 1989.

73. Rolls BJ, Phillips PA: Aging and disturbances of thirst and fluid balance, *Nutr Rev* 48:137, 1990.

74. Sahyoun NR and others: Dietary intakes and biochemical indicators of nutritional status in an elderly, institutionalized population, *Am J Clin Nutr* 47:524, 1988.

75. Sandstead H and others: Zinc nutriture in the elderly in relation to taste acuity, immune response, and wound healing, *Am J Clin Nutr* 36:1046, 1982.

76. Sheikh MS and others: Gastrointestinal absorption of calcium from milk and calcium salts, *N Engl J Med* 317:532, 1987.

77. Sherwood RA and others: Hypomagnesium in the elderly, *Gerontology* 32:105, 1986.

78. Snyder NA, Feigal DW, Arieff AI: Hypernatremia in elderly patients, *Ann Intern Med* 107:309, 1987.

79. Subar AF, Block G: Use of vitamin and mineral supplements: demographics and amounts of nutrients consumed, the 1987 Health Interview Survey, *Am J Epidemiol* 132:1091, 1990.

80. Svacha AJ, Waslien CI, Malvestuto PJ: Nutritional status of noninstitutionalized elderly Alabamians, *Nutr Res* 7:1321, 1987.

81. Swanson CA and others: Zinc status of healthy elderly adults: response to supplementation, *Am J Clin Nutr* 48:343, 1988.

82. Thomas PR: *Improving America's diet and health: from recommendations to action,* Washington, DC, 1991, National Academy Press.

83. Touitou Y and others: Prevalence of magnesium and potassium deficiencies in the elderly, *Clin Chem* 33/4:518, 1987.

84. Turnlund JR, Reager RD, Costa F: Iron and copper absorption in young and elderly men, *Nutr Res* 8:333, 1988.

85. Turnlund JR and others: Stable isotope studies of zinc absorption and retention in young and elderly men, *J Nutr* 116:1239, 1986.

86. US Department of Agriculture: Food and nutrient intakes of individuals in 1 day: low-income households, November 1977-March 1978, Nationwide Food Consumption Survey 1977-78, Preliminary Report No 11, Washington, DC, 1982, US Government Printing Office.

87. US Department of Health and Human Services, US Department of Agriculture: Nutrition monitoring in the United States: an update report on nutrition monitoring, DHHS Pub No (PHS) 89-1255, Washington, DC, 1989, US Government Printing Office.

88. Urberg M, Zemel MB: Evidence for synergism between chromium and nicotinic acid in the control of glucose tolerance in elderly humans, *Metabolism* 36:896, 1987.

89. Vaughan LA, Manore MM: Dietary patterns and nutritional status of low-income, free-living elderly, *Food Nutr News* 60(5):1, Nov.-Dec., 1988.

90. Virtamo J and others: Serum selenium and the risk of coronary heart disease and stroke, *Am J Epidemiol* 122:276, 1985.

91. Wood RJ, Zheng JJ: Milk consumption and zinc retention in postmenopausal women, *J Nutr* 120:398, 1990.

92. Zarkadas M and others: Sodium chloride supplementation and urinary calcium excretion in postmenopausal women, *Am J Clin Nutr* 50:1088, 1989.

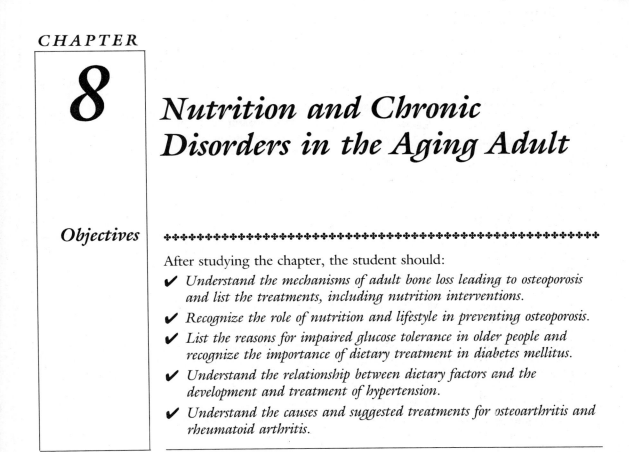

CHAPTER

8

Nutrition and Chronic Disorders in the Aging Adult

Objectives

✦✦✦

After studying the chapter, the student should:

✔ *Understand the mechanisms of adult bone loss leading to osteoporosis and list the treatments, including nutrition interventions.*

✔ *Recognize the role of nutrition and lifestyle in preventing osteoporosis.*

✔ *List the reasons for impaired glucose tolerance in older people and recognize the importance of dietary treatment in diabetes mellitus.*

✔ *Understand the relationship between dietary factors and the development and treatment of hypertension.*

✔ *Understand the causes and suggested treatments for osteoarthritis and rheumatoid arthritis.*

Introduction

Many chronic disorders that occur in older adults are influenced either directly or indirectly by food selection and nutritional status. Conversely, the drugs used to treat many disorders can also adversely affect nutritional health. Chronic disorders can be difficult to diagnose and treat because of our inability to separate physiologic changes associated with normal aging from those related to pathologic disease. The problem is complicated further by the differences in the rate and severity of age-related changes in different individuals. For example, all aging adults lose bone, but not all develop **osteoporosis** and suffer related bone fractures. Chronic disease may lead to changes in physiologic function that usually are associated with a nutrient deficiency, as occurs in the anemia of chronic disease. The nutrition professional working with older adults must recognize the role of nutrition intervention in delaying the progression of age- and nutrient-related disorders, ameliorating disease symptoms, and reducing the amount of medication required for management.

BONE DISORDERS IN THE AGING ADULT

Osteoporosis

Definition. Beginning about age 30 to 40, both men and women lose bone.[93] Losses accelerate in women after menopause and then slow or cease in advanced age. Although all people lose some bone as a consequence of aging, not all develop osteoporosis. Osteoporosis is a clinical disorder characterized by an absolute decrease in bone mineral and bone matrix. It results in bone fractures, despite minimal or no trauma; bone pain; and spinal deformity and loss of height.[59]

Public health aspects. Osteoporosis has enormous implications for both personal well-being and the health care system. By age 65 one in three women will have vertebral fractures; by age 90 one in three women and one in six men will have had a hip fracture.[92] A hip fracture often results in loss of independence; half of these patients are unable to return to their former residence and thus become dependent on nursing home care. The direct and indirect costs associated with osteoporosis are estimated to exceed $6 billion a year.[92]

Bone as a Tissue

Bone is composed of a protein and **collagen** matrix and minerals in the form of **hydroxyapatite** with a formula of $Ca_{10}(PO_4)_6OH_2$.[108] The hydroxyl group can be replaced by a fluoride ion to form **fluorapatite,** which is more resistant to resorption than hydroxyapatite. The matrix accounts for about one third of bone weight and the mineral deposits about two thirds of bone weight.

The mature skeleton has two types of bone. *Cortical bone* is dense and compact and has a slow turnover. It consists of circular layers arranged around a blood vessel. Cortical bone appears as a solid mineralized area on a normal x-ray. It is found in the skull, the jaw, and the shafts of the long bones. About 80% of the skeleton is cortical bone.[59,108] *Trabecular bone,* sometimes referred to as spongy or **cancellous bone,** has a greater surface area than cortical bone and is more metabolically active. It comprises numerous interwoven horizontal and vertical bars, called trabeculae, which form partitions filled with marrow and fat. Trabecular bone has a lacelike structure on magnification. It is found in the vertebrae, in the flat bones of the ribs and pelvis, and in the ends of the long bones such as the femur. Trabecular bone forms about 20% of the skeleton.[59,108]

Once thought to be relatively inert, bone is now recognized to be a dynamic tissue that undergoes constant remodeling throughout life. While old bone is being broken down at one location, new bone is being formed at another. **Osteoclasts** are the cells that are instrumental in bone resorption; these cells secrete acids that dissolve bone mineral and recruit **phagocytes** to remove remaining proteins. **Osteoblasts,** the active cells that form new bone, synthesize the protein matrix and accumulate the calcium and phosphorus deposited in the matrix.[98]

In young adults bone resorption and formation are tightly coupled. An advancing series of osteoclasts forms a cavity, which osteoblasts fill in with new bone. Under normal circumstances bone formation equals bone resorption, and bone mass is maintained. The first change to occur in bone remodeling is incomplete replacement of the bone that was resorbed, resulting in the age-related bone loss that begins about ages 30 to 40.[93] The accelerated bone loss that occurs in women immediately after menopause is associated with increased bone turnover. Both bone resorption and accretion escalate, but osteoclasts increase to a greater extent and create cavities in the bone that cannot be filled.[59,93] Loss of bone and the changing geometric pattern of the bone contribute to a loss in bone strength.

Bone Development and Loss

Factors influencing bone mass. Many factors contribute to bone formation and loss. Some of these are under an individual's control, whereas others are genetic or physiologic in nature. The characteristics listed in the accompanying box have been associated with lower bone mass.[53,98,108]

The most obvious predisposing factor for bone loss is being female. Over adult life women lose about 35% of their cortical bone and 50% of their trabecular bone; men lose only about two thirds as much.[93] Blacks have greater bone density compared to whites of similar age and sex, and blacks are less susceptible to bone loss and osteoporosis. Increased mechanical stress on the bone is believed to contribute to the higher bone density of obese women compared to lean women.[59] **Hyper-**

❖

CHARACTERISTICS ASSOCIATED WITH LOWER BONE MASS

GENETIC
Female
White or Asian race
Family history of bone disease
Extremely short or tall stature
PHYSIOLOGIC OR ENDOCRINE
Hyperparathyroidism
Hyperthyroidism
Diabetes mellitus
Premature menopause
Leanness
ENVIRONMENTAL
Low calcium intake
Little exposure to sunlight
Little physical activity
Use of alcohol
Smoking

---

parathyroidism and use of **glucocorticoids** accelerate urinary calcium losses and contribute to low bone mass. In contrast, **thiazide drugs** reduce the excretion of calcium, and users have a reduced incidence of hip fracture.[92] The impact of estrogen deficiency on bone mass has implications for bone health in young women in whom ovarian function is halted because of severely reduced caloric intake or extreme levels of physical exercise.

Bone development in early life. Bone density in older age is the sum total of bone acquired during the years of growth minus the bone lost after maturity. Because reduced bone mass is a major determinant of bone fracture, a high bone mass at maturity is believed to offer the best protection against age-related bone fractures.[93] An evaluation of two communities in Yugoslavia[74] having similar sun exposure, exercise patterns, and life-styles but differing in their consumption of dairy products suggests that a generous intake of calcium during the period of bone growth offers long-term benefits. Calcium intakes were about 450 and 1,000 mg in the men from the low- and high-calcium re-

gions and about 400 and 875 mg in the women. A difference in bone mass between the two populations was already apparent at age 30 (Fig. 8-1). Those with a greater bone mass at younger ages had a greater amount of bone remaining in later life despite bone loss. The rate of fractures was inversely proportional to bone mass, and differences in fracture rate existed in all age groups.

In the second National Health and Nutrition Examination Survey, (NHANES II), the mean calcium intake of teenage women ranged from 768 to 864 mg[24]; the recommended dietary allowance (RDA) for this age group is 1,200 mg.[38] These adolescent girls now developing their skeletal mass could be at high risk for low bone mass in later life.

Patterns of bone loss. Age of onset and patterns of bone loss differ between cortical and trabecular bone, and these differences contribute to the sequence of fractures associated with each type. Cortical bone loss begins about age 40 in men and women and proceeds slowly at a rate of about 0.3% to 0.5% a year. In women the rate of loss increases to 2% to 3% a year immediately after menopause and then gradually returns to lower levels. In some individuals cortical bone loss stops after age 70.[93] At the same time, hip fractures increase beyond age 70, suggesting that for some cortical losses continue.

The pattern of trabecular bone loss is less well understood. It generally is agreed that trabecular losses begin at least 10 years earlier than cortical losses in both sexes, with several studies suggesting age 30 to 35.[92] Although some researchers[93] have found continuous losses of trabecular bone of about 1.2% a year with no acceleration after menopause, others have reported excessive losses in younger women following **oophorectomy.** Losses may be less rapid in natural menopause, when estrogen withdrawal is more gradual. If trabecular bone loss does increase immediately after menopause, the duration of the increased loss is shorter than for cortical bone. The earlier onset of trabecular bone loss is paralleled by the earlier onset of vertebral fractures, fractures of the forearm, and tooth loss caused by changes in the **mandible.**[108]

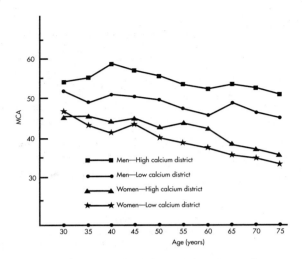

MCA

Men—High calcium district
Men—Low calcium district
Women—High calcium district
Women—Low calcium district

Age (years)

FIG. 8-1   Calcium intake and bone density by age and sex. Men at all ages have a greater metacarpal bone width than women, regardless of their calcium intake; women with higher calcium intakes have a greater metacarpal bone width than women with lower calcium intakes despite age-related bone loss.

(From Matkovic V and others: Bone status and fracture rates in two regions in Yugoslavia, *Am J Clin Nutr* 32:540, 1979. © American Society for Clinical Nutrition.)

Developing Osteoporosis

Two distinct syndromes of osteoporosis exist, and they differ in age of onset, relation to menopause, clinical symptoms, and hormonal patterns (Table 8-1).[92,93] **Postmenopausal osteoporosis (type I)** generally is found in women 15 to 20 years after menopause, although this type of osteoporosis does occur in men of similar age. The first clinical symptoms are fractures of the vertebrae, which cause spinal deformity, back pain, and a decrease in stature. The escalation in trabecular bone loss that occurs in type I osteoporosis is believed to result from the hormonal changes that accompany estrogen withdrawal. Accelerated bone mobilization and high serum calcium levels suppress parathyroid hormone (PTH) and elevate **calcitonin,** which in turn depresses **renal 1-α-hydroxylase activity,** the production of 1,25(OH)$_2$D, and calcium absorption. It is a fact, however, that although all women are deficient in estrogen after menopause, not all develop osteoporosis. The other factors that interact with or exacerbate the lack of estrogen are unknown.

Senile osteoporosis (type II) differs from postmenopausal osteoporosis in several respects.[93] First, it occurs later in life, at age 70 or after, and it is more common among men than type I osteoporosis. Two major characteristics that contribute to the deterioration in bone status are (1) a decrease in active osteoblasts, which widens the gap between bone resorption and formation, and (2) decreased production of 1,25(OH)$_2$D, which impairs calcium absorption and enhances bone calcium mobilization. Continued bone resorption leads to fractures of the hip and pelvis. Vertebral fractures form a wedge shape, resulting in **kyphosis,** or "dowager's hump."

Riggs and Melton[93] emphasize that all factors contributing to enhanced or decreased bone mass are cumulative; thus increased bone mass at maturity, increased bone loss related to smoking or use of alcohol, or the accelerated bone loss experienced at menopause all influence total bone density after age 70. With advancing age and continued bone loss, an increasing proportion of individuals will have bone mass levels that fall below the threshold associated with bone fracture.

Treating Osteoporosis

Many therapies are being examined with hopes of reversing excessive bone loss. Although particular regimens hold promise, many are both costly and experimental. Therapeutic agents act by decreasing bone resorption or stimulating bone formation.

Decreasing Bone Resorption

Estrogen replacement therapy. Bone resorption and loss after menopause can be effectively reduced with **estrogen replacement therapy.** Estrogen slows the activation of new osteoclasts, although it does not inhibit the activity of existing osteoclasts; nevertheless, the loss of both cortical and trabecular bone is reduced.[93] When initiated at menopause and continued for 5 years, estrogen replacement reduced subsequent hip and forearm fractures by 50% and vertebral fractures

TABLE 8-1 *Comparison of Postmenopausal and Senile Osteoporosis*

	Postmenopausal Osteoporosis	Senile Osteoporosis
Age of onset (years)	50 to 75	Over 70
Type of bone lost	Trabecular	Trabecular and cortical
Rate of bone loss	Rapid	Slow
Parathyroid hormone (PTH) level	Below normal	Above normal
Calcium absorption	Below normal	Below normal
Major cause	Menopause (estrogen withdrawal)	Aging (impaired bone remodeling and $1,25(OH)_2D$ production)

Adapted from Riggs BL, Melton LJ: Involutional osteoporosis, *N Engl J Med* 314:1676, 1986.

by 90%.[4] However, the benefits of estrogen replacement have not been demonstrated in women over age 70.

Current data relating risk of **endometrial** or breast cancer and estrogen replacement are conflicting. An expert panel reported that estrogen therapy extending beyond 10 years was associated with a small increase in diagnosed cases of breast cancer but not with an increase in cancer deaths.[4] In a 10-year prospective study of postmenopausal nurses, Colditz and colleagues[23] found about a 30% increase in the risk of breast cancer and an increased risk of endometrial cancer among current users of estrogen, and risk increased with age. Past use, even if long term, did not increase risk after 2 years. These authors recommended that estrogen be used with caution.

Calcitonin. Calcitonin is effective in preventing loss of trabecular bone in women with postmenopausal osteoporosis and may be an alternative to estrogen replacement therapy.[4] The effect of calcitonin on cortical bone loss or long-term prevention of fractures has not been established.

Biphosphonates. The **biphosphonate** compounds such as **etidronate** are known to inhibit the activity of osteoclasts.[101] These drugs are administered in a cyclical manner to alternately stimulate and depress osteoclastic activity and thereby synchronize bone resorption and formation. Each treatment cycle is expected to bring about a gain in bone mass. Research is needed to ascertain the long-term efficacy of this treatment.

Stimulating Bone Formation

Fluoride. Fluoride stimulates osteoblastic activity and at low levels increases trabecular bone mass. At higher levels, however, fluoride is very toxic, causing gastric distress and bone pain. A 4-year trial[94] conducted with 202 postmenopausal women given sodium fluoride or a placebo has proved to be disappointing. Although fluoride therapy increased trabecular bone density, it decreased cortical bone density, with an overall increase in skeletal fragility. Fractures of the hip and pelvis numbered 20 in the experimental group and 5 in the placebo group. In contrast, French women[77] given lower doses of fluoride experienced a 25% reduction in vertebral fractures with no change in nonvertebral fractures. A recent consensus conference[4] concluded that fluoride may have a very narrow therapeutic range and requires careful evaluation.

Calcitriol. Synthetic $1,25(OH)_2D$ (**calcitriol**) increases calcium absorption and improves calcium balance in osteoporotic patients and reduces the rate of fractures. An analysis of patient outcomes from several medical centers[39] indicated that fracture rates per 1,000 patient years were almost doubled in the group receiving the placebo compared to the group given calcitriol after 1 year of study (823 versus 450). Long-term studies focusing on bone density and potentially harmful side effects such as **hypercalcemia** or renal damage are necessary before calcitriol can be routinely prescribed.

Preventing Osteoporosis

Despite intensive research to evaluate the potential risks and benefits of new treatments for osteoporosis, major attention should also be directed toward preventing osteoporosis in younger and older adults. Primary factors to be considered in lifelong promotion of bone health include calcium intake, vitamin D status, exercise, and avoidance of smoking and alcohol.[92]

Calcium intake. Calcium intakes associated with improved bone status have ranged from 700 to 1,500 mg a day (see Chapter 7). However, efforts to relate calcium intake to the incidence of fractures have had mixed results. A 14-year prospective study[52] of 957 men and women from southern California who ranged in age from 50 to 79 years at time of entry found an increased incidence of hip fracture among those consuming less calcium. Smoking habits, alcohol use, and menstrual and reproductive history did not differ among groups. Those in the tertile consuming at least 765 mg of calcium a day had a 60% reduction in the risk of hip fracture compared to those consuming less than 470 mg or 470 to 764 mg per day. In contrast, a study of 900 British elderly[26] found no significant relationship between calcium intake and hip fracture in women, although risk was somewhat lower on intakes of at least 838 mg a day. After a comprehensive review, Wardlaw[108] concluded that evidence relating calcium intake and calcium balance in women ages 35 to 70 is weak; dietary calcium appears to explain only 4% of the variance in calcium balance. Intakes up to 1,500 mg a day have not been demonstrated to reduce the incidence of bone fracture. Resnick and Greenspan[92] pointed out that supplemental calcium is not only expensive but also can lead to side effects, including **digoxin toxicity** in older individuals with chronic disease and high drug use. An intake that meets the RDA of 800 mg[38] is a prudent measure for adults of all ages.

Vitamin D. An evaluation of nutrient intake and bone health in postmenopausal women conducted by Sowers and coworkers[100] found that bone density in the forearm was 4% greater in women with vitamin D intakes of at least 400 IU a day. Individuals who obtain a major portion of their calcium from vitamin D–fortified dairy products are likely to receive the recommended level. For those consuming their calcium in the form of supplements or nondairy foods, sun exposure on the face and arms for about 15 minutes three times a week should provide sufficient vitamin D.

Exercise. It has been known for some time that bed rest or immobilization precipitates the loss of mineral from the bones. Weightlessness, as experienced by modern astronauts, led to significant bone loss. The general explanation given for bone loss under these circumstances was the absence of gravitational pull and weight-bearing exercise acting on bone tissue.[59] Thus walking, jogging, and running have been prescribed to maintain bone health. However, current thought suggests that weight loads generated by the pull of muscles, as occurs in weight training, may stimulate bone formation to an even greater extent than weight loads that are generally distributed, as occurs in walking and running.[98] For example, the weight load exerted on the lower vertebrae while jogging is about two times body weight; the force exerted during weight lifting (usually considered a non-weight-bearing activity) can be five to six times body weight.

A comparison of the effects of exercise in postmenopausal women with a high-calcium intake (1,462 mg a day) versus a moderate-calcium intake (761 mg a day) suggests that calcium and exercise have different effects, depending on the type of bone.[84] In this double-blind study of 1 year,[84] the exercise group walked for 50 minutes four times a week. Trabecular bone in the spine increased by less than 1% in the exercise group but decreased by 7% in the sedentary group and was unaffected by calcium intake. In contrast, those with a high-calcium intake had a 2% increase in bone in the hip, whereas those with a moderate calcium intake lost about 1% of their bone at that site. It is important to advise clients that exercise programs must be continued for gains in bone mineral mass to be sustained. In older women who had achieved a 5% gain in lumbar bone mass with intensive exercise, bone mass returned to baseline levels within 13 months of discontinuing training.[30] Currently no data are available on the effects of weight training on bone mineral in older people.

A topic of current interest is the relationship between muscle mass, muscle strength, and bone mass in older people. Changes in skeletal mass over adult life are comparable to changes in muscle mass, since both decline 35% to 45%.[98] Muscle strength and bone mineral density appear to be related in older men and women. Cooper and coworkers[26] found that grip strength was inversely related to risk of hip fracture. An appropriate level of exercise in older adults may contribute to the preservation of bone mass and muscle mass.

Avoiding alcohol and cigarettes. Both alcohol and smoking have a toxic effect on bone. Ethanol directly inhibits osteoblastic activity and appears to exacerbate the deleterious effect of a low-calcium intake. The mechanism by which smoking adversely affects bone mass is unclear.[92]

Counseling the Osteoporotic Patient

Diet planning for an osteoporotic patient depends on the type and level of bone loss and associated chronic disease.[9] General dietary guidelines include:

- A high-calcium intake emphasizing food and/or supplements with high bioavailability
- An adequate level of vitamin D from food or sun exposure
- A prudent intake of protein, sodium, and fiber to minimize calcium losses
- Avoidance of alcohol, caffeine, and interfering vitamin or mineral supplements

Bales and Gold[9] call attention to the psychosocial well-being of the osteoporotic patient. This condition responds relatively slowly to dietary, medical, and exercise interventions. Patients can become depressed, since their prognosis is uncertain. An appropriate dietary pattern that includes calcium-rich foods may be a difficult adjustment if these items were not consumed previously. Continuing dietary care of osteoporotic patients within the context of their medical care is critical for successful management of this disease.

Diagnosis of Osteoporosis

Public awareness of the potentially debilitating effects of osteoporotic bone disease has led to the growth of storefront osteoporosis diagnostic centers whose methods and expertise are highly questionable. Older people who want to know their level of risk should be directed to established medical centers where appropriate diagnostic procedures (e.g., **dual photon** and **x-ray absorptiometry**) and treatment regimens are supervised by competent medical personnel.[7]

Osteomalacia

Developing osteomalacia. Osteomalacia, the adult form of **rickets,** occurs in older adults. Osteomalacia and osteoporosis are both characterized by an inadequate level of bone mineralization; however, their etiologies differ.[99] In osteomalacia a normal amount of protein matrix is present but is not mineralized because of vitamin D deficiency and inadequate calcium absorption. In contrast, osteoporotic bone has lost both mineral and matrix as a result of hormonal, nutritional, and life-style factors. In osteoporosis bone loss begins in the vertebrae or hip; in osteomalacia bone loss is most apparent in the peripheral skeleton. Sowers[99] suggests that both disorders can exist in the same individual, but techniques now being used to evaluate bone mineral mass cannot distinguish the presence of protein matrix. A bone **biopsy** and histologic examination of tissues are required to confirm osteomalacia.

In the young individual with vitamin D deficiency, newly formed bone matrix is not mineralized when calcium levels are insufficient. In the older individual, the situation is compounded by the fact that a fall in serum calcium and phosphate levels not only results in failure to mineralize the matrix formed in bone remodeling but also stimulates the secretion of PTH, which leads to the resorption of existing bone.[85] Nordin[85] suggests that the extensive bone loss observed in osteomalacia relates to the **secondary hyperparathyroidism.**

Clinical symptoms of osteomalacia include generalized pain, which in time becomes localized, and bones that become extremely sensitive to pressure. Changes in the vertebrae cause a loss in height, and the bones of the pelvis and sternum may become deformed. Muscle weakness becomes apparent in advanced osteomalacia and affects the pelvic and shoulder areas. Individuals may have trouble climbing stairs or raising their arms to comb their hair. Unfortunately, the pain often is assumed to be arthritic in origin, and muscle weakness tends to be rather common in older people.[85]

Causes of osteomalacia. Osteomalacia is less prevalent in the United States than in Great Britain, and this has been attributed to the vitamin D—fortification of milk and milk products. Nevertheless, institutionalized or homebound older people who do not go outdoors and do not consume vitamin D—fortified dairy products are at risk of vitamin D deficiency and osteomalacia. Liver or renal disease that interferes with the conversion of vitamin D to its active form can lead to osteomalacia.[99] In the United States osteomalacia is most likely to result from malabsorption, related chronic disease, or use of particular medications.[55]

Excessive use of antacids that contain **aluminum hydroxide** and bind dietary phosphate has been associated with this condition. In one clinical report[55] an earlier diagnosis based on radiologic findings had considered the bone problem to be osteoporosis and so the use of aluminum hydroxide—containing antacids had continued, with a further deterioration of bone health. A distinguishing biochemical feature associated with osteomalacia arising from excessive antacid ingestion and phosphate malabsorption is **hypercalciuria** accompanied by low urinary phosphate and low serum phosphate levels. Withdrawal of the antacids and a high-calcium intake with adequate vitamin D, will halt the bone loss.[55]

Despite the fact that osteomalacia could contribute to bone loss and hip fracture, it does not appear to be generally associated with osteoporosis. Examination of bone biopsy samples obtained from 49 patients ages 67 to 92 with hip fractures revealed only one patient with osteomalacia.[25] Nevertheless, vitamin D deficiency leading to secondary hyperparathyroidism can exacerbate the bone loss associated with osteoporosis. Older people should be cautioned against regular use of medications containing aluminum hydroxide.

CARBOHYDRATE METABOLISM AND GLUCOSE TOLERANCE

The ability to metabolize glucose deteriorates with age. It is estimated that 20% to 30% of people over age 60 have impaired glucose tolerance, and 10% to 35% have diabetes mellitus.[14] In a young adult abnormal **glucose tolerance** is associated with the development of overt diabetes. In an older adult, differentiating age-related changes from the pathologic sequence of disease is more difficult, as is deciding on appropriate treatment. Diabetes mellitus is a major chronic disorder among aging individuals, and older diabetics are more likely to have complications requiring hospitalization.[81]

Age and Changes In Glucose Tolerance

An elevated **plasma** glucose level after an oral dose of glucose occurs with increasing frequency across the adult years. In one study[81] that excluded all known diabetics, elevated plasma glucose levels in the glucose tolerance test were observed in 16% of those ages 45 to 54 and 42% of those ages 75 to 79. Morley and coworkers[81] estimate that 2-hour **postprandial** plasma glucose levels increase 5 to 10 mg/dl each decade over age 50. In contrast, **fasting** plasma glucose levels change very little over adulthood, increasing only 1 to 2 mg/dl each decade beyond middle age.[32]

Glucose Tolerance Test

For the **oral glucose tolerance test,** as defined by the **National Diabetes Data Group,**[82] 75 g of glucose are ingested in flavored water, and blood samples are taken every 30 minutes for 2 hours thereafter. Defined conditions include (1) a daily carbohydrate intake of 150 g or more for 3 days preceding the test; (2) a 10- to 16-hour fast before the test; and (3) the avoidance of exercise, coffee, or smoking before and during the test.

Caffeine, nicotine, and physical activity raise blood glucose levels, as do some drugs commonly used by older people, including aspirin and diuretics. A lack of physical activity or bed rest for several days before the test can result in abnormal glucose tolerance. Lack of adequate dietary preparation contributes to abnormal glucose tolerance.

Results obtained from the oral glucose tolerance test lead to a classification of normal glucose tolerance, impaired glucose tolerance, or diabetes mellitus.[82] As the number of older people increases, primary care physicians are being called upon to make decisions about the care of those demonstrating abnormal glucose tolerance. In younger individuals elevated plasma glucose leads to **microvascular** complications and disturbances in visual function, and glucose control retards these changes.[81] In older adults with somewhat elevated plasma glucose, it is not known if drug or dietary intervention that often requires a major change in life-style actually confers any benefit.[57]

Kahn and coworkers[57] emphasize that the current standards were established with data obtained from young and middle-aged adults. Using these criteria a greater proportion of older adults are judged to have impaired glucose tolerance or diabetes mellitus despite the absence of other symptoms. One approach to evaluating plasma glucose levels in older people could be age-corrected standards by which an individual's performance on the oral glucose tolerance test is judged according to that of peers of similar age.[2] This assumes, however, that age-related changes in glucose tolerance are a normal consequence of the aging process.[2] If impaired glucose tolerance is viewed as pathologic and predictive of diabetes mellitus, then any adjustment for age is inappropriate.[2,32]

The current standards for the classification of glucose tolerance in adults (see box) allow no adjustment for age. The higher the glucose levels observed, the more likely the individual is to develop overt diabetes mellitus. Elevated fasting glucose levels are viewed as more serious than elevated postprandial glucose levels in elderly adults.[57]

Hyperglycemia does increase cardiovascular risk independent of age, blood pressure, serum cholesterol levels, **body mass index (BMI),** or smoking. In a 14-year follow-up of 2,471 older adults, Barrett-Connor and coworkers[10] found that either a history of diabetes mellitus or a fasting plasma glucose of 140 mg/dl or higher resulted in a twofold increase in fatal **ischemic heart disease** in men and a threefold increase in women. These data suggested that diabetes

---

CRITERIA FOR CLASSIFYING GLUCOSE TOLERANCE (FASTING LEVELS AND AFTER A 75 G ORAL GLUCOSE CHALLENGE)

DIABETES MELLITUS
- Classic symptoms of diabetes (e.g., polyuria, polydipsia, ketonuria, extreme hyperglycemia)
- Fasting plasma glucose of 140 mg/dl or higher on at least two tests

or

- Plasma glucose of 200 mg/dl or higher at 120 minutes and at 30, 60, or 90 minutes

IMPAIRED GLUCOSE TOLERANCE
- Fasting plasma glucose below 140 mg/dl

and

- Plasma glucose of 200 mg/dl or higher at 30, 60, or 90 minutes

and

- Plasma glucose between 140 and 200 mg/dl at 120 minutes

NORMAL GLUCOSE LEVELS
- Fasting plasma glucose below 115 mg/dl
- Plasma glucose below 200 mg/dl at 30, 60, and 90 minutes
- Plasma glucose below 140 mg/dl at 120 minutes

Adapted from the National Diabetes Data Group: Classification and diagnosis of diabetes mellitus and other categories of glucose intolerance, *Diabetes* 28:1039, 1979.

mellitus or hyperglycemia set aside the natural resistance of women to fatal heart disease. In a longitudinal study of nursing home patients,[43] 31% with elevated plasma glucose levels became diabetic over time. These results would argue for dietary intervention for those with impaired glucose tolerance.

Basis for Change in Glucose Tolerance

Normal glucose regulation. The plasma glucose level is regulated by the hormones insulin and glucagon, which are secreted by the **beta** and **alpha islets** of the pancreas, respectively. Usually glucose is the primary energy source for the brain and red blood cells; thus it is important that adequate plasma levels be maintained between meals and overnight. Liver cells are very sensitive to the amounts of **insulin** and **glucagon** drained into the portal vein.[57] When plasma glucose levels fall, the secretion of glucagon will lead to a breakdown of liver glycogen and **gluconeogenesis** to restore plasma levels. After ingestion of food and a rise in plasma glucose, insulin is released, which suppresses hepatic glucose production and promotes glucose uptake by muscle and adipose cells. Glucose uptake and storage by the liver is not dependent on insulin. Glucose tolerance is altered by (1) reduced uptake of glucose in peripheral tissues; (2) inappropriate hepatic release of glucose; and (3) inappropriate release of glucagon or reduced release of insulin.

Insulin sensitivity of peripheral tissues. A decrease in the sensitivity of muscle and adipose cells to insulin has long been regarded as a major cause of impaired glucose tolerance in older people, although the mechanism leading to this change is unclear. The rate at which glucose enters these cells is reduced despite normal or in some cases elevated plasma insulin levels.[57] Reduced glucose movement into the cell could be related to a change in the number or effectiveness of cell receptor sites for binding insulin. However, Kahn and coworkers,[57] found similar numbers of receptors on cells from older and younger people, and the affinity of receptors for insulin was not changed by age.

Insulin sensitivity of hepatic tissues. Based on current evidence, it is unlikely that reduced hepatic **insulin sensitivity** contributes to impaired glucose intolerance in older people. In healthy elderly people,[15] hepatic release of glucose is rapidly suppressed by even small increases in insulin secretion. Changes in hepatic response to insulin do occur in **noninsulin-dependent diabetes mellitus (NIDDM),** also known as type II diabetes.

Pancreatic function. Changes in glucose tolerance could relate to hormonal secretion and control. Although some workers[15] have reported normal or increased serum insulin concentrations in older age, others have observed reduced levels. There does appear to be a reduction in the first phase of insulin secretion (the rapid release of insulin occurring immediately after ingestion of glucose), as well as an inability to sustain normal insulin secretion.[15] A defect in first-phase insulin secretion is associated with the inappropriate plasma glucose levels observed in those with NIDDM. These alterations in beta-cell function are believed to contribute to the decline in glucose uptake in the peripheral cells.[57]

Factors Contributing to Altered Glucose Metabolism

Changes in dietary pattern and life-style have been associated with the deterioration of glucose tolerance. Low carbohydrate intake, a high level of body fat, and limited exercise influence the disposal of a glucose load.

Carbohydrate intake. Chen and coworkers[19,21] evaluated glucose tolerance in younger men (ages 18 to 36) and older men (ages 65 to 82) on both self-selected diets and formulated diets containing different amounts of carbohydrate. The self-selected diets of the younger men contained a lower percentage of carbohydrate compared to that of the older men (41% versus 49%) but a higher absolute amount (292 versus 277 g). Plasma levels following a dose of glucose rose more rapidly and decreased more slowly in the older men (Fig. 8-2). **Insulin resistance,** as measured by the rate of disappearance of glucose per unit of insulin, was more than doubled in the older men. When dietary carbohydrate was increased from 49% to 85% of total kilocalories, the insulin sensitivity and the plasma glucose levels of the older men

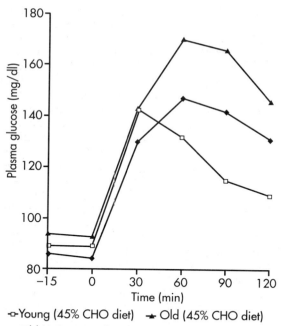

FIG. 8-2 Effect of age and carbohydrate intake on oral glucose tolerance. Plasma glucose levels in older men after a 75 g oral glucose challenge are significantly reduced when dietary carbohydrate is increased to 85% of total energy.

(With permission from Kahn SE and others: The glucose intolerance of aging: implications for intervention, *Hosp Pract* 26(4A):29, 1991.)

became more like those of the younger men. The mechanism by which dietary carbohydrate influences these responses is unknown.

A positive effect of complex carbohydrate in maintaining normal glucose tolerance was evident in a 4-year follow-up of 175 older people in Rotterdam.[35] Although total carbohydrate intake was similar in both groups, those who maintained normal glucose tolerance consumed more legumes compared to those whose glucose tolerance became impaired. Individuals with impaired glucose tolerance consumed more pastries, and high use of pastries more than tripled the risk of impaired glucose metabolism. Neither age nor intake of saturated fatty

acids was related to the detrimental effect of pastry on this function.

Body mass index. Obesity and enlarged adipose cells have been related to insulin resistance and impaired glucose tolerance in persons of all ages. An increased body mass index (BMI) (27 versus 24) was associated with a twofold increase in risk of impaired glucose tolerance in the older Rotterdam subjects described above.[35] With a higher BMI, both fasting and 2-hour postprandial plasma glucose levels were elevated. A loss of body fat may improve glucose homeostasis. Reaven and coworkers[91] reported that an average weight loss of 9 kg reduced the degree of hyperglycemia among 12 obese patients with an average age of 71 years. Improvement occurred despite the fact that none reached their ideal body weight. Conversely, a weight gain of even 10 pounds between ages 40 and 60 can double the risk of impaired glucose metabolism.[53]

Enlarged fat cells are less sensitive to insulin than smaller fat cells. It is important to recognize, however, that the impaired glucose tolerance observed in older people is at least in part independent of fat cell size. In older individuals glucose entry is enhanced at high plasma glucose concentrations, as is the case in normal young adults; the rate of glucose entry is not influenced by plasma glucose concentration in obese young adults.[20]

Exercise. Exercise improves insulin effectiveness through changes in the skeletal muscle. In 46 men ages 45 to 75 years, the fitness level, as measured by exercise time to exhaustion, was responsible for 47% of the variance in plasma insulin levels after a glucose load.[54] Insulin levels dropped by about one half in older men who participated in an intensive exercise program, although their glucose levels changed only slightly. Because elevated plasma insulin levels increase the risk of diabetes mellitus, a significant decrease in insulin secretion as a result of improved insulin sensitivity contributes significantly to health. In a follow-up study of 2,000 healthy people[53] over age 50, those using exercise as their means of avoiding weight gain reduced their risk of diabetes mellitus by one half.

Age. Despite other factors, age per se still exerts a significant effect on glucose tolerance.

Among 743 healthy men and recently added women in the Baltimore Longitudinal Study of Aging (BLSA),[97] fasting and 2-hour plasma glucose levels increased with age, although to a greater extent in men. The percentage of body fat and **waist-to-hip ratio** also increased with age and were positively related to plasma glucose levels; physical fitness, as measured by **maximum oxygen consumption,** was related to plasma glucose levels only in men. These associations did explain the age-related changes in glucose tolerance observed between the young (ages 17 to 39) and middle-aged (ages 40 to 59) men and women; however, they did not account for the further decline in glucose tolerance observed in the oldest age group (ages 60 to 92). Carbohydrate intake did not appear to influence these results, because intakes actually increased by 8 g a day per decade over this range.

The impairment in glucose tolerance that occurs with advancing age is poorly understood. Although increases in both fasting and postprandial blood glucose levels have been observed in healthy older adults, some workers[14] consider these changes to be disease related, not age related. NIDDM does increase in prevalence among older people, although the mechanisms underlying this disease differ from those associated with impaired glucose tolerance. Decreased hepatic sensitivity to insulin and impaired first-phase insulin secretion are primary factors in the development of NIDDM, whereas increased peripheral resistance to insulin and decreased ability of the beta-cells to sustain insulin secretion are of greater importance in impaired glucose tolerance.[14] It is likely, however, that these conditions act synergistically in promoting the development of overt diabetes mellitus. A diet high in complex carbohydrates, as currently recommended by the Food and Nutrition Board's Committee on Diet and Health,[24] coupled with regular exercise and the avoidance of inappropriate weight gain, can minimize the changes in glucose homeostasis.

Diabetes Mellitus in Older People

Most people who manifest diabetes mellitus in middle age or beyond have noninsulin-dependent diabetes mellitus (NIDDM). About half of all people with this disorder are over 65 years of age.[80] NIDDM is characterized by hyperglycemia uncomplicated by ketoacidosis. **Ketones** are present in the urine if the disease is poorly controlled, but they do not accumulate in the serum.[81] Insulin-dependent (type I) diabetes mellitus, with accompanying **ketoacidosis,** is less common in older individuals but does occur in those who no longer produce any significant amount of insulin. Morley and coworkers[81] emphasize that appropriate glucose control contributes significantly to the older patient's quality of life. Microvascular changes develop rapidly in older patients and lead to many problems, including ocular complications, with loss of color vision or total sight; neural complications, with increased pain, cognitive dysfunction, or depression; renal complications; increased susceptibility to infection; and impaired circulation in the lower extremities, with the risk of **gangrene** and the resulting amputations.

Management of the older diabetic patient. Management of the older individual with type II diabetes usually involves dietary modification, exercise, weight reduction if indicated, and a hypoglycemic drug if necessary.[80] Morley and Perry[80] recommend that treatment be implemented when fasting plasma glucose levels exceed 140 mg/dl on two separate occasions or when plasma glucose levels exceed 200 mg/dl at least 2 hours after the most recent meal.

Dietary modification. The American Diabetes Association recommends a diet high in carbohydrate (55% to 60%) and low in fat (less than 30%) to control blood glucose.[80] Other work indicates that a diet high in **monounsaturated fats** (50% of total kilocalories) and moderate in carbohydrate (35% of total kilocalories) may lower serum triglyceride and cholesterol levels as well as serum glucose levels, thus lowering the risk of **atherosclerotic lesions.**[80] Grundy[45] recommends the high-carbohydrate, low-fat regimen for obese individuals newly diagnosed with NIDDM who are attempting to lose weight or who may have been unsuccessful at losing weight but are maintaining good glucose control.

For those older nonobese individuals with a long-term history of NIDDM, a high-carbohydrate diet may aggravate elevated blood glucose levels. A reduced level of carbohydrate and an increased level of dietary fat in the form of monounsaturated fat may improve glycemic control.[45] In some older patients with NIDDM, a well-balanced, nondiabetic diet that excludes free sugar will maintain appropriate plasma glucose, plasma lipid, and **glycosylated hemoglobin levels.**[27] Coulston[27] pointed out that assignment to a regular diet provides older individuals with greater flexibility at mealtime and improves their psychologic outlook. A key to management of the older individual with NIDDM is individualization of the recommended diet.

Exercise and weight loss. Evidence obtained with younger individuals points to the beneficial effect of weight loss on glucose tolerance.[57] However, there is the risk of malnutrition in older individuals placed on diets that are low in kilocalories and that require many dietary changes.[80] Some clinicians[80] recommend weight reduction only for those elderly diabetics who are at least 20% above average weight using height-weight tables from individuals of similar age (see Chapter 11). An exercise program involving 20 to 30 minutes of brisk walking each day may improve glucose metabolism and cardiovascular fitness. Older diabetics undertaking a walking program need to be advised about proper footwear and care of their feet.

Oral hypoglycemic drugs. The **sulfonylureas,** such as **tolbutamide,** are prescribed in NIDDM.[80] Because these drugs stimulate the release of insulin from the beta-cells, they are not useful if all beta-cell function is lost. In contrast to insulin, oral hypoglycemic agents have no direct effect on plasma glucose levels. Individuals for whom plasma glucose levels cannot be controlled with diet, exercise, and oral hypoglycemic drugs, or those who have nonfunctional beta-cells, must be treated with insulin. (The management of insulin-dependent diabetes mellitus is beyond the scope of this book; interested readers should consult a therapeutic nutrition text.)

HYPERTENSION
Age and Blood Pressure

Blood pressure increases up to ages 50 to 60. Beyond age 60 **systolic blood pressure** tends to stabilize or decline in men but continues to increase in women. **Diastolic blood pressure** begins to stabilize somewhat earlier at about age 50.[109] Elevated blood pressure is more common in women and in black adults. Between the ages of 35 and 65, the prevalence of **hypertension** increases twofold in black women (from 29% to 59%) and fourfold in white women (from 10% to 42%). About one half of black men ages 65 to 74 have elevated blood pressure. In the **Framingham Heart Study,** 31% of the men and 43% of the women over age 70 had hypertension.[12]

At one time elevated blood pressure was considered a natural sequela of aging and of limited consequence.[109] It is now recognized that hypertension continues to be a significant risk factor into advanced age. **Systolic hypertension** adds to the risk of cardiovascular disease independently of any associated **arteriosclerosis.**[12] The definition of hypertension tends to be somewhat arbitrary. In general, a systolic blood pressure of 160 mm Hg or higher or a diastolic pressure of 90 mm Hg or higher is considered indicative of hypertension.

The two major types of hypertension most common in older people are **isolated systolic hypertension** and combined systolic-diastolic hypertension.[109] Isolated systolic hypertension is characterized by a systolic pressure over 160 mm Hg and a diastolic pressure that is normal or only minimally increased. In combined systolic-diastolic hypertension, both measurements are elevated. **Diastolic hypertension** appears to be responsible for the increase in cardiovascular risk associated with hypertension in younger age groups. In older age groups, however, systolic hypertension appears responsible for the added risk. Isolated systolic hypertension is the predominant form of hypertension in older people.

Weber and coworkers[109] argue that hypertension arises from different causes in older people than in younger people. Moreover, hypertension in an elderly individual usually is a newly developed condition, arising for the first time in the later years. Physiologic changes that contribute to the elevation of blood pressure in later life include (1) increased sodium retention related to excessive sodium intake, ineffective sodium excretion, or enhanced **aldosterone** secretion; (2) alterations in the sympathetic nervous system, leading to enhanced **vasoconstriction;** and (3) loss of elasticity of the large arteries.

Factors Contributing to the Development of Hypertension

Obesity. Body mass continues to influence blood pressure levels into advanced age. Among 255 Dutch elderly 65 to 79 years old,[70] BMI was positively associated with both systolic and diastolic blood pressures; in contrast, **creatinine** excretion, an indicator of lean body mass, was inversely related to systolic blood pressure. In that population a "normal" weight seemed to exert a protective effect against hypertension despite high sodium intakes. Not only the relative degree of adiposity but also its position may influence blood pressure. An increased waist-to-hip ratio was associated with the development of hypertension among nearly 42,000 women ages 55 to 69.[37] Women with a high degree of abdominal adiposity had a higher risk of hypertension even after accounting for body weight.

In young and middle-aged adults, loss of body weight is associated with a decrease in blood pressure, particularly during the period of active weight loss.[24] However, the efficacy of weight reduction as an antihypertensive therapy in older adults has not been evaluated.

Alcohol. Alcohol consumption exceeding 2 ounces a day is known to elevate blood pressure in adults of all ages.[24] Reducing alcohol consumption brings about reductions in both systolic and diastolic blood pressures in hypertensive individuals, and blood pressures return to their former levels when alcohol consumption is resumed. Alcohol abuse may contribute to the prevalence of hypertension in some older groups.

Exercise. Intervention studies suggest that **aerobic exercise** reduces blood pressure in hypertensive adults of middle age. However, in a recent clinical trial Blumenthal and coworkers[11] found no difference in systolic or diastolic blood pressure between mildly hypertensive subjects participating in supervised exercise sessions three times a week and nonexercising control subjects. These authors suggest that the positive effects of exercise reported by others may have resulted from a loss of body weight; body weight was unchanged in the exercise group that did not experience a decrease in blood pressure. Despite the uncertainty of the mechanism by which exercise may influence blood pressure, the overall benefits of exercise to health justify its use.

Dietary intake. Daily intakes of several minerals, including sodium, potassium, calcium, and magnesium, have been evaluated in respect to blood pressure. An excessive intake of sodium does lead to elevated blood pressure in sensitive individuals. It also appears that older people are more sensitive to sodium than younger people and often respond to moderate sodium restriction of 2 g of sodium a day (5 g of sodium chloride).[104] Sodium restriction to this level made it possible to control blood pressure with fewer medications.[110] Given the limited ability of aged kidneys to conserve sodium, clinicians advise against reducing sodium intake below 2 g a day.[104]

Potassium intake is inversely related to blood pressure. Löwik and coworkers[70] proposed that increased dietary potassium helped prevent hypertension among elderly Dutch men by increasing urinary sodium levels. A recent clinical trial[6] examined the effect of increased potassium intake from food sources on blood pressure in hypertensive adults. Potassium intake was increased from 1,500 to 2,400 mg in the experimental group. After 1 year, blood pressure and body weight were unchanged; however, 38% of those with an increased potassium intake no longer required drugs to control their hypertension as compared to only 9% of the control subjects. Physical symptoms related to elevated blood pressure or side effects of medications declined by almost half. How potassium acts to control blood pressure is still unclear; however, the fact that increasing one's intake of potassium-rich foods can reduce dependence on hypertension medication further supports the recommendation to eat more fruits and vegetables for long-term health benefits.

Dietary calcium is still of interest in relation to blood pressure. Although an evaluation of the NHANES I data[75] suggested that hypertensive individuals consumed less calcium than **normotensive** individuals, attempts to influence blood pressure using calcium supplements have yielded equivocal results. Gruchow and co-workers[44] suggest that a low calcium intake may enhance the pathologic effects of excessive sodium or depressed potassium levels on blood pressure. In light of the fact that systolic blood pressure was reduced in particular hypertensive individuals whose calcium intake met the recommended amount, it would make sense to encourage the consumption of 800 mg of calcium each day in the interest of general and bone health.

Treatment of Hypertension

Only in recent years has elevated blood pressure in older people been treated aggressively. Yet Tjoa and Kaplan[104] emphasize the need for caution in developing a care plan for the older individual, keeping in mind the physiologic characteristics of this group. Guidelines for nondrug intervention include:

- Initiating modest weight reduction if appropriate.
- Limiting sodium intake to 2 g (5 g of sodium chloride).
- Limiting alcohol consumption to 2 ounces a day or less.
- Initiating regular aerobic exercise if possible.
- Maintaining recommended daily intakes of potassium, calcium, and magnesium.

Drug therapy for treating hypertension in older people usually involves diuretics, but all classes of antihypertensive medications may be prescribed (see Chapter 9).

BODY WEIGHT MANAGEMENT

Obesity increases the risk of death from many causes (see Chapter 2), yet Durnin[33] proposes that a moderate degree of fatness is of nutritional benefit to the older individual should

food intake be reduced as a result of illness. **Unintentional weight loss** and low fat reserves are also associated with increased morbidity and mortality and a reduced ability to respond to a nutritional emergency. Situations involving extreme obesity or the loss of protein and fat tissues indicative of **protein-energy malnutrition,** leave no doubt as to the need for intervention, but implementation may prove difficult and the outcome uncertain. An unresolved question is the extent to which obesity or unintentional weight loss can be ameliorated in the older individual.

Weight Loss

Rapid, involuntary weight loss in an older adult is a sign of a deteriorating physical condition or serious disease.[33,36] The tissue lost is likely to include both lean body mass and body fat. An older individual with a substantial amount of body fat will lose a relatively small amount of lean tissue and a relatively large amount of fat when there is an energy deficit. Conversely, those with little body fat will be forced to break down lean tissue, resulting in muscular, cardiac, and visceral wasting.

Involuntary weight loss can have many causes. Physiologic and metabolic changes can reduce the absorption or assimilation of nutrients. Chronic disease, dementia, or disability may interfere with food intake.[89] Hyperthyroidism, causing an elevation in metabolic rate (see Chapter 3), results in weight loss. **Cytokinins,** released in the presence of tumors or infection, are elevated in cancer, uncontrolled diabetes, and pulmonary disease and contribute to the anorexia and **cachexia** associated with these problems.

Because of the vulnerability of older people to weight loss, body weight should be evaluated regularly, particularly in those with poor food intake or chronic disease. Fischer and Johnson[36] suggest the use of additional **anthropometric measurements,** since edema, tumor growth, or preexisting obesity can mask weight loss (see Chapter 11). Body weight should be measured once a month and the current weight compared to the previous weight. If an individual appears to be losing weight, weekly measurements may be required to identify the problem and define intervention strategies.

Involuntary weight loss is not uncommon among older people. In 1,200 consecutive admissions to a veterans' medical facility,[73] 91 individuals were identified for whom documented weight loss over the previous 6 months ranged from 3.2 to 45.4 kg. Psychiatric causes, including depression, were identified in eight patients. Physical causes of involuntary weight loss included cancer (18), gastrointestinal disease (13), cardiovascular disease (8), alcohol abuse (7), and pulmonary disease (5). In 24 cases no physical cause of weight loss could be found at the time of entry or for 1 year afterward. The patients with an identified physical cause of weight loss had an increased risk of death within 1 year (21 of 59 cases) compared to those with no identified physical disease (2 of 32 cases). It is equally important to note that 55 patients either maintained their level of functional capability or gained weight over that period. Several characteristics were associated with those who died or continued to lose weight compared to those with a favorable outcome (i.e., cancer as a physical cause of weight loss; age 80 or over; physical disability (unable to walk without help); body weight over 91 kg before weight loss; and abnormal laboratory values for blood or urine).

In people over 83 years of age, a BMI below 22 was associated with increased risk of mortality, permanent hospitalization, and decreased ability to cope with living at home.[90]

Institutionalized older adults are at particular risk of weight loss. In a 2-year follow-up of 335 institutionalized older people,[34] 30% experienced a weight loss of at least 4.5 kg from their admission weight. Several patients had extreme levels of weight loss, with one losing 12 kg the first year and 18 kg the second year. Six percent of the total population lost at least 9 kg over the 2-year period. The survival rate was lower among those losing at least 4.5 kg. Monitoring body weight is especially important in institutionalized patients with cognitive disorders or physical disabilities that lead to feeding problems.[36] Lewis and Bell[64] have defined significant weight loss as the loss of:

- 1% to 2% of body weight in 1 week
- 5% of body weight in 1 month
- 7.5% of body weight in 3 months
- 10% to 20% of body weight over time

Loss of body weight can be reversed in many older people with appropriate nutritional support.[22] Suggestions for using foods and supplement powders that can be added to liquid and soft foods can be found in Chapter 5. Enteral feeding procedures and appropriate formulas are discussed by Chernoff.[22]

Weight Gain

The general pattern of weight gain, as well as the absolute body weight, can influence health at older ages. A study published about 20 years ago[1] suggested that individuals who were underweight as children but gained weight rapidly in adulthood were more likely to have serious cardiovascular disease by age 50 than those who were somewhat overweight from childhood. Evaluation of the body weight history of participants in the Baltimore Longitudinal Study of Aging (BLSA)[68] suggested that variability in body weight was associated with a deterioration in glucose tolerance and a greater concentration of body fat on the trunk versus the limbs. The rate of weight change per year ranged from −4.3 to +2.6 kg, although the average change was −0.02 kg a year. Among 89 patients with osteoarthritis[111] who ranged in age from 60 to 89 years, weight gain, common over adulthood, averaged about 26.6 kg, or almost half a kilogram a year after age 20. Substantial weight gain over adulthood may influence functional capacity and the ability to remain independent.

Another aspect of disease risk is the pattern of weight loss followed by weight gain observed in overweight individuals. It is estimated that 90% of those who lose about 11 kg or more will regain that weight within 2 years.[86] If continued, this pattern may actually increase the risk of earlier death. In a 25-year follow-up[46] of more than 2,100 men ages 40 to 56 when the study began, the risk of coronary death was about doubled in the men who had gained and lost at least 10% of their body weight during any 5-year period compared to men with a similar weight gain but no further fluctuation in weight. Findings were similar in the Framingham Heart Study.[69] Individuals with a high degree of fluctuation in their BMI had a higher risk regardless of their level of obesity or overall trend in body weight. In fact, the Framingham workers concluded that the relative risk associated with continued fluctuations in body weight was as great as that associated with static obesity.

It is evident that either body weight fluctuation itself or the dietary patterns or life-style associated with loss and regain of body weight has a deleterious effect on general health. The physiologic or psychologic stress associated with weight gain and loss may have especially adverse effects on an older individual with a diminished reserve capacity and chronic disease.

Basis for Weight Loss Intervention

A recent consensus development conference[83] concluded that weight reduction should be recommended to individuals of all ages who are more than 20% overweight based on the 1983 Metropolitan Life Insurance Co. standards. In the NHANES II study, the standards used to designate overweight were a BMI above 27.8 for men and 27.3 for women. Morley and Glick[79] propose that weight reduction be initiated in anyone over 65 years of age who is more than 30% above average weight. However, these approaches do not allow for an age-related increase in body weight. Andrus and co-workers[3] maintain that some increase in body weight is a normal accompaniment of the aging process, and they have published the average heights and weights of healthy BSLA participants to provide a basis for evaluation. Weight reduction, with a loss of body fat, may be especially desirable for people with NIDDM, hypertension, heart disease, or pulmonary disease. Weight reduction could also benefit those with osteoarthritis.

The possible advantages of weight loss must be evaluated against the possible physical and emotional stress imposed by a weight loss program. Severely limiting caloric intake when protein, vitamin, and mineral status is already precarious may further compromise general well-being. Also, even modest caloric restriction results in a loss of 1 g of lean body tissue for every 3 g of fat in healthy young adults.[102]

Very-low-calorie diets, which lead to severe **negative nitrogen balance,** or **anorectic drugs** are not appropriate for the older individual.[79]

In older people with chronic illness, an improvement in metabolic or physiologic status is a more appropriate goal than actual weight lost.[29] A decrease in blood glucose or insulin levels, an increase in high-density lipoprotein (HDL) cholesterol, or a positive change in waist-to-hip ratio is of greater importance to health goals than weight loss per se. A reasonable approach is a well-balanced diet, more exercise, and life-style changes as appropriate.

Caloric intake and food selection. Little information exists describing weight reduction programs in older people. It is suggested that diets provide at least 1,000 kcal daily,[79] and even this level is likely to reduce the **resting metabolic rate.**[28] It is difficult to provide adequate vitamins and minerals on this caloric intake, and a supplement providing the RDA for these nutrients is recommended. For individuals who are bedridden or chairbound and have a low lean body mass, an intake of 1,000 kcal may not result in weight loss, although it may prevent weight gain.

A well-balanced diet that is lower in fat and higher in carbohydrate may reduce caloric intake. A recent intervention trial[42] with women ages 45 to 69 indicated that decreasing dietary fat from 39% to 22% of total energy resulted in a loss of about 2.4 kg over 3 months. This is particularly noteworthy because the women were not counseled to reduce their total dietary intake, merely their intake of fat. Their decrease in fat intake was substantial and lowered daily caloric intake from 1,738 to 1,300 kcal. This was achieved in part by substituting lower fat dairy products and salad dressings for higher fat products and pretzels and similar low-fat grain products for potato chips and other high-fat grain products. Overall, intakes of fruit and grain products increased. Reducing the use of fat as a flavoring can also lower total dietary fat.[62] Lowering fat intake to 22% of total energy is not recommended for older adults; however, some decrease in dietary fat can, over time, contribute to weight loss or help prevent weight gain.

Exercise program. Creating a caloric deficit

with consistent exercise allows a higher intake of food and necessary nutrients and reduces the loss of lean body mass. Walking for 30 minutes has been estimated to use 186 kcal in a 76.5 kg man and 141 kcal in a 58.5 kg woman.[5] A walk of 2 to 3 miles several times a week is a reasonable goal for older people in good health. Swimming, jogging, or square dancing are other alternatives. Even a short daily walk at a slow pace will assist in weight control. Although **aerobic exercises** burn the most kilocalories and improve cardiovascular fitness, strength training also adds to energy expenditure and is beneficial in preserving muscle mass.[5] Implementing an exercise program for sedentary older adults requires professional supervision (see Chapter 3).

Life-style. Active participation in a variety of activities helps prevent unwanted weight gain. Spending an afternoon walking around the mall expends more energy than sitting in a favorite chair. Among employed adult men, those who watched television more than 3 hours a day were twice as likely to be obese as those who watched television only 1 to 2 hours a day.[106] This held true regardless of age, level of physical fitness, and hours of exercise weekly. Efforts to develop spare time pursuits involving some physical activity should begin early in adult life.

NUTRITIONAL ANEMIA
Causes of Anemia

Anemia results from a change in either the number or characteristics of the **erythrocyte.** A progressive anemia that leads to a decrease in the oxygen-carrying capacity of the blood and an oxygen deficit in the tissues can cause an increase in heart rate, shortness of breath, and weakness. **Nutritional anemias** are most commonly related to deficiencies of iron, folate, or vitamin B_{12} and are reversed when the nutrient is restored. In older people an **anemia of chronic disease** is associated with protein-energy malnutrition and chronic disease and may involve various nutrients. The anemia of chronic disease can occur with **rheumatoid arthritis** or **osteoarthritis, myocardial infarction, inflammatory bowel disease,** renal disease, and low-grade infection.[51]

Iron-Deficiency Anemia

Basis of problem. The nutritional anemia most easily identified and corrected in older people is **iron-deficiency anemia,** although vitamin deficiencies may complicate the problem. In 100 consecutive older people admitted to a hospital[103] with deficient **hemoglobin** levels, 45 were deficient in iron, 25 were deficient in vitamin B_{12} or folate, and 27 were deficient in all three nutrients.

Iron-deficiency anemia is caused by (1) poor iron intake, (2) poor iron absorption, or (3) increased **erythropoiesis** resulting from chronic blood loss. **Occult blood** loss through the gastrointestinal tract is a frequent and critical cause of iron-deficiency anemia in older people.[50] Excessive blood in the stool may go unnoticed, discovered only on examination for anemia or other problems. Normal blood loss in the stool is less than 3 ml a day; losses above this level are pathologic. Blood losses of 50 to 75 ml impart a dark red or black color to the stool; however, significant losses below this level are not usually obvious and require chemical analysis for detection.[103]

Conditions associated with gastrointestinal bleeding include gastric or duodenal ulcers, **diverticulitis, hiatus hernia,** hemorrhoids, and cancer. Long-term use of aspirin, with irritation of the gastric mucosa, can lead to significant blood loss. Many times individuals are free of symptoms and do not seek medical attention until the condition has progressed and the anemia is severe. One milliliter of blood from an individual with a hemoglobin level of 15 g/dl contains about 0.5 mg iron; consequently, extended losses will severely deplete iron stores.

Prevalence of iron-deficiency anemia. The prevalence of anemia varies according to age, sex, socioeconomic status, race, and general health.[18,40,67] Among healthy, economically advantaged older people in New Mexico,[40] only 2.3% of the men and 1.2% of the women had hemoglobin levels below 14 and 12 g/dl, respectively. Fewer than 2% of the group had low plasma iron levels, and fewer than 3% had low **transferrin saturation.** None had a deficient serum **ferritin** level. In a survey of 80 older Canadians (ages 59 to 88)[72] living in the community, 21% of the women and 27% of the men had hemoglobin levels in the deficient range; however, a similar number also had deficient serum vitamin B_{12} levels. Fewer than 4% had abnormally low ferritin levels, suggesting that a vitamin B_{12} deficiency rather than a lack of iron was responsible for the anemia.

Institutionalized individuals with chronic disease are more likely to be anemic. A study of 50 independent-living and 50 institutionalized older people[18] revealed that only 4% of the men and 8% of the women living in the community had iron-deficiency anemia, whereas this was true of 40% of the institutionalized group. Of 50 older men in a long-term care facility,[13] eight had biochemical evidence of iron-deficiency anemia, and seven of the eight were over age 80. Within a group of homebound elderly in Arkansas,[71] 11% to 20% of the white women and men were anemic, compared with 31% to 44% of the black women and men. These data suggest that older people with a limited food supply or several chronic diseases are at greater risk of anemia.

Age and Hematologic Parameters

Currently there is no evidence to suggest that standards used to identify anemia should differ for older and younger people. An evaluation of healthy elderly[116] age 84 or over revealed that hematologic values are remarkably stable into advanced age. All mean values were within the normal range. In the 20 older participants for whom hemoglobin levels were available over a 5-year period, the variation within individual subjects was only 0.55 g/dl.

Schultz and Freedman[96] maintain that anemia is one of the first signs of illness in older people and that lowering the normal range of values could delay recognition and treatment. Unfortunately, a recent survey[31] indicated that many clinicians assume an age-related decline in the parameters used to assess anemia. About half of the 232 physicians responding were willing to tolerate a difference of up to 2 g/dl from the established standard for hemoglobin before initiating a stool test for occult blood.[31] After extensive review, Lynch and coworkers[71] concluded that simple iron-deficiency anemia is uncommon among healthy older people. It is critical that the nutritional and physiologic factors contributing to low hemoglobin levels be identified.

Parameters for Evaluating Iron Status

Recent population studies[88] evaluating iron and hematologic status have used several parameters, since different methods provide clues to the severity or cause of an existing anemia. Individual methods and their general limitations for use with older people are described in Table 8-2.

Hemoglobin levels in older people relate to sex, age, and health. Among 267 healthy Danes,[78] men ages 60 to 79 years had higher hemoglobin levels than men ages 80 to 93 years (14.4 g/dl versus 13 g/dl). The hemoglobin level of women across this age range was 13.8 g/dl. In older institutionalized women, hemoglobin levels below 12 g/dl occurred in 32% of those with known inflammatory conditions compared to only 11% of those free of such conditions. Lipschitz[67] considering a hemoglobin level of 14 g/dl to represent the lower level of normal in men noted that a large percentage of the men ages 65 to 74 in the NHANES II study were anemic. A reduction in mean corpuscular volume appears less frequently in older people than a low hemoglobin level. Fewer than 3% of those ages 65 to 74 in the NHANES II study had a mean corpuscular volume below normal.[88]

Serum iron and transferrin levels are influenced more by body iron stores than by sex or age but are significantly lower in elderly people with inflammatory diseases. In the NHANES II study,[88] fewer than 10% of older adults had a transferrin saturation below the normal range (less than 16%), although black men were most likely to have low levels.

Erythrocyte protoporphyrin levels have become recognized as indicators of faulty erythropoiesis. Protoporphyrin is a precursor of **heme;** if iron is unavailable for incorporation into hemoglobin, protoporphyrins will accumulate; thus high levels indicate a developing anemia. Inflammatory processes also elevate the erythrocyte protoporphyrin level, limiting its usefulness in older people with such conditions. In the NHANES II study,[88] 10% of all men ages 65 to 74 had protoporphyrin levels suggestive

TABLE 8-2 *Parameters Used to Identify Anemia*

Parameter	Advantages and Limitations With Older People
Hemoglobin level	Does not support early intervention, because levels drop relatively late in the development of anemia; low levels do not distinguish between iron deficiency or other anemias; levels are reduced by inflammation or infection and in folic acid or vitamin B_{12} deficiency; levels are increased by dehydration
Mean corpuscular volume	Does not support early intervention, because volume decreases only when iron deficiency has become severe; folic acid or vitamin B_{12} deficiency will cause an increase in volume; when both iron and vitamin B_{12} deficiencies are present, there may be no change in red cell volume
Serum iron, transferrin and transferrin saturation levels	Serum iron levels decrease fairly early in the development of iron-deficiency anemia; serum iron levels exhibit diurnal variation and are also decreased by infection and inflammation; transferrin levels are reduced by chronic disease, infection, inflammation, and protein-energy malnutrition
Erythrocyte protoporphyrin level	Levels increase fairly early in the development of iron-deficiency anemia; levels are increased by infection
Serum ferritin level	Decrease in level is an early indicator of declining iron status; extremely high levels indicate iron overload; levels are increased by chronic disease, liver disease, and inflammation
Red blood cell count	Does not support early intervention, because the total number of erythrocytes declines late in the development of iron-deficiency anemia; age-related changes in the bone marrow can reduce production of red blood cells

of a problem in hemoglobin synthesis. In an institutionalized population,[51] 59% of those with inflammatory conditions had elevated levels compared to only 19% of older controls.

Serum ferritin levels provide a good estimate of iron stores (see Chapter 7). Unfortunately, inflammation and disease processes raise serum ferritin levels and thus may mask a true iron deficiency. In the general population relatively few older adults (2% to 3%) have low serum ferritin levels (below 12 ng/ml). Conversely, about 5% appear to have iron overload, as indicated by serum ferritin levels above 300 to 400 ng/ml, the upper limits of normal in women and men, respectively.[88]

The number of red blood cells seems to decrease in advanced age even in healthy individuals. In the NHANES II study,[107] 15% to 21% of white adults over age 64 and 25% to 36% of older black adults had red cell counts below recommended levels, although hemoglobin concentrations were normal in the erythrocytes that were present.

Diagnosing Anemia

Both iron-deficiency anemia and the anemia of chronic disease are characterized by iron-deficient erythropoiesis; however, their etiologies are vastly different.[67] In iron-deficiency anemia, iron stores have been depleted as a result of blood loss or long-term deficient intake. In the anemia arising from chronic disease, the **reticuloendothelial cells** are unable to retrieve the iron from degraded erythrocytes. Consequently, inadequate iron is delivered to the bone marrow for incorporation into newly forming erythrocytes.[67] In the anemia of chronic disease, tissue iron stores are normal or may actually be increased. In infection, body iron stores become unavailable for hemoglobin synthesis, thus making iron less available to the disease organism as well.

The anemia of chronic disease and iron-deficiency anemia usually can be distinguished on the basis of erythrocyte and biochemical parameters (Table 8-3).[50,51,67] Both conditions are characterized by low serum iron, low transferrin saturation, and high erythrocyte protoporphyrin levels, although Lipschitz[67] considers a low transferrin saturation level to more likely

TABLE 8-3 *Hematologic Parameters in Iron-Deficiency Anemia and the Anemia of Chronic Disease*

	Iron-Deficiency Anemia	Anemia of Chronic Disease
Hemoglobin levels	<12 g/dl	<12 g/dl
Serum iron levels	<40 µg/dl	<60 µg/dl
Serum transferrin levels	>375 µg/dl	<250 µg/dl
Transferrin saturation (%)	<20%	<20%
Serum ferritin levels	<20 ng/ml	>100 ng/ml

indicate an iron deficiency. Iron stores are high in an anemia of chronic disease, and serum ferritin levels may exceed 100 ng/ml. In individuals with inflammatory disorders and gastrointestinal iron loss, both types of anemia may be present.[50]

The effect of inflammation in lowering serum iron and transferrin saturation levels and raising erythrocyte protoporphyrin levels could lead to an inappropriate diagnosis of iron-deficiency anemia.[51] Conversely, the effect of inflammation in raising serum ferritin levels could result in a lack of treatment for iron-deficiency anemia when it is present. Hercberg and coworkers[51] consider plasma transferrin levels to be the parameter least influenced by inflammatory processes. In their opinion, a high erythrocyte protoporphyrin level, a high plasma transferrin level, and a low transferrin saturation level suggest the presence of iron deficiency despite accompanying inflammatory processes. The presence of inflammation does not in itself cause transferrin levels to rise.

An analysis of the NHANES I and II data[114] concluded that inflammation is the predominant cause of anemia in elderly individuals. Of those with anemia, more than 66% reported the presence of inflammatory conditions. Less than 10% of the anemia in those over age 60 was related to iron deficiency. Those authors suggest that changes in hematologic parameters in apparently healthy individuals may reflect subclinical chronic disease rather than normal aging.

Age and Bone Marrow Function

Bone marrow is a tissue with a high cellular turnover and thus is particularly sensitive to nutritional deprivation. At the same time, age-related changes diminish **hematopoietic** capacity. Although the **stem cells** of the bone marrow appear to retain their ability to divide throughout the lifespan, stem cells from older human donors have a reduced capacity to proliferate compared to cells from younger human donors.[67] This is particularly evident under conditions of stimulation; cells from older donors are less able to increase their production of hematopoietic cells.

Changes in bone marrow function become significant under physiologic or nutritional stress and contribute to anemia. Elderly people with unexplained anemia were found to have fewer bone marrow stem cells than healthy people of similar age, and healthy older people had lower levels than young controls.[67] Impaired nutrient delivery to proliferating cells may contribute to reduced erythrocyte production. Bone marrow stem cells respond to high levels of erythropoietin by producing mature cells in shorter intervals of time. Decreased release of or response to erythropoietin may also contribute to anemia in older people.[58]

Treating Iron-Deficiency Anemia

Treatment of iron-deficiency anemia should be preceded by careful evaluation, and the regimen should be supervised by a physician. Administering supplemental iron to individuals who actually are vitamin B_{12} deficient has serious consequences, since the vitamin B_{12} deficiency eventually will lead to neural damage. Equally unwise is supplementation with iron and all necessary vitamin cofactors. Excessive or inappropriate supplementation can cause gastrointestinal distress or excessive iron storage and may mask occult blood loss. In diagnosed anemia, 60 mg of iron daily as **ferrous sulfate** divided across the three meals should result in an increase in hemoglobin of 0.5 g/dl a week.[67] A lower level of iron may be necessary to minimize common side effects, including nausea, vomiting, constipation, and diarrhea. Self-medication with iron can lead to **hemochromatosis** or can mask a pathologic condition causing gastrointestinal blood loss.

Pernicious Anemia

Basis of the problem. Pernicious anemia is a progressive, **macrocytic anemia** that results from a lack of **intrinsic factor** and subsequent **vitamin B_{12}** deficiency. Pernicious anemia occurs in only 1% to 2% of the population, but the incidence increases with age.[76] The average age of onset is 60 years. Pernicious anemia is more common in women and rarely occurs in black adults.[67] The pathological aspects of this condition relate to both the anemia and the role of vitamin B_{12} in maintaining neural tissue. Although the macrocytic anemia associated with a lack of vitamin B_{12} disappears when the vitamin is restored, the damage to the **myelin** covering of the spinal nerves cannot be reversed (see Chapter 6).

The underlying cause of the pernicious anemia that results from **atrophic gastritis** and the virtual absence of intrinsic factor is not known.[76] Pernicious anemia was associated with **hypothyroidism** and a family history of pernicious anemia among people over age 75 admitted to a long-term care facility.[17] There is also evidence that an **autoimmune reaction** may cause pernicious anemia. **Parietal cell** antibodies that lead to atrophic gastritis have been identified in most patients with pernicious anemia, suggesting that the loss of both gastric acid and intrinsic factor secretion are related.[115]

Criteria for diagnosis. A major issue in current clinical practice is appropriate criteria for identifying pernicious anemia. At one time it was believed that hematologic changes occurred early in the disorder and neurologic changes rather late and never before the classic macrocytic anemia.[50,76] There is now evidence that the neurologic damage associated with pernicious anemia can occur in the absence of anemia or extremely low serum vitamin B_{12} levels. Carmel[16] proposes that true vitamin B_{12} deficiency is not only more common than is generally believed, but that it also develops in a more subtle fashion. Among 80 consecutive patients diagnosed with pernicious anemia, 36% had serum vitamin B_{12} levels above the deficient range; 19% had hemoglobin levels in the normal range; and 33% had normal-sized erythrocytes.

Of the 10 patients with neither anemia nor macrocytic cells, six had neurologic abnormalities, including numbness of the hands and feet, confusion, or bizarre behavior.

These findings about the early appearance of neurologic damage were confirmed in a series of 141 consecutive patients[66] with neuropsychiatric abnormalities related to vitamin B_{12} deficiency. Forty had normal hemoglobin, hematocrit, and mean cell volume measurements despite sensory losses and psychiatric disturbances. Thirty-eight of these 40 patients were treated with vitamin B_{12}. All but 10 became free of symptoms, and all showed improvement. In some cases a correct diagnosis of the condition had been delayed for months or even years because vitamin B_{12} deficiency was believed to be unlikely in the absence of anemia.

It is unclear why some older individuals develop neuropsychiatric rather than hematologic abnormalities in vitamin B_{12} deficiency. It has been suggested[16,50] that iron deficiency in combination with vitamin B_{12} deficiency prevents the development of macrocytic cells. Folic acid supplements administered inappropriately may also alter the progression of symptoms in pernicious anemia.[66]

Although it is agreed that low serum vitamin B_{12} levels indicate the need for further evaluation, the usual standard of deficiency (74 pmol/L) does not effectively identify older people with pernicious anemia, and subtle changes in the morphology of red blood cells can be difficult to ascertain.[66] Lindenbaum and coworkers[66] reported elevated serum levels of **methylmalonic acid** and **homocysteine** in untreated patients with pernicious anemia. These metabolic intermediates accumulate because subsequent reactions require vitamin B_{12} as a cofactor. Upon supplementation with vitamin B_{12}, serum levels of both metabolites dropped markedly. A critical need is a sensitive and cost-

effective protocol for evaluating vitamin B_{12} status in elderly individuals.

Treating pernicious anemia. The usual treatment for pernicious anemia is intramuscular injection of 1,000 µg of vitamin B_{12} every 1 to 3 months. Oral intakes of 500 to 1,000 µg a day carry little risk of toxicity and appear to be adequate to maintain normal function in patients with pernicious anemia.[47] Also, oral **cobalamin** is relatively inexpensive when compared to the cost associated with injections that must be administered in a clinic or by a home health nurse.[63] Lederle[63] emphasizes that oral supplementation should be considered with appropriate monitoring and follow-up. Patients must also be advised of the need for continuing supplementation. Symptoms of deficiency were found to reoccur in older people with pernicious anemia who discontinued treatment when they began to feel well.[95]

ARTHRITIS AND BONE JOINT DISEASE

Arthritis with inflammation of the joints and pain and swelling is a major cause of functional disability in older people. The most common form of arthritis is osteoarthritis, believed to exist in about 80% of adults over age 65.[65] Rheumatoid arthritis, on the other hand, usually appears first in middle age and is marked by periods of acute intensity and remission.[105]

Osteoarthritis

The etiology of osteoarthritis is unclear. Because it increases in prevalence and severity with age, these changes in the bone joint were considered to be the result of years of wear and tear. It now appears that both genetic and mechanical factors contribute to degenerative joint disease.[65] Under normal conditions cartilage, consisting of proteins, **mucopolysaccharides,** and fluid, covers the ends of the bones and provides a cushion that prevents the bones from rubbing against one another. As degenerative changes lead to cracking and the wearing away of the cartilage, friction and inflammation in the joint increase, and swelling and pain result. The finger, hip, and knee joints are particularly susceptible, and such changes can cause problems with food preparation, locomotion, and self-care.

Treatment of osteoarthritis usually involves medications that control pain and thereby encourage normal activity and movement. Surgery to replace a hip or knee joint with an artificial joint may become necessary. Aspirin, **acetaminophen,** and **nonsteroidal antiinflammatory drugs (NSAIDs)** such as ibuprofen are in general use.[112] (See Chapter 9 for nutrition-related side effects.) Weight control or, if possible, weight loss to reduce the stress on the weight-bearing joints is an important component of treatment. Among elderly men and women in Goteborg, Sweden,[8] the highest grade of osteoarthritic degeneration of the knee was found in those with the highest BMI. Wolman[112] emphasizes the vulnerability of older people with pain and stiffening joints to dietary regimens touted to relieve arthritis. Diets that exclude all grain products, all dairy products, or most fruits, or regimens that advocate the use of extreme levels of vitamin supplements (e.g., 200,000 IU of vitamin D, 2,000 mg of vitamin B_6, or 4 to 10 g of ascorbic acid) carry the potential for serious interactions and toxicities.

Rheumatoid Arthritis

Rheumatoid arthritis is a systemic rather than a localized inflammatory disorder and influences both functional and metabolic status.[105] Destruction of the cartilage, ligaments, and bone results from the recurring episodes of inflammation exacerbated by mechanical stress on the damaged tissues. Joints most affected are those of the upper extremities including the hand, wrist, elbow, and shoulder. Jaw movement and chewing can be impaired. The usual treatment of rheumatoid arthritis involves the use of aspirin and NSAIDs to reduce inflammation. Glucocorticoids are sometimes prescribed, and these lead to loss of body protein, reduced calcium absorption, and electrolyte disturbances. Sodium restriction, potassium supplementation, and fluid monitoring may be required.

Recent work has focused on dietary strategies for controlling this disorder.[61,105] **Leukotrienes,** which are biologically active compounds found in the **leukocytes,** appear to promote inflammatory reactions. **Omega-3 fatty acids** inhibit the production of leukotrienes, and populations that consume high amounts of fish have a lower incidence of this disease. A 24-week, double-blind study[61] of patients with rheumatoid arthritis found a significant reduction in joint swelling, tenderness, stiffness, and pain in those supplemented with 90 mg/kg of omega-3 fatty acids. Kremer and coworkers[61] note that further evaluation is necessary to discern possible toxic effects of this intake of fatty acids. At the same time, any side effects of the omega-3 fatty acids must be evaluated within the context of the deleterious side effects of the drugs currently used to treat this disorder.

A more controversial intervention for rheumatoid arthritis now being studied is a **vegan, gluten**-free diet for 3 to 5 months followed by gradual adoption of a lactovegetarian diet.[60] After 1 year patients on this regimen continued to demonstrate improvement as compared to control subjects. Food allergy or intolerance can aggravate rheumatoid arthritis, and fasting is an effective means of suppressing symptoms, although they return when food intake is resumed. Although adoption of a vegan diet without supervision and appropriate supplementation for even a short period is dangerous to nutritional health and should be vigorously discouraged, further study of dietary influences on inflammatory responses is justified.

Summary

Age-related degenerative changes exacerbated by chronic disease make the older individual increasingly vulnerable to nutrient-related chronic disorders, regardless of health status. Decreased response of the beta-cells of the pancreas to increased plasma glucose levels and alterations in the sensitivity of peripheral tissues to insulin have been implicated in the deterioration in glucose tolerance observed in even healthy older individuals. At the same time, increased intakes of carbohydrate and increased physical exercise appear to reverse these age-related changes to some extent, although the mechanism is unknown. Continued deterioration in glucose tolerance coupled with disease-related alterations in glucose metabolism can lead to overt diabetes mellitus.

Osteoporosis, characterized by a loss of bone matrix and mineral with a loss of bone strength, is a major cause of bone fracture and associated disability, particularly in older women. Bone mass at maturity, intakes of calcium and vitamin D, genetic disposition, level of physical activity, presence of metabolic disorders that enhance PTH secretion and urinary calcium loss, as well as estrogen status, all influence bone health at older ages. Attention to recommended intakes of calcium and potassium and avoidance of excessive intakes of sodium contribute to the effective management of hypertension with a reduced dependence on drugs. Avoidance of inappropriate weight gain and the appropriate loss of even small amounts of excessive body weight can improve glucose tolerance and reduce the stress on osteoarthritic joints. Repeated episodes of weight gain and loss, however, appear to enhance the risk of disease. Unintentional weight loss in older adults can be an indicator of serious disease and requires careful diagnosis and intervention.

Nutritional anemia in the aged person can have many different causes. Although iron-deficiency anemia is most often the result of occult blood loss, chronic infection, disease, protein-energy malnutrition, or changes in the bone marrow can impair erythropoiesis. Pernicious anemia, uncommon in younger people, is associated with macrocytic anemia, neural damage, and behavior changes in older people. A strategy for identifying vitamin B_{12} deficiency in the absence of anemia is urgently needed. Hematologic parameters falling below normal ranges in older adults demand aggressive evaluation and intervention.

REVIEW QUESTIONS

1. Why are chronic disorders hard to diagnose and treat in older persons? Why is osteoporosis so "costly?" What factors influence bone density? Do cortical bone and trabecular bone differ in patterns of loss? What is the difference between osteoporosis and osteomalacia?
2. What are the differences between Type I and Type II osteoporosis? What treatments are currently being used for osteoporosis? What health

risks are associated with the use of estrogen replacement therapy? What nutritional factors are important in preventing osteoporosis? How can exercise be beneficial in preserving or increasing bone mass?
3. Is the change in glucose tolerance seen with aging a physiologic or normal age change, or is it a pathologic age change? How does weight gain, weight loss, and body mass index influence glucose tolerance? What are the differences between impaired glucose tolerance and noninsulin–dependent diabetes mellitus? What is the most appropriate dietary management of the older person with diabetes?
4. Why is hypertension a significant risk factor for heart disease, even into advanced age? What physiologic changes contribute to altered blood pressure with aging? What dietary and lifestyle factors contribute to the development of hypertension? What role do the minerals sodium, potassium, and calcium play in the management of hypertension?
5. Why are institutionalized elderly at risk for unintentional weight loss? What changes in body weight are considered significant? Why is the pattern of weight loss or gain considered significant to disease risk? Why are older people at greater risk for iron deficiency anemia? What is the significance of the inflammatory process to anemias?

SUGGESTED LEARNING ACTIVITIES

1. Your 86-year-old uncle has recently been diagnosed with osteoporosis. He tells you that men do not get osteoporosis—that it is a "woman's disease." How would you respond to him? Plan a 3-day diet program for your uncle including calcium-rich foods, even though he is also lactose intolerant.
2. Go to the library and look up some of the work of William J. Evans and his colleagues from the USDA Human Nutrition Research Center on Aging at Tufts University. Abstract three articles from their research on exercise and bone density as applied to older adults.
3. Practice calculating waist-to-hip measurements with your classmates and calculate risk of hypertension, diabetes, and heart disease based on your ratios. Ask the physician or nurse at your school's health clinic if you can conduct a clinic to measure waist-to-hip ratios on students as part of a health fair.
4. Your elderly neighbor suffers from osteoarthritis. She knows you are studying nutrition and she tells you she started taking primrose oil and vita-

min E capsules to cure her arthritis. In addition, she tells you she avoids "nightshade" vegetables and wears a copper bracelet to treat her condition. What would you tell her about these habits and their relationship to osteoarthritis?

Key Terms

Provided here for review is a list of the major terms in this chapter. The definitions can be found in the Glossary, which begins on p. 336. To help you understand how these terms are applied, the page number is given for the first mention of each term in the chapter.

REFERENCES

1. Abraham S, Collins G, Nordsieck M: Relationship of childhood weight status to morbidity in adults, *Public Health Rep* 86:273, 1971.
2. Andres R: Aging and carbohydrate metabolism. In Carlson LA, editor: Nutrition in old age, Symposia Swedish Nutrition Foundation X, Stockholm, 1972, Almqvist & Wiksell.
3. Andres R and others: Impact of age on weight goals, *Ann Intern Med* 103:1030, 1985.
4. Anonymous: Consensus development conference: prophylaxis and treatment of osteoporosis, *Am J Med* 90:107, 1991.
5. Anonymous: No-sweat guide to designing a fitness plan, *Tufts Diet Nutr Letter* 10(2):3, April, 1992.
6. Anonymous: Supplemental dietary potassium reduced the need for antihypertensive drug therapy, *Nutr Rev* 50:144, 1992.
7. Anonymous: Techniques for assessing bone density, *Nutr and the MD* 18:1, 1992.

8. Bagge E and others: Factors associated with radiographic osteoarthritis: results from the population study of 70-year-old people in Goteborg, *J Rheumatol* 18:1218, 1991.
9. Bales CW, Gold DT: Nutrition education for osteoporosis patients: an innovative approach to care of the chronically ill elderly, *J Nutr Educ* 23:120, 1991.
10. Barrett-Connor E and others: Why is diabetes mellitus a stronger risk factor for fatal ischemic heart disease in women than in men?: the Rancho Bernardo study, *JAMA* 265:627, 1991.
11. Blumenthal JA, Siegel WC, Appelbaum M: Failure of exercise to reduce blood pressure in patients with mild hypertension; results of a randomized controlled trial, *JAMA* 266:2098, 1991.
12. Bots ML, Grobbee DE, Hofman A: High blood pressure in the elderly, *Epidemiol Rev* 13:294, 1991.
13. Brody JP and others: Study of nutritional anemia in male residents of a chronic care facility, *Nutr Res* 5:1167, 1985.
14. Broughton DL, Taylor R: Review: deterioration of glucose tolerance with age: the role of insulin resistance, *Age Ageing* 20:221, 1991.
15. Broughton DL and others: Peripheral and hepatic insulin sensitivity in healthy elderly human subjects, *Eur J Clin Invest* 21:13, 1991.
16. Carmel R: Pernicious anemia: the expected findings of very low serum cobalamin levels, anemia, and macrocytosis are often lacking, *Arch Intern Med* 148:1712, 1988.
17. Catania J and others: Hypothesis: a history of hypothyroidism or a family history of pernicious anaemia are useful in identifying masked pernicious anaemia in elderly patients with microcytic hypochromic anaemia, *Age Ageing* 18:279, 1989.
18. Chen LH, Cook-Newell ME: Anemia and iron status in the free-living and institutionalized elderly in Kentucky, *Int J Vitam Nutr Res* 59:207, 1989.
19. Chen M, Bergman RN, Porte D: Insulin resistance and β-cell dysfunction in aging: the importance of dietary carbohydrate, *J Clin Endocrinol Metab* 67:951, 1988.
20. Chen M and others: Pathogenesis of age-related glucose intolerance in man: insulin resistance and decreased β-cell function, *J Clin Endocrinol Metab* 60:13, 1985.
21. Chen M and others: The role of dietary carbohydrate in the decreased glucose tolerance of the elderly, *J Am Geriatr Soc* 35:417, 1987.
22. Chernoff R: Nutritional support in the elderly. In Chernoff R, editor: *Geriatric nutrition: the health professional's handbook,* Gaithersburg, Md, 1991, Aspen Publishers.
23. Colditz GA and others: Prospective study of estrogen replacement therapy and risk of breast cancer in postmenopausal women, *JAMA* 264:2648, 1990.
24. Committee on Diet and Health, Food and Nutrition Board: *Diet and health: implications for reducing chronic disease risk,* Washington, DC, 1989, National Academy Press.
25. Compston JE, Vedi S, Croucher PI: Low prevalence of osteomalacia in elderly patients with hip fracture, *Age Ageing* 20:132, 1991.
26. Cooper C, Barker DJ, Wickham C: Physical activity, muscle strength, and calcium intake in fracture of the proximal femur in Britain, *Br Med J* 297:1663, 1988.
27. Coulston AM: Nutrition management in nursing homes. In Morley JE, Glick Z, and Rubenstein LZ, editors: *Geriatric nutrition: a comprehensive review,* New York, 1990, Raven Press.
28. Council on Scientific Affairs: Treatment of obesity in adults, *JAMA* 260:2547, 1988.
29. D'Eramo-Melkus G, Hagan JA: Weight reduction interventions for persons with a chronic illness: findings and factors for consideration, *J Am Diet Assoc* 91:1093, 1991.
30. Dalsky GP and others: Weight-bearing exercise training and lumbar bone mineral content in postmenopausal women, *Ann Intern Med* 108:824, 1988.
31. Daly MP, Sobal J: Anemia in the elderly: a survey of physicians' approaches to diagnosis and workup, *J Fam Pract* 28:524, 1989.
32. Davidson MB: The effect of aging on carbohydrate metabolism: a review of the English literature and a practical approach to the diagnosis of diabetes mellitus in the elderly, *Metabolism* 28:688, 1979.
33. Durnin JVGA: Anthropometric methods of assessing nutritional status. In Horwitz A and others, editors: *Nutrition in the elderly,* New York, 1989, Oxford University Press.
34. Dwyer JT and others: Changes in relative weight among institutionalized elderly adults, *J Gerontol* 42:246, 1987.
35. Feskens EJM, Bowles CH, Kromhout D: Carbohydrate intake and body mass index in relation to the risk of glucose intolerance in an elderly population, *Am J Clin Nutr* 54:136, 1991.
36. Fischer L, Johnson MA: Low body weight and weight loss in the aged, *J Am Diet Assoc* 90:1697, 1990.

37. Folsom AR and others: Incidence of hypertension and stroke in relation to body fat distribution and other risk factors in older women, *Stroke* 21:701, 1990.

38. Food and Nutrition Board: *Recommended dietary allowances,* ed 10, Washington, DC, 1989, National Academy of Sciences.

39. Gallagher JC and others: The effect of calcitriol on patients with postmenopausal osteoporosis with special reference to fracture frequency, *Proc Soc Exp Biol Med* 19:287, 1989.

40. Garry PJ, Goodwin JS, Hunt WC: Iron status and anemia in the elderly: new findings and a review of previous studies, *J Am Geriatr Soc* 31:389, 1983.

41. Goldberg JP: Aging and the cardiovascular system. In Chernoff R, editor: *Geriatric nutrition: the health professional's handbook,* Gaithersburg, Md, 1991, Aspen Publishers.

42. Gorbach SL and others: Changes in food patterns during a low-fat dietary intervention in women, *J Am Diet Assoc* 90:802, 1990.

43. Grobin W: A longitudinal study of impaired glucose tolerance and diabetes mellitus in the aged, *J Am Geriatr Soc* 37:1127, 1989.

44. Gruchow HW, Sobocinski KA, Barboriak JJ: Calcium intake and the relationship of dietary sodium and potassium to blood pressure, *Am J Clin Nutr* 48:1463, 1988.

45. Grundy SM: Dietary therapy in diabetes mellitus: is there a single best diet? *Diabetes Care* 14:796, 1991.

46. Hamm P, Shekelle RB, Stamler J: Large fluctuations in body weight during young adulthood and twenty-five-year risk of coronary death in men, *Am J Epidemiol* 129:312, 1989.

47. Hathcock JN, Troendle GJ: Oral cobalamin for treatment of pernicious anemia, *JAMA* 265:96, 1991.

48. Helmrich SP and others: Physical activity and occurrence of non-insulin-dependent diabetes mellitus, *N Engl J Med* 325:147, 1991.

49. Herbert V: Don't ignore low serum cobalamin (vitamin B_{12}) levels, *Arch Intern Med* 148:1705, 1988.

50. Herbert V: Nutritional anemias in the elderly. In Prinsley DM, Sandstead HH, editors: *Nutrition and aging,* New York, 1990, Alan R Liss.

51. Hercberg S and others: Influence of inflammation on laboratory indicators of iron deficiency in the elderly, *Nutr Res* 6:1259, 1986.

52. Holbrook TL, Barrett-Connor E, Wingard DL: Dietary calcium and risk of hip fracture: 14-year prospective population study, *Lancet* 2(8619):1046, 1988.

53. Holbrook TL, Barrett-Connor E, Wingard DL: The association of lifetime weight and weight control patterns with diabetes among men and women in an adult community, *Int J Obes* 13:723, 1989.

54. Houmard JA and others: Effects of fitness level and the regional distribution of fat on carbohydrate metabolism and plasma lipids in middle- to older-aged men, *Metabolism* 40:714, 1991.

55. Insogna KL and others: Osteomalacia and weakness from excessive antacid ingestion, *JAMA* 244:2544, 1980.

56. Kahn SE and others: Effect of exercise on insulin action, glucose tolerance, and insulin secretion in aging, *Am J Physiol (Endocrinol Metab)* 21:E937, 1990.

57. Kahn SE and others: The glucose intolerance of aging: implications for intervention, Hosp Pract 26(4A):29, 1991.

58. Kario K, Matsuo T, Nakao K: Serum erythropoietin levels in the elderly, *Gerontology* 37:345, 1991.

59. Kiebzak GM: Age-related bone changes, *Exp Gerontol* 26:171, 1991.

60. Kjeldsen-Kragh J and others: Controlled trial of fasting and 1-year vegetarian diet in rheumatoid arthritis, *Lancet* 338:899, 1991.

61. Kremer JM and others: Dietary fish oil and olive oil supplementation in patients with rheumatoid arthritis, *Arthritis Rheum* 33:810, 1990.

62. Kristal AR and others: Long-term maintenance of a low-fat diet: durability of fat-related dietary habits in the Women's Health Trial, *J Am Diet Assoc* 92:553, 1992.

63. Lederle FA: Oral cobalamin for pernicious anemia: medicine's best-kept secret, *JAMA* 265:94, 1991.

64. Lewis EJ, Bell SJ: Nutritional assessment of the elderly. In Morley JE, Glick Z, Rubenstein LZ, editors: *Geriatric nutrition: a comprehensive review,* New York, 1990, Raven Press.

65. Liang MH: Osteoarthritis: a joint endeavor, *Harvard Health Letter* 17(6):1, 1992.

66. Lindenbaum J and others: Neuropsychiatric disorders caused by cobalamin deficiency in the absence of anemia or macrocytosis, *N Engl J Med* 318:1720, 1988.

67. Lipschitz DA: Impact of nutrition on the age-related declines in hematopoiesis. In Chernoff R, editor: *Geriatric nutrition: the health professional's handbook,* Gaithersburg, Md, 1991, Aspen Publishers.

68. Lissner L and others: Body weight variability in men: metabolic rate, health and longevity, *Int J Obes* 14:373, 1989.

69. Lissner L and others: Variability of body weight and health outcomes in the Framingham population, *N Engl J Med* 324:1839, 1991.

70. Löwik MR and others: Nutrition and blood pressure among elderly men and women (Dutch Nutrition Surveillance System), *J Am Coll Nutr* 10:149, 1991.

71. Lynch SR and others: Iron status of elderly Americans, *Am J Clin Nutr* 36:1032, 1982.

72. Martinez OB: Indices of vitamin, iron, and hematological status of a selected sample of elderly Canadians, *Nutr Res* 8:1345, 1988.

73. Marton KI, Sox HC, Krupp JR: Involuntary weight loss: diagnostic and prognostic significance, *Ann Intern Med* 95:568, 1981.

74. Matkovic V and others: Bone status and fracture rates in two regions of Yugoslavia, *Am J Clin Nutr* 32:540, 1979.

75. McCarron DA and others: Blood pressure and nutrient intake in the United States, *Science* 224:1392, 1984.

76. McRae TD, Freedman ML: Why vitamin B_{12} deficiency should be managed aggressively, *Geriatrics* 44:70, 1989.

77. Meunier PJ: Fluoride therapy for vertebral osteoporosis. In Munro H, and Schierf G, editors: *Nutrition of the elderly, Nestle Nutrition Workshop Series,* vol 29, New York, 1992, Raven Press.

78. Milman S, Andersen HC, Pedersen NS: Serum ferritin and iron status in healthy elderly individuals, *Scand J Clin Lab Invest* 46:19, 1986.

79. Morley JE, Glick Z: Obesity. In Morley JE, Glick Z, Rubenstein L, editors: *Geriatric nutrition: a comprehensive review,* New York, 1990, Raven Press.

80. Morley JE, Perry HM: The management of diabetes mellitus in older individuals, *Drugs* 41:548, 1991.

81. Morley JE and others: Diabetes mellitus in elderly patients: is it different? *Am J Med* 83:533, 1987.

82. National Diabetes Data Group: Classification and diagnosis of diabetes mellitus and other categories of glucose intolerance, *Diabetes* 28:1039, 1979.

83. National Institutes of Health Consensus Development Panel on the Health Implications of Obesity: Health implications of obesity, *Ann Intern Med* 103:1073, 1985.

84. Nelson ME and others: A 1-year walking program and increased dietary calcium in postmenopausal women: effects on bone, *Am J Clin Nutr* 53:1304, 1991.

85. Nordin BE: Metabolic bone and stone disease, Baltimore, Md, 1973, Williams & Wilkins.

86. Pace PW, Bolton MP, Reeves RS: Ethics of obesity treatment: implications for dietitians, *J Am Diet Assoc* 91:1258, 1991.

87. Pacini G and others: Insulin sensitivity and beta-cell responsivity are not decreased in elderly subjects with normal OGTT, *J Am Geriatr Soc* 36:317, 1988.

88. Pilch SM, Senti FR, editors: Assessment of the iron nutritional status of the US population based on data collected in the second National Health and Nutrition Examination Survey, 1976-1980, Bethesda, Md, 1984, Life Sciences Research Office, Federation of American Societies for Experimental Biology.

89. Rabinovitz M and others: Unintentional weight loss: a retrospective analysis of 154 cases, *Arch Intern Med* 146:186, 1986.

90. Rajala SA and others: Body weight and the 3-year prognosis in very old people, *Int J Obes* 14:997, 1990.

91. Reaven GM and others: Beneficial effect of moderate weight loss in older patients with non-insulin-dependent diabetes mellitus poorly controlled with insulin, *J Am Geriatr Soc* 33:93, 1985.

92. Resnick NM, Greenspan SL: Senile osteoporosis reconsidered, *JAMA* 261:1025, 1989.

93. Riggs BL, Melton LJ: Involutional osteoporosis, *N Engl J Med* 314:1676, 1986.

94. Riggs BL and others: Effect of fluoride treatment on the fracture rate in postmenopausal women with osteoporosis, *N Engl J Med* 322:802, 1990.

95. Savage D, Lindenbaum J: Relapses after interruption of cyanocobalamin therapy in patients with pernicious anemia, *Am J Med* 74:765, 1983.

96. Schultz BM, Freedman ML: Iron deficiency in the elderly, *Baillieres Clin Haematol* 1:291, 1987.

97. Shimokata H and others: Age as an independent determinant of glucose tolerance, *Diabetes* 40:44, 1991.

98. Snow-Harter C, Marcus R: Exercise, bone mineral density, and osteoporosis, *Exerc Sport Sci Rev* 19:351, 1991.

99. Sowers MF: Osteoporosis and osteomalacia. In Brown ML, editor: *Present knowledge in nutrition,* ed 6, Washington DC, 1990, Interna-

tional Life Sciences Institute, Nutrition Foundation.

100. Sowers MF, Wallace RB, Lemke JH: Correlates of mid-radius bone density among postmenopausal women: a community study, *Am J Clin Nutr* 41:1045, 1985.

101. Storm T and others: Effect of intermittent cyclical etidronate therapy on bone mass and fracture rate in women with postmenopausal osteoporosis, *N Engl J Med* 322:1265, 1990.

102. Stunkard AJ: Conservative treatments for obesity, *Am J Clin Nutr* 45:1142, 1987.

103. Thomas JH, Powell DE: *Blood disorders in the elderly,* Bristol, 1971, John Wright & Sons.

104. Tjoa HI, Kaplan NM: Treatment of hypertension in the elderly, *JAMA* 264:1015, 1990.

105. Touger-Decker R: Nutritional considerations in rheumatoid arthritis, *J Am Diet Assoc* 88:327, 1988.

106. Tucker LA, Friedman GM: Television viewing and obesity in adult males, *Am J Public Health* 79:516, 1989.

107. United States Department of Health and Human Services: *Hematological and nutritional biochemistry reference data for persons 6 months—74 years of age: United States, 1976-1980,* DHHS Publication No (PHS) 83-1682, Washington, DC, 1982, US Government Printing Office.

108. Wardlaw G: The effects of diet and life-style on bone mass in women, *J Am Diet Assoc* 88:17, 1988.

109. Weber MA, Neutel JM, Cheung, DG: Hypertension in the aged: a pathophysiologic basis for treatment, *Am J Cardiol* 63:25H, 1989.

110. Weinberger MH and others: Dietary sodium restriction as adjunctive treatment of hypertension *JAMA* 259:2561, 1988.

111. White-O'Connor B, Sobal J, Muncie HL: Dietary habits, weight history, and vitamin supplement use in elderly osteoarthritis patients, *J Am Diet Assoc* 89:378, 1989.

112. Wolman PG: Management of patients using unproven regimens for arthritis *J Am Diet Assoc* 87:1211, 1987.

113. Working Group on Hypertension in the Elderly: Statement on hypertension in the elderly, *JAMA* 256: 70, 1986.

114. Yip R, Dallman PR: The roles of inflammation and iron deficiency as causes of anemia, *Am J Clin Nutr* 48:1295, 1988.

115. Young EA, Urban E: Aging, the aged, and the gastrointestinal tract. In Young EA, editor: *Nutrition, aging, and health,* New York, 1986, Alan R Liss.

116. Zauber NP, Zauber AG: Hematologic data of healthy very old people, *JAMA* 257:2181, 1987.

Drugs and Nutritional Considerations in the Aged

Connie E. Vickery

✦✦✦

After studying the chapter, the student should:

✔ *Recognize the reasons why older persons take 31% of all prescription medications.*

✔ *Define polypharmacy and list the factors contributing to polypharmacy in the elderly.*

✔ *Identify reasons for heavy drug use in long-term care populations.*

✔ *List the age-related changes in drug metabolism.*

✔ *Recognize the most common drug-nutrient interaction in the elderly.*

Introduction

Older adults in this country take substantial amounts of prescription and **over-the-counter (OTC) drugs.** Although older adults make up about 12% of the population, they take 31% of all prescription medications.[45,86] This figure is expected to reach 50% by the year 2000.[45] By 2030, it is projected that approximately 40% of total drug expenditures in developed countries will be attributed to those over age 65.[16] From 1977 to 1980, prescription drug expenditures in the United States increased 100%.[44] As a group, the elderly are the primary consumers of prescribed drugs. The use of nonprescription drugs is unknown, but speculation suggests it is sevenfold that for the general adult popula-

tion.[52] It has been estimated that OTC drugs account for 40% of all drugs used in nursing homes and 80% of all drugs used by community-dwelling older people.[99]

Today a physician has approximately 10,000 drugs available for use in diagnosis or treatment.[22] Stewart and colleagues[87] reported that based on a survey of the Pharmaceutical Manufacturers Association, 221 drugs were in some stage of clinical development to treat 23 diseases commonly affecting the older adult. This fact, coupled with a public attitude that "there is a pill for every complaint and ill," makes the older population particularly vulnerable to the undesirable consequences that can occur with drug therapy.

There is a fine line between the therapeutic and the detrimental effects of drugs. The consequences of doing nothing must be compared with the potential benefits of an intervention tempered by the adverse effects that almost invariably accompany drugs.[49] Different approaches should also be considered, because the primary goal of improving the quality of life for an older person may be accomplished by simple measures without using drugs.[100]

DRUG USE BY THE ELDERLY
Basis for Use

The prevalence of symptoms and disease increases with age, and life expectancy has increased. Elderly people commonly have several health problems. More than 80% of elderly individuals have one chronic disease or more.[23] Consequently, drugs are prescribed by the physician or self-prescribed by the older individual to resolve or manage chronic conditions. Older adults frequently report several vague and nonspecific symptoms, posing difficulties for the physician attempting to diagnose correctly and prescribe appropriate treatment. Some symptoms are so common among the older age group that diagnostic significance is lost. Several drugs may be prescribed for treatment, further complicating a clinician's attempts to establish an accurate diagnosis. The adverse side effects of medications rarely raise suspicion that new symptoms are drug related. It is more likely that new drugs will be prescribed to treat symptoms attributed to a new disease, to exacerbation of an existing condition, or simply to the aging process.[26]

Self-prescription of medications can also pose problems for the elderly. OTC drugs may relieve an individual's symptoms, and the older adult may hesitate to seek medical attention in a timely manner or may feel unable to afford a visit to the doctor. Self-medication may be achieved from former prescriptions, from drugs borrowed from others, or from nonprescription preparations. Nonprescription drugs frequently are viewed as harmless, because a physician's prescription is not required. However, many OTC drugs have active ingredients that would require a prescription if taken in greater amounts. An older adult may neglect to tell the physician about OTC drugs he or she is taking, believing that these drugs are harmless.

Neither the use of prescription drugs nor self-medication by older adults is expected to decline, because sophisticated diagnostic techniques have enabled physicians to identify more diseases amenable to drug treatment. The patterns of drug use among ambulatory elderly, as assessed through population-based household surveys, underscore this premise.

Currently, even though the number of new drugs approved by the U.S. Food and Drug Administration (FDA) is increasing, research on drug therapy in the elderly is limited.[17,34,49,100] There is no mandate for drug testing in the elderly, and drug studies typically are conducted on large populations without specific attention to the elderly.[17] A physician is likely to be prescribing drugs for the elderly according to guidelines based only on healthy young adults. Most studies fail to identify which conditions are the result of normal aging itself and which are caused by multiple diseases and multiple drug regimens.[34] Difficulties in research design and administration, and the cost of longitudinal studies on drugs and the elderly exacerbate the problem of limited research.

An increase in the use of drugs to treat the elderly also means an increase in cost. As noted before, the amount spent on prescription medicines in the United States increased 100% between 1977 and 1980.[44] The average drug bill for a nursing home resident is about $300 a year; the bill for an elderly individual living in the community is almost $100 a year.[12] Drug costs are expected to continue to rise.

Polypharmacy in the Elderly

Factors contributing to polypharmacy. As the number of older adults increases, in concert with the growing number of drugs available to treat and prevent their health problems, concern about **polypharmacy** is becoming acute. Polypharmacy is the use of several medications by an individual, whether prescribed or OTC drugs.[56] Polypharmacy may be related to a host of symptoms, including weakness, unsteadiness, confusion, anorexia, incontinence, and immobility.[53] Some authors use the term "polyphar-

macy" to describe only excessive and unnecessary use of medications.[51] Simpson[82] identified several features associated with polypharmacy:
- Use of medications without a defined need or condition
- Use of duplicate medications
- Concurrent use of interacting medications
- Use of a contraindicated medication
- Use of inappropriate doses of a medication
- Use of drugs to treat **adverse drug reactions**
- Improvement following discontinuation of medications

This pattern of taking medications can have several causes.[42,51,56] An older person may improperly use drugs that have been appropriately prescribed by the physician, or the individual may select from formerly prescribed drugs that have been stored or even hoarded for future need. The older person seeking information about nutritional supplements may heed advice from clerks in health food stores or from television commercials. The physician may be inappropriately prescribing medications, partly because the suitability of drug therapy for the elderly can be difficult to predict. Elderly individuals frequently are seen in several clinics, and they may fail to inform each physician of the drugs they are taking. Compounding the problem with prescribed medications, some older people may be self-prescribing OTC drugs and may neglect to tell the physician about these drugs.

Other factors contribute to polypharmacy among the elderly.[8,22,44] Unintentional errors in drug use may be attributed to unclear directions. Instructions may be given when the patient is particularly anxious or in physical discomfort. Also, just when the elderly need more time to learn about the medicines they will be taking, they actually receive less.[44] Errors can occur when instructions are delivered hastily, particularly when medical jargon is used. Elderly people whose hearing is impaired may not fully comprehend what is being said about the medicines prescribed. Many elderly people have impaired sight and are also vulnerable to problems associated with packaging and labeling. A person with arthritis may have difficulty opening childproof drug containers, and special in-

structions may be written in print that is too small to be read clearly and understood.

Polypharmacy in the elderly occurs in community-living, hospitalized, and long-term care populations. Those at home are likely to take between two and four different drugs each day; institutionalized elderly commonly take on average between five and 10 different drugs.[96]

Drug use among community-living elderly. One 10-year, cross-sectional study indicated that the average number of drugs used increased significantly among 4,509 older people living in the community studied.[87] Use of prescription and nonprescription medications increased by 0.52 and 0.21 per person, respectively, from 1978-79 to 1987-88. The four most common types of therapeutic drugs reported (as a percentage of all drugs used for the 1978-79 period) were **antihypertensives, analgesic-antipyretics, antirheumatics,** and **cathartics;** by 1987-88 the most common were antihypertensives, analgesic-antipyretics, **anticoagulants,** and antirheumatics. An overall decline in all drug classes was attributed to the availability of new classes of drugs and the effects of aging on the population. Participants were typically white, upper middle class, retired volunteers and thus not representative of all older people in the country.

The Iowa 65+ Rural Health Study involved 3,467 older people living in rural areas.[35] The three most common types of prescription drugs used were cardiovascular agents, central nervous system agents, and **analgesics;** the three most commonly used OTC drugs were analgesics, vitamins and minerals, and laxatives. Not surprisingly, average prescription and overall drug use increased significantly with age; use of OTC drugs remained relatively unchanged. Conversely, the number of individuals reporting no drug use declined with increasing age. When the participants were asked about the purpose of each medication they took, 10% of the responses were either inappropriate or showed that the person did not know the purpose of the medication.[80]

Opdycke and associates[63] reported on 70 individuals, ages 61 to 94, who participated in the **Focused Drug Therapy Review Program** conducted by the University of Michigan College of Pharmacy and Institute of Gerontology. Pharmacists were surveyed to identify medication-related education problems in this group of elderly. The most common problem was inadequate understanding of the purpose of medications, followed by noncompliance, inappropriate use of medications, and inadequate communication with health professionals.

In an investigation of drug use in a group of relatively healthy and functional individuals ages 76 to 96, most of the 61 subjects were able to name their medications and identify their use.[17] Also, drug use was not excessive. Almost half of the OTC drugs were vitamin and mineral supplements.

Drug use among hospitalized elderly. Gosney and Tallis[30] examined drug orders for 573 elderly patients, on admission to the hospital and daily thereafter through discharge or death, to establish how often contraindicated and interacting drugs were prescribed. On admission, patients reported using an average of about two drugs. During hospitalization they were taking about six drugs, and on discharge about three or four. The drugs most commonly prescribed (in descending order) were **antibiotics** (70% of all patients), analgesics (65%), **diuretics** (51%), hypnotics or sedatives (36%), **potassium salts** (24%), **digoxin** (16%), and antacids (15%). Of the 6,160 prescriptions analyzed, 200 drugs were contraindicated or had the potential for adverse reactions. The study did not consider OTC drugs or dosage errors. The authors concluded that 66% of the contraindicated prescriptions were avoidable.

Beers and associates[3] studied the effect of hospitalization on medications used by the elderly after discharge. They reviewed the medical and pharmacologic records of 197 patients, age 65 or older, who were admitted to a large Veterans' Hospital. On admission these individuals were taking 4.5 drugs each, with a range of none to 16 drugs. On discharge little change was seen in the average number of drugs taken per person (4.8; range, none to 12). Most subjects (71%) had at least one admission drug deleted before discharge. The 29% of admission drugs not continued at discharge were replaced with a similar type of drug. Patients who were taking an above-average number of drugs on admission were discharged with fewer drugs. Although the overall number of drugs taken before and after hospitalization did not change significantly, the types of drugs prescribed did change. At discharge the use of narcotic analgesics, laxatives, and antibiotics had increased. These findings support the thesis that polypharmacy may be influenced by hospitalization.

Drug use in long-term care patients. Approximately 5% of those age 65 or older in this country are institutionalized. Two recent review articles on multiple drug use in nursing home residents[51,56] noted that although the elderly in long-term care facilities suffer from the same maladies as their community-dwelling counterparts, nursing home residents are among the heaviest users of drugs. Nursing home placement frequently involves a person with altered mental status, for whom required medications result in altered central nervous system (CNS) function. Nursing home residents are most likely to be recipients of excessive **psychotherapeutic drugs,** and the need for chronic use of these drugs has been questioned. Depression, anxiety, insomnia, and agitation are symptoms frequently seen in the nursing home, and drugs may be indiscriminately prescribed to control them. Although changes in staffing patterns and commitment to therapeutic interaction with the nursing home resident may lessen the need for psychotherapeutic drugs, medications are likely to be used because they are easy to prescribe and quickly satisfy both resident and care-giver.

In 1976 almost one third of nursing home residents were given eight to 16 medications a day.[18] An average of about six drugs per resident was reported in a study based on a sample of nursing home residents covered by Medicaid and Medicare.[61] Lamy and Michocki[46] noted that 12% of nursing home residents are prescribed one drug; 14%, two drugs; 15%, three drugs; 14%, four drugs; and 45%, five drugs or more.

Beers and colleagues[2] monitored 12 intermediate-care facilities in Massachusetts for 1 month. Geriatric residents received an average of almost six drugs given at least once; about 50% of these drugs were prescribed prn, or for use as needed. Approximately 40% of all drugs prescribed in nursing homes are to be given pro re nata (**prn**) (on average, three drugs per resident).[2,36,41] Prn drugs tend to be primarily sedatives, hypnotics, analgesics, and laxatives.

Patrick and coworkers[64] compared drug prescription patterns of 21 nursing homes with **gerontologic nurse practitioners (GNP)** and 21 without a GNP. The drug records of 210 elderly residents were selected for review. Significantly fewer drugs and doses of drugs were prescribed in the nursing homes with gerontologic nurse practitioners. Residents of these nursing homes were prescribed an average of about eight drugs. Residents of nursing homes without gerontologic nurse practitioners were given an average of 10 drugs. A similar finding was noted with OTC drugs. Annually, projected drug costs were $120,192 for GNP nursing homes and $156,828 for the non-GNP facilities.

Adverse Drug Reactions

An adverse drug reaction is defined as any drug-induced, undesirable or unwanted consequence that necessitates treatment, a decrease in dosage or cessation of a drug, and/or selection of an alternate drug or treatment.[8] Adverse drug reactions in the elderly are related to (1) the increasing number of drugs they take; (2) the diminished functional capacity of organs involved in drug absorption, distribution, and elimination; and (3) noncompliance with medication regimens.[11,29] Aging itself is an independent risk factor for adverse drug reactions.[12,34] The most important reason for adverse drug reactions, however, is polypharmacy.[49]

Drug-induced **iatrogenic** health problems are a major concern for the elderly, although the frequency of adverse drug reactions in the elderly is unknown.[55] It has been estimated that 10% to 15% of hospital admissions of older people are the result of adverse drug reactions.[49,100,101] The figure may reach 31% when the definition is broadened to a "drug-related problem." Among elderly hospitalized patients, 20% of adverse drug reactions are associated with a patient's receiving an average of 10 different drugs.[45] Within 6 months of discharge from the hospital, approximately 22% to 36% of elderly individuals are readmitted.[5] Bero and coworkers[5] observed that 24% of the 706 elderly individuals they followed were readmitted because of adverse drug reactions.

Twenty percent of admissions for drug-induced iatrogenesis are attributable to OTC preparations.[10] In nursing homes 22% of drug reactions occur in residents taking four to nine drugs a day, and adverse drug reactions affect 23% to 53% of all residents.

Drugs frequently implicated in adverse reactions among the elderly are those used to treat high blood pressure, **congestive heart failure, cardiac arrhythmias,** lung disease, arthritis, and blood clots.[49,55,56] Most of these drugs have a narrow **therapeutic index,** which means there is only a slight difference between therapeutic and toxic doses.[56] Thus dose-related toxicity is a heightened concern.

A number of factors make the elderly particularly vulnerable to iatrogenic illness caused by adverse drug reactions. Just as increasing drug use is correlated with increasing age, reactions are more likely to occur in the very young and the very old.[8] Women are more likely than men to have adverse drug reactions. People being treated with several drugs are at greater risk of adverse reactions. Reactions are also associated with certain diseases, such as those of the gastrointestinal tract, liver, and kidneys, as well as with increased severity of disease resulting from age-related changes in tissue responsiveness to drug therapy and the influence of associated diseases.[29,51] Compensatory mechanisms seen in the young are not as effective in the elderly at buffering the body against troublesome side effects.

AGE-RELATED CHANGES IN DRUG METABOLISM

Increased intolerance to drugs is a characteristic identified with increasing age, and it is attributed to the diminished functional capacity of many body organs.[29] Under normal conditions a drug is absorbed from the gastrointestinal tract into the bloodstream and distributed to various body compartments. Some drugs may be further broken down into intermediate compounds for excretion, which occurs primarily in urine, but certain drugs may also be eliminated through the bile, feces, sweat, and saliva. Differences in the elderly person's drug distribution and response to drugs can be attributed to age-related changes in **pharmacokinetics** and **pharmacodynamics.**[22]

Pharmacokinetics

"Pharmacokinetics" refers to how the body absorbs, distributes, metabolizes, and excretes a drug and its metabolites.[100] The most commonly prescribed route of drug administration is the **oral** route, or through the mouth. Drug absorption depends on two factors: the rate of absorption and the extent of absorption.

Drug absorption. With age gastric pH increases as a result of a decrease in the secretion of gastric acid (see Chapter 4).[92] Drugs designed to dissolve in an acid environment may dissolve poorly and therefore may not be absorbed as well.[8] In the elderly, **splanchnic blood flow** is reduced 40% to 45%, which may delay drug absorption. A longer intestinal transit time may actually enhance absorption because of increased exposure of the mucosal surface to the drug. The number of mucosal cells and cell types can change as a person ages, resulting in some loss of absorptive surface and a decrease in the amount of drug that enters the **systemic circulation.**

There appears to be a lack of conclusive evidence that drug absorption is significantly affected in the elderly; that is, it is unlikely that drugs are less **bioavailable** in the healthy elderly than in the healthy young.[96]

Drug disposition. Changes in body composition that occur with normal aging can affect drug disposition, depending on the chemical nature of the drug. However, it is important to remember that an age-related effect on a pattern of drug disposition is difficult to differentiate from changes caused by chronic diseases. The percentage of body water decreases by 10% to 15% between 20 and 40 years of age.[90] Lean body mass and muscle decrease. As lean tissue decreases with age, fat content increases. These

changes are more marked in women than men. In men body fat increases from 18% to 35%. In women body fat increases from 33% to 48%.

The blood levels of drugs that are distributed primarily in body water and those distributed in lean body tissues will increase. Also, water-soluble drugs may not be adequately distributed because of the decline in relative body water. Conversely, highly lipid-soluble drugs may be stored in adipose tissue, thus prolonging or possibly increasing their effects.[8,29]

Changes in blood flow associated with aging may be another cause of altered pharmacokinetics. Cardiac output is reduced, and overall circulation becomes sluggish, favoring the brain, heart, and kidneys.[29,90] Drug arrival at target receptors is delayed, and drug release from storage tissues is impaired. As noted earlier, splanchnic blood flow declines 40% to 45%. The **glomerular filtration rate** declines, as does renal blood flow; the rate at which a drug or its byproducts is excreted is decreased. Blood concentrations of flow-dependent drugs rise.

Changes in drug binding to plasma proteins, red blood cells, and other body tissues can also affect drug distribution. Aging sometimes is accompanied by a reduction in **plasma albumin** available for binding. The result is an increase in unbound or free drug available for pharmacologic action. A small reduction in plasma protein available for drug binding could mean a twofold or threefold increase in the concentration of free, and hence active, drug available.[29,92] For example, **warfarin,** an anticoagulant, is a protein-bound drug whose action is enhanced when albumin is decreased. Thus the potential for serious bleeding is heightened. Small reductions in serum albumin in the healthy elderly do not appear to be clinically significant, based on epidemiologic studies.[9] However, in an older adult with a chronic disease or an individual taking several drugs simultaneously, the incidence of adverse drug reactions is likely to increase.

Drug metabolism. After the drug has been distributed to body tissues, it is removed from the body through metabolism and excretion. The site of metabolism for most drugs is the liver.[8] Age-related changes in hepatic drug metabolism are difficult to separate from other factors that can influence the liver's ability to process drugs. These other factors include chronic diseases, environmental factors, multiple drug therapies, and possibly genetic factors.[55,102] The liver's capacity to metabolize drugs is reduced with advancing age. The liver loses 35% of its weight between early adulthood and late old age.[102] Disintegration of hepatocytes is evident; thus a reduction in the liver's capacity to metabolize drugs may be related to the number of functioning liver cells. A slower metabolic rate suggests that the drug remains in the body longer, increasing the risk of drug toxicity.

Drug Excretion. Drugs may be eliminated via the liver through the bile and into the feces. The predominant route of drug elimination is through the kidneys into the urine, and this involves three processes: glomerular filtration, **active tubular secretion,** and passive tubular resorption.[8] In the renal tubular fluid, the drug concentration is increased as water is passively reabsorbed via the **nephron.** Fluid excretion by the kidneys is enhanced.

The best documentation of altered pharmacokinetics and aging is the decreased rate of drug elimination by the kidneys.[57] Diminished renal function, attributable to changes in renal vascular hemodynamics and in the nephrons, is common among the elderly and may well be the most important factor responsible for altered drug levels in this group.[7,29] The glomerular filtration rate may diminish by as much as 50% between the ages of 20 and 90. Renal blood flow declines 1.9% a year after age 30. The body's ability to concentrate urine declines, particularly with water deprivation, and renal sodium conservation is also retarded with age. The overall effect of diminished renal function is less-efficient drug clearance, leading to higher circulating blood levels of a drug.[8,29] Slow renal excretion, drug accumulation, and the potential for toxicity resulting from renal changes are aggravated by dehydration, congestive heart failure, renal disease, hypotension, and diabetes.[7,22]

The older person's impaired ability to concentrate urine means that more fluid is lost. The thirst sensation of the elderly is not a reliable mechanism for water maintenance, and diuret-

ics can aggravate the condition. The Food and Nutrition Board[25] suggests a water requirement based on energy expenditure of 1 ml/kcal under average conditions. Although a specific requirement has not been suggested for the elderly, strict monitoring of water maintenance is imperative, because older people are prone to dehydration. (See Chapter 7 for a discussion of fluid requirements and related issues.)

Pharmacodynamics

"Pharmacodynamics" refers to the effect of drugs on a target organ.[8,57] Studies on pharmacodynamics in the elderly are more limited than those on pharmacokinetics in aging.

Receptor sites in a target organ may be altered by a change in number, function, or sensitivity with increasing age.[98] For example, **receptor sensitivity** usually increases, which explains the high incidence of toxic drug reactions in this age group. However, decreased receptor sensitivity may develop, resulting in a reduced therapeutic response to a drug. A larger dose is required to achieve a therapeutic response, which puts the elderly person at risk of drug toxicity. Age differences in responsiveness vary with the drug studied, emphasizing the need for caution in prescribing medications according to guidelines based on research using young, healthy adults.

DRUG-NUTRIENT INTERACTIONS

Drugs can influence the nutritional status of an individual by exerting physiologic and biochemical actions that alter patterns of absorption, utilization, and excretion of nutrients. Conversely, profound changes in drug metabolism and efficacy can be affected by changes in a person's diet. Drug-nutrient interactions are significantly more problematic in the elderly, particularly the frail elderly and those on marginal diets who are already at increased nutritional risk. Nutritional risk increases with chronic and multiple drug use. The symptoms of a nutrient deficiency resulting from drug-nutrient interactions may be more severe than those resulting from a dietary deficiency.[66] Unfortunately, drug-induced nutritional side effects are often subtle in manifestation and slow to be identified. Frequently they escape detection.

Drug Effects on Nutrition

Short-term drug use is unlikely to have a significant impact on nutritional status. However, chronic use of some drugs may have a substantial effect and may exacerbate existing dietary deficiencies.[103] Drugs can interfere with nutritional status through their effect on food intake, nutrient absorption, metabolism, and excretion.

Drugs and food intake. Drug-induced changes in appetite or the senses of taste or smell may influence the dietary intake of an older person. The adverse gastrointestinal side effects of a drug may also influence food intake. For example, many **antineoplastic** drugs can cause anorexia by evoking an adverse response such as nausea or vomiting when food is consumed, thus reducing food intake.[66] **Cardiac glycosides** also cause anorexia accompanied by nausea.[7] Nausea, vomiting, and diarrhea are common side effects of several antihypertensive drugs, such as **hydralazine** and **diazoxide,** and act to suppress the appetite.

Not all effects on the appetite are negative. **Psychotropic** medications used to treat anxiety and depression can stimulate the appetite and may result in weight gain.[66] Another example of a **hyperphagic** drug is **tolbutamide,** an oral diabetic agent.

Blumberg and Suter[7] note that although some drugs may be classified as **hypophagic** or hyperphagic, the effect on appetite is influenced by situation factors. For example, an improvement in appetite frequently accompanies an improvement in mood in older people, whose rate of drug metabolism is slowed. However, the typical improvement in mood and psychologic function and increase in food intake associated with some psychotropic agents is not seen in older patients. To the contrary, they may cause drowsiness and disinterest in food. And, although **amitriptyline hydrochloride** is a hyperphagic drug, the result in the aged may be behavioral agitation, which interferes with eating.

Drugs and nutrient absorption. The effect of drugs on nutrient absorption is the most common type of drug-nutrient interaction known and the best described.[7] Drug-induced changes in absorption and utilization appear to have more significant influence on micronutrients than macronutrients.[103]

Drugs can interact with nutrients in several ways to compromise nutrient absorption.[66] For example, the environment of the gastrointestinal lumen may be affected by changes in the composition of bacterial flora. Laxatives may change gastrointestinal transit time, resulting in loss of calcium and potassium.[43] Generalized malabsorption can occur with the change in gastrointestinal motility associated with **anticholinergic drugs.** Antacids may change gastrointestinal pH, leading to thiamin deficiency. Nutrient bioavailability may be decreased through inactivation of bile salts, impairing the intraluminal phase of fat digestion and absorption.[7] For example, **cholestyramine** disrupts the formation of micelles and prevents the reabsorption of bile salts, thus decreasing absorption of the fat-soluble vitamins.[72] Cholestyramine also binds to **intrinsic factor,** preventing uptake of vitamin B_{12}, as does **paraaminosalicylic acid.** Some medications may form **insoluble** precipitates or chelate with a nutrient and impair absorption. The classic example of the latter type of drug-nutrient interaction is the interaction between **tetracycline** and various minerals, including calcium and magnesium; chelates are formed, and absorption of these nutrients decreased.

Certain drugs may damage the intestinal mucosa and destroy villi and microvilli, leading to inhibition of brush border enzymes and intestinal transport systems.[43,66] **Colchicine,** an antiinflammatory drug used in the treatment of gout, can damage the intestinal mucosa and inhibit the intestinal enzyme lactase, resulting in decreased absorption of fat, vitamin B_{12}, carotene, sodium, and potassium and a reduced breakdown of lactose. Enzyme inactivation is a possible mechanism of **neomycin,** an antibiotic, and **clofibrate,** a lipid-lowering drug, resulting in decreased carbohydrate absorption.[94] Some drugs may produce a physical barrier to absorption. Laxatives containing **emollients** such as mineral oil or phenolphthalein dissolve fat and fat-soluble vitamins. The nutrients are then excreted in the feces.

Blumberg and Suter[7] have identified secondary mechanisms that can interfere with nutrient absorption. Digestion of food may be affected by adverse effects on gastric or intestinal secretions, pancreatic exocrine function, or hepatic bile secretion. For example, **cimetidine,** an H_2-receptor **antagonist** used in the treatment of **peptic ulcers** to decrease gastric secretions, can induce vitamin B_{12} deficiency by inhibiting the production of gastric acid. Release of the vitamin from its protein-bound form is decreased, and less of the active free form is available for association with intrinsic factor. Further, the effect of a drug on one nutrient may have secondary consequences for yet another.

Drugs and nutrient metabolism. Drugs may affect nutrient status by altering the intermediary metabolism of a nutrient or by promoting catabolism of a nutrient.[66] In some instances this action may be a deliberate and desired therapeutic effect. Oral anticoagulants such as warfarin act as vitamin K antagonists to depress blood clotting mechanisms. Similarly, the therapeutic advantage of **methotrexate** is to antagonize the metabolism of folic acid, which is necessary for DNA and amino acid metabolism, making the drug useful as an antineoplastic agent.

Drugs may increase the rate of metabolism of certain vitamins by enhancing the production of catabolic enzymes or inhibiting controlling enzymes.[58] Although the anticonvulsant **phenytoin** is believed to interfere with folate absorption, the folate depletion observed may also relate to enhanced activation and destruction of folate.[72]

Isoniazid, a drug used in the treatment of **tuberculosis,** can interfere with the hydroxylation of vitamin D and ultimately result in a secondary impairment of calcium absorption.

Drugs and nutrient excretion. Drugs may affect nutrient status through hyperexcretion accomplished by replacing nutrients on carrier protein binding sites, by chelation, or by disturbances in renal excretion.[66] Aspirin enhances the plasma clearance of folic acid by competing for the vitamin's binding sites. A zinc deficiency is possible in those receiving long-term administration of **penicillamine.** This antiinflammatory drug, used in the treatment of **rheumatoid arthritis,** chelates with zinc and copper, resulting in increased urinary excretion of the minerals.

The desired effect of diuretic therapy, decreased reabsorption of sodium, generally is accompanied by hyperexcretion of potassium, magnesium, and zinc, particularly with long-term administration of diuretics.[66] Increased renal excretion of thiamin is also an effect of **furosemide,** a **loop diuretic.** The cardiovascular abnormalities associated with thiamin deficiency are important considerations when these diuretics are prescribed for older people with chronic congestive heart failure.

Effect of Food on Drugs

Just as drugs can affect nutrient status, so may food and dietary patterns affect the activity of a drug. Foods or specific components in food can decrease the effectiveness or increase the hazards of drug therapy. Diet can influence drug activity in one of several ways. First, dietary constituents may affect absorption of the drug. Through enzyme induction or inhibition, food may alter drug metabolism. Foods may also cause hyperexcretion of a drug as a consequence of excessive acidification or alkalization of urine attributed to a particular composition of the diet. Pharmacologically active substances in foods may alter the response of a particular drug if it is administered at the same time the food is eaten.

Food and drug absorption. Drug absorption may be enhanced, reduced, delayed, or unaffected by a concomitant feeding, by particular foods, by specific nutrient constituents, or by nonnutrient constituents of the diet. For food to have a clinically significant effect on a drug, the impact on drug absorption must be substantial and the drug must have a narrow therapeutic range.[66] Nutrients that enhance drug absorption may result in life-threatening drug intoxication. Conversely, concurrent administration of nutrients that reduce absorption of a drug with a narrow therapeutic range may minimize the drug's efficacy.

Food may affect drug absorption by altering the rate of gastric emptying and drug dissolution.[96] Absorption is likely to be most efficient when a drug has had sufficient time to dissolve in the stomach and empties quickly into the intestine, or provided it can dissolve rapidly in the proximal small intestine. Increasing the viscosity of gastric secretions reduces the rate of drug diffusion to mucosal absorptive sites. Solid meals, particularly with a high fat content, tend to slow stomach emptying by activating receptors in the duodenum. Conversely, light, liquid meals activate stretch receptors in the stomach, thereby speeding up the emptying rate. A drug may be barred access to the mucosal surface by foods that act as mechanical barriers. The bioavailability of a drug may be markedly compromised by chelation with specific food components and nutrient supplements.

Food and drug metabolism. Drugs are metabolized by mucosal enzymes and by microflora in the intestines. Although a change in the diet may affect the overall rate of drug metabolism, studies of older populations are limited. After a drug has been absorbed, its therapeutic effect is influenced by how quickly the drug is extracted from the bloodstream. Dietary components (carbohydrates, proteins, and fats) regulate splanchnic blood flow and the rate of hepatic extraction and thus may alter the therapeutic efficacy of drugs. For example, the short-term **postprandial effect** of a protein-rich diet (more than 20% of kilocalories) is an increase over fasting levels in splanchnic blood flow.[66] A high-fat diet (more than 50% of kilocalories) also enhances the rate of hepatic perfusion. A diet with more than 70% of kilocalories from carbohydrates has little or no effect.

A change in the diet may alter the composition of microflora and influence the intestinal metabolism of drugs. Manipulating sources of dietary fiber may affect the gut microflora and intestinal transit time.

Food and drug excretion. Changes in dietary patterns can result in changes in urinary pH. For example, fruits such as prunes, plums, rhubarb, and cranberries contain large amounts of quinic acid which, instead of being completely oxidized in the body, is converted to hippuric acid. Hippuric acid is eliminated through the urine and increases urinary acidity.

Diet-induced alkalization or acidification of the urine may change the excretion rates of certain drugs and influence the therapeutic effect.

Drugs may be classed as either weak acids or weak bases.[66] In an acid urine, excretion of weak acids is retarded and their effective concentration is prolonged. Conversely, excretion of drugs that are weak bases is increased in a decreasing urinary pH and their effective concentration is lessened. **Quinidine** is an antiarrhythmic drug classed as a weak base. Reabsorption by the kidneys is enhanced in an alkaline urine, which may result from a large intake of fruit juices (more than 1 L a day), thereby increasing the plasma concentration of the drug.[84]

Pharmacologically active foods. A number of foods contain pharmacologically active substances; that is, substances that exert druglike actions or alter drug action in the body. The classic example of this type of food-drug interaction occurs between foods that contain tyramine or other high pressor amines and **monoamine oxidase (MAO) inhibitors.**[54] MAO inhibitors are prescribed as antidepressants, and although experience with these drugs in the elderly is limited, attention is warranted. Foods and beverages containing **tyramine** stimulate the release of **norepinephrine** from storage sites within neurons. Normally, monoamine oxidase inactivates dietary tyramine, and the release of excessive norepinephrine is prevented. The tyramine–MAO inhibitor interaction may result in severe headaches and acute hypertensive attacks, which can be fatal. Restricted foods include those that are spoiled, decayed, fermented, overripe, old, or aged.[39] Examples of excluded items include aged cheeses (bleu, Swiss, and cheddar), aged or smoked meats (herring, sausage, and corned beef), sour cream, and ripe bananas and avocados. Red wines are prohibited, although other forms of alcohol may be consumed in moderation. Broad bean pods and fava beans are restricted foods. MAO inhibitors are not recommended for the elderly because of the possibility of interactions with other drugs that may be prescribed[6] and because it is difficult to ensure that restricted foods will not be consumed.

Licorice imported from European countries

contains a substance, **glycyrrhizic acid,** that has pharmacologic action. The active ingredient has mineralocorticoid activity, and when this licorice is consumed in excessive amounts by people taking antihypertensive drugs, hypokalemia, sodium retention, and edema may result.

NUTRITIONAL CONSIDERATIONS OF PRESCRIPTION DRUGS

A significant number of drugs pose a particular risk for the elderly. A few of the most frequently prescribed drugs have been selected for elaboration. Table 9-1 offers some examples of the possible drug-nutrient interactions of chronic drugs commonly used by the elderly.

Drug Management of Cardiovascular Disease

Digitalis glycosides. The digitalis glycosides increase **myocardial contractility.** In the failing heart, such as in congestive heart failure, these drugs increase overall cardiac efficiency. The drugs also are used in the treatment of certain cardiac arrhythmias, including **atrial fibrillation** and **atrial tachycardia.**

Because digoxin has a narrow therapeutic range, digitalis toxicity is more likely.[84] Absorption of the drug can be delayed by the presence of food in the gastrointestinal tract or by delayed gastric emptying. In these cases more of the drug is likely to be metabolized, leaving less of the unchanged drug available for absorption.[7] The result is an erratic therapeutic response. Because the distribution of digoxin is closely related to lean body mass, the elderly require lower-than-normal doses. Furthermore, because renal function and renal clearance are reduced in the elderly, the serum concentration of digoxin is elevated.[57,68] **Digitalis intoxication** commonly occurs in as many as 30% of those for whom the drug is prescribed. Digoxin also may increase urinary excretion of magnesium and calcium.[12] The drug's effects may be potentiated by concurrent administration of calcium or vitamin D supplements.[84]

The clinical manifestations of digitalis toxic-ity include anorexia, nausea, vomiting, diarrhea, and diet- or drug-induced changes in plasma electrolytes.[84] High doses of the drug may lead to **digitalis cachexia.** Gastrointestinal disturbances may also affect food intake, resulting in compromised nutritional status. Because many of the symptoms of digitalis toxicity are similar to those associated with conditions for which the drug is prescribed (e.g., nausea and vomiting attributable to heart failure, arrhythmias), it is important to know the elderly person's dietary habits.

Antiarrhythmic drugs. Antiarrhythmic drugs are used to treat irregularities in the rate and rhythm of heart contractions, disturbances that pose the risk of cardiac failure. Quinidine, an antiarrhythmic agent, is another drug with a low therapeutic index.[57] Because of altered pharmacokinetics in the elderly, elimination of the drug is prolonged. Thus older people are at increased risk of toxic effects, including **cinchonism,** a cluster of adverse effects characterized by gastrointestinal distress, headache, **tinnitus,** dizziness, blurred vision, and mild tremors.[84] Cinchonism is more commonly associated with low body weight. An older adult taking quinidine should be cautioned to avoid drinking large amounts of citrus fruit juices (more than 1 L a day), because these juices increase urinary pH.[84] Renal clearance of the drug is reduced in alkaline urine, and therefore serum concentration of the drug is increased.

Anticoagulants. Anticoagulant therapy is directed toward preventing the development of **intravascular** thromboses. The **hypoprothrombinemic** effect of oral anticoagulants may be enhanced by drugs that decrease vitamin K levels, such as antibiotics.[84] The older person who drinks herbal teas containing naturally occurring **coumarin** should also be counseled that the anticoagulant action of his or her medications may be increased. Alcohol inhibits the metabolism of anticoagulant drugs. Conversely, a decreased anticoagulant effect may be observed in those who currently consume large amounts of green tea and foods high in vitamin K, such as green, leafy vegetables; liver; cheese; egg yolks; tomatoes; meat, and cereal. It is essential to know the patient's habits so as to provide appropriate counseling.

TABLE 9-1   Drug-Nutrient Interactions Possible With Some Prescription Drugs Commonly Used by the Elderly

Type of Drug*	Mechanism/Risk of Interference	Nutritional Considerations
Antiarrhythmic drug Quinidine	Vitamin K deficiency if given with anticoagulants.	With high intake of fruit, juices: quinidine toxicity.
Anticoagulant Warfarin	Antagonism of anticoagulant effects by vitamin K.	Large amounts of vitamin K–containing foods (cabbage, green peas, turnip greens, broccoli) should be avoided.
Anticonvulsants Phenytoin	Impaired nutrient metabolism and utilization: folate deficiency. Increases activation of 25-OH-vitamin D: osteomalacia (long-term use).	Should be taken with food or immediately after meals to minimize gastric irritation. Folic acid supplement may be prescribed (limit 1 mg/day).
Primidone	Impaired nutrient metabolism and utilization: folate deficiency; neurologic complications. May interfere with bone mineralization via interruption of vitamin K–dependent bone proteins.	Supplementation with vitamin K may be considered.
Antidepressants Imipramine	Possible inducement of riboflavin deficiency; interferes with assessment of riboflavin status. Acidifies urine. Causes gastric discomfort; constipation.	Should be administered with or immediately after food to reduce gastric irritation. May require increase in dietary fiber and fluid to overcome drug-induced constipation.
Phenelzine	MAO antidepressant: concomitant intake of tyramine foods can precipitate sudden hypertensive crisis. Can cause GI distress, dry mouth, and appetite changes.	Foods and beverages high in tyramine and other pressor amines should be avoided. Body weight should be checked and any unusual changes reported. Sugarless candy or gum may help stimulate salivary flow.
Antigout drug Colchicine	Damage to intestinal mucosa: decreased absorption of vitamin B_{12}, carotene, fat, cholesterol, lactose, D-xylose. Long-term administration leads to megaloblastic anemia.	To reduce gastric irritation, should be taken with water immediately before or after meals. Encourage adequate fluid intake.

*Drug classes are included in the Glossary.

Continued.

TABLE 9-1—CONT'D **Drug-Nutrient Interactions Possible with Some Prescription Drugs Commonly Used by the Elderly**

Type of Drug*	Mechanism/Risk of Interference	Nutritional Considerations
Antihypertensive drug Hydralazine	Administration with food: increased drug bioavailability. Vitamin B_6 deficiency: risk vitamin B_6 deficiency, causing neuritis.	Medication should be taken with food. Diet restricted in kilocalories and sodium may be warranted. Supplementation with vitamin B_6 may be considered.
Antiinfective drugs Isoniazid	Altered nutrient excretion and vitamin B_6 antagonist: vitamin B_6 deficiency; pellagra secondary to vitamin B_6 deficiency. Interferes with vitamin D metabolism: risk of osteomalacia. Administration with food: decreased drug absorption.	Supplementation with vitamin B_6, niacin, and vitamin D may be considered. Risk of osteomalacia is greatest in homebound or institutionalized elderly who do not drink milk. Should be taken on an empty stomach with water.
Sulfadiazine (a sulfonamide)	Impaired folacin absorption. Anorexia. Administration with food alters GI motility and transit time: decreased drug absorption rate.	Foods rich in folacin should be encouraged. Supplementation with folic acid may be considered. To minimize gastric irritation, drug should be taken with food or water or after meals. Adequate fluid intake should be encouraged.
Tetracycline	Impaired nutrient metabolism and utilization. Interferes with vitamin K intestinal synthesis. Milk, dairy products, and iron supplements decrease drug absorption.	Supplementation with riboflavin, ascorbic acid, and calcium may be considered. Should be taken on an empty stomach with water. No milk, dairy products, or iron-containing foods should be taken within 3 hours of drug administration. Adequate fluids should be encouraged.
Antiinflammatory drug Penicillamine	Appetite suppression: weight loss.	Supplementation with multivitamin and mineral pill may be advised, because the drug can increase need for vitamin B_6 and zinc. Should not be administered with iron or other mineral supplements. Should be taken 1 hour before or 3 hours after meals. Adequate fluid intake is necessary.

*Drug classes are included in the Glossary.

Type of Drug*	Mechanism/Risk of Interference	Nutritional Considerations
Antiparkinson drug Levodopa	Vitamin B_6 causes accelerated conversion of levodopa to dopamine: decreased dopamine penetration of blood-brain barrier.	Intake of vitamin B_6 in diet and supplements should be restricted. Foods high in amino acids should be limited.
Cardiac stimulant Digoxin	Anorexia and nausea: weight loss. Low potassium intake: digoxin toxicity. Bran cereal: slows drug absorption.	Well-balanced meals and adequate potassium intake should be encouraged. High-sodium foods should be avoided. Bran should be avoided in the meal that accompanies or follows drug administration.
Diuretics Furosemide	Enhances excretion of sodium, chloride, potassium, magnesium, calcium, and water.	High-sodium foods should be restricted. Foods rich in potassium, calcium, and magnesium should be encouraged.
Spironolactone	Enhances excretion of sodium, chloride, and water. Reduces excretion of potassium.	Potassium supplements should not be used, nor should a salt substitute.
Thiazides	Enhances excretion of sodium, potassium, magnesium, and water.	High-sodium foods should be restricted. Foods rich in potassium and magnesium should be encouraged.
Lipid-lowering drug Cholestyramine	Interferes with bile acid activity: vitamins A, D, E, K, and folate deficiencies.	Supplementation is recommended with vitamins A, D, K (if hypoprothrombinemia occurs) and folic acid (for those with reduced serum or red cell folacin). Low-cholesterol diet is indicated. A high-bulk diet and increased fluid intake should be encouraged as tolerated.
Tranquilizers Chlorpromazine	Increases appetite. Possible inducement of riboflavin deficiency; interferes with assessment of riboflavin status. May result in constipation, fecal impaction; sore mouth and gums.	May require increase in dietary fiber and fluid to overcome drug-induced constipation. Sore mouth may be relieved by rinsing mouth or frequent sips of water. Sugarless candy or gum may also help stimulate salivary flow.

Antihypertensive drugs. Drug therapy of hypertension is directed toward reducing elevated **arterial pressure.** Antihypertensive drugs exert their effects through numerous mechanisms and on many sites in the body. Drugs indicated in the management of hypertension include **adrenergic inhibitors, vasodilators,** and diuretics.

Adrenergic inhibitors. Beta-adrenergic blocking agents are the preferred antihypertensive drugs for older adults, although there are greater risks of adverse reactions to drugs such as **propranolol.**[69] Beta-blockers reduce or block **myocardial stimulation,** vasodilation, and **bronchodilation.**[99] Ventricular and myocardial contractility are decreased; blood pressure and heart rate are reduced. The bioavailability of these drugs is enhanced in the presence of food because of food-related increases in splanchnic blood flow.[71,84] Because renal clearance rates are reduced in the elderly and almost all beta-blockers are excreted by the kidneys, drug excretion may be retarded. The risk of prolonged retention is also significant in elderly people with **hypoalbuminemia.**[73] Having less albumin available to bind the drug means that more of the medication can diffuse into nervous tissue and give rise to CNS side effects.

Vasodilators. Hydralazine is a nondiuretic antihypertensive vasodilator whose primary effect is dilation of the blood vessels, particularly the arterioles.[84] The bioavailability of hydralazine is enhanced in the presence of food. **Peripheral neuropathy** in individuals taking hydralazine may be attributable to its antipyridoxine effect, which results because the drug combines with pyridoxine coenzymes, making them unavailable.[12] Thus the patient may have an increased need of vitamin B_6, and supplementation (25 mg a day) may be prescribed to counter this side effect.[71] Older patients should be cautioned against taking vitamin B_6 in amounts above that found in a daily multivitamin pill unless advised to do so by their physician.[74]

Diuretics. Retention of excess fluid by the body depends primarily on sodium retention. The effectiveness of a diuretic is related to its ability to excrete excess sodium, which usually is accomplished by interfering with reabsorp-

tion of sodium ions in the renal tubules. The elderly are more susceptible to fluid and electrolyte disorders.

Loop diuretics such as furosemide and **ethacrynic acid** decrease sodium and chloride absorption in the ascending loop of Henle.[71] It is important to monitor electrolyte levels carefully, because low blood levels of sodium, potassium, magnesium, and calcium are possible side effects. Although the patient should be counseled to avoid foods high in sodium and indiscriminate use of OTC medications, a restricted sodium diet (less than 1.5 g of sodium a day) is contraindicated. A strong argument for sodium restriction in these situations is that potassium loss is directly proportional to sodium excretion, which increases with dietary intake.[98] Wilber[98] suggests limiting sodium intake to 75 mEq, which can be accomplished by eliminating highly salted, prepared foods from the diet and by not adding salt at the table. This approach enhances the effectiveness of the oral diuretic and may eliminate the need for potassium supplements or the relatively expensive potassium-sparing diuretic combinations. To compensate for the increased urinary excretion of calcium, which can speed up the development of osteoporosis, an older patient should be encouraged to drink milk each day.[73]

Thiazide diuretics, which decrease sodium reabsorption in the distal tubules, are also associated with the risk of fluid and electrolyte imbalances. The risk of magnesium and potassium loss is increased. Calcium retention has been observed, and elevated blood levels of calcium may occur with prolonged thiazide therapy.[73,103] The potential for **hyperglycemia** is heightened for people with diabetes.

Not all diuretics increase the risk of potassium loss. Potassium-sparing diuretics conserve potassium by reducing distal tubular secretion in conjunction with sodium reabsorption. The principal use of potassium-sparing drugs is in combination with other diuretics. If potassium-sparing drugs are used as single agents, significant hyperkalemia can result. For an elderly person taking potassium-sparing drugs, using potassium supplements or salt substitutes can exacerbate the problem.

Lipid-lowering drugs. The National Cholesterol Education Program–Adult Treatment Program[24] supports the use of lipid-lowering medications as adjunctive therapy to dietary changes but does not approve the use of these drugs as a substitute for such changes.

Cholestyramine is an effective plasma cholesterol-lowering drug that combines with bile acids in the intestines. Bile acid reabsorption is prevented, and excretion in the feces is increased. **Bile acid sequestrants** such as cholestyramine should be used cautiously in the elderly, because gastrointestinal discomfort, severe constipation, and nutrient malabsorption are likely.[84] Long-term therapy with bile acid sequestrants, including **colestipol**, has been shown to depress the absorption of fat-soluble vitamins, folate, and vitamin B_{12} by inhibiting absorption or decreasing the availability of bile acids.[71,84] Nutrition counseling should encourage the incorporation of dietary fiber to counter the constipating effects of the diet.

In pharmaceutical doses, niacin may be prescribed to decrease serum lipids by decreasing **very-low-density lipoproteins (VLDL)** and **low-density lipoproteins (LDL).**[90] However, the use of niacin as a lipid-lowering drug is limited by the adverse effects of flushing and itching. In addition, any ulcers present may be aggravated, and vomiting, diarrhea, and **dyspepsia** may result. Liver function may be impaired, increasing serum **transaminase** activity, and **jaundice** has been reported. **Niacin** in the form of **nicotinamide** (rather than as nicotinic acid) does not produce flushing. Since tolerance frequently develops after a few weeks, increasing the dosage gradually may minimize the adverse side effect.

Niacin is available without a prescription and has become a well-known therapeutic agent. Its popularity has been enhanced by numerous lay articles and books. However, because of the potential for hepatotoxicity and other side effects and contraindications in those with diabetes mellitus, active peptic ulcer disease, and acute gout, older people should be cautioned against self-medicating with niacin.

Pulmonary Drugs

A number of changes occur with increasing age, such as a 50% increase in residual lung volume between early adulthood and age 70.[99] A decrease in **vital capacity** is the result of a stiffer chest wall. Weaker respiratory muscles, impaired ciliary action, and a less effective cough further predispose an older person to a variety of pulmonary diseases and disorders. Pulmonary conditions commonly seen in the elderly include **pneumonia, chronic obstructive pulmonary disease, pulmonary embolism,** and tuberculosis.

Bronchodilators. Bronchodilators relax the **bronchioles. Theophylline** is a xanthine-derivative bronchodilator indicated for the treatment of a variety of chronic pulmonary obstructive diseases common in the elderly.[73,84] The presence of food has little effect on theophylline availability, although absorption may be somewhat slower when food is present than from an empty stomach. However, variations in food components can affect the drug's efficacy. A high-protein, low-carbohydrate diet may decrease the effect of the drug by increasing drug metabolism and clearance. Conversely, a high-carbohydrate, low-protein diet slows theophylline metabolism and predisposes the individual to undesirable side effects such as dizziness, flushing, and headache.[73] A high-fat diet potentiates the risk of dizziness because of rapid absorption. Taking theophylline with beverages containing caffeine may result in additive CNS stimulation.[84]

Antitubercular drugs. Isoniazid, a vitamin B_6 antagonist, may produce clinical symptoms of vitamin deficiency by inhibiting **pyridoxal kinase.**[103] As many as 40% of those taking the drug may have this side effect. The adverse effect is increased in those given concurrent antitubercular drugs, in individuals with a low vitamin B_6 intake, and in patients not given supplementation. Roe[73] recommends vitamin B_6 supplementation of 25 mg a day. The high histamine content of foods such as sardines, skipjack, and tuna predisposes the individual taking isoniazid to severe headaches, itching of the eyes and face, chills, palpitations, and loose stools.[43]

Gastrointestinal Disease

H_2-receptor antagonists. Long-term administration of cimetidine coupled with a high-fiber diet may result in the formation of gastric phytobezoars, or hard balls of fiber.[60] A diet low in cellulose may need to be considered for the elderly person receiving long-term therapy with cimetidine or for those with chewing problems. Antacids may impair oral absorption of H_2-blockers if administered concurrently.[6] Vitamin B_{12} depletion can be induced by cimetidine, particularly in vegans who take the drug for a prolonged time (longer than 1 year).

Psychotherapeutic Drugs

The number of psychotherapeutic drugs prescribed for the elderly appears to be increasing.[22] Unfortunately, there is also evidence that these drugs are being misused in this segment of the population. The problem may be an improper diagnosis, but these drugs are also being prescribed as a panacea against problems of daily living, such as to quiet an individual in an institution or even within the family. Psychotherapeutic drugs such as sedatives or antidepressants frequently are prescribed for the elderly to control disruptive behavior. Older people are especially sensitive to the intended pharmacologic effects and the undesirable adverse effects of psychotherapeutic drugs.

Tranquilizers. The side effects of many tranquilizers may include nausea and vomiting, which may cause loss of appetite and lead to malnutrition.[12] However, **phenothiazine antipsychotic drugs,** which include chlorpromazine, may actually stimulate the appetite to the point that the individual with free access to food may grossly overeat.[70] Obesity may then become a concern. **Chlorpromazine** may also induce riboflavin depletion.[74] In rats interaction has been observed between the drug and the metabolism of riboflavin, which has a similar chemical structure.[103]

Antidepressants. The reported incidence of depression in the elderly is approximately 10%. Tricyclic antidepressants (amitriptyline and **imipramine**) frequently are prescribed for the elderly and are accompanied by potentially serious side effects such as arrhythmias, **orthostatic hypotension,** and anticholinergic effects.[95] Consequently, constipation may be a severe problem, and the importance of including an adequate amount of fiber in the diet

should be stressed. These drugs are also known to alter metabolism and induce riboflavin depletion.[74,103]

Enhanced appetite may be seen in some people taking tricyclic antidepressants, and this may lead to weight gain.[84] This development may be due to improved mental state or improved taste perception. Dry mouth is a possible side effect with tricyclic antidepressants. To cope with the problem, the patient should be counseled to avoid drinking more high-calorie beverages; rather, low-calorie beverages, sugarless gum, candy, or ice should be selected.

Drug therapy in Alzheimer's disease. Senile dementia of the Alzheimer type (SDAT) is the most common type of dementia in the United States, and the number of cases is increasing.[13] Treatment is primarily supportive, although drug therapy has been helpful in some cases. Currently between 10 and 20 drugs are undergoing trials before gaining final approval from the FDA. The drugs used in the treatment of SDAT are divided into two broad categories: drugs directed at improving abnormal behavior and those directed at improving cognitive function.

Numerous drugs are available to treat behavioral problems (although none is specific for SDAT), and these drugs may be useful in dementia of any origin. **Neuroleptics** are the most widely prescribed drugs to treat abnormal behavior, although their mode of action in controlling psychotic behavior has not been established. No one drug in this category has been shown to have greater effectiveness than another. Chlorpromazine, once a favorite, has largely been replaced by **thioridazine hydrochloride,** because the latter is less likely to cause adverse symptoms such as immobility, rigidity, restlessness, and tremors.[20] Other side effects associated with neuroleptic drugs include seizures, inappropriate secretion of antidiuretic hormone, jaundice, and weight gain.[13] Sedatives or minor tranquilizers are indicated for use in short-term treatment of anxiety or in less severe cases, but they may increase the risk of falling. The exact mechanism of effectiveness of drugs such as propranolol and **carbamazepine** (used to treat agitation and violent behavior) is unknown, and the role of these drugs is largely undefined.[13,65,93]

More recent drug development has centered on attempts to improve cognitive function. Because SDAT is recognized as a deficiency in the neurotransmitter **acetylcholine,** researchers have sought to increase brain levels of acetylcholine. Because the enzyme **cholinesterase** degrades acetylcholine, drugs that inhibit the enzyme's action could potentially increase acetylcholine levels. A second category of drugs, nootropic drugs, is also used to improve cognitive function. Although the way in which they affect memory is unknown, nootropic drugs act to improve nerve cell function. The third subcategory of drugs used to improve cognitive function is the **calcium channel blockers,** which act on the vascular system. In addition to their vasodilating properties, these drugs have the ability to block calcium entry into injured or hypoxic brain neurons, which may be a key to their effectiveness.

At best drugs may slow the progression of the disorder; none has yet been discovered that will reverse the course of this disease. Multiple-drug therapy may be the best line of treatment for SDAT, a disease characterized by multiple defects.

Antiparkinsonian Drugs

Drug treatment of **Parkinson's disease** is directed toward augmenting dopaminergic function or reducing cholinergic activity. Clinical manifestations of the incurable disease include **bradykinesia,** rigidity, and tremors. Difficulties with mastication and swallowing may also be observed.[84]

Levodopa, an antiparkinsonian drug, has a structure similar to that of amino acids and therefore competes with amino acids for absorption sites in the small intestine.[74,84] If the drug is taken concurrently with a high-protein diet, its bioavailability may be significantly compromised. The suggested daily protein intake of individuals taking levodopa is 0.5 g/kg body weight, which should be adequate if protein foods of high biologic value are stressed. Eating protein foods later in the day is another strategy to suggest. The patient should also be counselled to avoid multivitamin supplements containing pyridoxine (vitamin B_6), because this vitamin enhances the peripheral conversion of levodopa to dopamine, and the drug's effects will be reduced.

Antineoplastic Drugs

Whether the elderly as a group are less likely to receive vigorous, potentially beneficial **chemotherapy** treatment for cancer has received considerable attention.[4,33,75,81] In a comparison of toxicity from chemotherapy in individuals under age 70 and those age 70 or older, no significant difference was observed between the two groups in important prognostic factors such as functional status, weight loss, and previous therapy.[4] Toxicity was similar for both groups, with the exception of hematologic toxicity. A significantly greater number of elderly adults experienced hematologic toxicity. An increase in toxicity with age may be associated with the age-related physiologic decline in a specific organ system.

Essentially all neoplastic drugs cause nausea and vomiting, resulting in a reduced food and fluid intake and electrolyte imbalance and leading to weight loss. The drugs' effects on the gastrointestinal tract may induce anorexia. Antineoplastic drugs, particularly methotrexate, cause malabsorption through desquamation of intestinal epithelial cells and inflammation of the mucous membrane lining the mouth, throat, and esophagus; **stomatitis;** and **glossitis.** Malabsorption may continue after chemotherapy has been discontinued. If a person tries to eat when the drug is causing side effects, he or she may develop an aversion to those foods by associating them with the unpleasant side effects.[72] Roe[70] states that it is unlikely that a change in appetite associated with the drug alone will induce a nutritional deficiency.

NUTRITIONAL CONSIDERATIONS OF OVER-THE-COUNTER DRUGS

The use of nonprescription drugs is high, although reports vary as to its extent. Almost one third of drug expenditures by the elderly goes to OTC drugs.[55] Further, use of nonprescrip-

TABLE 9-2 **Nutritional Considerations with Over-the-Counter Drugs Commonly Used by the Elderly**

Classification/Drug	Examples	Nutritional Considerations
Analgesics Aspirin	Bayer, Bufferin, Excedrin	Chronic ingestion may be associated with depressed plasma ascorbic acid and folate levels; supplemental therapy may be indicated. May cause iron-deficiency anemia as a result of gastrointestinal (GI) blood loss.
Acetaminophen	Datril, Tylenol	Coadministration with a high-carbohydrate meal may significantly retard absorption. Individuals with poor nutrition or who have ingested alcohol over prolonged periods are prone to liver disease, and drug may cause anorexia, nausea, vomiting, dyspepsia, constipation, or diarrhea. May increase urinary loss of ascorbic acid.
Antacids Aluminum hydroxide	Amphojel	Large doses for prolonged periods along with a diet low in phosphorus and protein can develop phosphorus-deficiency syndrome—the elderly person in poor nutritional status is at high risk. Vitamin A and thiamin deficiencies can occur as a result of reduced absorption. Constipation occurs commonly, and intestinal obstruction has been reported.
Magnesium hydroxide	Milk of Magnesia	Excessive dosage can cause nausea, abdominal cramps, diarrhea, alkalinization of urine, and dehydration. Magnesium toxicity can develop in those with kidney failure.
Antidiarrheal drugs	Lomotil, Kaopectate	May cause nausea, vomiting, abdominal discomfort, constipation, and fecal impaction. Caffeine beverages and alcohol should be avoided, since both increase peristalsis. Prolonged use may interfere with intestinal absorption of nutrients and promote constipation.
Antiemetics	Dramamine, Bonine	May cause dry mouth, nose, and throat; epigastric distress; and constipation.
Antihistamines	Benedryl, Chlor-Trimeton	GI side effects may be lessened by administration of drug with meals or milk. Dry mouth may be relieved by sugarless candy or gum or rinses with water. Elderly people are especially likely to experience dizziness, sedation, and hypotension.

Classification/Drug	Examples	Nutritional Considerations
Cold preparations	Robitussin	Fluid intake should be increased to 2 to 3 L daily to help thin and mobilize respiratory secretions, but the elderly should be monitored closely to avoid fluid overload.
Laxatives		
Bulk-forming	Metamucil, Mitrolan	Adequate fluid intake must be maintained; fecal impaction can occur if fluid intake by mouth is insufficient. Can decrease appetite through abdominal fullness. Products contain varying amounts of sugar and salt. Electrolyte imbalance is possible with chronic use.
Fecal softeners	Colace	Adequate fluid intake must be maintained.
Stimulants	Bisacolax, Correctol, Dulcolax, Ex-Lax	Abuse can cause electrolyte imbalance, including potassium depletion; malabsorption, with weight loss, can also occur. Frequent use may result in laxative dependence.

tion drugs among the elderly is expected to continue to increase in concert with the expansion of home health care, the fastest growing segment of the health care market.[47] Lamy[47] reports that the most frequently used OTC drugs are analgesics, followed by cough and cold preparations, vitamins, antacids, and laxatives. Use of nonprescription medicine is more likely with advancing age, particularly among women. However, elderly adults are not likely to discuss the use of OTC drugs with the physician, and the physician is not likely to ask about their use. Unfortunately, indiscriminate use of these therapeutically valuable drugs can lead to unexpected consequences. The elderly are particularly at risk for the hazards associated with nonprescription drugs for several reasons.[47] Additive effects and interactions with prescribed drugs can develop in people undergoing complex drug regimens. In self-prescribing OTC drugs, the elderly person may not be able to correctly diagnose the condition, select an appropriate drug, and follow directions. In this era of increasing self-care, more prescription drugs are being changed to nonprescription status, increasing the potential for further adverse effects. Table 9-2 offers some nutritional con-siderations for OTC drugs commonly used by the elderly.

Analgesics

Individuals age 65 or older are the greatest users of analgesics.[15] The mostly commonly used analgesic in the United States is aspirin, followed by **acetaminophen.** Because aspirin and other derivatives of **salicylic acid** have anal-gesic, antipyretic, and antiinflammatory effects, they frequently are prescribed to relieve mild to moderate pain, to reduce elevated body temperature, and to treat the symptoms of certain in-flammatory conditions (e.g., rheumatoid arthritis and osteoarthritis). Aspirin is also prescribed to reduce the risk of heart attack or stroke.

Common side effects of aspirin include gastric distress, dyspepsia, and nausea.[31,48] Salicylate toxicity can occur at high doses or with prolonged use.[43] Symptoms include confusion, irritability, tinnitus, impaired hearing or vision, nausea, vomiting, and diarrhea. Because of aspirin's antipyretic action, subnormal body temperatures can occur. **Gastritis,** ulceration of the gastric mucosa, and hemorrhaging are harmful side effects experienced by the elderly who, because of inadequate diets and poor nutritional status, are less able to compensate for even a small blood loss.[15] Iron-deficiency anemia may be induced. Folic acid deficiency and **macrocytic anemia** are also associated with chronic aspirin therapy, particularly those with a marginal intake of the vitamin. Vitamin C depletion has also been observed.

Aspirin can also affect prescribed drug therapy.[15] By competing for protein binding sites, aspirin may enhance the actions and toxicity of oral anticoagulants and oral **hypoglycemic** drugs. Through this action and by competitively inhibiting the renal secretion of methotrexate, plasma concentrations of free methotrexate may increase, as may the risk of a serious toxic reaction.

Acetaminophen is a paraaminophenol derivative with analgesic and antipyretic action. It is a commonly used aspirin substitute.[15] The drug has several advantages over aspirin. A lower incidence of gastrointestinal upset and bleeding has been observed, as well as fewer reports of hypersensitivity reactions. No significant interaction with oral anticoagulants is evident. However, unlike aspirin, acetaminophen has no significant antiinflammatory activity. The major concern is that acetaminophen can induce hepatotoxicity when ingested as an acute massive overdose. Further, liver damage is a possible occurrence with long-term use in alcoholics and those with impaired liver function.

Antacids

Antacids frequently are used to treat upper gastrointestinal disorders ranging from mild indigestion and **heartburn** to peptic ulcer. Appropriate antacid therapy should be selected cautiously, because indiscriminate use of the widely available and easily obtainable preparations result in serious, harmful effects. This is particularly important for the susceptible elderly (e.g., those with altered bowel habits, severe organ-system disease, or renal impairment).[28]

With antacid therapy, the absorption of acidic drugs may be increased; the absorption of basic drugs, decreased.[43] If possible, other drugs should not be administered within 1 to 2 hours of antacid ingestion. By delaying gastric emptying, absorption of a number of drugs may be delayed and elimination of others may be influenced by the antacid's effect on urinary pH.

Some antacids have a significant amount of sugar. The sodium content of antacids should also be explored, especially for patients who have been advised to restrict sodium in their diets because of hypertension, edema, or congestive heart failure. Antacids with more than 5 mEq of sodium per dose carry a precautionary warning on the label, but sodium bicarbonate and effervescent forms are exempt.[28]

Antacids with calcium ions may induce a rebound hyperacidity.[28] **Milk-alkali syndrome** is a possible complication associated with high doses over several years. Symptoms include **metabolic alkalosis, hypercalcemia,** vomiting, confusion, headache, and **renal insufficiency.** Development of **renal calculi** has also been reported in elderly people undergoing calcium carbonate therapy. More acute problems have been observed with calcium-containing antacids at lower doses. Constipation and fecal impaction may be promoted.

Antacids containing aluminum may be constipating and may result in intestinal obstruction, particularly in a bedridden individual.[43] This type of antacid has also been implicated in dementia observed in elderly uremic patients. Phosphate depletion is likely, since aluminum antacids bind phosphate ions in the intestine. Accelerated elimination of the nonabsorbable phosphates follows. Symptoms include anorexia, muscle weakness, impaired reflexes, depression, and osteomalacia.

Aluminum hydroxide is sometimes paired with magnesium hydroxide to reduce the occurrence of constipation associated with aluminum and the diarrhea frequently associated with magnesium alone. Antacids containing magnesium can cause profound diarrhea, leading to dehydration and significant losses of vitamins and electrolytes, particularly potassium. Magnesium toxicity, characterized by nausea, vomiting, impaired reflexes, hypotension, and respiratory depression, can develop in people with impaired renal function.[74]

Preparations containing sodium carbonate are indicated for short-term therapy only because of the potential for sodium overload, which is significantly enhanced during prolonged treatment. The pH of the jejunum may be sufficiently increased to decrease the absorption of folic acid. Milk-alkali syndrome and rebound acid hypersecretion are also possible.

Laxatives

A laxative is an agent that facilitates evacuation of the bowel. It has been estimated that 90% of the elderly who are laxative dependent or laxative abusers are women.[28] Laxative use among the elderly is similar to the use of analgesics. Laxatives can be classified by their respective mechanisms of action.

Stimulant laxatives increase intestinal propulsion, which may produce excessive **catharsis,** leading to the development of fluid and electrolyte disturbances. The intensity of the response to the drug is directly proportional to the dose. Side effects may include intestinal cramps, increased secretion of mucus, and excessively fluid evacuations. Castor oil is an example of a stimulant laxative, and it should be used cautiously in the elderly because of its potential for dehydration. Prolonged use can result in laxative dependency and may result in severe malabsorption, with **steatorrhea** and **protein-losing enteropathy.**[7] Decreased absorption of glucose, calcium, potassium, and vitamin D has been observed.

Saline or **osmotic cathartics** should also be used with caution in the elderly because of potential side effects. These drugs mechanically stimulate **peristalsis** and alter stool consistency by retaining water in the intestinal lumen. The older individual should be encouraged to drink sufficient water to prevent dehydration.

Emollient laxatives soften the fecal mass by reducing surface tension of interfacing liquid bowel contents.[99] Fluid accumulation in the bowel is promoted. Stool softeners are relatively safe and are recommended for conditions in which hard or dry stool might prove painful or in which straining is undesirable, such as with heart disease. Potassium deficiency, attributable to gastrointestinal losses and lack of colonic reabsorption, has been observed with some stool softeners.[19]

Bulk-producing laxatives are cellulose derivatives that swell in intestinal fluid and stimulate peristalsis by retaining water in the stool. The size of the stool is increased, and transit time is decreased. These laxatives are the preferred type for short-term treatment of most types of mild constipation. However, they should be administered with and followed by large amounts of water. Bulk-forming laxatives are contraindicated for individuals prone to intestinal ulcerations or disabling **adhesions** because of the danger of impaction.[28]

The preferred measures for maintaining a soft, formed stool and regular bowel habits are a sufficient fluid intake and a well-balanced diet rich in high-fiber foods. Important sources of dietary fiber include whole-grain cereals and breads, fruits and vegetables, and nuts. Cereals are preferable sources of fiber, because they are high in **soluble fiber,** which has proved to be more effective in producing bulk. Bran has been shown to be particularly effective in decreasing constipation and maintaining bowel function. Adding in high-fiber foods to the diet should be done slowly to prevent **flatulence** and abdominal cramps. Excessive fiber intake can interfere with the absorption of minerals and may lead to intestinal obstruction.

ALCOHOL USE IN OLDER PEOPLE

Alcohol is one of the most pervasive drugs in our society.[78] Its use or abuse places the elderly at risk for a variety of adverse and life-threatening effects, including liver disease, gastritis, peptic ulcer disease, heart muscle disorder, malnutrition, and changes in mental status.[22,84]

Until recently, use and abuse of alcohol by the elderly did not receive a great deal of attention. This may have been partly due to an attitude that abusers would "mature out" of their habits.[97] Also, symptoms associated with a problem drinker (tremors, impaired memory, disturbed sleep patterns, peripheral neuropathy, unsteady gait, depression) may be mistakenly identified as common problems of aging.[22] However, with the population as a whole aging, current interest in the use of alcohol by the aged is heightened.

Use of Alcohol

Using data from the National Health and Nutrition Examination Surveys (NHANES I and II) Iber and coworkers[37] suggest that alcohol consumption is widespread, although more common among men than women. Alcohol ingestion peaks between ages 40 and 60 and then declines. In Iber's study, the highest intakes were 5% and 6% of total kilocalories. In a random sample of 239 British elderly, 76 (32%) identified themselves as drinkers, and 161 (68%) identified themselves as nondrinkers.[38] As with other community studies, men were more likely to drink than women.

Sulsky and associates[89] observed that alcohol consumption decreased with age among 611 noninstitutionalized, nonalcoholic elderly people ages 60 to 95. Once again, men were more likely to drink than women; men were also more likely to consume large quantities of alcohol than women. Among 270 healthy older people in New Mexico, 46% of the men and 41% of the women consumed alcohol at least once over a 3-day period.[27] Mean daily intake was higher for men than women (12 versus 6 g) and also decreased with age.

Although a significant number of older people appear to consume alcoholic beverages regularly, the number of alcohol abusers is not clear. Widner and Zeichner[97] purport that a significant number go undetected and that drinking behavior may be underreported by as much as 50%. In an investigation of 310 older residents of a community in Dade County, Florida, 68% described themselves as "abstainers"; yet, 28% identified themselves as "moderate to heavy drinkers."[21] In a Canadian study of the drinking behavior of 142 elderly people, 62% reported that they abstained or drank infrequently.[83] Almost 11% showed the symptoms of problem drinkers.

Of 280 consecutive admissions of men age 65 or older requiring medical or surgical care in a veterans' facility, 11% were alcoholics.[77] Approximately 7% of 3411 individuals over age 55 admitted to a proprietary hospital were diagnosed as being alcoholics. Estimates of alcoholism among institutionalized elderly may be as high as 44%.[97]

Although the elderly population cannot be described as a homogenous group based on behavioral characteristics, they do fall into two classes: the early-onset and the late-onset problem drinker.[97] The early-onset problem drinker has a long history of heavy alcohol consumption before age 40. The support network of family and friends is less likely to be as strong as that of the late-onset problem drinker, whose history of heavy drinking began after age 40. The latter group usually has fewer alcohol-related physical problems and appears more responsive to treatment. Late-onset problem drinkers account for one third of all geriatric problem drinkers, and onset seems to be related to depression, loneliness, retirement, and bereavement.

Underreporting true alcohol consumption by the elderly may be associated with isolation from an active support network of people who typically would recognize and report alcohol-related problems.[97] On the other hand, family members may hesitate to report the older person's drinking problem in an attempt to protect the dignity of the individual.[78]

Nutritional Aspects

Tolerance to alcohol decreases and adverse side effects increase with age, even in chronic alcoholics.[79] The risk of nutritional deficiency arising from use of other drugs is markedly increased by excessive use of alcohol or when prior alcoholism has depleted nutrient stores. Moreover, alcohol interacts with some drugs to exacerbate negative effects. Both alcohol and aspirin irritate the stomach mucosa and can lead to **gastrointestinal bleeding.** When both drugs are combined, the anticoagulant effect of aspirin can result in serious hemorrhage.[79]

A high alcohol intake decreases potassium levels. This presents a serious danger to the cardiac patient taking digoxin, since both cardiac arrhythmias and digoxin toxicity can result. The insulin-dependent diabetic may become hypoglycemic following high alcohol intake, since alcohol interferes with **gluconeogenesis.**[73,79] The non-insulin-dependent diabetic taking an oral antidiabetic agent such as tolbutamide may experience hyperglycemia, because alcohol can shorten the drug's period of action.[73] **Chlorpropamide,** another **oral antidiabetic agent,** can result in a chlorpropamide-alcohol flush reaction in some non-insulin-dependent diabetics when the drug is mixed with alcohol in beverages, food, or other drugs.

Thiamin deficiency. Alcohol interferes with thiamin absorption. At the low concentrations in which it normally is found in the intestine, thiamin is absorbed against a concentration gradient by an active transport mechanism requiring both oxygen and energy. Although alcohol does not inhibit thiamin uptake by the mucosal cell, the vitamin is not released into the blood as a result of alcohol inhibition of the enzyme required for this step (sodium-potassium ATPase).[37]

Thiamin absorption is impaired in alcoholics with or without liver disease and returns to normal when use is discontinued (within 8 weeks).[91] The direct effect of alcohol on the absorption mechanism is confirmed by the observation that absorption is similarly depressed in normal individuals given alcohol before thiamin ingestion. As a result of ineffective absorption, thiamin deficiency is common among alcohol abusers. In one report nearly half of a group of chronic alcoholics (n = 50) had below-normal **red blood cell transketolase** activity, compared to only 2% of healthy adults (n = 1,152).[37]

Neurologic disorders marked by visual disturbances, abnormal gait **(ataxia)**, mental confusion, and memory loss (e.g. **Wernicke-Korsakoff syndrome**) occur in thiamin deficiency regardless of associated alcoholism.[37,50] Degeneration of the peripheral nerves, with loss of normal reflexes and burning sensations, weakness, and pain in the lower extremities are classic signs of inadequate thiamin. Clinical **beriberi** with disturbed cardiac function, edema, and eventual cardiac failure has been described in both experimental and accidental thiamin deficiency. As pointed out by Iber and coworkers,[37] cardiac disease, loss of memory, and loss of vibratory sense in the lower extremities, suggestive of thiamin deficiency, frequently occur with advancing age. The diagnostic problem is complicated further by the fact that older people may have several vitamin deficiencies regardless of alcohol abuse.[50]

Although older alcoholics or individuals with poor thiamin intake (over at least 3 months) often respond to thiamin therapy, both behavior changes and cardiac symptoms in older people can result from a variety of disease conditions. Long-term neurologic and psychologic follow-up of older people whose thiamin status was restored to normal is needed to provide information about both physiologic and behavioral changes pertinent to thiamin problems in this age group.

VITAMIN AND MINERAL SUPPLEMENTS IN OLDER PEOPLE
Extent of Use

A large number of older people use vitamin and mineral supplements. Block and associates[6] analyzed previously uncoded data from NHANES I to study the use of these supplements. People age 65 or older regularly took supplements twice as often as any other age group with the exception of vitamin E, iron, and multiple vitamins. More recent studies have corroborated this, with estimates that approximately 33% to 69% of the geriatric population regularly use vitamin and mineral supplements.* In addition, the data indicate that the elderly frequently take supplements in potentially toxic doses,[32,62,85] overestimate the benefits of the products,[76] and do not select supplements that will correct existing dietary deficiencies.

Data from the 1987 **National Health Interview Survey** reported estimates of supplement use in a large representative sample of the U.S. population.[88] The survey involved 2,498 respondents from ages 65 to 74, and 1,742 respondents age 75 or older. In the 65 to 74 age group, multivitamin-mineral supplements were the most commonly used supplement (22%), followed in decreasing order of daily use by calcium (12%), vitamin C (11%), vitamin E (7%), and vitamin A (2%). In those age 75 or older, the order changed somewhat: multivitamin-mineral supplement (22%), vitamin C

---

*References 14, 32, 35, 62, 76, and 85.

(10%), calcium (9%), vitamin E (7%), and vitamin A (2%).

Elderly people taking vitamins and minerals tend to have misperceptions about vitamin and mineral supplements. More than half of 102 elderly subjects from rural congregate meal programs believed that taking supplements makes one feel better physically, 64% believed that most elderly people need dietary supplements, and 70% believed that a "run down" feeling indicates a need for vitamins and minerals.[62] Almost half of the subjects in the study were taking supplements inappropriately, interpreted as the use of a multivitamin/mineral with more than 150% of the U.S. Recommended Dietary Allowance (USRDA) or taking three or more individual supplements not prescribed by a physician.

Potentially toxic doses of vitamin A (25,000 IU or more) were being taken by 3.2% of 11,888 residents of a retirement community in southern California.[32] More than one fourth of those who took vitamin E supplements and 23% of those who took vitamin C supplements were taking at least 10 times the RDA.

Twenty "overusers" of nutrient supplements (defined as taking at least one vitamin or mineral supplement usually exceeding 200% of the RDA without medical recommendation) took 44 types of products.[67] Supplement intakes greater than 25 times the RDA were reported for many overusers for vitamin E, vitamin B_{12}, thiamin, riboflavin, and vitamin C. One person took excess amounts of calcium (3 g a day) and vitamin D (25,000 IU a day); another took a potentially toxic amount of iron (400 mg a day). Inappropriate reasons cited for taking supplements included preventing arthritis and infections by taking vitamin C, improving memory with niacin, and preventing constipation by taking vitamin E.

Nutrient Toxicities

A panel of experts evaluating the potential danger of excessive ingestion of vitamins or minerals concluded that toxicities are unlikely to occur as a result of food intake except in those adopting the most unusual food pattern.[59] However, indiscriminate or inappropriate consumption of vitamin and mineral preparations predisposes the elderly to real hazards. Currently we do not know the maximum blood levels reached following ingestion of high-potency supplements nor the period of time such levels are maintained. It is likely, however, that the kinetics of tissue disposal or excretion differ in older as compared to younger individuals based on the former group's reduced glomerular filtration rate and **renal tubular secretion** of metabolites. The fact that the aged adult is more susceptible to drug overdose and toxicity than a younger adult lends credence to such an argument.

ROLE OF THE NUTRITION PROFESSIONAL

Food and drug interactions are of increasing concern to nutrition professionals. This may be partly because of the 1985 mandate by the **Joint Commission on Accreditation of Healthcare Organizations** that a patient education plan for drug-nutrient interactions be implemented by dietetic services.[40] The responsibility of monitoring and providing information-potential food-drug interactions is shared by all health care professionals. However, the nutrition professional has the expertise to screen for medications with the potential for drug-nutrient interactions and to evaluate the elderly person's dietary pattern and nutritional status, which can affect a drug.

A complete diet history is essential. In addition to the usual meal pattern, the nutrition professional needs to ask about any **food idiosyncracies** the person may have, any known allergies or **food intolerances,** and what food or nutrient supplements are currently being used. Armed with knowledge of the more common and more serious drug-nutrient interactions, the nutrition professional can ask more meaningful questions.

The nutrition professional must also question the person about currently prescribed and OTC medications being taken, what he or she knows about the drugs, and any drug-related problems the patient may have experienced. If the older person is taking medications known to interact with nutrients or if nutritional status is likely to interfere with drug therapy, the pharmacist and physician should be consulted so that appropriate intervention can be planned. The older person needs to be educated about the possible side effects of drugs he or she is taking, including the effect diet may have on drug therapy.

The nutrition professional should be aware of his or her own limitations. A patient is more likely to know the brand name than the generic name of a drug. The nutrition professional has the responsibility to identify any drug from its brand name and its generic name. This information is available from sources such as the **American Hospital Formulary,** the **Physician's Desk Reference (PDR),** and the **U.S. Pharmacopeia Dispensing Information** (USPDI). The clinical pharmacist is a tremendous resource for drug information. The nutrition professional must keep current on newly discovered uses, side effects, and interactions of drugs that are already on the market.

Summary

Using prescription and OTC drugs can be deleterious to nutritional status. The older adult population, with attendant multiple health problems and chronic conditions, is particularly vulnerable. They are the chief users of drugs in the United States. Vitamin and mineral supplements and alcohol can act as drugs and, if used in excess, are detrimental to nutritional and physical health. Supplements are often taken at higher-than-recommended levels, and, unfortunately, these supplements do not always supply the nutrients lacking in the diet.

Multiple drug intake can lead to drug-drug interactions and compromise nutritional status. The problem is exacerbated when the elderly person is consuming a marginal diet and/or when drugs are misused, whether intentional or unintentional. Drugs can interfere with nutrient intake, absorption, and metabolism, or they can enhance nutrient excretion. Conversely, food and dietary patterns can jeopardize drug activity and increase the hazards of drug therapy. Monitoring and providing counseling about potential food and drug interaction is a challenge for the nutrition professional.

REVIEW QUESTIONS

1. Why do older people take more prescription and over-the-counter drugs than do younger people? What factors contribute to multiple drug use in older people? What are the most common drugs used by the elderly living in the community and those living in long-term care facilities?
2. Why are older persons more vulnerable to adverse drug reactions? What physiologic, sociologic, and psychologic factors influence drug use in the elderly? How does drug metabolism change as we age?
3. Define pharmacokinetics and pharmacodynamics and discuss how each influences drug metabolism in the elderly. Which organ systems are most important in metabolizing drugs? How does serum albumin influence drug transport?
4. What are the effects of drugs on nutritional status? What are the effects of nutritional status on drugs? What drugs can cause an increase in nutrient excretion? What effect does food have on drugs?
5. What are some of the most common drugs used to treat cardiovascular disease in the elderly and what are the most common drug-nutrient interactions? Why are the number of psychotherapeutic drug prescriptions increasing? What nutritional effects do these types of drugs have in an elderly population?

SUGGESTED LEARNING ACTIVITIES

1. You are counseling a 68-year-old female patient who was recently admitted to the hospital with mild congestive heart failure. The patient is taking Lanoxin and Lasix. During the nutritional assessment she complains of a decreased appetite, nausea, and an increasing sense of weakness. Write a SOAP note, indicating the possible drug-nutrient interactions and suggestions for improving food intake.
2. Visit a drug store and record the sodium level of the following over-the-counter (OTC) medications: antacids, cough/cold remedies, and enema preparations. Prepare a 1-page information sheet on sodium-containing OTC medications that can significantly contribute to sodium intake.
3. Write a lesson plan for a 20-minute talk for older persons on high-fiber foods, including easy-to-prepare recipes. Emphasize the dangers of laxatives and how fiber-containing foods and water intake can often correct constipation.
4. Interview two drug store pharmacists and one health food store clerk about vitamin/mineral preparations targeted at older consumers. After

this assignment, do you think these products are useful?

5. Go the library and find three articles about the nutrient-drug interactions with MAO inhibitor drugs. Prepare a comprehensive list of foods to be avoided while taking these medications.

Key Terms

Provided here for review is a list of the major terms in this chapter. The definitions can be found in the Glossary, which begins on p. 336. To help you understand how these terms are applied, the page number is given for the first mention of each term in the chapter.

REFERENCES

1. Aycock EK: PRN drug use in nursing homes, *Am J Hosp Pharm* 38(1):105, 1981.
2. Beers M and others: Psychoactive medication use in intermediate-care facility residents, *JAMA* 260:3016-3020, 1988.
3. Beers MH and others: Influence of hospitalization on drug therapy in the elderly, *J Am Geriatr Soc* 37:679-683, 1989.
4. Begg CB, Carbone PP: Clinical trials and drug toxicity in the elderly: the experience of the Eastern Cooperative Oncology Group, *Cancer* 52:1986-1992, 1983.
5. Bero LA, Lipton HL, Bird JA: Characterization of geriatric drug-related hospital readmissions, *Med Care* 29(10):989-1003, 1991.
6. Block G and others: Vitamin supplement use by demographic characteristics, *Am J Epidemiol* 127(2):297-309, 1988.
7. Blumberg JB, Suter P: Pharmacology, nutrition, and the elderly: interactions and implications. In Chernoff R, editor: *Geriatric nutrition: the health professional's handbook,* Gaithersburg, Md, 1991, Aspen Publishers.
8. Cadieux RJ: Drug interactions in the elderly, *Postgrad Med* 86(8):179-184, 186, 1989.
9. Campion EW, deLabry LO, Glynn RJ: The effect of age on serum albumin in healthy males: report from the Normative Aging Study, *Geriatrics* 43(1):M18-M20, 1988.
10. Caranassos G, Stewart RB, Cluff LE: Drug-induced illness leading to hospitalization, *JAMA* 228(6):713-717, 1974.
11. Castleden CM, Pickles H: Suspected adverse drug reactions in elderly patients reported to the Committee on Safety of Medicines, *Br J Clin Pharmacol* 26:347-353, 1988.
12. Chen LH and others: Survey of drug use by the elderly and possible impact of drugs on nutritional status, *Drug-Nutrient Interactions* 3:73-86, 1985.
13. Cooper JK: Drug treatment of Alzheimer's disease, *Arch Intern Med* 151:245-249, 1991.
14. Cotugna N: Predictors of nutrition supplement use in the elderly. II. The role of beliefs, attitude, subjective norm, and intention, *J Nutr Elderly* 8:15-33, 1989.
15. Cupit GC: The use of nonprescription analgesics in an older population, *J Am Geriatr Soc* 30:S76-S80, 1982.
16. Cusack BJ: Polypharmacy and clinical pharmacology. In Beck J, editor: *Geriatrics review syllabus: a core curriculum in geriatric medicine,* New York, 1989, American Geriatric Society pp. 127-136.
17. Delafuente JC and others: Drug use among functionally active, aged, ambulatory people, *Drug Intell Clin Pharm* 26(2):179-193, 1992.
18. Department of Health, Education, and Welfare, Long-Term Facility Improvement Campaign: Physicians drug prescribing patterns in skilled nursing facilities, Monograph No 2, Pub No (OS) 76 50050, Washington, DC, 1976, Department of Health, Education, and Welfare, Office of Long-Term Care.
19. Donowitz M, Binder HJ: Effect of dioctylsulfosuccinate on colonic fluid and electrolyte movement, *Gastroenterology* 69:941-950, 1975.
20. Drugs for psychiatric disorders, *Med Lett* 31:13-20, 1989.
21. Dunham RG: Aging and changing patterns of alcohol use, *J Psychoactive Drugs* 13(2):143-151, 1981.
22. Ebersole P, Hess P: Drug use and abuse. In *Toward healthy aging: human needs and nursing response,* ed 3, St Louis, 1990, Mosby—Year Book.
23. Eraker SA, Kirscht JP, Becker MH: Understanding and improving patient compliance, *Ann Intern Med* 100(2):258-267, 1984.
24. Expert Panel: Report of the National Cholesterol Education Program Expert Panel on detection, evaluation, and treatment of high blood cholesterol in adults, *Arch Intern Med* 148:36-69, 1988.
25. Food and Nutrition Board: *Recommended di-*

etary allowances, ed 10, Washington, DC, 1989, National Academy of Sciences.

26. Friesen AJD: Adverse drug reactions in the geriatric client. In Pagliaro LA, Pagliaro AM, editors: *Pharmacologic aspects of aging,* St Louis, 1983, Mosby–Year Book.

27. Garry PJ and others: Nutritional status in a healthy elderly population: dietary and supplemental intakes, *Am J Clin Nutr* 36(2):319-331, 1982.

28. Gerbino PP, Gans JA: Antacids and laxatives for symptomatic relief in the elderly, *J Am Geriatr Soc* 30:S81-S87, 1982.

29. Goldberg PB, Roberts J: Pharmacologic basis for developing rational drug regimens for elderly patients, *Med Clin North Am* 67(2):315-331, 1983.

30. Gosney M, Tallis R: Prescription of contraindicated and interacting drugs in elderly patients admitted to hospital, *Lancet* 1:564-567, 1984.

31. Govoni LE, Hayes JE: *Drugs and nursing implications,* ed 5, Norwalk, Conn, 1985, Appleton-Century-Crofts.

32. Gray GE and others: Vitamin supplement use in a Southern California retirement community, *J Am Diet Assoc* 86(6):800-802, 1986.

33. Greenfield S and others: Patterns of care related to age of breast cancer patients, *JAMA* 257(20):2766-2770, 1987.

34. Gurwitz JH, Avorn J: The ambiguous relation between aging and adverse drug reactions, *Ann Intern Med* 114(11):956-966, 1991.

35. Helling DK and others: Medication use characteristics in the elderly: the Iowa 65+ Rural Health Study, *J Am Geriatr Soc* 35(1):4-12, 1987.

36. Howard JB, Strong Sr, KE, Strong Jr, KE: Medication procedures in a nursing home: abuse of prn orders, *J Am Geriatr Soc* 25(2):83-84, 1977.

37. Iber FL and others: Thiamin in the elderly: relation to alcoholism and to neurological degenerative disease, *Am J Clin Nutr* 36(5):1067-1082, 1982.

38. Iliffe S and others: Alcohol consumption by elderly people: a general practice survey, *Age Ageing* 20:120-123, 1991.

39. Jenike MA: The use of monoamine oxidase inhibitors in the treatment of elderly depressed patients, *J Am Geriatr Soc* 32:571-575, 1984.

40. Joint Commission on Accreditation of Hospitals: *Accreditation manual for hospitals 1985,* Chicago, 1984, The Commission.

41. Kalchthaler T, Coccaro E, Lichtiger S: Incidence of polypharmacy in a long-term care facility, *J Am Geriatr Soc* 25(7):308-313, 1977.

42. Kroenke K, Pinholt EM: Reducing polypharmacy in the elderly, *J Am Geriatr Soc* 38(1):31-36, 1990.

43. Lamy PP: Effects of diet and nutrition on drug therapy, *J Am Geriatr Soc* 30(11):S99-S111, 1982.

44. Lamy PP: Hazards of drug use in the elderly, *Postgrad Med* 76(1):50-52; 56-57; 60-61, 1984.

45. Lamy PP: Drug interactions and the elderly, *J Gerontol Nurs* 12(2):36-37, 1986.

46. Lamy PP, Michocki RJ: Medication management, *Clin Geriatr Med* 4(3):623-638, 1988.

47. Lamy PP: Nonprescription drugs and the elderly, *Am Fam Physician* 39(6):175-179, 1989.

48. Lamy PP: Nonprescription drugs and the elderly. In *Handbook of nonprescription drugs,* ed 9, Washington, DC, 1990, The American Pharmacological Association.

49. Lamy PP: Adverse drug effects, *Clin Geriatr Med* 6(2):293-307, 1990.

50. Leevy CM: Thiamin deficiency and alcoholism, *Ann NY Acad Sci* 378:316-326, 1982.

51. LeSage J: Polypharmacy in geriatric patients, *Nurs Clin North Am* 26(2):273-289, 1991.

52. Levine MA: Rational and pharmacologically sound drug therapy for the elderly patient, *Geisinger Bull* 37(2):34-39, 1988.

53. Lile JL, Hoffman R: Medication-taking by the frail elderly in two ethnic groups, *Nurs Forum* 26(4):19-24, 1991.

54. Lippmann S: Monoamine oxidase inhibitors, *Am Fam Physician* 34(1):113-119, 1986.

55. Miller MJ: Drug use and misuse among the elderly. In Young RF, Olson EA, editors: *Health, illness, and disability later in life: practical issues and interventions,* Newbury Park, Calif, 1991, Sage Publications.

56. Montamat SC, Cusack B: Overcoming problems with polypharmacy and drug misuse in the elderly, *Clin Geriatr Med* 8(1):142-158, 1992.

57. Montamat SC, Cusack BJ, Vestal RE: Management of drug therapy in the elderly, *N Engl J Med* 321:303-309, 1989.

58. National Dairy Council: Diet-drug interactions, *Dairy Council Digest* 48(2): 1977.

59. National Nutrition Consortium: *Vitamin-mineral safety, toxicity, and misuse,* Chicago, 1978, The American Dietetic Association.

60. Nichols TW: Phytobezoar formation: A new complication of cimetidine therapy, *Ann Intern Med* 95(1):70, 1981.

61. Nolan L, O'Malley K: Prescribing for the elderly. II. Prescribing patterns: differences due

to age, *J Am Geriatr Soc* 36(3):245-254, 1988.

62. Oakland MJ, Thomsen PA: Beliefs about and usage of vitamin/mineral supplements by elderly participants of rural congregate meal programs in central Iowa, *J Am Diet Assoc* 90(5):715-716, 1990.

63. Opdycke RAC and others: A systematic approach to educating elderly patients about their medications, *Patient Educ Couns* 19(1):43-60, 1992.

64. Patrick M and others: Prescription for the high cost of drugs in nursing homes, *Geriatr Nurs* 12(2):88-89, 1991.

65. Petrie WM, Ban TA: Propranolol in organic agitation, *Lancet* 1:324-327, 1981.

66. Pinto JT: The pharmacokinetic and pharmacodynamic interactions of food and drugs, *Topics Clin Nutr* 6:14-33, 1991.

67. Ranno BS, Wardlaw GM, Geiger CJ: What characterizes elderly women who overuse vitamin and mineral supplements? *J Am Diet Assoc* 88(3):347-348, 1988.

68. Roberts J, Turner N: Pharmacodynamic basis for altered drug action in the elderly, *Clin Geriatr Med* 4:127-149, 1988.

69. Robertson D: Pharmacology and aging: pharmacokinetics and pharmacodynamics. In Brocklehurst JC, editor: *Textbook of geriatric medicine and gerontology*, ed 3, Edinburgh, 1985, Churchill Livingstone.

70. Roe DA: Drug-nutrient interactions in the elderly, *Geriatrics* 41(3):57-74, 1986.

71. Roe DA: Drug and nutrient interactions in elderly cardiac patients, *Drug-Nutrient Interactions* 5(4):205-212, 1988.

72. Roe DA: *Diet and drug interactions,* New York, 1989, Van Nostrand Reinhold.

73. Roe DA: Drug-nutrient interactions in the elderly. In Munro HN, Danford DE, editors: *Nutrition, aging, and the elderly,* New York, 1989, Plenum Press.

74. Roe DA: *Handbook on drug and nutrient interactions: a problem-oriented reference guide,* ed 4, Chicago, 1989, The American Dietetic Association.

75. Samet J and others: Choice of cancer therapy varies with age of patient, *JAMA* 255(24): 3385-3390, 1986.

76. Schneider CL, Nordlund DJ: Prevalence of vitamin and mineral supplement use in the elderly, *J Fam Pract* 17:243-247, 1983.

77. Schuckit MA and others: A 3-year follow-up of elderly alcoholics, *J Clin Psychiatry* 41(12):412-416, 1980.

78. Scott RB, Mitchell MC: Aging, alcohol, and

the liver, *J Am Geriatr Soc* 36(3):255-265, 1988.

79. Seixas FA: Drug/alcohol interactions: avert potential dangers, *Geriatrics* 34(10):89-94; 101-102, 1979.

80. Semla TP and others: Perceived purpose of prescription drugs: the Iowa 65+ Rural Health Study, *Drug Intell Clin Pharm* 25(4):410-413, 1991.

81. Silliman RA and others: Age as a predictor of diagnostic and initial treatment intensity in newly diagnosed breast cancer patients, *J Gerontol* 44:M46-50, 1989.

82. Simpson W: *Medication and the elderly: a guide for promoting proper use,* Rockville, Md, 1984, Aspen Publishers.

83. Smart RG, Liban CB: Predictors of problem drinking among elderly, middle-aged, and youthful drinkers, *J Psychoactive Drugs* 13:153-162, 1981.

84. Smith CH: Drug-food/food-drug interactions. In Morley JE, editor: *Geriatric nutrition,* New York, 1990, Raven Press.

85. Stewart ML and others: Vitamin/mineral use: a telephone survey of adults in the United States, *J Am Diet Assoc* 85:1585-1590, 1985.

86. Stewart RB: Polypharmacy in the elderly: a fait accompli? *Drug Intell Clin Pharm* 24(3): 321-323, 1990 (editorial).

87. Stewart RB and others: Changing patterns of therapeutic agents in the elderly: a 10-year overview, *Ageing* 20:182-188, 1991.

88. Subar AF, Block G: Use of vitamin and mineral supplements: demographics and amounts of nutrients consumed: the 1987 Health Interview Survey, *Am J Epidemiol* 132:1091-1101, 1990.

89. Sulsky SI and others: Descriptors of alcohol consumption among noninstitutionalized nonalcoholic elderly, *J Am Coll Nutr* 9(4): 326-331, 1990.

90. Thornburg JE: Gerontological pharmacology. In Wingard Jr LB and others, editors: *Human pharmacology molecular-to-clinical,* St Louis, 1991, Mosby-Year Book.

91. Tomasulo PA, Kater RM, Iber FL: Impairment of thiamin absorption in alcoholism, *Am J Clin Nutr* 21(11):1341-1344, 1968.

92. Tregaskis BF, Stevenson IH: Pharmacokinetics in old age, *Br Med Bull* 46(1):2-21, 1990.

93. Tunks ER: Carbamazepine in the dyscontrol syndrome associated with limbic system dysfunction, *J Nerv Ment Dis* 164:56-60, 1977.

94. Vestal RE: Pharmacology and aging, *J Am Geriatr Soc* 30:191-200, 1982.

95. Vestal RE, Dawson GW: Pharmacology and aging. In Finch CE, Schneider EL, editors: *Handbook of the biology of aging,* ed 2, New York, 1985, Van Nostrand Reinhold.
96. Welling P: Nutrient effects on drug metabolism and action in the elderly, *Drug-Nutrient Interactions* 4:173-207, 1985.
97. Widner S, Zeichner A: Alcohol abuse in the elderly: review of epidemiology research and treatment, *Clin Gerontologist* 11(1):3-18, 1991.
98. Wilber JA: The role of diet in the treatment of high blood pressure, *J Am Diet Assoc* 80:25, 1982.
99. Williams BR, Baer CL: *Essentials of clinical pharmacology in nursing,* Springhouse, Pa, 1990, Springhouse.
100. Williams L, Lowenthal DT: Drug therapy in the elderly, *South Med J* 85:127-131, 1992.
101. Williamson J, Chopin JM: Adverse reactions to prescribed drugs in the elderly: a multicentre investigation, *Age Ageing* 9(2):73-80, 1980.
102. Woodhouse KW, James OFW: Hepatic drug metabolism and ageing, *Br Med Bull* 46(1):22-35, 1990.
103. Young RC, Blass JP: Iatrogenic nutritional deficiencies, *Annu Rev Nutr* 2:201-227, 1982.

10

Nutritional Status of Older Adults

Marie Fanelli Kuczmarski

Objectives

✦✦

After studying this chapter, the student should be able to:

✔ *Understand the difference between nutritional status and dietary status, and recognize the factors that contribute to nutritional status*

✔ *Apply the information gained from national nutrition surveys to the nutritional care of older people*

✔ *Understand the physical and biochemical markers used to assess nutritional status in older people*

✔ *Recognize the differences in nutritional status between institutionalized older people and those living in the community.*

Introduction

Nutritional status encompasses **anthropometric,** biochemical, clinical, dietary, and socioeconomic factors. Although the term "nutritional status" sometimes is used interchangeably with **"dietary status,"** these terms do have different connotations. Dietary status is a more limited term that refers to intake of foods, beverages (both nonalcoholic and alcoholic), and nutrients, including supplements.

The data on dietary and nutritional status representative of noninstitutionalized older adults in the United States are derived from the 1977-1978 **Nationwide Food Consumption Survey (NFCS),** conducted by the U.S. Depart-

ment of Agriculture, and the **Second National Health and Nutrition Examination Survey (NHANES II)** 1976-1980, conducted by the Department of Health and Human Services. In addition, the **Hispanic Health and Nutrition Examination Survey (HHANES),** a survey of three Hispanic subgroups consisting of Mexican Americans, Cubans, and Puerto Ricans from selected areas of the United States, was conducted from 1982 to 1984.

Although this information may appear dated, it is the most current available. The 1987-1988 NFCS has been completed; however, the findings have not yet been released by the Department of Agriculture. NHANES III, a 6-year survey, was fielded in 1988. The data should be released for analysis approximately 2 years after completion of this survey.

This chapter presents selected data from the 1977-1978 NFCS, NHANES II, and HHANES to provide a descriptive picture of the dietary and nutritional status of noninstitutionalized older Americans. Where possible, data are stratified by age, ethnic group, and sex. Reports from smaller surveys are used to describe the nutritional status of institutionalized older adults. Even though older adults typically are defined as individuals age 65 or older, data for people over age 50 are presented for comparison purposes.

OVERVIEW OF NATIONAL SURVEYS*

Nationwide Food Consumption Survey

The Nationwide Food Consumption Survey (NFCS) was designed to provide a **probability sample** representative of the 48 conterminous states. Information on food consumed by individuals both at home and away from home was collected by trained interviewers for 3 consecutive days using a 24-hour dietary recall and a 2-day food record. Dietary data were collected on all days of the week and during all seasons of the year.[23] There were 4,983 people age 55 or older who satisfactorily completed both the dietary recall and food record. There was no upper age limit for inclusion in this survey, and the sample included 159 people age 85 or older.

The Second National Health and Nutrition Examination Survey

The Second National Health and Nutrition Examination Survey (NHANES II) used **probability cluster sampling** to select a representa-

tive sample of the civilian population living in households from all 50 states in the United States. This survey collected data on nutritional and health status through interviews and direct physical examinations. Food intake data were gathered with a 24-hour dietary recall, food frequency questionnaire, and questions relating to eating habits and nutrition-related practices. Physical examinations included components such as anthropometric measurements, hematologic and biochemical assessments, and physical and dental examinations.[10,16]

Trained dietary interviewers administered the 24-hour recall. This recall contained information on specific food items consumed by the respondent from midnight to midnight preceding the interview. Because the interviews generally were scheduled on Tuesdays through Saturdays, excluding most holidays, intakes reflected weekday consumption.

The upper age limit for this survey was 74 years. The sample included 9,179 people ages 50 to 74, or 33% of the total NHANES II sample. Of those older adults selected, 7,920 (86%) were interviewed and 5,919 (64%) were examined.[10]

The Hispanic Health and Nutrition Examination Survey

The Hispanic Health and Nutrition Examination Survey (HHANES) was a probability sample survey whose target population consisted of civilian, noninstitutionalized eligible Hispanics age 6 months to 74 years. The Mexican-origin population resided in five Southwestern states (Arizona, California, Colorado, New Mexico and Texas) and represented approximately 84% of the 1980 Mexican population in the United States and 97% in the five selected states.[9] The total Mexican American sample age 50 years or older was 1,413. Of those selected, 1,110 (79%) were interviewed, and 928 (66%) were examined.[10]

The Cuban-origin population resided in Dade County, Florida, and included about 57% of the 1980 Cuban population in the United States and 96% in the Dade County area.[9] The total Cuban sample age 50 years or older was 679. Of those selected, 528 (78%)

---

*Descriptions of data collection procedures and all data collection instruments have been published for the Nationwide Food Consumption Survey[23]; the Second National Health and Nutrition Examination Survey[10,16]; and the Hispanic Health and Nutrition Examination Survey.[9,10,17]

were interviewed, and 400 (59%) were examined.[10]

The Puerto Rican–origin population resided in the New York City metropolitan area and represented about 59% of the 1980 Puerto Rican population in the United States and 90% in the New York City metropolitan area.[9] The total Puerto Rican sample age 50 years or older was 575. Of those selected, 498 (87%) were interviewed, and 378 (66%) were examined.[10]

Similar to NHANES II, HHANES information was collected in two stages, during an interview conducted in the home and during a physical examination conducted in mobile examination centers. A 24-hour dietary recall and food frequency questionnaire were administered by trained, bilingual dietary interviewers.[17] The energy and nutrient intake data were released to the public in late 1990, and physical examination and biochemical assessment data were available earlier.

Because the samples of Cuban and Puerto Rican older adults were relatively small, some statistics cannot be produced. When the sample consisted of fewer than 25 individuals, no statistic was calculated (see Figs.). If the sample numbered between 25 and 44, a statistic was generated. However, it was considered an unstable estimate, indicating that it may not meet the reliability standard because the distribution of the sampling error may not be normal (see Figs.). Unlike the statistics generated from NHANES II, the statistics generated from HHANES reflect only the Hispanic populations examined, not the entire U.S. population.

DIETARY INTAKE

Dietary intake data can be used to describe the actual foods eaten and the level of energy nutrients consumed for the development of nutritional intervention and education programs and for policy-making decisions.

Food Intakes

The 1977-1978 NFCS data have been used to identify the **core foods** in the diets of older American men and women.[7] Core foods are those routinely consumed by a population group. They can be determined by a variety of different approaches, such as frequency tallies or weighted formulas. Individuals age 55 or older reported consuming approximately 2,500 different foods over the 3-day dietary collection period. However, only 30 foods were identified as core items by Fanelli and Stevenhagen.[7]

The core foods were not markedly different between the sexes or among the three age groupings (55 to 64, 65 to 74, and 75 or older). The core items derived from a weighted formula approach were categorized by the major food groups as follows: grains (white and whole-wheat bread, cereals, and crackers); fruits (orange juice, bananas, and apples); vegetables (lettuce, potatoes, and tomatoes); dairy (whole and low-fat milk, natural and processed cheese, and ice cream); protein foods (eggs and luncheon meats); and fats and oils (margarine, butter, salad dressing, and bacon). Sugar was among the top five core foods for all sex and age groups. The nondairy, nonalcoholic beverages consumed by all six population groups included coffee, tea, and cola. Beer was the only alcoholic beverage in the core food listing, and it was reported once, for men age 55 to 64.

Many of the core food items were those generally associated with breakfast—eggs, bacon, bread, jam or jelly, ready-to-eat cereals, orange juice, tea, coffee, and milk. This finding is not surprising, since 87% of older Americans, or nearly nine out of 10, eat breakfast.[1] The inclusion of items high in fat and cholesterol should be noted. It should also be recognized that red meat, fish, poultry, legumes, mixed dishes, and dessert type items were not among the core items.

Even though the income levels for the age and sex groups varied substantially, the core food listings did not vary greatly, indicating that the core foods appeared to have low income elasticity. It should be noted that the results describe food consumption patterns of older Americans in the late 1970s. The list of core foods consumed by older adults in the 1990s may differ because of the increased number and variety of products available on the retail market, because of increased awareness of the role of diet in health, and because of changes in personal health habits. Core foods also may vary as different individuals compose these age cohorts. However, the top core foods (i.e., bread, milk, coffee, sugar, and margarine) probably will remain the same, because they are staple items in the U.S. diet.

The quality of the diets consumed by people over age 65 who were interviewed in the 1977-1978 NFCS has also been determined.[14] A better quality diet was defined by Murphy and colleagues[14] as a diet that provided two thirds or more of the recommended dietary allowance (RDA) for at least five of the nine selected nutrients (i.e., vitamins A, C, B_6, B_{12}, thiamin, riboflavin, calcium, iron, and magnesium). More older men had better quality diets than did women. About 88% of men ages 65 to 84 and 81% of those age 85 or older had better quality diets, compared to 82% of women age 65 to 74 and 78% of women age 85 or older. These data document an increase in the proportion of people age 85 or older with poorer quality diets than those in the 65 to 84 age group. Thus the group at greatest risk of inadequate intakes was women age 85 or older. The nutrients that tended to be low in the diets of these older adults were calcium, magnesium, and vitamin B_6. Thirty-one percent of the 65 to 84 age group and 21% of the 85 or older group reported consuming diets with intakes of all nine nutrients above 67% of the RDAs.

Another study using NFCS 1977-1978 data identified the characteristics of older Americans with increased risk of poor quality diets.[5] The diet was considered to be poor quality if an individual reported low intakes (below two thirds of the RDAs) for five of the nine selected nutrients (vitamins A, C, B_6, B_{12}, thiamin, riboflavin, calcium, iron, and magnesium). Living alone, particularly for men over age 75, was a risk factor for dietary inadequacy. The researchers found that the increased risk of dietary inadequacy for older people living alone was not the result of choosing poor quality foods but rather of eating too little food. Older Americans with low incomes, low food expenditures, and poor health, and unemployed men were at higher risk of poor quality diets.

Energy and Nutrient Intakes

Mean calorie and nutrient intakes for 16 nutrients derived from 24-hour dietary recalls obtained from white and black men and women, age 50 or older, who were interviewed in NHANES II, are presented in Tables 10-1 and 10-2, respectively. Dietary supplements were not included in these calculations. The mean caloric intake of both white and black men ages 50 to 59 was significantly higher than that of men ages 60 to 69 and 70 to 74 (Table 10-1). The decline in reported caloric intakes across the age groups was generally accompanied by a decrease in nutrient intakes, such that the 70 to 74 age group had the lowest values. However, this observation was not seen for intakes of vitamins A and C reported by white men. Vitamin A intake was highest for the 70 to 74 age group, whereas vitamin C was essentially the same for all three age groups.

As shown in Table 10-1, for 12 of the 16 nutrients, intakes of white men age 60 to 69 were significantly greater than those of white men age 70 to 74. For black men, a comparison of these two age groups indicated that only the carbohydrate, iron, thiamin, and riboflavin intakes were significantly different (Table 10-1).

Similar to the findings for men, the mean caloric intakes reported by older women were significantly higher for the 50 to 59 age group than for either the 60 to 69 or the 70 to 74 age group (Table 10-2). Mean nutrient intakes tended to be higher for younger age groups. When comparing the 60 to 69 age group to the 70 to 74 group, mean intakes were significantly higher for seven nutrients for the white women and for three nutrients for the black women. As shown in Table 10-2, a reverse trend was observed for white women in the 70 to 74 age group, who reported higher intakes of vitamins A and C than women age 50 to 59 or 60 to 69. The mean intakes of calcium, iron and vitamin C of black women age 70 to 74 were higher than those reported by black women in the younger two age groups.

The mean caloric intakes of black individuals were lower than those of white people for each age group; and consequently, mean nutrient intakes appeared lower (Tables 10-1 and 10-2). T-tests were performed for each age group to

TABLE 10-1   Mean Energy and Nutrient Intakes of Older Men Examined in NHANES II

	White Men						Black Men					
Age	50-59		60-69		70-74		50-59		60-69		70-74	
n	575		1,354		427		77		151		56	
	X	± SEM*	X	± SEM	X	± SEM	X	± SEM	X	± SEM	X	± SEM
Energy (kcal)	2,232	± 79[a]†	1,991	± 25[a]	1,757	± 39[a]	2,025	± 191[a,b]	1,691	± 77[a]	1,503	± 99[b]
Protein (g)	90.1	± 3.8[a]	80.3	± 1.4[a]	68.4	± 1.9[a]	79.2	± 9.4[a,b]	66.4	± 3.5[a]	64.2	± 5.3[b]
Carbohydrate (g)	231.3	± 10.7[a,b]	213.1	± 3.2[a]	202.4	± 5.1[b]	201.7	± 22.9[a]	181.8	± 10.4[b]	155.7	± 10.9[a,b]
Fat (g)	92.6	± 3.3[a]	83.6	± 1.1[a]	71.5	± 1.8[a]	80.8	± 7.6[a]	69.1	± 3.4	64.0	± 5.0[a]
Saturated fatty acids (g)	33.8	± 1.3[a]	30.0	± 0.4[a]	25.1	± 0.7[a]	28.6	± 2.9	24.6	± 1.3	22.8	± 1.9
Oleic acid (g)	34.6	± 1.5[a]	31.6	± 0.5[a]	26.8	± 0.9[a]	30.9	± 3.6[a]	26.9	± 1.6	24.9	± 2.3[a]
Linoleic acid (g)	12.5	± 0.7[a]	11.1	± 0.2[a]	9.9	± 0.4[a]	10.2	± 1.3[a]	8.7	± 0.6	7.8	± 0.9[a]
Cholesterol (mg)	443	± 23[a]	413	± 9[b]	357	± 13[a,b]	436	± 58	434	± 25	411	± 43
Calcium (mg)	866	± 49[a]	780	± 15[a]	677	± 24[a]	641	± 103	577	± 43	589	± 72
Iron (mg)	15.5	± 0.5[a]	15.0	± 0.2[b]	13.6	± 0.3[a,b]	12.8	± 1.1	12.6	± 0.6[a]	10.3	± 0.6[a]
Sodium (mg)	3,343	± 129[a,b]	3,036	± 46[a]	2,882	± 77[b]	2,652	± 302	2,560	± 137	2,269	± 154
Potassium (mg)	2,844	± 99[a]	2,635	± 36[a]	2,363	± 58[a]	2,231	± 253[a]	2,008	± 110	766	± 132[a]
Vitamin A (IU)	6,051	± 539	6,148	± 278	7,079	± 593	6,648	± 1,175	6,590	± 681	5,078	± 841
Vitamin C (mg)	103	± 9	104	± 3	103	± 6	117	± 30[a]	81	± 10[a]	92	± 19
Thiamin (mg)	1.43	± 0.05	1.43	± 0.02	1.32	± 0.05	1.24	± 0.12[a]	1.16	± 0.06[b]	0.98	± 0.05[a,b]
Riboflavin (mg)	2.07	± 0.09[a]	1.96	± 0.04[a]	1.83	± 0.08[a]	1.58	± 0.19[a]	1.48	± 0.09[a]	1.32	± 0.11[a]
Niacin (mg)	23.8	± 0.9[a]	21.8	± 0.3	19.4	± 0.6[a]	18.5	± 1.8	16.3	± 0.8	13.5	± 0.1

*Mean plus standard error of the mean.
†Numbers with the same superscript are significantly different ($p < 0.05$) from those on same line.

TABLE 10-2 *Mean Energy and Nutrient Intakes of Older Women Examined in NHANES II*

Age (years) n	White Women						Black Women					
	50-59 649		60-69 1,487		70-74 533		50-59 101		60-69 170		70-74 64	
	X	± SEM*	X	± SEM	X	± SEM	X	± SEM	X	± SEM	X	± SEM
Energy (kcal)	1,430	± 52[a]†	1,346	± 17[a]	1,281	± 24[a]	1,393	± 113[a,b]	1,228	± 46[a]	1,149	± 71[b]
Protein (g)	56.6	± 2.8[a]	53.4	± 0.9[a]	49.4	± 1.2[a]	54.6	± 5.3[a]	50.3	± 2.4	46.2	± 3.4[a]
Carbohydrate (g)	158.9	± 6.6	158.7	± 2.3	160.7	± 3.8	159.9	± 15.3	146.6	± 7.1	143.4	± 11.5
Fat (g)	59.0	± 2.3[a]	53.9	± 0.7[a]	48.7	± 1.0[a]	57.6	± 5.3[a,b]	48.6	± 1.9[a]	43.0	± 3.3[b]
Saturated fatty acids (g)	20.7	± 0.9[a]	18.5	± 0.3[a]	16.5	± 0.4[a]	19.9	± 2.0[a]	16.8	± 0.7	14.2	± 1.0[a]
Oleic acid (g)	21.6	± 1.0[a]	19.8	± 0.3[a]	17.7	± 0.5[a]	21.4	± 2.4[a,b]	18.3	± 0.9[a]	15.7	± 1.7[b]
Linoleic acid (g)	8.3	± 0.4[a]	7.9	± 0.2[b]	7.3	± 0.3[a,b]	8.4	± 1.0	7.1	± 0.4	6.9	± 0.8
Cholesterol (mg)	261	± 15[a]	258	± 6[b]	219	± 9[a,b]	286	± 43	295	± 18[a]	166	± 19[a]
Calcium (mg)	589	± 37	561	± 11	549	± 17	446	± 57	455	± 27	489	± 50
Iron (mg)	10.6	± 0.4	10.7	± 0.2	10.2	± 0.3	9.3	± 0.7	8.9	± 0.3	9.5	± 0.7
Sodium (mg)	2,230	± 92[a]	2,126	± 33[b]	1,922	± 43[a,b]	2,114	± 223	1,862	± 88	1,753	± 141
Potassium (mg)	2,051	± 81	2,026	± 26	1,997	± 44	1,714	± 134	1,669	± 77	1,679	± 126
Vitamin A (IU)	5,150	± 508	5,376	± 201	5,398	± 390	7,074	± 1,915	5,136	± 457	6,296	± 882
Vitamin C (mg)	102	± 9	101	± 3	112	± 5	104	± 20	99	± 12	120	± 17
Thiamin (mg)	1.01	± 0.04	1.02	± 0.02	0.96	± 0.02	0.88	± 0.08	0.90	± 0.04	0.86	± 0.09
Riboflavin (mg)	1.38	± 0.08	1.38	± 0.03	1.34	± 0.05	1.23	± 0.20	1.11	± 0.06	1.17	± 0.15
Niacin (mg)	15.4	± 0.6	15.0	± 0.2	14.3	± 0.4	14.1	± 1.2	12.3	± 0.6	12.5	± 0.9

*Mean plus standard error of the mean.
†Numbers with the same superscript are significantly different ($p < 0.05$) from those on same line.

determine if differences in intakes between whites and blacks within each sex were significant. There were no consistent findings, but some differences were statistically significant (P ≤ 0.05). Intakes of carbohydrate, linoleic acid, calcium, sodium, iron, potassium, thiamin, riboflavin, and niacin were significantly higher for white men age 50 to 59 than for black men in the same age group. Except for cholesterol and vitamin A, caloric and nutrient intake differences between white and black men age 60 to 69 were significant. Intakes of energy, carbohydrate, sodium, iron, potassium, vitamin A, thiamin, riboflavin, and niacin were significantly greater for white men age 70 to 74 than for black men in the same age group.

For women, few significant differences were found. Among the 50 to 59 age group, calcium, iron, potassium, and thiamin intakes of white women were significantly higher than those of black women. The energy, fat, saturated fatty acid, calcium, sodium, iron, potassium, riboflavin, and niacin intakes of white women were significantly greater than those of black women in the 60 to 69 age group. In the 70 to 74 age group, only cholesterol and potassium intakes were significantly different between white and black women.

When nutrient intakes were compared to recommendations published by the National Research Council's Committee on Diet and Health,[18] the population group age 50 to 74 got more than 30% of their caloric intake from total fat and more than 10% from saturated fatty acids; they got less than 10% from polyunsaturated fatty acids and less than 55% from carbohydrates. Linoleic acid levels were used as an estimate for polyunsaturated fatty acid intake. Protein intakes did not exceed twice the RDA, as recommended by the Committee on Diet and Health. The cholesterol intakes of only the men, regardless of race, exceeded the recommended level of 300 mg a day.

The caloric and nutrient intakes presented in Tables 10-1 and 10-2 were compared to the 1989 RDAs.[19] Two thirds of the RDA was used as a cut-off point for nutrients to identify people whose intakes may be below an average requirement level. With one exception, the nutrient intakes of the older adults examined in NHANES II exceeded 67% of the RDA for protein, vitamin C, thiamin, riboflavin, niacin, calcium, and iron. The calcium intake of black women was less than 536 mg (67% of 800 mg). The caloric intakes of both the older men and women were less than that recommended. In addition, the potassium intakes of black men and women age 50 to 74 and of white women age 70 to 74 fell below the minimum requirement of 2,000 mg a day.[19]

The population group age 50 or older surveyed in NHANES II showed a wide range of caloric and nutrient intakes. Thus even though mean intakes may appear adequate, many older people may be at risk for malnutrition. Income has been shown to influence dietary intake and thereby overall dietary quality.[2,14] Tables 10-3 and 10-4 reveal the range of intakes (5th, 50th, and 95th percentiles) for energy and seven selected nutrients by income status.[8]

Income status was determined by the **poverty income ratio (PIR),** a measure of the income of the household relative to the average poverty level. A PIR below 1 indicated that a sample individual was below the poverty level; a PIR of 1 or higher indicated that a sample individual was at or above the poverty level. No significance testing was done, because no statistical software was available to test medians in surveys such as NHANES II with complex designs.

The median (50th percentile) caloric intakes of men and women with an income below the poverty level were lower than those of people with a PIR of 1 or higher (Tables 10-3 and 10-4). Caloric intake at the 5th percentile for all age and sex groups fell below 1,000 kcal. At this calorie level, it is difficult to obtain adequate amounts of essential nutrients without supplementation. The difference in caloric intakes reported at the 5th and 95th percentiles was approximately fourfold.

For vitamin C, the 5th and 95th percentile values could vary as much as 100-fold. Older people with a PIR of 1 or higher had notably higher median vitamin C intakes than those for people with a PIR below 1. This finding was also true for vitamin A, suggesting that intakes of these vitamins may be related to income.

Median iron intakes for older women regardless of poverty status were lower than those for men of comparable ages (Tables 10-3 and 10-

4). The median iron intakes of men and women age 55 to 64 whose income was below the poverty level were 11.1 mg and 7.8 mg, respectively. In contrast, the median iron intakes of men and women of similar ages who were at or above the poverty level were 13.6 mg and 9.6 mg, respectively. For men age 65 to 74, the median iron intake was 10.4 mg for those with a PIR below 1 and 12.5 mg for those with a PIR of 1 or higher. The median intake values for women with a PIR of 1 or higher were almost identical—9.6 mg for the group age 55 to 64 and 9.3 mg for those age 65 to 74.

Median calcium intakes for all people over age 55 fell below the RDA of 800 mg. The median values did not appear to be related to poverty status or age.

Sodium intakes reflect the sodium in foods and do not account for sodium added to foods in cooking or at the table. For older men, median sodium intakes ranged from 2,070 to 2,782 mg (Table 10-3). For older women, median intakes ranged from 1,738 to 2,005 mg (Table 10-4).

Median sodium intakes tended to be slightly higher in groups with a PIR of 1 or higher.

Median dietary cholesterol intakes of older men were greater than 300 mg a day, whereas median intakes of women were 170 to 196 mg a day (Tables 10-3 and 10-4). For the 55 to 64 age group, median intakes for people with a PIR of 1 or higher were slightly higher than those for people with a PIR below 1. A reverse trend was seen in both sexes in the 65 to 74 age group.

Vitamin and Mineral Supplements

For the most accurate dietary assessment, intake from supplements should be added to the nutrient intake from food. The nutrient intakes presented in Tables 10-1, 10-2, 10-3, and 10-4 would be higher if supplements had been included. However, no quantifiable supplement data were available.

In the 65 and older age group, approximately 41% of Hispanics, 40% of whites and 14% of blacks reported taking nonprescription vitamin

TABLE 10-3 *Energy and Selected Nutrient Intakes for Men Age 55 to 74 by Poverty Status*

	5th Percentile		50th Percentile		95th Percentile	
	PIR <1	PIR ≥1	PIR <1	PIR ≥1	PIR <1	PIR ≥1
Men 55 to 64 years (n = 1,227)						
Energy (kcal)	548	978	1,715	1,979	3,456	3,521
Vitamin C (mg)	2	9	52	86	275	273
Vitamin A (IU)	319	906	3,433	3,682	23,457	16,565
Calcium (mg)	135	205	638	686	1,595	1,839
Iron (mg)	3.3	6.2	11.1	13.6	24.9	28.3
Sodium (mg)	561	1,079	2,536	2,782	5,488	5,731
Cholesterol (mg)	57	83	341	363	903	975
Men 65 to 74 years (n = 1,199)						
Energy (kcal)	667	859	1,495	1,744	2,623	3,137
Vitamin C (mg)	2	6	45	85	222	274
Vitamin A (IU)	252	1,088	2,722	4,013	14,890	17,593
Calcium (mg)	119	197	595	597	1,560	1,563
Iron (mg)	3.5	5.9	10.4	12.5	21.8	28.3
Sodium (mg)	707	1,171	2,070	2,623	4,790	5,720
Cholesterol (mg)	58	66	319	307	1,014	898

Data from Fanelli MT, Woteki CE: Nutrient intakes and health status of older Americans, *Ann NY Acad Sci* 561:94, 1989.

TABLE 10-4   *Energy and Selected Nutrient Intakes for Women Age 55 to 74 by Poverty Status*

	5th Percentile		50th Percentile		95th Percentile	
	PIR <1	PIR ≥1	PIR <1	PIR ≥1	PIR <1	PIR ≥1
Women 55 to 64 years (n = 1329)						
Energy (kcal)	503	623	1,204	1,352	2,361	2,466
Vitamin C (mg)	4	7	47	93	223	285
Vitamin A (IU)	408	720	2,912	3,493	12,450	16,028
Calcium (mg)	115	146	388	490	1,251	1,255
Iron (mg)	3.8	4.4	7.8	9.6	21.7	21.2
Sodium (mg)	540	745	1,738	2,005	3,612	4,446
Cholesterol (mg)	41	48	172	196	805	702
Women 65 to 74 years (n = 1416)						
Energy (kcal)	464	649	1,163	1,231	2,030	2,191
Vitamin C (mg)	5	8	71	92	265	261
Vitamin A (IU)	710	893	3,137	3,383	15,502	15,182
Calcium (mg)	110	147	477	473	1,258	1,137
Iron (mg)	3.8	4.4	8.0	9.3	22.9	19.6
Sodium (mg)	676	664	1,825	1,830	4,057	3,883
Cholesterol (mg)	24	39	171	170	671	582

Data from Fanelli MT, Woteki CE: Nutrient intakes and health status of older Americans, *Ann NY Acad Sci* 561:94, 1989.

and mineral supplements in the 1986 **National Health Interview Survey.**[13] Of the older adults taking supplements, approximately 57% of the women and 62% of the men reported taking a broad-spectrum product, whereas about 70% of the women and 62% of the men reported taking a specialized product. Broad-spectrum products were defined as those containing at least three of the following vitamins: A, B complex vitamins, C, D, and E, plus one or more of the following minerals: calcium, phosphorus, iodine, iron, magnesium, copper, zinc, and manganese. All the remaining products, such as single vitamin or mineral supplements, were defined as specialized products. Among supplement users, vitamin C was the most common vitamin supplement taken by both elderly men (84%) and women (79%).[13] The most prevalent minerals taken were calcium, by older women (62%), and iron, by older men (51%).[13]

The median daily intake for vitamins from supplements was 100% to 300% of the RDA,

and for minerals 15% to 270% of the RDA.[13] These findings indicate that nonprescription supplements are commonly used by older Americans and that intakes of selected vitamins and minerals from supplements can exceed 100% of the RDA. Therefore it seems prudent to use information on supplement usage when evaluating the adequacy of older adults' diets.

ANTHROPOMETRIC EVALUATION

Several body measurements were performed by specially trained health technicians in the NHANES II and the HHANES. Height and weight data were used to calculate **body mass index (BMI)**—the ratio of weight (kg) to height squared (m²). A BMI equal to or greater than 27.8 defined overweight for men and a BMI equal to or greater than 27.3 defined overweight for women.[10] These values represented the 85th percentile for men and nonpregnant

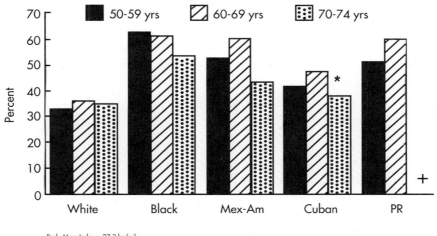

Body Mass Index > 27.3 kg/m²
*Unreliable statistic; + inadequate sample

FIG. 10-1 Percentage of overweight older American women. A higher percentage of older black, Mexican American, and Puerto Rican women are overweight (BMI over 27.3 kg/m²) compared to older white and Cuban women. Overweight tends to decrease among those ages 70 to 74.

(From US Department of Health and Human Services: Second National Health and Nutrition Examination Survey, 1976-80, and Hispanic Health and Nutrition Examination Survey, 1982-84.)

women age 20 to 29 examined in NHANES II. The cut-off points were chosen on the basis of a statistical approach and are not based on morbidity or mortality data from the survey population. The 20 to 29 age group was selected as a reference because these individuals are considered relatively lean, and the increases in weight observed with age generally reflect increased accumulation of fat. Thus overweight is a condition in which a person's body weight substantially exceeds a reference population value.

The prevalence of overweight was higher in older women than men, regardless of race or ethnicity or poverty status (Figs. 10-1 and 10-2). Among older women, the prevalence was highest in black women, followed by Mexican American, Puerto Rican, Cuban, and white women (Fig. 10-1). A different trend was observed for men (Fig. 10-2). The prevalence of overweight was highest for Mexican American

men. White and black men had similar rates. For both sexes and most race and ethnic groups, fewer individuals between age 70 and 74 were defined as overweight compared to people age 50 to 59 or 60 to 69. In older men, the prevalence of overweight is lower in groups below the poverty level, whereas the reverse is seen in older women.[8,10]

CLINICAL ASSESSMENTS
Hypertension

In the NHANES II and the HHANES, duplicate readings of **systolic** and **diastolic blood pressure** were obtained during the physicians' examination, and the results were averaged. If mean systolic pressure was 140 mm Hg or higher and/or average diastolic pressure was 90 mm Hg or higher, or if the person reported taking antihypertensive medications, the indi-

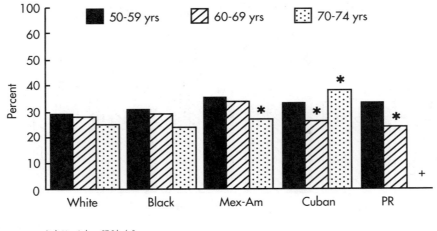

Body Mass Index > 27.3 kg/m²
*Unreliable statistic;+ inadequate sample

FIG. 10-2   Percentage of overweight older American men. A higher percentage of older Mexican-American men are overweight (BMI over 27.3 kg/m²) compared to older white and black men.

(From US Department of Health and Human Services: Second National Health and Nutrition Examination Survey, 1976-80, and Hispanic Health and Nutrition Examination Survey, 1982-84.)

vidual was classified as **hypertensive.**[10] In general, hypertension was more prevalent in the oldest age groups for both sexes (Figs. 10-3 and 10-4).

More than half of those age 60 or older were hypertensive. By race or ethnicity, black men and women age 60 to 74 had the highest prevalence. The prevalence of hypertension among Hispanics age 50 to 59 and 60 to 69 was lower than that of whites and blacks of similar ages (Figs. 10-3 and 10-4). The prevalence of hypertension was greater in the groups below the poverty level than in the groups above it.[8,10]

Physical Limitations

Most older people in their earlier retirement years are relatively healthy and not limited in activity, even though they may have chronic illnesses. The likelihood of activities becoming limited increases by the eighth and ninth decades of life.

In 1984 the National Health Interview Survey included a supplemental survey on aging that collected information about the physical limitations of older Americans living in the community.[15] This survey indicated that approximately 23% of those age 65 or older had difficulty with one or more of the seven **activities of daily living (ADLs),** and 27% had difficulty with at least one of the six **instrumental activities of daily living (IADLs).**[25] (For a review of the ADLs and IADLs, see Chapter 1.) The percentage of individuals experiencing difficulty increased with age. For example, approximately 1.5% of men and 0.9% women age 65 to 74 had difficulty eating, compared to 2.5% of those age 75 to 84 and 4.4% of those age 85 or older.[15] The statistics on preparing meals were more striking; this activity posed some diffi-

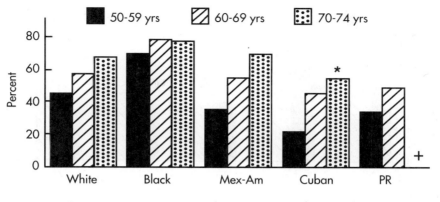

FIG. 10-3 Percentage of older American women with hypertension. The percentage of older women with hypertension (systolic pressure over 140 mm Hg and/or diastolic pressure over 90 mm Hg or taking antihypertensive drugs) tends to increase with age.

(From US Department of Health and Human Services: Second National Health and Nutrition Examination Survey, 1976-80, and Hispanic Health and Nutrition Examination Survey, 1982-84.)

culty for 3% of men and 4.8% of women age 65 to 74, 6% of men and 10.5% of women age 75 to 84, and 18.4% of men and 29.5% of women age 85 or older.[15]

BIOCHEMICAL MEASUREMENTS
Serum Cholesterol

The mean serum cholesterol levels of older Americans (age 50 to 74) who were examined in NHANES II and HHANES have been published in *Nutrition Monitoring in the United States: An Update Report on Nutrition Monitoring.*[10] Regardless of race or ethnic group, the mean serum cholesterol levels of older women were higher than those of older men of similar ages. Since heart disease is the leading cause of death in the United States and elevated serum cholesterol is a risk factor for coronary heart disease (CHD), the prevalence of high-risk serum cholesterol was determined. The criterion for high-risk serum cholesterol levels recom-

mended by the **National Cholesterol Education Program** (over 240 mg/dl) was used to identify people at increased risk of CHD.

As shown in Figure 10-5, *A* and *B*, regardless of race or ethnicity, women age 60 to 74 had the highest prevalences for elevated serum cholesterol. The range for women was 19% to 37%. Among women age 60 to 74, white women had the highest prevalences and Cuban women the lowest (Fig. 10-5, *A*). This finding was also true for men age 60 to 69 (white men, 21%; Cuban men, 8%) (Fig. 10-5, *B*). However, prevalences did not vary markedly among men age 70 to 74. The prevalence of high-risk serum cholesterol levels was higher in groups at or above the poverty level than in groups below it. Regardless of income status, women had the highest prevalences.[8,10]

Iron Status

Iron deficiency is the most common single nutrient deficiency in the United States.[10] Iron

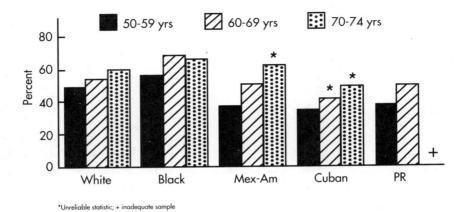

*Unreliable statistic; + inadequate sample

FIG. 10-4   Percentage of older American men with hypertension. The percentage of older men with hypertension (systolic pressure over 140 mm Hg and/or diastolic pressure over 90 mm Hg or taking antihypertensive drugs) tended to be highest among those ages 70 to 74.

(From US Department of Health and Human Services: Second National Health and Nutrition Examination Survey, 1976-80, and Hispanic Health and Nutrition Examination Survey, 1982-84.)

deficiency among older adults is frequently the result of disorders characterized by gastrointestinal bleeding and frequent use of aspirin.

The iron status of older adults examined in NHANES II and HHANES was assessed by the **mean corpuscular volume (MCV)** model, an indicator of iron-deficiency anemia. Three parameters of iron nutriture—**transferrin saturation, erythrocyte protoporphyrin content,** and MCV—were determined. Impaired iron status was defined as having abnormal values for at least two of the three parameters. For people in the 15 to 74 age group, the criteria for abnormal values were less than 19% transferrin saturation, more than 70 μg/dl erythrocyte protoporphyrin, and less than 80 fl MCV.[10] It should be recognized that transferrin saturation and erythrocyte protoporphyrin are also affected by inflammatory disease. Using the MCV model, older men were less likely than older women to be iron deficient. The percentage of men age 70 to 74 with impaired iron status (3% to 6%) appeared to be greater than that of men age 60 to 69 (2% to 3%).[10] Black men had the highest prevalences—3% for ages 60 to 69 and 6% for ages 70 to 74. No similar finding was observed for women. The highest prevalences among older women were for black women age 60 to 69 (7.9%) and Cuban women age 70 to 74 (8.4%) (Fig. 10-6).

Because many older people may have inflammatory diseases, which influence serum transferrin levels and erythrocyte protoporphyrin content, the estimation of iron deficiency prevalence by the MCV model may be inflated. When an alternate model for assessing iron deficiency was used, based on measures of MCV or **serum ferritin,** transferrin saturation, and erythrocyte protoporphyrin content, approximately 1% of the men and women age 70 to 74

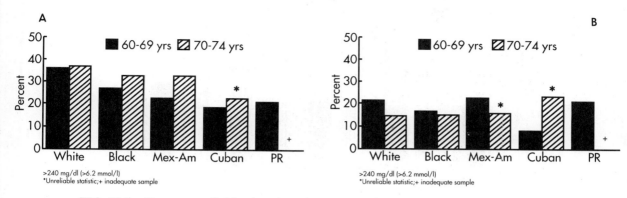

FIG. 10-5 Percentage of older American **A,** women and **B,** men with high-risk serum cholesterol levels. A lower percentage of older men as compared to older women have high-risk serum cholesterol levels (over 240 mg/dl; over 6.2 mmol per L).

(From US Department of Health and Human Services: Second National Health and Nutrition Examination Survey, 1976-80, and Hispanic Health and Nutrition Examination Survey, 1982-84.)

examined in NHANES II were categorized as iron deficient.[10] Regardless of the method of evaluation, the percentages of older men and women with impaired iron status were higher for those below the poverty level than for those at or above it.[8,10]

Serum Albumin

Serum albumin typically composes 50% to 65% of total serum proteins and is an indicator of protein nutritional status. A low serum albumin (less than 3.5 g/dl) can indicate protein-calorie malnutrition. Data from NHANES II indicated the prevalence of low serum albumin among people age 55 to 74 to be extremely small. Among these individuals, the prevalence was 0.3% for white men and black women and 1.2% for black men.[24] The prevalence of low serum albumin was greater for those below the poverty level than for those at or above it. For example, the prevalence was 1.6% for men age 55 to 74 with incomes below the poverty level and 0.2% for men of similar age with incomes above the poverty level.[24]

Serum Ascorbic Acid

In the NHANES II study, serum vitamin C was used to indicate vitamin C status. Low serum vitamin C was defined as less than 0.25 mg/dl (less than 14 μmol/L). The prevalence of low serum vitamin C was 6.5% for white men, 16.2% for black men, 1.8% for white women, and 5.3% for black women.[24] Low serum vitamin C was more prevalent among those below the poverty level than among those at or above it. Approximately 20% of men and 5% of women age 55 to 74 with incomes below the poverty level had low serum vitamin C.[24] For older people of similar ages above the poverty level, the percentage of men with low serum levels (6%) exceeded that of women (2%). Individuals at higher risk for poor vitamin C nutritional status include those whose diets are low in vitamin C because of infrequent consumption of vitamin C–rich foods, cigarette smokers, and the poor.[27]

Serum Zinc

Serum zinc was the only assessment of zinc status measured in NHANES II, even though

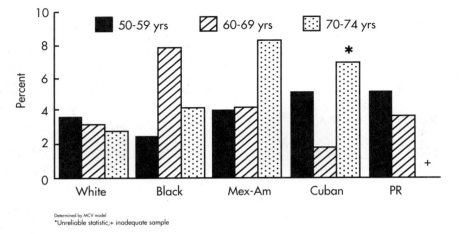

Determined by MCV model
*Unreliable statistic;+ inadequate sample

FIG. 10-6   Percentage of older American women with iron-deficiency anemia. Iron-deficiency anemia was most prevalent among black women ages 60 to 69 and Mexican American and Cuban women ages 70 to 74. Iron deficiency was determined by the MCV model (see text).

(From US Department of Health and Human Services: Second National Health and Nutrition Examination Survey, 1976-80, and Hispanic Health and Nutrition Examination Survey, 1982-84.)

the limitations of using serum zinc as an indicator of zinc nutritional status were recognized. Serum zinc may be influenced by such factors as **diurnal variation,** fasting status, consumption of a meal, infections, and hypoalbuminemia. An expert scientific working group defined low serum values for the NHANES II population based on the time of collection and the fasting state of the subject.[20] Specifically, the cut-off values chosen were less than 70 μg/dl (less than 10.7 μmol/L) for samples collected from fasting subjects in the morning, less than 65 μg/dl (less than 9.9 μmol/L) for samples from nonfasting subjects collected in the morning, and less than 60 μg/dl (less than 9.2 μmol/L) for all samples collected after noon. Using these definitions, the prevalence of low serum zinc among people age 55 to 74 was as follows: 1.9% for white men, 3.3% for black men, 2.4% for white women, and 3.8% for black women.[24] Within this older age group, the prevalence of low se-

rum zinc was not consistently associated with poverty status. It was noted that 3.7% of men and 1.8% of women below the poverty level had low serum zinc, whereas 2% of the men and 2.5% of the women at or above the poverty level had low values.[8,24]

NUTRITIONAL STATUS OF NONINSTITUTIONALIZED OLDER ADULTS

Data derived from the 1977-1978 NFCS, NHANES II, and HHANES suggest that the oldest-old, older adults with incomes below the poverty level, and individuals living alone may be at greater risk of nutritional problems. These noninstitutionalized people tend to have lower food intakes and an increased prevalence for hypertension and suboptimum blood levels of vitamin C and iron. A positive finding among poor older adults was that they had a lower prevalence of elevated serum cholesterol. Conversely, older adults with incomes above the poverty level are at higher risk for elevated serum cholesterol and overweight (for men only). Differences in dietary and nutrition status do exist among various race and ethnic groups. The information currently available suggests that older blacks are at higher risk for poor nutritional status.

Although national data suggest that malnutrition exists, no national estimates are available. A study of 2,986 ambulatory older people age 60 or older found the prevalence of malnutrition to be 3.25% (98 people).[11] People were considered moderately malnourished if they were between the 5th and 15th percentiles of weight for height based on NHANES II data, and severely malnourished if they were below the 5th percentile of weight for height. Of the 98 malnourished individuals, 63.3% (62 persons) had an underlying disease that contributed to the malnutrition, but one third did not.[11] Thus malnutrition can be present without a major comorbid illness.

Data from NFCS and NHANES II provide a picture of the dietary and nutritional status of the civilian, noninstitutionalized population in the United States. These surveys use complex, stratified probability methods of sampling. This method either limits the size of the subgroup or eliminates some subgroups that may be at high risk for nutritional problems. For example, although Native Americans residing on reservations were included in the survey design of the 1987-1988 NFCS, the number of individuals interviewed was not large enough to produce reliable statistics. To capture high-risk populations, alternate approaches such as oversampling or conducting specialized surveys must be implemented.

A study was conducted by the Indian Health Service, U.S. Public Health Service, to determine the prevalence of protein malnutrition among elderly Navajo Indians.[26] Protein deficiency was prevalent, as evidenced by both anthropometric and biochemical markers and by **structural proteins** (midarm muscle area and midarm muscle circumference) and **visceral proteins** (serum albumin and transferrin). The

malnutrition was more prevalent among men than women and in those age 75 or older.[26] The investigators indicated that the prevalence of malnutrition may be attributable to such factors as poverty, limited knowledge of nutrient needs, and replacement of nutritionally adequate traditional diets with commodity foods, as well as a lack of refrigeration and running water.

INSTITUTIONALIZED OLDER ADULTS

Approximately 5% of the older adult population in the United States is institutionalized. It is estimated that 20% of Americans will require chronic institutionalization in their later years.[21] Among the nursing home population, 40% require assistance in eating. Approximately 3.5% of institutionalized people age 80 to 84 and 6.5% of those over age 85 have eating disabilities.[6] In addition, studies indicate that 30% to 40% of nursing home residents experience **dysphagia,** or difficulty in swallowing.[6] Dysphagia can result in malnutrition and **aspiration pneumonia,** which can increase morbidity and mortality. About 70% of older adults in nursing homes have chronic brain disease, usually with dementia.[21] Malnutrition is commonly found in institutionalized, severely demented individuals.[12,22]

Nutritional deficiencies are common in the nursing home population. Estimates of caloric intake indicated that 5% to 18% of nursing home patients are below the RDA.[21] Approximately half of these individuals are underweight and have substandard adipose mass. Up to 30% consume less than 0.8 g of protein per kilogram of body weight per day, and 15% to 60% have substandard midarm muscle circumference and/or serum albumin.[21] Thus protein-calorie malnutrition is prevalent, ranging from 30% to 60%.[3,21,22] In addition, low dietary intakes of zinc, iron, calcium, folate, thiamin, riboflavin, and vitamins A, B$_6$, C, and D have been reported.[4,21] Subnormal blood values have also been found for these micronutrients.[21] For example, 40% of an institutionalized elderly population in Kentucky had iron-deficiency anemia.[4]

In geriatric populations, the incidence of infection and the mortality rate have been shown to be higher in malnourished patients than in patients judged to be adequately nourished.[3,22] The annual mortality rate in the nursing home population is 10% to 40%.[21] In general, among the institutionalized population, the individuals most likely to die soon have low serum albumin, low serum cholesterol, a small triceps skinfolds, low BMI, and low hemoglobin and hematocrit.[21]

NUTRITIONAL STATUS OF INSTITUTIONALIZED OLDER ADULTS

The findings on the nutritional status of nursing home residents show a considerable range. This diversity can be partly explained by the heterogeneity of this population. In any nursing home, the residents can differ substantially with respect to the reason for institutionalization, the mode of feeding, functional capabilities, and the degree of **cognitive impairment.** Many nursing home residents are unable or unwilling to eat, despite their higher nutritional needs for recovery from infection, surgery, and illness. Thirty to 80% of nursing home patients are **edentulous** and depressed.[21] Loss of manual dexterity is common. As mentioned previously, dysphagia is prevalent and often associated with dementing illnesses. Low food intakes in long-term care facilities can also be the result of **anorexigenic drugs** and chronic medical disorders. Another factor for diminished food intake may be a low level of physical activity. Regardless of the cause, reduced caloric intakes can result in suboptimum intakes of essential nutrients, increasing the risk of malnutrition. Malnutrition adversely affects not only the length but also the quality of life.

SUMMARY

In conclusion, national nutrition and dietary survey data suggest that, among older adults living in the community, individuals who live alone and have incomes below the poverty level are at greatest risk for poor nutritional status. Malnutrition is more prevalent among the institutionalized population as compared with the elderly population living in the community. The challenge to nutritionists, dietitians, and other health professionals is to improve or maintain the nutritional health of all older Americans, thereby improving their quality of life.

REVIEW QUESTIONS

1. Why are data from national surveys useful to the study of the nutritional status of older people? How do the surveys differ in their data collection methods, and what do they reveal about the nutritional status of older people?
2. What are core foods? What core foods comprise the diets of older people in the United States? Do these core foods differ from the foods eaten by younger adults?
3. How is the quality of a diet assessed? What is the dietary quality of older people in the United States? Are there any differences in the quality of diets consumed by older people of different races, ethnic backgrounds, or socioeconomic status? Which nutrients are consumed in insufficient quantities by older people?
4. Do older people use vitamin and mineral supplements? If so, what supplements are used and for what reasons? Is there a sex difference in vitamin and mineral consumption patterns among older people?
5. What is the prevalence of hypertension in the older population? How many older people have physical disabilities, and how do these disabilities affect nutritional status?
6. Does nutritional status differ between institutionalized and noninstitutionalized older people? If so, in what ways?

SUGGESTED LEARNING ACTIVITIES

1. Visit your library, and find statistics on how many Hispanic older people live in your community. Discover what core foods are likely to be consumed in their diets, and plan a 3-day diet for an older Hispanic person, using preferred cultural foods.
2. Instruct an older person on keeping a 3-day food diary. Obtain the diary after it has been completed and analyze it, using a computer dietary analysis program. Compare your results to data found in NHANES II.
3. Plan a 20-minute lecture on vitamin and mineral supplements for an audience of older adults. Develop a survey instrument on vitamin and mineral

use, and distribute the survey after your lecture. Stratify the results by age group, sex, and race. Compare your findings to those found in the national surveys.

4. Telephone a nursing home near your house, and obtain the name of the consulting dietitian. Set up an appointment with the dietitian, and interview her on the nature of her work at the nursing home, the nutritional status of the residents, and the nutrition care plan process for the residents.

5. Plan a 3-week cycle menu for residents of a personal care home. The residents are men, over age 75, ambulatory, and many are edentulous.

Key Terms

Provided here for review is a list of the major terms in this chapter. The definitions can be found in the Glossary, which begins on p. 336. To help you understand how these terms are applied, the page number is given for the first mention of each term in the chapter.

activities of daily living (ADLs), 246

anthropometric, 236

anorexigenic drugs, 252

aspiration pneumonia, 251

body mass index (BMI), 244

cognitive impairment, 252

core foods, 238

diastolic blood pressure, 245

dietary status, 236

diurnal variation, 250

dysphagia, 251

edentulous, 252

erythrocyte protoporphyrin content, 248

Hispanic Health and Nutrition Examination Survey (HHANES), 236

hypertensive, 246

instrumental activities of daily living (IADLs), 246

mean corpuscular volume (MCV), 248

National Cholesterol Education Program (NCEP), 247

National Health Interview Survey, 244

Nationwide Food Consumption Survey (NFCS), 236

nutritional status, 236

poverty income ratio (PIR), 242

probability cluster sample, 237

probability sample, 237

Second National Health and Nutrition Examination Survey (NHANES II), 236

serum albumin, 249

serum ferritin, 248

structural proteins, 251

systolic blood pressure, 245

transferrin saturation, 248

visceral proteins, 251

REFERENCES

1. Adler M, Kitchen S, Irion A: *Databook on the elderly: a statistical portrait,* Washington, DC, 1987, US Department of Health and Human Services.

2. Bianchetti A and others: Nutritional intake, socioeconomic conditions, and health status in a large elderly population, *J Am Geriatr Soc* 38:521, 1990.

3. Bienia R and others: Malnutrition in the hospitalized geriatric patient, *J Am Geriatr Soc* 30:433, 1982.

4. Chen LH, Cook-Newell ME: Anemia and iron status in the free-living and institutionalized elderly in Kentucky, *Int J Vitam Nutr Res* 59:207, 1989.

5. Davis MA and others: Living arrangements and dietary quality of older US adults, *J Am Diet Assoc* 90:1667, 1990.

6. Dwyer J, Coletti J, Campbell D: Maximizing nutrition in the second fifty, *Clin Appl Nutr* 1:19, 1991.

7. Fanelli MT, Stevenhagen KJ: Characterizing consumption patterns by food frequency methods: core foods and variety of foods in diets of older Americans, *J Am Diet Assoc* 85:1570, 1985.

8. Fanelli MT, Woteki CE: Nutrient intakes and health status of older Americans, *Ann NY Acad Sci* 561:94, 1989.

9. Fanelli-Kuczmarski M, Woteki CE: Monitoring the nutritional status of the Hispanic population: selected findings for Mexican Americans, Cubans, and Puerto Ricans, *Nutrition Today* 25:6, 1990.

10. Life Sciences Research Office, Federation of American Societies for Experimental Biology: *Nutrition monitoring in the United States: an update report on nutrition monitoring,* DHHS Pub No (PHS) 89-1255, Washington, DC, 1989, US Government Printing Office.

11. Manson A, Shea S: Malnutrition in elderly ambulatory medical patients, *Am J Public Health* 81:1195, 1991.

12. Morley JE, Silver AJ: Anorexia in the elderly, *Neurobiol Aging* 9:9, 1988.

13. Moss AJ: Uses of vitamin and mineral supplements in the United States: current users, types of products, and nutrients, Vital and Health Statistics, advance data, No 174, Hyattsville, Md, 1989, National Center for Health Statistics.

14. Murphy SP and others: Factors influencing the dietary adequacy and energy intake of older Americans, *J Nutr Ed* 22:284, 1990.

15. National Center for Health Statistics: Health statistics on older persons, United States, 1986, Vital and Health Statistics, Series 3, No 25, DHHS Pub No (PHS) 87-1409, Washington, DC, 1987, US Government Printing Office.

16. National Center for Health Statistics: Plan and operation of the Second National Health and Nutrition Examination Survey, 1976-80, Vital and Health Statistics, Series 1, No 15, DHHS Pub No (PHS) 81-1317, Washington, DC, 1981, US Government Printing Office.

17. National Center for Health Statistics: Plan and operation of the Hispanic Health and Nutrition Examination Survey, 1982-84, Vital and Health Statistics, Series 1, No 19, DHHS Pub No (PHS) 85-1321, Washington, DC, 1985, US Government Printing Office.

18. National Research Council: *Diet and health: implications for reducing chronic disease risk,* Washington, DC, 1989, National Academy Press.

19. National Research Council: *Recommended dietary allowances,* ed 10, Washington, DC, 1989, National Academy Press.

20. Pilch SM, Senti FR, editors: *Assessment of zinc nutritional status of the US population based on data collected in the Second National Health and Nutrition Examination Survey, 1976-80,* Bethesda, Md, 1984, Life Sciences Research Office.

21. Rudman D, Feller AG: Protein-calorie undernutrition in the nursing home, *J Am Geriatr Soc* 37:173, 1989.

22. Sandman P and others: Nutritional status and dietary intake in institutionalized patients with Alzheimer's disease and multiinfarct dementia, *J Am Geriatr Soc* 35:31, 1987.

23. US Department of Agriculture: Food intakes: individuals in 48 states, year 1977-78, Nationwide Food Consumption Survey 1977-78, Rep No 1-1, Hyattsville, Md, 1983, The Department.

24. US Department of Health and Human Services and US Department of Agriculture: *Nutrition monitoring in the United States: a progress report from the joint nutrition monitoring evaluation committee,* DHHS Pub No (PHS) 86-1255, Washington DC, 1986, US Government Printing Office.

25. US Senate Special Committee on Aging: *Aging America: trends and projections,* 1987-88 ed (LR3377[188].D12198), Washington, DC, 1989, US Department of Health and Human Services.

26. Williams R, Boyce WT: Protein malnutrition in elderly Navajo patients, *J Am Geriatr Soc* 37:397, 1989.

27. Woteki CE, Johnson C, Murphy R: Nutritional status of the US population: iron, vitamin C, and zinc. In: *What is America eating?* Washington, DC, 1986, National Academy Press.

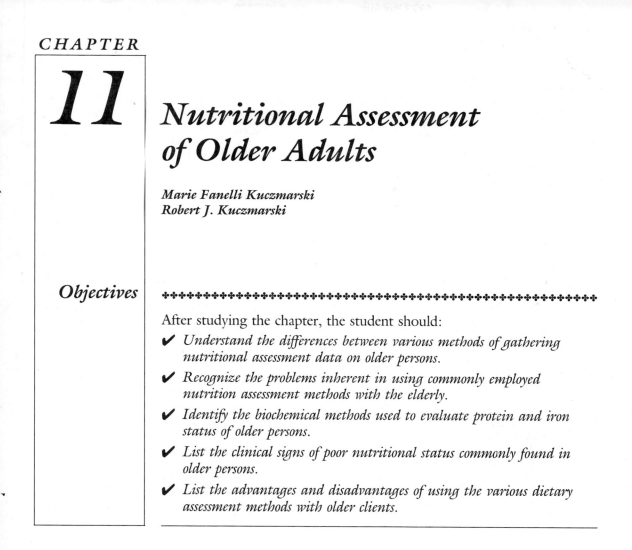

11

Nutritional Assessment of Older Adults

Marie Fanelli Kuczmarski
Robert J. Kuczmarski

Objectives

After studying the chapter, the student should:

✔ *Understand the differences between various methods of gathering nutritional assessment data on older persons.*

✔ *Recognize the problems inherent in using commonly employed nutrition assessment methods with the elderly.*

✔ *Identify the biochemical methods used to evaluate protein and iron status of older persons.*

✔ *List the clinical signs of poor nutritional status commonly found in older persons.*

✔ *List the advantages and disadvantages of using the various dietary assessment methods with older clients.*

It is recognized that many older adults in the United States are at risk for nutritional deficits, excesses, and imbalances. Inadequate quantity and/or quality of food intake, poverty, social isolation, chronic diseases or conditions, disability, chronic prescription drug use, and advanced age (80+ years) are associated with increased risk of poor **nutritional status.** Nutritional indicators to assess an individual's status are quantitative and have been classified historically as **anthropometric,** biochemical, clinical,

and dietary. The various applications of each of these four components are identified in Table 11-1.[52] Examples of indicators within each component are listed in the accompanying box. In addition, information concerning relevant economic and sociodemographic data, cultural food practices and habits, and food beliefs should be collected because these factors are known to affect nutritional status.

Measures of nutritional status are used in applied settings at (1) the individual level in pa-

TABLE 11-1 Nutritional Assessment Methods and Their Purpose

Method	Purpose
Anthropometric	• Determine and monitor body weight to detect changes in weight • Determine and monitor body composition, especially body fat and water • Determine body fat distribution to assess risk for selected chronic conditions
Biochemical	• Determine and monitor nutritional risk for selected chronic conditions such as heart disease • Determine and monitor the level of recent dietary intakes of selected nutrients • Determine and monitor nutrient stores • Obtain functional measures of nutritional adequacy or deficiency • Confirm or refute nutritional diagnoses based on other assessment measures • Determine immune function
Clinical	• Determine presence of signs or symptoms diagnostic of nutritional deficiency or toxicity • Determine and monitor ability to perform ADLs • Evaluate and monitor dental health • Evaluate cognitive status • Determine whether signs or symptoms indicative of nutritional problems are reversed by nutritional intervention
Dietary	• Obtain actual food and beverage intakes to determine quality of diet • Monitor food consumption patterns of individuals or groups to identify changes and trends over time • Determine usage of supplements and their effect on nutrient intake • Evaluate feeding practices of institutionalized older adults

tient diagnosis, screening, intervention, and monitoring, and at (2) the population level for setting policy, in program evaluation, and in **nutritional surveillance.** Nutritional status indicators are used by a diverse group of professionals such as researchers, clinical practitioners, program managers, and policy makers. Consequently, it should be recognized that no single indicator for a given nutrient will meet the needs of all users. Selecting the best indicator depends on the purpose of the nutritional evaluation.

When a nutritional evaluation is initiated by an older adult's physician, it is with the consent of that individual. Informed consent must be obtained from an older adult when the evalua-

❖

COMPONENTS OF NUTRITIONAL ASSESSMENT FOR OLDER ADULTS

• *Anthropometric*
Weight
Stature/knee height
Circumferences
Skinfolds
Bioelectrical impedance
• *Biochemical*
Cholesterol levels
Folate status
Iron status
Protein status
• *Clinical*
Signs and symptoms
Functional status
Cognitive status
Oral health
Use of drugs
• *Dietary*
Food and beverage intake
Food preferences
Food security/insecurity
Use of supplements

---

tion is part of a research, intervention, or planning program, which could be initiated by a university/college, government agency, or nonprofit community agency. Older adults should be informed as to who is conducting the evaluation, the objective of the study, how the data will be used, how confidentiality of information will be protected, and exactly what is expected of the participant.

NUTRITIONAL ASSESSMENT

Nutritional assessment is the integration and interpretation of anthropometric, biochemical, clinical, and dietary data to determine the nutritional and health status of individuals and population groups. A nutritional assessment can take one of three forms—surveys, surveillance, or screening. With nutrition surveys, data are collected in specified population groups either crossectionally or sequentially over specified pe-

riods. This information is used to establish baseline information, and also identify subgroups at risk for malnutrition, for the purpose of ascertaining the nutritional status of the population examined. Nutritional surveillance is the continuous monitoring of nutritional status indicators for the purpose of detecting changes so as to initiate or evaluate intervention measures as necessary. Nutrition screening programs are more targeted and generally less comprehensive than are surveys or surveillance systems. Nutrition screening is the process of determining characteristics or risk factors known to be associated with dietary or nutritional problems and then identifying individuals who either have the condition or are at high risk for the condition. Surveys and surveillance represent nutritional assessment approaches that are used at the community level for population groups, whereas screening applies to individuals in clinical settings, as well as to more narrowly defined population subgroups.

Our knowledge of the complex relationships between nutrition and aging is still evolving. Assessment of older adults presents special challenges to health professionals because evidence that may indicate a nutritional problem can also result from nonnutritional causes. Interpretation of nutritional status data is sometimes difficult because selected references for older adults' have not been established. Some of the physiologic changes that occur with age are indistinguishable from clinical signs of nutrient deficiencies. Finally, the frequent use of prescription drugs by older persons can affect the interpretation of biochemical assays and may influence clinical signs and symptoms. This chapter provides an overview of the commonly used methods of nutritional assessment and also information on resources for appropriate references.

DEFINITIONS

The terms described below were defined by various panels of experts in nutrition.[2,30,58] These definitions are currently being used in the **Nutrition Screening Initiative** (NSI),[16] which is discussed in the next section.

Nutritional status is defined as the health

condition of a population or an individual as influenced by the ingestion and utilization of nutrients and nonnutrients. Measures of nutritional status reflect the processes of dietary intake and digestion, absorption, transport, metabolism and storage, and the excretion of food components and their metabolic products. *Marginal nutritional status* is a condition in which nutrient stores may be low; however, performance, health, or longevity may not be impaired. Individuals with marginal nutritional status are at risk for nutritional deficiency, particularly if subjected to physical, social, or emotional stressors that may further increase requirements or deplete stores of nutrients or energy.

Malnutrition is a condition that results from an excess, deficit, or imbalance of nutrients or energy in relation to metabolic and tissue needs. *Overnutrition,* a form of malnutrition, results from an excess of nutrient availability in relation to tissue needs. Obesity, an excess of body fat, is an example of energy overnutrition from fat, carbohydrate, protein, or alcohol sources. Another form of malnutrition is *undernutrition,* which results from a deficit of nutrient availability with respect to tissue needs. An example of undernutrition that is prevalent among institutionalized elderly persons is **protein-energy malnutrition.** *Nutritional imbalance* is a condition arising from insufficient or excessive intakes of one nutrient or nonnutrient (such as dietary fiber) relative to another, and it may be associated with adverse health consequences, especially in older adults.

NUTRITION SCREENING

Nutrition screening is important for older adults. Nearly 50% of the elderly population have undetected dental disease, and over 50% have some undetected disease or condition such as colon cancer, breast cancer, cardiovascular disease, impaired physical functioning, or nutritional problems.[4] Approximately 2% to 3% of older adults who have an undetected condition or disease can be diagnosed by routine laboratory tests. The most commonly undetected nutrition-related conditions for which screening methods are available include **anemia, hyperlip-**idemia, diabetes, and electrolyte disturbances caused by **diuretics** and **nonsteroidal antiinflammatory agents.**[4] Onset of diseases and subsequent complications can be lessened by early detection of risk factors or conditions and initiation of nutritional intervention measures. As a result, older adults may maximize their independence in carrying out activities of daily living and lessen the number of illness-related days of restricted activity. Ultimately, nutrition services can contribute substantial savings in health care costs.

Panels of experts from various fields specializing in the care of elderly persons have recommended various screening procedures.[4] The following section discusses two instruments focused on nutrition—the **Nutritional Risk Index (NRI)**[60] and the **Determine-Your-Nutritional-Health checklist.**[45] These screening instruments are not intended to replace standard clinical or biochemical indicators, nor are they to replace accepted diagnostic approaches. They are devices to be used to identify older individuals who are candidates for more detailed and extensive nutritional assessment measurements.

The NRI consists of 16 questions (see accompanying box) that focus on the mechanics of food intake, prescribed dietary restrictions, morbid conditions affecting food intake, discomfort associated with food intake, and significant changes in dietary habits. The NRI can be administered in various settings by personnel with limited training, paraprofessionals, or allied health professionals. It is also suitable for use in telephone surveys.

Clinical validation studies have shown that the NRI is significantly correlated with established clinical and biochemical indicators of nutritional status, such as **body mass index (BMI),** abdominal circumference, **hemoglobin,** and hydration status. Individuals scoring 7 or more on the NRI are considered to be at greater risk for poor nutritional status, poor health status in general, and greater use of health services than are individuals scoring less than 7.[60] The value of the NRI is its ability to assist professionals in identifying older adults in need of nutritional interventions and/or in-depth nutritional status assessment.

The checklist shown in Fig. 11-1 was devel-

❖

NUTRITIONAL RISK INDEX (NRI): QUESTIONS

Do you wear dentures?

In the past month, have you taken any medicines prescribed by a doctor?

Have you ever had an operation in your abdomen?

In the past month, have you taken any medicines that were not prescribed by your doctor?

Do you have any troubles with your bowels that make you constipated or give you any diarrhea?

Are there any types of foods that you do not eat because they disagree with you?

Do you have trouble biting or chewing any type of food?

Do you now have an illness or condition that interferes with your eating?

Do you smoke cigarettes regularly now?

Are you on any type of a special diet?

Have you ever been told by a doctor that you were anemic (had iron-poor blood)?

Have you had any spells of pain or discomfort lasting 3 days or more in your abdomen or stomach in the past month?

Do you have an illness that has cut down on your appetite?

Have you had any trouble swallowing for at least 3 days in the last month?

Have you had any vomiting at for least 3 days in the last month?

Have you gained or lost any weight in the last 30 days? (NOTE: net gain/loss must exceed 10 pounds.)

Modified from Wolinsky FD, et al: *J Nutr* 120:1549, 1990.

oped as part of the Nutrition Screening Initiative, a 5-year, multifaceted national effort to promote routine nutrition screening.[45] This initiative, which began in 1990, is under the direction of the **American Academy of Family Physicians,** the **American Dietetic Association,** and the **National Council on the Aging.** The statements in the checklist provide a vehicle for the older adult or caregiver to determine risk factors associated with the elderly person and a starting point for a general discussion about nutrition and health. Individuals receiving higher scores are more likely to have (1) low nutrient intakes when compared to the **Recommended Dietary Allowances** (RDAs) and (2) increased risk of adverse health conditions.[59] These individuals may need health or social services intervention as well as further assessment of nutritional status.

A score above 6 on the checklist indicates the need for more in-depth assessment, specifically the administration of either the Level 1 or Level 2 Screening Tool.[44] The Level 1 Screen is designed to be administered in community settings by professionals such as dietitians, trained caregivers, and health and social services professionals. The screening questions address body weight, body mass index, changes in weight, eating habits, living environment, and functional status. The Level 1 Screen is designed to distinguish between two categories of older adults—those with a documented, significant change in body weight that requires immediate referral to a health professional for more intensive nutritional assessment; and those who do not have a quantifiable nutritional deficit severe enough to require a referral for specific medical care. The latter group may benefit from preventive interventions such as participating in a **congregate** or a **home-delivered meal program,** shopping or transportation assistance, dietary counseling, socialization activities, and participating in food or economic assistance programs.

For individuals requiring more specific diagnostic information on nutritional status, the Level 2 Screening Tool should be administered. The Level 2 Screen is designed for use by physicians and other medical professionals to identify older adults with common nutrition-related problems, such as protein-energy malnutrition, obesity, hyperlipidemia, and **osteoporosis.** It includes the indicators from the Level 1 Screen plus the following measurements.

- Anthropometric measures: **mid-arm circumference, triceps skinfold, mid-arm muscle circumference.**
- Biochemical tests: **serum albumin,** total serum cholesterol.

The Warning Signs of poor nutritional health are often overlooked. Use this checklist to find out if you or someone you know is at nutritional risk.

Read the statements below. Circle the number in the yes column for those that apply to you or someone you know. For each yes answer, score the number in the box. Total your nutritional score.

DETERMINE YOUR NUTRITIONAL HEALTH

	YES
I have an illness or condition that made me change the kind and/or amount of food I eat.	2
I eat fewer than 2 meals per day.	3
I eat few fruits or vegetables, or milk products.	2
I have 3 or more drinks of beer, liquor or wine almost every day.	2
I have tooth or mouth problems that make it hard for me to eat.	2
I don't always have enough money to buy the food I need.	4
I eat alone most of the time.	1
I take 3 or more different prescribed or over-the-counter drugs a day.	1
Without wanting to, I have lost or gained 10 pounds in the last 6 months.	2
I am not always physically able to shop, cook and/or feed myself.	2
TOTAL	

Total Your Nutritional Score. If it's —

0-2   **Good!** Recheck your nutritional score in 6 months.

3-5   **You are at moderate nutritional risk.** See what can be done to improve your eating habits and lifestyle. Your office on aging, senior nutrition program, senior citizens center or health department can help. Recheck your nutritional score in 3 months.

6 or more   **You are at high nutritional risk.** Bring this checklist the next time you see your doctor, dietitian or other qualified health or social service professional. Talk with them about any problems you may have. Ask for help to improve your nutritional health.

These materials developed and distributed by the Nutrition Screening Initiative, a project of:

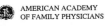
AMERICAN ACADEMY OF FAMILY PHYSICIANS

THE AMERICAN DIETETIC ASSOCIATION

NCOA   NATIONAL COUNCIL ON THE AGING, INC.

Remember that warning signs suggest risk, but do not represent diagnosis of any condition. Turn the page to learn more about the Warning Signs of poor nutritional health.

FIG. 11-1   Nutrition screening initiative checklist.
Used with permission of the Nutrition Screening Initiative.

- Cognitive assessment: minimental status exam.
- Emotional status assessment: **Geriatric Depression Scale, Beck Depression Index.**
- Chronic medication use: number and name of prescription and nonprescription drugs.
- Clinical signs of nutrient deficiency: skin changes, bone pain or fractures, oral tissue changes.[59]

Information obtained from the Level 2 Screen can be used in developing nutritional support interventions for older adults in various settings, such as nursing homes, adult day care centers, doctors' offices, and hospitals.

ANTHROPOMETRIC ASSESSMENT

Anthropometry is the art and science of measuring the human body, which can be done in several ways (see Chapter 3). Anthropometric measurements that are frequently used in clinical settings and nutrition surveys include weight, height, skinfolds, and circumferences. They are used to estimate or predict amounts of various components of the body, which can be more definitively defined in a research body composition laboratory. Anthropometric measurements are particularly useful in detecting moderate and severe degrees of malnutrition, notably imbalances of protein and energy. Detailed descriptions of the procedures for anthropometric methods have been published in the *Anthropometric Standardization Reference Manual.*[32]

Body Weight

The most accurate body weight of ambulatory adults is obtained with a calibrated scale. However, as people enter their 80s and 90s, they often become bed-bound or chair-bound. For **nonambulatory persons,** a calibrated wheelchair or bed beam–type scale should be used. In a clinical setting, the individual should be weighed wearing either a hospital gown or minimal underclothing. In community settings, persons should be dressed in minimal light indoor clothing. Heavy sweaters, jackets, handbags, pocket contents, and shoes should be removed before the person is weighed. The individual who records body weight should not only document the date of the measurement, but also the type of clothing worn and the hydration status of the older adult. **Edema** or severe dehydration can distort actual body weight measurements and lead to misinterpretation of relative weight for height values and weight changes.

Body Height

In comparison to body weight measurements, height or stature measurements can be more complicated. Stature of older adults capable of standing upright can be measured with a stadiometer or against a calibrated, nonstretchable tape attached to a vertical surface. Ideally, the person's heels, buttocks, shoulders, and head should be touching the stadiometer, and his or her eyes should look straight ahead so that the line of vision is perpendicular to the body. Ideally, the person should also be barefoot; however, height can be measured in stocking feet. For some older adults with large amounts of adipose tissue, not all four body parts previously mentioned will come in contact with the stadiometer.

It is impossible to obtain an accurate height measurement with a stadiometer in older adults with **kyphosis (dowager's hump)** or **scoliosis** (curvature) of the spine, or in nonambulatory older adults. **Recumbent** length, the distance from the crown of the head to the heel, can serve as a proxy measure of height, provided head and foot boards are available. Because the length of the long bones remains stable with aging, when a standing height cannot be measured, alternate methods such as measuring arm length,[38] arm span,[29] or knee height[11, 12] can be used to predict stature. Total arm length, the distance from the tip of the right **acromial process** of the scapula to the end of the styloid process of the ulna with the elbow bent at a 45° angle, is measured with a caliper. Knee height is the distance from the sole of the foot at the heel to the anterior surface of the thigh with the ankle and knee each flexed to a 90° angle. None of these alternative methods to estimate stature is flawless. Bowed legs, which are seen in cases of progressive bone loss, can affect the accuracy of knee height measurements, whereas kyphosis can influence arm span measurements.

Knee height measurement is highly recommended because it is an easier measure for health professionals to obtain and it has a low interobserver error. Knee height can be measured with a broad-blade caliper with the person either in a sitting or in a recumbent position. The shaft of the caliper should be parallel to the shaft of the tibia and pass over the anklebone and just behind the head of the fibula. One of the blades of the caliper is positioned under the heel of the foot and the other over the anterior surface of the thigh above the **condyles** of the **femur** just proximal to the **patella** (Fig. 11-2). Stature can be estimated from knee

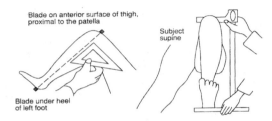

FIG. 11-2   Measurement of knee height.

Used with permission from Gibson RA: *Principles of nutritional assessment,* New York, 1990, Oxford University Press.

height measurement using the following formulas[11]:

White men—Stature = 59.01 + (2.08 × knee height [cm])

Black men—Stature = 95.79 + (1.37 × knee height [cm])

White women—Stature = 75.00 + (1.91 × knee height [cm]) − (0.17 × age [yrs])

Black women—Stature = 58.72 + (1.96 × knee height [cm])

These equations were derived from data obtained from a nationally representative sample of ambulatory persons (438 white men, 453 white women, 50 black men, 60 black women), 60 to 80 years of age.[11] The equations for whites were cross-validated using two independent samples of elderly white men and women. Thus, these equations will probably yield acceptable results with other groups of white older persons. However, the sample of black older adults was limited, so use caution in interpreting results when applying these equations to other black populations.

Relative Weight for Height

Relative weight for height, the ratio of an individual's present weight to a reference weight based on the individual's height, is a parameter used to assess anthropometric data. The most widely used weight references are the Metropolitan Life Insurance Company height and weight tables,[36] the table of average weight for height published by Master, Lasser, and Beckman,[35] and tables of weight for height derived from data from the National Health and Nutrition Examination Surveys (NHANES).[17]

All these references have limitations. The **Metropolitan Company's weight-for-height tables** do not include values for persons above 59 years. The table by Master et al.[35] is based on a sample of about 5600 **ambulatory,** disease-free, noninstitutionalized white persons in the U.S. and provides reference weights for persons 65 to 94 years old. Although regarded by many as the best data currently available for the older adult population, these measurements were recorded 30 years ago by many observers and with pieces of equipment that were not uniformly standardized. The NHANES data were collected by trained technicians following standardized protocols from a representative national sample, but data were restricted to persons aged 79 years and younger.

A more recently published reference table is based on data from the NHANES I Epidemiological Follow-up Survey and includes the fifteenth, fiftieth, and eighty-fifth percentiles of body weight for each inch of height for men and women, ages 55 to 84 years[13] (Table 11-2). This study population consisted of 562 black persons (272 men and 290 women) and 2777 white persons (1314 men and 1463 women). These reference data provide three useful categories for distinguishing underweight, average weight, and overweight: <15% (underweight or lean), 15% to 84% (average), and ≥85% (overweight or obese). Recognizing the need for more extensive weight and height data for older adults, the NHANES III will measure an estimated 5180 persons, aged 60 years and older, representative of the noninstitutionalized elderly population in the U.S.[28] When available, these data may provide the best reference values for older adults.

Weight Changes

A person's usual weight and history of recent weight changes are important. Generally, the shorter the period for a given weight loss, the more likely nutritional health is compromised (see Chapter 8). A significant weight change is a loss of 1% to 2% in a week, 5% in a month, 7.5% in 3 months, or 10% in 6 months.[6,25] Weight losses greater than these percentages indicate severe malnutrition.[6] Before defining the severity of malnutrition, accuracy of the weight

TABLE 11-2   *Percentiles of Body Weight for Each Inch of Height, by Age and Sex: USA 1982-1984*

	Age														
	60-64 yr			65-69 yr			70-74 yr			75-79 yr			80-84 yr		
Percentile:	15th	50th	85th	15th	50th	85th	15th	50th	85th	15th	50th	85th	15th	50th	85th
Height (in.)															
Women															
58	103	130	166	103	128	164	101	126	160	100	122	154	98	118	148
59	107	133	169	106	132	167	105	129	163	104	126	158	102	121	151
60	111	137	172	110	135	170	109	133	166	107	130	161	105	125	154
61	115	140	176	114	139	173	113	137	169	111	133	164	109	129	157
62	118	144	179	118	142	176	117	140	173	115	137	167	113	132	161
63	122	147	182	121	146	180	120	144	176	119	140	170	117	136	164
64	126	151	185	125	149	183	124	147	179	122	144	174	120	139	167
65	130	154	188	129	153	186	128	151	182	126	147	177	124	143	170
66	133	158	192	133	157	189	132	154	185	130	151	180	128	146	173
67	137	161	195	136	160	192	135	158	188	134	154	183	132	150	176
68	141	165	198	140	164	196	139	161	192	137	158	186	135	153	180
69	145	168	201	144	167	199	143	165	195	141	161	190	139	157	183
70	148	172	204	148	171	202	147	168	198	145	165	193	143	160	186
Men															
60	128	142	161	123	140	158	120	138	154	118	135	149	116	131	143
61	131	146	166	126	144	163	123	142	159	121	139	154	119	135	147
62	134	150	170	129	148	168	126	146	164	124	143	158	122	139	152
63	137	154	175	132	152	172	129	150	168	127	147	163	125	142	157
64	140	158	180	136	156	177	132	154	173	130	151	168	128	146	161
65	143	162	184	139	160	182	135	158	178	133	155	173	131	150	166
66	146	166	189	142	164	186	138	162	183	136	159	177	134	154	171
67	149	170	194	145	168	191	141	166	187	139	163	182	137	158	176
68	152	174	198	148	172	196	144	170	192	142	166	187	140	162	180
69	155	178	203	151	176	201	147	174	197	145	170	191	143	166	185
70	158	182	208	154	180	205	150	178	201	148	174	196	146	170	190
71	161	186	213	157	184	210	153	182	206	151	178	201	150	174	194
72	164	190	217	160	188	215	156	186	211	154	182	206	153	178	199

Modified from Cornoni-Huntley JC, et al: An overview of body weight of older persons, including impact on mortality, *J Clin Edidemiol* 44:743, 1991.

NOTE: based on weighted linear regression models using common slope with intercepts for each age group fitted by quadratic model.

Separate models for men and women.

history and interpretation of the weight measurements with respect to the hydration status of the individual at the time of the measurements must be carefully considered.

Body Mass Index

If weight and stature measures are valid, BMI can be computed or determined from a nomogram (Fig. 11-3). The BMI has been shown to

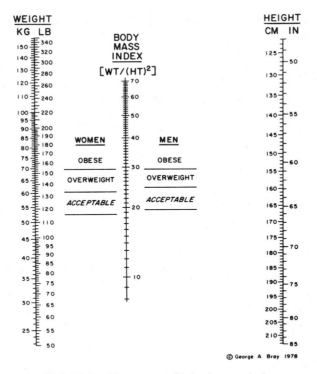

FIG. 11-3   Nomogram for body mass index.

Courtesy of George A. Bray.

have a reasonable correlation with body fat in young adults. However, because of the progressive decrease in lean body mass and increase in body fat, along with a decrease in height, the BMI may result in miscalculated estimates of body fat in older adults.

The NSI is currently recommending intervention for older adults with a BMI of less than 24 or greater than 27.[44] Individuals with a BMI of less than 24 may be at risk for poor nutritional status. Individuals with a BMI of more than 27 are obese and consequently are at risk for several conditions, including hypertension, diabetes, and **osteoarthritis.**

Similar to the adjustments made for kyphosis that were discussed for height measurements, weight references must be adjusted for persons who have lost a body part because of surgery or trauma. Figures for adjusting body weight according to the type of amputation are available.[43]

Circumference Measurements

Circumference measurements are emerging as increasingly important data to collect on elderly persons for several reasons. First, a shift in fat patterning from peripheral to central occurs with increasing age (i.e., a shift from the extremities to the trunk, notably in women, and from **subcutaneous** to deep adipose tissue in both men and women). The **abdominal fat** accumulation seems to be greater in men than in women, as shown by larger waist circumferences in men, and increases progressively with age. Fat patterning is an important determinant of **HDL,** triglyceride, and HDL: total cholesterol ratio.[46]

The second reason to measure circumferences in older adults is because of the ties between fat distribution and health outcomes.[27] Prospective studies have shown that the risk of disease increases steeply when the waist-to-hip ratio rises above 1.0 for men and 0.8 for women.[5]

Thirdly, circumference measurements require minimal expertise and very unsophisticated equipment—a calibrated, nonstretchable tape. The greatest problem is agreement on where the circumference tape should be placed.

The mid-upper arm circumference reflects both the subcutaneous fat and muscle of the arm. Therefore, a change in this circumference reflects a gain reduction in muscle mass, a gain/reduction in subcutaneous tissue, or both. Changes in mid-upper arm circumference measurements in adults can be used to monitor progress of nutritional interventions.

The circumference of the upper arm is measured at its midpoint, the distance halfway between the acromion and olecranon processes. The arm is bent at a 90° angle with the palm of the hand facing upward. Percentiles for mid-upper arm circumference measurements have been published for persons aged 55 to 74 years of age who were examined in NHANES II.[39] (Table 11-3). The fiftieth percentile represents the average value of a measurement, and the ninety-fifth and fifth percentiles are the upper and lower limits, respectively, of normal values for a measurement. Persons at the extremes, (i.e., less than fifth or more than ninety-fifth percentiles) are more likely to have a nutritional disorder or disease than are persons closer to the fiftieth percentile. Serial measurements can help to detect abnormal change and to monitor the effectiveness of nutritional intervention.

Skinfold Assessments

Skinfold measurements have several inherent limitations when used in any age group. When coupled with the physical changes experienced by older persons (including the apparent redistribution of fat, the decreased elasticity of the skin, marked alterations in skin thickness, and atrophy of subcutaneous adipocytes contributing to increased tissue compression), the caliper measurements may have a limited potential to reliably assess subcutaneous fat and accurately predict total body fat using regression equations. As mentioned in Chapter 3, body density equations typically used to predict total body fat may not apply to older persons because of the noted changes in body composition.

The triceps skinfold thickness is measured on the back of the mid-upper arm over the triceps

TABLE 11-3 *Mid-Upper Arm Circumference for Older Males and Females by Race*

Age	Percentile		
	5th (cm)	50th (cm)	95th (cm)
White			
Males			
55-64 yrs	27.5	32.3	37.6
65-74 yrs	25.5	31.6	36.8
Females			
55-64 yrs	25.1	30.8	39.4
65-74 yrs	24.3	30.5	38.8
Black			
Males			
55-64 yrs	27.2	32.6	39.6
65-74 yrs	24.6	30.6	38.2
Females			
55-64 yrs	25.5	33.5	45.1
65-74 yrs	26.1	32.7	39.1

Modified from Najjar MF, Rowland M: *Anthropometric reference data and prevalence of overweight, United States, 1976-1980*, Vital and Health Statistics, Series 11, No 238, DHHS Publication No (PHS) 87-1688, Washington, DC, 1987, US Government Printing Office.

muscle. A calibrated **skinfold caliper** such as the Lange, Harpenden, or Holtain should be used for the measurement. The triceps skinfold represents a double fold of subcutaneous fat thickness. Table 11-4 presents the fifth, fiftieth and ninety-fifth percentile values obtained from NHANES II.[39] Individuals with a triceps skinfold measurement above the ninety-fifth percentile are generally considered obese, whereas those below the fifth percentile are considered underweight. In addition, the triceps skinfold measurement, along with the mid-upper arm circumference measurement, can be used to estimate body muscle mass. The formula for muscle area is:

$$(\text{Midarm circumference} - (3.14 \times \text{Triceps skinfold})^2 \div 12.56.[23]$$

TABLE 11-4   *Triceps Skinfold for Older Males and Females by Race*

Age	Percentile		
	5th (mm)	50th (mm)	95th (mm)
White			
Males			
55-64 years	5.5	12.0	24.5
65-74 years	5.0	12.0	25.0
Female			
55-64 yrs	12.5	26.0	43.1
65-74 yrs	12.0	25.0	41.1
Black			
Male			
55-64 years	3.5	10.5	29.0
65-74 years	4.0	10.0	27.5
Female			
55-64 yrs	12.0	28.5	46.0
65-74 yrs	11.5	29.0	47.5

Modified from Najjar MF, Rowland M: *Anthropometric reference data and prevalence of overweight, United States, 1976-1980*, Vital and Health Statistics, Series 11, No 238, DHHS Publication No (PHS) 87-1688, Washington, DC, 1987, US Government Printing Office.

Bioelectrical Impedance

Bioelectrical impedance analysis (BIA) appeals greatly as an approach to measuring body composition because it is quick (less than 2 minutes), simple, relatively inexpensive, safe, and highly reproducible. It has an added attraction for older persons because no physical demands are placed on the subjects. In addition, BIA measures body water, which is of interest in older adults because of their increased risk for dehydration.

The limitation of BIA at the moment is that the quantification of fat-free mass and fat mass by this method are based on prediction formulas used by manufacturers of the BIA equipment, which in turn are based on measurements in younger populations. These equations can overestimate fat-free mass by approximately 6 kg[14] and therefore underestimate fat mass and are not applicable to elderly populations. These errors in estimation result in part from the variability in hydration levels occurring with aging. Regression equations for older adults have been published in the literature[14,56] and could be used in place of the equations supplied by BIA manufacturers.

The assessment of fat-free mass from BIA in older adults seems to be reliable, provided age-specific prediction formulas are used.[14] Further research is needed in developing and cross-validating prediction equations from impedance in older adults, as compared with estimates obtained from multicompartmental models (see Chapter 3).

BIOCHEMICAL ASSESSMENT

Biochemical methods are more sensitive than are anthropometric and clinical methods and reflect alterations in nutritional status before the same changes can be detected using these other methods. When a nutrient deficiency occurs, tissue stores are gradually depleted. This depletion results in reductions in the levels of nutrients in reserve stores and body fluids, in the levels of metabolic products, and in the activity of nutrient-dependent enzymes.

Blood samples for biochemical analysis can be obtained by either fingerprick or venipuncture, depending on the biochemical test selected. The number of assays available from a fingerprick sample are limited. In addition, this technique is subject to problems with hemodilution, hemoconcentration, and environmental contamination. A sufficient volume of blood can almost always be obtained with a venipuncture, so analysis is not compromised. However, this procedure can be difficult in obese individuals whose veins in the upper arm are inaccessible or in elderly persons in whom accessible veins may collapse. It is also necessary to recruit a qualified professional such as a phlebotomist to perform venipuncture.

Plasma and serum transport newly absorbed nutrients to the tissues and therefore provide an index of current dietary intake. Conversely, tissue stores reflect long-term nutrient status. The effect of recent dietary intake on plasma or serum nutrient levels can be reduced by collecting fasting blood samples.

Among older adults, protein-energy malnutrition, hyperlipidemia, and iron and folate deficiency anemias are common nutritional problems. The following section focuses on the biochemical indicators used to diagnose these problems. Selected criteria for biochemical measures are given in Table 11-5.

Protein Status

The most reliable diagnostic indicators of protein energy malnutrition in older adult populations include levels of serum albumin, **transferrin,** hemoglobin, and serum cholesterol, and total **lymphocyte** count. Serum albumin and transferrin are good markers for evaluating visceral protein status. Visceral proteins include serum proteins, **erythrocytes, granulocytes, lymphocytes,** and solid tissue organs such as the liver, kidneys, pancreas, and heart. Total lymphocyte count is an indicator of **immunocompetence.** Hemoglobin can be used to detect anemia, which is commonly associated with malnutrition.

Serum albumin concentrations do not decrease with age to a significant degree in healthy older persons (1% to 6%).[16] Serum albumin has a long half-life of 14 to 21 days. Thus alterations of serum albumin take several weeks. Hypoalbuminemia or low serum albumin levels may be the consequence of a nutrition-related decrease in protein synthesis. However, various factors can influence serum albumin levels. Hypoalbuminemia may result from certain gastrointestinal and renal diseases, liver disease, **hypothyroidism, congestive heart failure,** infection, or zinc deficiency. In normally hydrated older adults, serum albumin levels should not be lower than 3.5 g/dl.[16] Lipschitz and Mitchell[31] suggest that a serum albumin value of less than 3.0 g/dl can be used to differentiate malnourished from well nourished older adults.

Serum transferrin is located almost totally intravascularly and serves as an iron transport protein. In comparison to serum albumin, serum transferrin has a short half life of 8 to 10 days and a smaller body pool. Therefore it responds more rapidly to changes in protein status over short periods. Like serum albumin, serum transferrin concentrations are affected by other factors such as **pernicious anemia;** iron overload; gastrointestinal, renal, and liver diseases; congestive heart failure; and inflammation. In concomitant protein-energy malnutrition and iron deficiency, a decrease in transferrin levels may be masked because transferrin synthesis is increased in response to increased iron absorption. Therefore serum transferrin is not an appropriate index of protein status when both **iron-deficiency anemia** and protein-energy malnutrition are present. Serum transferrin values of less than 200 mg/dl can be used to detect protein deficiency in older adults.[31]

Total lymphocyte count (TLC) declines and lymphocyte response to **antigens** is impaired in malnutrition. TLC is determined using the following formula:

$$\text{TLC} = (\% \text{ lymphocytes} \times \text{ white blood cell count}) - 100.$$

Unfortunately, the specificity (the ability of the index to identify and classify those persons who are genuinely well nourished) and sensitivity (the extent to which the index reflects nutritional status or predicts changes in nutriture) is low for TLC. This is because other factors such as stress, **sepsis, neoplasia,** and the administration of steroids affect the absolute lymphocyte count. The similarity between the effects of normal aging and the effects of protein-energy malnutrition also make the interpretation of routine immunologic testing difficult. A TLC of less than 1200/mm^3 suggests moderate protein depletion, and a count of less than 800/mm^3 suggests severe malnutrition.[6]

There is much controversy about cut-off values for hemoglobin to define anemia in older adults. It seems that a normal physiologic response to aging is a decline in hemoglobin. Mitchell and Lipschitz[37,38] recommend hemoglobin values of less than 12 g/dl and less than 10 g/dl be used to identify anemia in older men and women, respectively.

Evidence exists showing that low total serum cholesterol levels are predictive of excess mortality, independent of cancer incidence.[53] In ad-

TABLE 11-5   *Guidelines for Interpreting Biochemical Data*

Blood Biochemistries	Biochemical Values			Source
Cholesterol	*High*			
Total	$\geq$240 mg/dl			40
LDL	$\geq$160 mg/dl			40
Protein	*Deficient*			
Serum albumin	<3.0 g/dl			30
Serum transferrin	<200 mg/dl			30
Total lymphocyte count	<800 to 1200 cells/mm^3			6
Hemoglobin				37
Men	<12 g/dl			
Women	<10 g/dl			
Cholesterol	<160 mg/dl			53
Selected minerals				
Iron	*Depletion*	*Deficient erythropoiesis*	*Anemia*	21
Serum ferritin	<20 µg/dl	10 µg/dl	<10 µg/dl	
Plasma iron	<115 µg/dl	<60 µg/dl	<40 µg/dl	
Total iron binding capacity	>360 µg/dl	>390 µg/dl	>410 µg/dl	
Transferrin saturation	30%	<15%	<15%	
Erythrocyte protoporphyrin	30 µg/dl RBC	>100 µg/dl RBC	>200 µg/dl RBC	
Zinc	*Deficient*			18
Serum zinc*	<70 µg/dl			
Selected vitamins				
Folate	*Depletion*	*Deficient erythropoiesis*	*Anemia*	21
Serum folate	<3 ng/ml	<3 ng/ml	<3 ng/ml	
Erythrocyte folate	<160 ng/ml	<120 ng/ml	<100 ng/ml	
Vitamin B$_{12}$	*Depletion*	*Deficient erythropoiesis*	*Anemia*	21
Serum vitamin B$_{12}$	<150 pg/ml	<100 pg/ml	<100 pg/ml	
Vitamin A	*Low*	*Deficient*		
Plasma retinol	10-20 µg/dl	<10 µg/dl		18, 50
Vitamin C	*Low*	*Deficient*		
Serum ascorbic acid	0.20-0.29 mg/dl	<0.20 mg/dl		18, 50
Leukocyte ascorbic acid	8-15 mg/dl	<8 mg/dl		18, 50
Vitamin B$_6$		*Deficient*		
Serum vitamin B$_6$		<3.0 ng/ml		50
Red cell vitamin B$_6$		<12.0 ng/ml		50

*AM + fasting sample.

dition, low total cholesterol levels in elderly persons are associated with an increased risk of hemorrhagic **stroke.**[16] A total serum cholesterol value of less than 160 mg/dl is also a marker for protein-energy malnutrition. This latter value is being used in the Level II Screen of the Nutrition Screening Initiative[44] to indicate the need for nutritional counseling or support intervention.

Hypercholesterolemia

High blood cholesterol, especially elevated **LDLs (low-density lipoproteins)** and decreased HDLs (high density lipoproteins), is a risk factor for coronary artery disease. The **National Cholesterol Education Program** screening guidelines are considered appropriate for use with older adults. A total cholesterol level above 240 mg/dl and a LDL level above 160 mg/dl are viewed as high risk.[40] The total cholesterol value is being used in the Level II Screen of the Nutrition Screening Initiative.[44]

Iron Status

Iron deficiency is considered the most common nutrient deficiency in the world. Clinical manifestations of iron deficiency are provided in Table 11-6. Iron deficiency among older persons is generally associated with increased blood loss, excessive intake of aspirin or antiinflammatory drugs for relief of arthritic pain, or achlorhydria.

Three stages have been used to characterize the development of iron-deficiency anemia.[21, 26] The first stage, **iron depletion,** is characterized by progressive reduction in the amount of storage iron, reflected by a decline in serum/plasma ferritin concentrations. The second stage, **iron-deficient erythropoiesis,** is characterized by complete depletion of iron stores. **Microcytic hypochromic anemia** is the third and final stage of iron deficiency. This stage is characterized by a reduction in the concentration of hemoglobin in the red blood cells and by decreases in the hematocrit and **mean corpuscular volume (MCV).** The biochemical cutoff values used to defined each stage are provided in Table 11-5.

Hemoglobin levels are probably the most widely used screening test for iron-deficiency anemia because it is inexpensive. However, this index has several limitations. Cigarette smoking is associated with higher concentrations of hemoglobin, whereas chronic infections, inflammation, hemorrhage, protein-energy malnutrition, vitamin B_{12} or **folate** deficiency, and overhydration can result in low hemoglobin concentrations. In addition, regardless of age or income, black individuals may have hemoglobin values lower than those of white persons. Hence, they may be misdiagnosed as having iron deficiency if the reference values are based on white population values.

As noted above, several factors can affect an index of iron status. Chronic disease states such as infection, inflammation, and certain neoplastic diseases lead to an anemia of disease.[18, 26] Its hallmark is normal or elevated iron stores in the presence of **hypoferremia** (see Chapter 8).[26] Elevated concentrations of **serum** ferritin can occur with liver disease, leukemia, or **Hodgkin's disease,** whereas serum ferritin may display normal or even slightly above-normal levels in vitamin B_{12} or folate deficiency. Vitamin B_{12} or folate deficiency can increase transferrin saturation and elevate MCV.

No single biochemical indicator has proven to be diagnostic of iron deficiency. To provide the best measure of iron status, several indices should be used simultaneously. In general, two or more abnormal values are considered indicative of impaired iron status. The selection of the most appropriate combination depends on the health of the individuals and the objectives of the assessment. Several combinations have been proposed.[47, 58] A panel of experts in nutrition proposed a 4-variable model for assessing iron status, especially for older adults.[58] The 4-variable model includes erythrocyte protoporphyrin, transferrin saturation, serum ferritin, and MCV. With this model, either the ferritin or MVC value (or both) plus one additional value (either **erythrocyte protoporphyrin** or **transferrin saturation**) must be abnormal. This model may reduce the contribution of inflammatory conditions to prevalence estimates of iron deficiency.

Folate Status

Folate deficiency in older adults can be caused by low dietary intakes of folate, malab-

TABLE 11-6 *Clinical Signs and Possible Nutrient Deficiency in Adults*

Clinical Signs	Consider Deficiency	Definition/Comment
Hair		
Easily pluckable, sparse	Protein, biotin	
	Protein	
Straight, dull	Protein	
Coiled, corkscrewlike	Vitamin A, vitamin C	Caused by follicular and keratinization change
Skin		
Xerosis	Essential fatty acid	Dryness of skin/aging, loss of skin lubricants
Petechiae	Vitamin A, vitamin C	Pin-headed sized hemorrhages
Pigmentation	Niacin	Sign of pellagra distributed symmetrically in sun-exposed areas; also seen in hemochromatosis
Follicular keratosis	Vitamin A, possibly essential fatty acid	Keratin plugs in follicles, "goose flesh"
"Flaky-paint" dermatitis	Protein	
Subcutaneous fat loss, fine wrinkling	Protein-energy	Aging process
Poor tissue turgor	Water	Aging process
Edema	Protein, thiamin	Seen in protein-energy malnutrition with hypoalbuminemia and in wet beriberi resulting from to thiamin deficiency
Purpura	Vitamin C, vitamin K	Also seen in vitamin E toxicity
Perifollicular hemorrhage	Vitamin C	
Pallor	Folacin, iron, vitamin B12, copper, biotin	
Tendency toward excessive bruising (ecchymoses)	Vitamin C, vitamin K	Caused by increased fragility of capillary walls; aging process
Pressure sores	Protein-energy	
Seborrheic dermatitis	Essential fatty acid, pyridoxine, zinc, biotin	
Poor wound healing	Protein-energy, zinc, and possibly essential fatty acids	
Thickening of skin	Essential fatty acid	
Eyes		
Dull, dry (xerosis) conjunctiva	Vitamin A	Can lead to xerophthalmia in severe deficiency
Keratomalacia	Vitamin A	Softening of cornea
Bitot's spot	Vitamin A	Early evidence of deficiency
Corneal vascularization	Riboflavin	
Photophobia	Zinc	

Adapted from Heymsfield SB, Williams PJ: Nutritional assessment by clinical and biochemical methods. In Modern nutrition in health and disease, ed 7, Philadelphia, 1988, Lea & Febiger.

Clinical Signs	Consider Deficiency	Definition/Comment
Lips and oral structures		
Angular fissures, scars, or **stomatitis**	B-complex, iron, protein, riboflavin	Also seen with ill-fitting dentures
Cheilosis	B_6, niacin, riboflavin, protein	Also seen with ill-fitting dentures, exposure to sun or cold
Ageusia, dysgeusia	Zinc	Also associated with altered sense of smell
Swollen, spongy, bleeding gums	Ascorbic acid	If not edentulous
Tongue		
Magenta tongue	Riboflavin	
Fissuring, raw	Niacin	
Glossitis	Pyridoxine, folacin, iron, vitamin B_{12}	Also seen with food irritants, antibiotic administration, uremia
Fiery red tongue	Folacin, vitamin B_{12}	Seen if anemia is not pronounced
Pale	Iron, vitamin B_{12}	Seen in severe cases
Atrophic papillae	Riboflavin, niacin, iron	Also seen with ill-fitting dentures, food irritants, aging
Nails		
Spoon-shaped nails (**koilonychia**)	Chromium, iron	
Brittle, ridged, lined nails	Nonspecific	May be protein undernutrition
Heart		
Tachycardia, cardiomegaly, congestive heart failure	Thiamin	"Wet" beriberi associated with high output congestive heart failure
Decreased cardiac function	Phosphorus	
Cardiac arrhythmias	Magnesium, potassium	
Small heart, decreased output, bradycardia	Protein-energy	Prone to congestive heart failure during refeeding
Abdomen		
Hepatomegaly	Protein	Fatty liver/commonly seen in alcoholics
Wasting	Energy	Found in marasmus
Enlarged spleen	Iron	Found in 15% to 25% subjects with a significant degree of iron-deficiency anemia
Bones		
Bone pain	Calcium, vitamin D, phosphorus, vitamin C	Seen in osteomalacia

Continued.

TABLE 11-6 *Clinical Signs and Possible Nutrient Deficiency in Adults—cont'd*

Clinical Signs	Consider Deficiency	Definition/Comment
Muscles, extremities		
Wasting	Protein-energy	
Pain in calves, weak thighs	Thiamin	
Edema	Protein, thiamin	Also seen with sodium toxicity and hypertension
Muscular twitching	Pyridoxine	
Muscular pains	Biotin, selenium	
Muscular weakness	Sodium, potassium	
Muscle cramps	Sodium, chloride	
Neurologic		
Ophthalmoplegia, footdrop	Thiamin	Wernicke's encephalopathy
Disorientation	Thiamin, sodium, water	Korsakoff's psychosis; fabrication occurs in thiamin-deficient alcoholics
Decreased position, vibratory sense, ataxia, optic neuritis	Vitamin B_{12}	Subacute spinal cord degeneration
Weakness, paresthesia of legs (burning and tingling)	Thiamin, pyridoxine, pantothenic acid, vitamin B_{12}	Nutritional polyneuropathy, especially with alcoholism; "burning foot" syndrome with pantothenic acid deficiency
Hyporeflexia	Thiamin	Aging process
Mental disorders	Niacin, magnesium, vitamin B_{12}	In untreated B_{12} deficiency, mental disorders may progress to severe psychosis
Convulsions	Pyridoxine, calcium, magnesium, phosphorus	
Depression, lethargy	Biotin, folacin, vitamin C	Aging process
Sleep disturbances	Pantothenic acid	Aging process
Peripheral neuropathy	Pyridoxine	
Other		
Diarrhea	Niacin, folacin, vitamin B_{12}	Also seen in vitamin C toxicity
Delayed wound healing and tissue repair	Vitamin C, zinc, protein-energy	
Anemia, pallor	Vitamin E, pyridoxine, vitamin B_{12}, iron, folacin, biotin, copper	
Anorexia	Vitamin B_{12}, chloride, sodium, thiamin, vitamin C	Also seen with vitamin A, zinc, or iron toxicity
Nausea	Biotin, pantothenic acid	
Fatigue, lassitude, apathy	Energy, biotin, pantothenic acid, magnesium, phosphorus, iron, potassium, sodium	

sorption syndrome, or selected drugs, such as chronic aspirin use and alcohol ingestion. Serum and erythrocyte folate concentrations are the most frequently used biochemical indicators of folate status. Serum levels reflect recent intake and acute folate status. Erythrocyte folate levels reflect body stores and are a more reliable index of folate status.

Similar to iron, there are three stages of folate deficiency—folate depletion, folate deficiency erythropoiesis, and folate deficiency anemia.[21] The cutoff values for serum and erythrocyte folate are provided in Table 11-5. Low folate intake for more than a month may gradually reduce folate stores, resulting in folate depletion. Erythrocyte folate levels continue to decline as the stages of folate deficiency progress.

CLINICAL ASSESSMENT

Clinical assessment can include a medical history; physical examination to determine which physical signs and symptoms of nutritional disease are present; assessment of functional status, particularly skills related to purchasing, preparing, and eating foods; and an oral examination. When interviewing and examining older adults, health professionals should remember that (1) many elderly persons may not report symptoms or changes in functional status because they accept their condition as a problem resulting from aging, and (2) some may be mentally confused and not able to clearly describe signs and symptoms. Clinical signs and symptoms are generally nonspecific and develop in the advanced stages of a nutritional deficiency.

Clinical Signs

A comprehensive listing of clinical signs indicating nutritional disease are in Table 11-6.[22] An abbreviated checklist of clinical appearances suggesting nutritional problems includes the following: wasted appearance, edema, pale color, bruises, general weakness, apathy, tremors, skin lesions, rashes, scaly skin, and cracks or sores around the mouth. Remember that the symptoms and signs commonly found in the elderly population can have nonnutritional etio-

logic causes. For example, purpura (subcutaneous skin hemorrhages) is more commonly the result of aging of the skin and not the result of scurvy (a vitamin C deficiency) or vitamin K deficiency. Furthermore, **night blindness** may result from **cataracts** rather than vitamin A deficiency; and angular stomatitis can be caused by drooling of saliva rather than a riboflavin deficiency. In addition, clinical signs and symptoms are not diagnostically specific and should be confirmed by other components of nutritional status assessment.

Functional Status

Changes in functional status represent an important symptom of nutritional status that needs to be monitored. Two measures of independence/dependence commonly used to assess functional status are (1) activities of daily living (ADLs) and (2) **instrumental activities of daily living (IADLs).** Dependence is defined as needing assistance for an activity most of the time, whereas independence implies that the activity can be performed without assistance. The inability to perform any of the ADLs and the nutrition-related IADLs signals the potential presence of poor nutritional status.[16]

Feeding is considered one of the six ADLs. Independent feeding is evidenced by the ability to get food from the plate into the mouth, whereas dependence implies the need for assistance in the act of feeding because the person is not eating at all, or requires parenteral feeding.[16]

IADLs measure home management activities essential to independent living, including three nutrition-related activities—shopping, food-preparation, and mode of transportation. Independence with respect to shopping means the individual takes care of all shopping needs and shops independently for small purchases. An individual who must be accompanied on any shopping trip or is completely unable to shop is dependent. An independent older adult is able to plan, prepare, and serve adequate meals independently or prepare adequate meals if the ingredients are supplied. Dependence implies that a person is able to prepare meals or heat and serve prepared meals but does not maintain an adequate diet, or that a person must have his or her meals prepared and served. With respect to mode of transportation, a dependent individual would travel on public transportation accompanied by another person, limit travel to automobile or taxi with assistance, or not travel at all. An independent living older person would travel on public transportation unaccompanied, drive his or her own car, or arrange his or her travel via taxi.[16]

Oral Status

Not only is the ability to select, secure, and prepare foods important, but adequate oral health is also essential for the ingestion of these foods. Therefore an assessment of the oral status of older adults is considered a critical feature of a nutritional status evaluation. The most common dental diseases and conditions in older persons are **dental caries,** advanced **gingivitis,** inflammation of the periodontium because of dryness of the mouth, and oral lesions, including oral cancer.[4]

Oral screening can define the presence or absence of difficulties in chewing and/or swallowing food. The screening instrument chosen can be used to determine reasons for chewing difficulties, such as poorly fitting dentures, absence of teeth, a sore mouth, swollen gums, glossitis (red tongue without papillae), ulcers in the mouth, paralytic disease involving the face, and/or dry mouth. A more comprehensive assessment of both dentition and oral mucosa requires a dentist, preferably one who specializes in geriatric dentistry.

Mental/Cognitive Status

In general, nearly 4% of older adults suffer from unrecognized dementia or chronic cognitive impairment.[4] **Cognitive status** refers to an individual's intellectual capability and includes areas such as memory, language, reading, and writing, and orientation to time, place, and person. Changed or diminished cognitive status can serve as an indicator of a nutritional problem.[19] The **Folstein Mini-Mental State Examination** is considered by expert panels as the best screening procedure.[4] This validated instrument has been used to detect **dementia,** which is responsible for most of the loss of cognitive function. Unfortunately, it is useful only in English-speaking populations.

Depression should also be regarded as an indicator of malnutrition because it can result in loss of appetite and inadequate food intake. It can be caused by metabolic disorders; drug toxicity; dehydration; protein-energy malnutrition; loss of spouse, sibling, and/or child; and/or change in lifestyle. Several useful screening instruments for depression are available.* Few data are available on either the best methods for screening for depression in the elderly or the accuracy of screening.

METHODS OF DIETARY ASSESSMENT
Prospective versus Retrospective Methods

With a **prospective** method of dietary assessment, records of food intake are obtained at the time food is consumed. **Retrospective** methods, however, rely on the ability of the person to recall food intake in the past and therefore rely on memory.[15]

Prospective Method

Food diary or record. A **food diary** is a record of what is eaten made at the time of consumption. The errors associated with memory laspe are less with this method than with retrospective methods. This method requires more motivated and literate older adults who are able to hold a pen or pencil and write. The older adult needs to be instructed on how to record food intake and estimate portion sizes. Providing measuring aids to assist in estimating portions is recommended. Records must be checked by trained interviewers for completeness before nutrient analysis. With the food diary, food intakes may be altered during reporting periods. In fact, underreporting is common. In a study conducted by Abernethy and Fanelli Kuczmarski,[1] a group of 36 women, ages 65 to 88 years (mean age = 72.5), recorded 4 days of food intake successfully. This group was highly educated, with 36% completing more than 17 years of education and another 36% completing

---

*References 3,7,48,49,61,62.

14 to 16 years of education. These women stated that they did not feel this method was burdensome or time consuming.

Although 7-day records are considered to provide the most representative summary of usual food intake, obtaining usable records beyond 4 days is often difficult because of respondent burden. Hence, the validity of the 7-day record to assess usual intakes of elderly persons is questioned.[18]

Retrospective Methods

24-hour food recall. The 24-hour recall method is one in which an individual recalls all the foods and beverages consumed in the previous 24 hours. Because the **respondent** burden is low and the time for administration is short, this method is widely accepted. Unlike the food diary, intakes are not consciously altered. Typically, individuals forget snack items, sweets, and alcohol. Therefore trained interviewers need to be able to probe without leading the respondent. In general, the 24-hour recall record tends to underestimate mean intakes of older adults.[9,33] A recent study[10] reported that recall of foods eaten was significantly improved when elderly persons were notified that they would be asked to report intake from the previous day.

It is widely recognized that a single 24-hour recall record does not represent an individual's usual intake. Serial 24-hour recall records are needed to provide an estimate of usual intakes of individuals.

Food Frequency Questionnaires

Generally, **food frequency questionnaires** provide a qualitative description of how often foods are eaten in a specific period. They are easy to standardize and do not require highly trained interviewers for administration. In fact, many are self-administered by persons who can read. Respondent burden is low, provided the number of food items listed is limited.

Food frequency questionnaires are extremely useful for describing food intake patterns for diet and meal planning, for studying the associations of types of foods and disease, and for developing nutrition education programs. However, they provide only limited information about energy and selected nutrient in-

takes because portion sizes usually are not obtained. Despite this limitation, Smiciklas-Wright and associates[55] noted the need for a valid and reliable food frequency questionnaire for assessing food intake of homebound older adults.

Obtaining information on total food consumption is difficult with food frequency questionnaires because some foods are not included on the lists. A controversial issue is the length of time that can be recalled. Food frequency questionnaires probably should not go beyond 30 days. As with the 24-hour recall method, the individual's ability to remember affects the accuracy of this method.

Semiquantified food frequency questionnaires (or simplified dietary history) include an estimate of the amounts of foods consumed, along with their frequency of use. This method can be administered by professional nutritionists or other health workers, or it can be self-administered. Development of a semiquantified food frequency questionnaire for older adults has been described in detail by Hankin.[20] Photographs of small-, medium-, and large-portion sizes of foods were used to estimate quantities. She has demonstrated that this method produces both valid and reliable results for this population group.

Dietary History

The Burke-type **dietary history** method provides a more complete and detailed description of both qualitative and quantitative aspects of food intake than do food diaries, 24-hour recall records, or food frequency questionnaires. Dietary intakes obtained by this method correlate well with other measures of nutritional status. Unfortunately, it is time consuming (1 to 2 hours) and requires a highly trained nutritionist or dietitian and highly motivated participants. The required in-depth interview includes describing a typical's day eating pattern, occasional alternative foods, usual portion sizes, and any irregularities. A detailed list of foods is then reviewed as a cross-check to verify the eating pattern. The respondent also keeps a 3-day measured food record. All of this information is used to derive a usual daily food intake. This method is vunerable to memory lapses and psychologic tendencies to exaggerate or minimize self-described behavior.[34]

DIETARY ASSESSMENT

The first stage of a nutrient deficiency is generally identified by a dietary evaluation. The dietary evaluation should not only assess food consumption patterns, but also assess food security/insecurity, food storage and cooking facilities, and use of therapeutic diets. **Food insecurity** is defined either as the limited or uncertain availability of nutritionally adequate and safe foods or as the limited or uncertain ability to acquire acceptable foods in socially acceptable ways.[2] In contrast, food security means all people have access to enough food for an active, healthy life at all times.[2] Roe[51] recommended that food insecurity be assessed when surveying homebound older adults because Title III-C meals usually are not available on weekends. Examples of questions that can be asked to judge food security are found in the accompanying box.

Before selecting a dietary assessment method, the following basic questions need to be answered.

- What is the objective of the assessment?
- Why is the dietary assessment being conducted?
- What needs to be assessed—foods and/or energy and selected nutrients?
- How precise does the assessment need to be?

If the objective of the assessment is to determine whether the diet of a group of free-living older adults is meeting the Dietary Guidelines for Americans, a quantified food frequency questionnaire would be satisfactory. However, if the objective is to compare the energy and nutrient intakes of individuals who participate in a congregate meal program with nonparticipants, 24-hour dietary recalls would be the preferred method. Dietary records of multiple days would be appropriate when studying the relationship between nutrient intakes and food-related attitudes.

Several issues related to the target audience also need to be considered when selecting a method. These issues include respondent burden, level of education and literacy of the individuals, and the degree of willingness and motivation of the individuals to cooperate. Respondent burden refers to the time spent for all aspects of the assessment, including the time required to be interviewed or to complete questionnaires and travel time to the site where the measurements are taken, if not in the home.

Obviously, the method chosen should be both reliable and valid, as well as cost-effective. A reliable method is one that generates typical intake patterns that are representative of the individual or group. **Validity** refers to accuracy. A valid method will generate a "true" estimate of intake. Except in a metabolic laboratory setting where all food can be weighed and consumption levels closely monitored, measurement of food intake tends to be imprecise. It depends highly on the skill and patience of the interviewer and the understanding and cooperation of the individual being interviewed. Natow and Heslin[43] have published guidelines for dietary assessment interviewing that help ensure a successful session. A skilled interviewer will listen carefully, not interrupt the older adult unnecessarily, and allow sufficient time for the older adult to think and respond fully. The interviewer must not be judgemental or express ei-

---

❖

SAMPLE FOOD SECURITY QUESTIONS

1. During the past month, did you skip any meals because there was not enough food or money to buy food?
2. How many days in the past month did you skip any meals because there was not enough food or money to buy food?
3. Which of the following reasons explain why you had this problem?
   a. You did not have transportation.
   b. You did not have working appliances for storing or preparing foods, such as a stove or refrigerator.
   c. You did not have access to a congregrate meal site or home meal delivery program.

ther approval or disapproval at the older adult's responses. Another aspect to remember when interviewing older adults is to speak slowly and loudly if the elderly person has a hearing impairment. In addition, the interviewer should use simple and easy-to-understand language and take time to explain unfamiliar terms.

Information obtained during a dietary assessment may be incomplete or not reflect usual intakes. Regardless of the method used, some persons may attempt to please the interviewer rather than report his or her actual intake. For example, persons may underreport desserts and sweets or forget to mention alcoholic beverages. In addition, sometimes the foods consumed, particularly ethnic foods, may not be included in the nutrient data bases used to analyze diets for energy and nutrient content.

Assessing dietary intakes of older adults can be difficult because of impaired memory, reduced appetite, language barriers in selected ethnic groups, and low educational level. In some instances, reliable information must be obtained from a caregiver.[54] No firm evidence exists that long-term memory of diet is affected adversely in advancing age. Hankin[20] and Byers[8] reported that older adults, 70 years of age and older, performed as well as those less than 70 years of age in recalling food intakes. The ability to recall past dietary intakes may depend more on the person's awareness of what is consumed than age per se. Some persons eat almost mechanically, without thought to the types and amounts of food items consumed. This phenomenon has been suggested to occur more in men than in women, who plan, prepare, and serve meals. When interviewing older men at home, it is beneficial to have the spouse present to assist in providing details about foods eaten at home.

Evaluation of Dietary Data

The food intake of individuals or groups can be evaluated against various standards of adequacy. The **Dietary Guidelines for Americans**[57] and the report entitled, "Diet and Health: Implications for Reducing Chronic Disease Risk"[41] included recommendations to achieve an optimal and highly desirable dietary pattern

for maintaining good health. This diet should provide the following.

- $< 30\%$ of energy from total fat
- $< 10\%$ of energy from saturated fat
- $\leq 10\%$ of energy from polyunsaturated fatty acids
- < 300 mg/day of cholesterol
- $> 55\%$ of energy from carbohydrates, especially complex sources
- < 6 g salt/day
- < 1 ounce alcohol/day

Food practices can be evaluated against the **Food Guide Pyramid.**[24] As shown in Fig. 11-4 and the accompanying box, the pyramid is an outline of the types and amounts, (i.e., number of servings) of foods to eat each day. The actual

---

❖

FOOD GUIDE PYRAMID: SERVING SIZES

- *Bread, Cereal, Rice, and Pasta*
1 slice of bread
1 ounce of ready-to-eat cereal
½ cup of cooked cereal, rice, or pasta
- *Vegetable*
1 cup of raw, leafy vegetables
½ cup of other vegetables, cooked or chopped raw
¾ cup of vegetable juice
- *Fruit*
1 medium apple, banana, orange
½ cup of chopped, cooked, or canned fruit
¾ cup of fruit juice
- *Milk, Yogurt, and Cheese*
1 cup of milk or yogurt
1½ ounces of natural cheese
2 ounces of process cheese
- *Meat, Poultry, Fish, Dry Beans, Eggs, and Nuts*
2 to 3 ounces of cooked lean meat, poultry, or fish
½ cup of cooked dry beans, 1 egg, or 2 tablespoons of peanut butter count as 1 ounce of lean meat

From Human Nutrition Information Service: *USDA's food guide pyramid, Home and Garden Bull 249* Hyattsville, 1992, U.S.D.A.

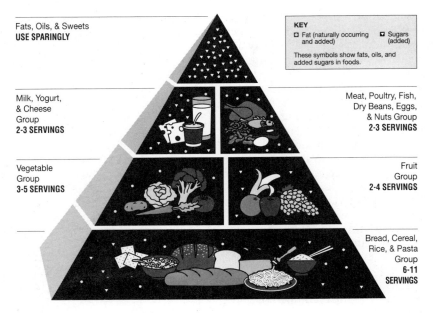

KEY
- □ Fat (naturally occurring and added)
- ☑ Sugars (added)

These symbols show fats, oils, and added sugars in foods.

Fats, Oils, & Sweets
USE SPARINGLY

Milk, Yogurt, & Cheese Group
2-3 SERVINGS

Meat, Poultry, Fish, Dry Beans, Eggs, & Nuts Group
2-3 SERVINGS

Vegetable Group
3-5 SERVINGS

Fruit Group
2-4 SERVINGS

Bread, Cereal, Rice, & Pasta Group
6-11 SERVINGS

FIG. 11-4   Food guide pyramid.

From Human Nutrition Information Service: USDA's food guide pyramid, *Home and Garden Bull 249,* Hyattsville, 1992, United States Department of Agriculture.

number of servings a person should consume depends on his or her energy needs. Consuming the lowest number of servings for each food group provides approximately 1600 kcal. This energy level is appropriate for some older adults. Consuming the midpoint of the range of servings for each major food group provides about 2200 kcal, and the highest number of servings provides approximately 2800 kcal.[24]

Energy and nutrient intakes can be compared to the RDA.[42] Except for energy, most of the recommended levels for essential nutrients provide a margin of safety. Some researchers compare nutrient intakes from dietary assessments to 100% of the RDA. If an older adult has nutrient intakes at or above 100% of the RDA, it is very likely that his or her nutrient needs are being met. Other researchers consider 67% of the RDA value to be adequate. An older adult consuming between 67% and 100% of the

RDA may be at risk for inadequate intakes. Consuming less than 67% of the RDA increases one's risk for nutritional problems and, in that situation, additional measures of nutritional status should be evaluated to verify a suspected nutritional problem.

APPLICATIONS OF NUTRITIONAL ASSESSMENT

Selecting nutritional indicators to assess nutritional status depends on several factors. These include the objective of the assessment, the amount of time available for the assessment, and the level of personnel and money available to support the evaluation. Biochemical assessments generally involve invasive techniques and can be time-consuming and expensive because of the cost related to the personnel required to

TABLE 11-7 *Recommended Indicators for Nutritional Status for Various Settings*

	Free-Living*	Adult Day Care Center	Congregate Feeding Site	Long-Term Care Facilities	Hospital
Anthropometric					
Weight	X	X	X	X	X
Height	X	X	X	X	X
Biochemical	X			X	X
Clinical					
Signs and symptoms				X	X
Functional status	X	X	X	X	X
Cognitive status	X	X	X	X	X
Drug use	X	X	X	X	X
Dietary					
Intake	X	X	X	X	X
Food security	X		X		
Supplement use	X	X	X	X	X
Food preferences	X	X	X	X	X

*Older adults residing in community but not participating in congregate meal site program or adult day care centers.

draw blood samples and to perform the assays. In comparison, anthropometric measurements can be easily obtained by trained personnel with relatively inexpensive tools. In addition, scales, calipers, height boards, and measuring tapes are transportable. If the objective is to obtain baseline data and then monitor the nutritional status of older adults in a day-care facility on a limited budget, the choice of indicators could be a 24-hour food recall, body weight and height measurements, and questionnaires dealing with eating practices, food preferences, presence of chronic diseases, and use of prescription drugs. Table 11-7 identifies indicators for assessments for nutritional status in various settings.

In summary, remember the special considerations when performing nutritional assessments of older adults. The normal process of aging, the presence of chronic conditions or diseases, and the frequent use of prescription drugs can affect the interpretation of nutritional assessment data. Selected nutritional status methods and standards are available for older adults, al-

though they may require some refinement to meet the special considerations of some older adults, as documented in this chapter.

REVIEW QUESTIONS

1. What are the definitions of nutrition assessment, nutrition surveillance, and nutrition screening? When is it appropriate to use each method? Why does nutrition assessment pose a problem for practitioners in collecting and evaluating data on older persons?
2. What is the Nutrition Screening Initiative? What are the definitions of nutritional status, marginal nutritional status, malnutrition, undernutrition, overnutrition, and nutritional imbalance? Why is nutrition screening important?
3. What is anthropometry and what anthropometric techniques are useful in assessing the elderly? How can aging influence body measurements? What is relative weight for height? Why are circumference measurements useful in nutritional assessment of older persons?
4. What are the most reliable biochemical indicators of protein-energy malnutrition in the elderly? Why is the identification of iron deficiency impor-

tant in older persons? What laboratory tests are most useful for identification of iron-deficiency anemia? Why is functional and cognitive assessment an important part of clinical assessment in the elderly?

5. What are the differences between prospective and retrospective methods for collecting and assessing food intake information? What are the advantages and disadvantages of each type of method? What guidelines are useful for evaluating dietary intake information?

SUGGESTED LEARNING ACTIVITIES

1. Ask the director of a senior center if you may conduct a nutrition screening clinic. Half of the class should use the Nutritional Risk Index (the box on pg. 259) and half of the class should use the Determine Your Nutritional Health checklist (Fig. 11-1). Debate the benefits of each in a formal class debate.

2. As part of your nutrition screening clinic, obtain heights and weights using the various methods discussed in this chapter. Record the difficulties you had in obtaining these data in an older population. With these data, calculate body mass index and identify which participants were at risk for health problems associated with being underweight or overweight.

3. Go to the library and find all the reference tables for triceps skinfolds, mid-arm circumferences, and mid-arm muscle circumferences that have been published. Prepare a report with a copy of the tables to use as a reference for future work with older populations.

4. Using the guidelines for interviewing older people, interview one older person using two of the methods for collecting dietary intake data discussed in this chapter. Ask permission to record the interview session and have your instructor critique your interviewing skills.

Key Terms

Provided here for review is a list of the major terms in this chapter. The definitions can be found in the Glossary, which begins on p. 336. To help you understand how these terms are applied, the page number is given for the first mention of each term in the chapter.

abdominal fat, 264
acromial process, 261
Activities of Daily Living (ADLs), 273

ambulatory, 262
American Academy of Family Physicians, 259
American Dietetic Association, 259
angular stomatitis, 271
anemia, 258
anthropometric, 255
antigen, 267
Beck Depression Index, 260
bioelectrical impedance analysis (BIA), 266
Body Mass Index (BMI), 258
cataract, 273
cognitive status, 274
condyles, 261
congestive heart failure, 267
congregate meal program, 259
dementia, 274
dental caries, 274
Determine Your Nutritional Health checklist, 258
Dietary Guidelines for Americans, 277
dietary history, 275
diuretic, 258
dowager's hump, 261
edema, 261
erythrocyte, 267
erythrocyte protoporphyrin, 269
femur, 261
ferritin, 269
folate, 269
Folstein Mini-Mental State Examination, 274
food diary, 274
food frequency questionnaire, 275
Food Guide Pyramid, 277
food insecurity, 276
Geriatric Depression Scale, 260
gingivitis, 274
glossitis, 271
granulocytes, 267
hemoglobin, 258
high-density lipoprotein (HDL), 264
Hodgkin's disease, 269
home delivered meals program, 259
hypoferremia, 269

REFERENCES

1. Abernethy MM, Fanelli Kuczmarski M: Food intake and food-related attitudes of older women: implications for nutrition education, *J Nutr Ed* (in press).

2. Anderson SA: *Core indicators of nutritional state for difficult-to-sample populations,* Besthesda, MD, 1990, Life Sciences Research Office, Federation of American Societies for Experimental Biology.

3. Beck AT, Beck RW: Screening depressed patients in family practice: a rapid technique, *Postgrad Med* December, page 81, 1972.

4. Beers MM, Fink A, Beck JC: Screening recommendations for the elderly, *Am J Public Health* 81:1131, 1991.

5. Bjorntorp P: Obesity and the risk of cardiovascular disease, *Ann Clin Res* 17:3, 1985.

6. Blackburn GL, et al: Nutrition in metabolic assessment of the hospitalized patient, *J Parenteral and Enteral Nutr* 1:11, 1977.

7. Burman MA, et al: Development of a brief screening instrument for detecting depressive disorders, *Med Care* 26:775, 1988.

8. Byers TE, et al: Dietary history from the distant past: a methodological study, *Nutr Cancer* 5:69, 1983.

9. Campbell VA, Dodds ML: Collecting dietary information from groups of older people, *J Am Diet Assoc* 51:29, 1967.

10. Chianetta MM, Head MK: Effect of prior notification on accuracy of dietary recall by the elderly, *J Am Diet Assoc* 92:741, 1992.

11. Chumlea WC, Guo S: Equations for predicting stature in white and black elderly individuals, *J Gerontol* 47:197, 1992.

12. Chumlea WC, Roche AF, Steinbaugh ML: Estimating stature from knee height for persons 60 to 90 years of age, *J Am Geriat Soc* 33:116, 1985.

13. Chumlea WC, Roche AF, Mukherjee D: Some anthropometric indices of body composition for elderly adults, *J Gerontol* 41:36, 1986.

14. Cornoni-Huntley JC, et al: An overview of body weight of older persons, including impact on mortality, *J Clin Epidemiol* 44:743, 1991.

15. Deurenberg P, et al: Assessment of body composition by bioelectrical impedance in a population aged >60 yrs, *Am J Clin Nutr* 51:3, 1990.

16. Dwyer, JT: Assessment of dietary intake. In Shils ME, Young VR, eds: *Modern nutrition in health and disease*, ed 7 Philadelphia, 1988, Lea & Febiger.

17. Dwyer JT: *Screening older American's nutritional health: current practice and future possibilities*, Washington, DC, 1991, Nutrition Screening Initiative.

18. Frisancho AR: New standards of weight and body composition by frame size and height for assessment of nutritional status of adults and elderly, *Am J Clin Nutr* 40:808, 1984.

19. Gibson RA: *Principles of nutritional assessment*, New York, 1990, Oxford University Press.

20. Goodwin JS, Goodwin JM, Garry PJ: Association between nutritional status and cognitive functioning in a healthy elderly population, *J Am Med Assoc* 249:2917, 1983.

21. Hankin JH: Development of a diet history questionnaire for studies of older persons, *Am J Clin Nutr* 50:1121, 1989.

22. Herbert V: The 1986 Herman Award Lecture. Nutrition science as a continually unfolding story: the folate and vitamin B_{12} paradigm, *Am J Clin Nutr* 46:387, 1987.

23. Heymsfield SB, Williams PJ: Nutritional assessment by clinical and biochemical methods. In Shils ME, Young VR, eds: *Modern nutrition in health and disease*, ed 7, Philadelphia, 1988, Lea & Febiger.

24. Heymsfield SB, et al: Anthropometric assessment of adult protein-energy malnutrition. In Wright RA, Hemysfield S, McMan CB, eds: *Nutritional assessment*, Boston, 1984, Blackwell Scientific Publications.

25. Human Nutrition Information Service: *USDA's food guide pyramid, Home and Garden Bull 249*, Hyattsville, MD, 1992, US Department of Agriculture.

26. Jeor ST, Scott BJ: "Weight" as a clinical indicator: adults, *Top Clin Nutr* 7:44, 1991.

27. Johnson MA: Iron: nutrition monitoring and nutrition status assessment, *J Nutr* 120:1486, 1990.

28. Kubena KS, et al: Anthropometry and health in the elderly, *J Am Diet Assoc* 91:1402, 1991.

29. Kuczmarski RJ: Need for body composition information in elderly subjects, *Am J Clin Nutr* 50:1150, 1989.

30. Kwok T, Whitelaw MN: The use of armspan in nutritional assessment of the elderly, *J Am Geriatr Soc* 39:492, 1991.

31. Life Sciences Research Office, Federation of American Societies for Experimental Biology: *Nutrition monitoring in the United States: an update report on nutrition monitoring*. DSSH Publication No (PHS) 89-1255, Washington, DC, 1989, US Government Printing Office.

32. Lipschitz DA, Mitchell CO: Nutritional assessment of the elderly—special considerations. In Wright RA, Hemysfield S, McMan CB, eds: *Nutritional assessment*, Boston, 1984, Blackwell Scientific Publications.

33. Lohman TG, Roche AF, Martorell R, eds: *Anthropometric standardization reference manual*, Champaign, Ill, 1988, Human Kinetics Books.

34. Madden JP, Goodman SJ, Guthrie HA: Validity of the 24-hr. recall: analysis of data obtained from elderly subjects, *J Am Diet Assoc* 68:143, 1976.

35. Mahalko JR, et al: Comparison of dietary histories and seven-day food records in a nutritional assessment of older adults, *Am J Clin Nutr* 42:542, 1985.

36. Master AM, Lasser RP, Beckman G: Tables of average weight and height of Americans aged 65 to 94 years, *J Am Med Assoc* 172:658, 1960.

37. *1983 Metropolitan height and weight tables, Statistical Bull* 64:2, 1983, Metropolitan Life Insurance Company.

38. Mitchell CO, Lipschitz DA: Detection of protein-calorie malnutrition in the elderly, *Am J Clin Nutr* 35:398, 1982.

39. Mitchell CO, Lipschitz DA: The effect of age and sex on the routinely used measurements to assess the nutritional status of hospitalized patients, *Am J Clin Nutr* 36:340, 1982.

40. Najjar MF, Rowland M: *Anthropometric reference data and prevalence of overweight, United States, 1976-80*, Vital and Health Statistics, Series 11, No 238, DHHS Publication No (PHS) 87-1688, Washington, DC, 1987, US Government Printing Office.

41. *National Institutes of Health expert panel on detec-*

tion, evaluation, and treatment of high blood cholesterol in adults, Bestheda, MD, 1987, National
Heart, Lung and Blood Institute.
42. National Research Council: *Diet and health: implications for reducing chronic disease risk*, Washington, DC, 1989, National Academy Press.
43. National Research Council: *Recommended dietary
allowances*, ed 10, Washington, DC, 1989, National Academy Press.
44. Natow AB, Heslin J: *Nutritional care of the older
adult*, New York, 1986, Macmillan Publishing.
45. *Nutrition interventions manual for professionals
caring for older Americans*, Washington, DC,
1992, The Nutrition Screening Initiative.
46. *Nutrition screening manual for professionals caring
for older Americans*, Washington, DC, 1991, The
Nutrition Screening Initiative.
47. Ostlund RE, et al: The ratio of waist-to-hip circumference, plasma insulin level, and glucose intolerance as independent predictors of the HDL_2
cholesterol level in older adults, *N Engl J Med*
322:229, 1990.
48. Pilch SM, Senti FR, eds: *Assessment of the iron
nutritional status of the US population based on
data collected in the second National Health and
Nutrition Examination Survey, 1976-80*, Besthesda, MD, 1984, Life Sciences Research Office, Federation of the American Societies for
Experimental Biology.
49. Radloff LS: The CES-D scale: a self-report depression scale for research in the general population, *Appl Psychiatr Meas* 1:385, 1977.
50. Robins LN, et al: National Institute of Mental
Health diagnostic interview schedule: its history,
characteristics and validity, *Arch Gen Psychiatry*
38:381, 1981.
51. Roe DA: *Geriatric nutrition*, ed 3, Englewood
Cliffs, NJ, 1992, Prentice Hall.
52. Roe DA: In-home nutritional assessment of in-
ner-city elderly, *J Nutr* 120:1538, 1990.
53. Roe D: Nutritional assessment of the elderly,
World Rev Nutr Diet 48:85, 1986.
54. Rudman D, Feller AG: Protein-calorie undernutrition in the nursing home. *J Am Geriatr Soc*
37:173, 1989.
55. Samet JM: Surrogate measures of dietary intake,
Am J Clin Nutr 50:39, 1989.
56. Smiciklas-Wright H, et al: Nutritional assessment of homebound rural elderly, *J Nutr*
120:1535, 1990.
57. Svendsen OL, et al: Measurement of body fat in
elderly subjects by dual-energy-x-ray absorptiometry, bioelectrical impedance, and anthropometry, *Am J Clin Nutr* 53:1117, 1991.
58. United States Department of Agriculture and
Department of Health and Human Services:
*Nutrition and your health: dietary guidelines for
americans*, ed 3, Washington, DC, 1990, US
Government Printing Office.
59. United States Department of Health and Human Services and Department of Agriculture:
*Nutrition monitoring in the United States: a
progress report from the joint nutrition monitoring
evaluation committee*, DSSH Publication No
(PHS) 86-1255, Washington, DC, 1986, US
Government Printing Office.
60. White JV, et al: Nutrition screening initiative:
development and implementation of the public
awareness checklist and screening tools, *J Am
Diet Assoc* 92:163, 1992.
61. Wolinsky FD, et al: Progress in the development
of a nutritional risk index, *J Nutr* 120:1549,
1990.
62. Yesavage JA, et al: Development and validation
of a geriatric depression screening scale: a preliminary report, *J Psychiat Res* 17:37, 1983.
63. Zung WW: A self rating depression scale, *Arch
Gen Psychiatr* 12:63, 1965.

12 Food Selection Patterns Among the Aged

Marsha Read
Eleanor D. Schlenker

Objectives

✛✛

After studying the chapter, the student should:

✔ *Recognize how the aging process influences food selection.*

✔ *Identify changes in the marketplace that affect food choices by older persons.*

✔ *Understand the psychologic, physiologic, and sociologic factors influencing food selection by the elderly.*

✔ *Identify the effect of income on food choice in the elderly.*

✔ *List methods of feeding and nutrition support practices for the functionally impaired elderly.*

Introduction

Many aspects of people's lives change as they grow older. They retire from full-time employment, allowing time for new interests, social activities, and recreational pursuits. They may develop health problems necessitating changes in their dietary, exercise, or living patterns. They may move to a senior housing complex offering a wide variety of social opportunities. Food patterns and resources change and adapt, just as other components of the older adult's life-style respond to changes in leisure time, income, health status, and personal needs. All these factors are important in helping older individuals select appropriate foods.

FOOD SELECTION AS A CONTINUUM

Influences on Food Selection

Although food intake has nutritional significance, it has great social and emotional significance as well. Angulo[1] puts forth the idea that not only do we eat to live, we also eat to achieve health, to derive pleasure, and to express our cultural or ethnic heritage. Our selection, preparation, and consumption of food are shaped by psychological and social values. Food takes on meaning other than as mere substance; food is transformed into such categories as "edible" or "healthy."[1] Such food meanings appear to translate into action. McIntosh and coworkers[67] found that elderly individuals who assigned a health value to foods and compared "health foods" to "regular foods" actually had higher vitamin intakes than those who did not hold such health food beliefs. In an older person, food patterns reflect lifelong attitudes and habits as influenced by the changing environment. To better understand the influence of life-style, health, and economic status on food choices, individual factors have been identified and evaluated in older adults. Such factors are in the accompanying box.

Although each of these factors may be considered singly, all act in combination. The older woman who has enjoyed food preparation and prided herself on "cooking from scratch" will face a dilemma as worsening arthritis makes it more difficult to shop for and prepare food. Possible alternatives for her are using the motorized carts available in many larger supermarkets, substituting more preprepared items that require less work, relying on home-delivered meals, or relocating to another type of living situation where communal dining opportunities are afforded. If a spouse is present, he or she may be able to take over some food responsibilities. Helping older people solve their food problems often involves seeking alternatives and doing things differently from the usual practice.

Changes in Lifelong Food Patterns

From a life span perspective, human behavior, including nutrition behavior, is constantly undergoing transition, adaptation, and change.[1] Consequently, the later years can be characterized as a period of continual adjustment to new situations, such as a changing family size as children leave home and establish their own households. With the change in family size, food patterns may also change. The mother who traditionally prepared a large batch of spaghetti sauce for her active family of four

---

❖

INFLUENCES ON FOOD CHOICES

- *Psychological factors*
Social activity
Self-esteem
Nutrition knowledge
Perceived health benefit
Loneliness
Bereavement
Symbolism of food
Mental awareness
Food aversion
Food faddism
- *Physiologic factors*
Appetite
Taste acuity
Olfactory acuity
Dental status
Prescribed diets
Chronic disease
Food intolerance
Health status
Physical status (based on activities of daily living [ADLs] and instrumental activities of daily living [IADLs])
Physical exercise
Use of drugs (prescribed and over the counter)
- *Socioeconomic factors*
Age
Sex
Income
Cooking facilities
Daily schedule
Retirement/leisure time
Education
Distance to food store
Availability of transportation
Availability of familiar foods

---

children may not have the inclination to reduce the recipe to accommodate just herself and her spouse once the children have left home.

Loss of income at retirement or upon the death of a spouse also imposes a period of transition and adaptation. Alternatively, retirement allows time for participating in hobbies or rewarding community service. Retirement may also open up opportunities for more socialization involving food, such as taking part in a **congregate meal program** or regularly meeting other retirees or friends for a simple breakfast at a local fast food restaurant "now that we don't have to punch a clock and be at work at a certain time." Social interaction may actually increase and result in more snacking, with a higher overall food intake or a higher intake of particular types of food.

For older people, life is more a continuation of previous habits than a change.[96] Kivett and Scott[46] found that elderly people who perceived themselves as being in good health had not significantly altered their food habits since midlife. Yet elderly individuals who had expressed concern about their health had changed their diets in such ways as to reduce fats and total quantities of food. For them, changes in health status motivated changes in lifelong food habits. Other writers[56] have discussed the potential for change in food habits and food patterns brought about by technology. In light of the new options presented by microwave ovens, food processors, and more and more prepared foods, Letsou and Price[56] pose the question, "Will some older people have to be retaught to cook?"

The diet of the older individual reflects traditional food patterns and the current food supply. Contrary to popular opinion, older people do try new foods and adapt to changing food situations. The mere fact of their survival points to their ability to select a reasonably adequate diet over a period of time.[96] Advancing age, however, does lead to changes in food intake. Although these changes can be detrimental to nutritional status, this is not always the case. Some older individuals consume very limited types and amounts of food, but such a pattern is not typical of this age group, and when it does occur, it usually is the result of very extenuating circumstances. For most older people, there are positive aspects of the diet to serve as a foundation for any further improvement required.

AGE AND FOOD INTAKE
Level of Food Intake

Normal aging brings about a decrease in both calorie requirements and the quantity of food consumed.[25,100-102] The National Food Consumption Survey (NFCS)[101] confirmed these observations. For men, peak caloric consumption occurred between the ages 20 and 29, with a mean intake of 2,501 kcal, and declined to 1,875 kcal by age 70. The highest caloric consumption among women, 1,634 kcal, occurred between the ages of 20 and 29 and declined to 1,386 kcal by age 70 (Fig. 12-1). Blacks had lower caloric intakes than their white counterparts at all ages.

A recent evaluation of diet records gathered from the **Baltimore Longitudinal Study of Aging (BLSA)**[39] between 1960 and 1987 indicated changing trends in energy intake. In the 1960s older men had lower caloric intakes than younger men, but this was not evident in the 1970s and 1980s. In these men protein intake remained fairly stable, at about 15% to 16% of total energy, although kilocalories obtained from fat declined from 42% to 34%, and kilocalories from carbohydrate increased from 39% to 44%. Cholesterol intake declined by 255 mg a day over this period. This finding implies that older as well as younger individuals are attempting to reduce their intake of fat and adopt more positive dietary practices. However, the men who participated in the BLSA tended to be well educated and economically advantaged and were not necessarily representative of the general population.

In contrast to the BLSA, the NFCS data[101] indicate little change over adulthood in the contribution of particular macronutrients to total caloric intake. Among both sexes the percentage of kilocalories from protein was relatively consistent, ranging from 16% to 17% from ages 19 to 75 and older. The percentage of kilocalories from carbohydrate rose slightly in both sexes, from 42% to 43% in men and from 43% to 45% in women. The percentage of kilocalories from fat remained at approximately 41% in all male cohorts. Women demonstrated a slight decline in fat intake, from 40% to 39%, between ages 19 to 22 and 75 and over. These

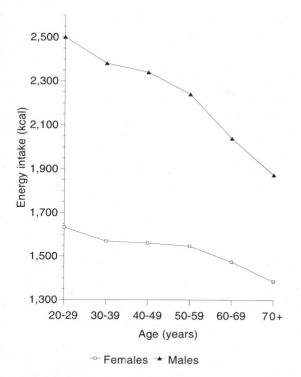

‑‑□‑‑ Females ‑‑▲‑‑ Males

FIG. 12-1 Energy intakes decline in both sexes over adulthood but decrease to a greater extent in males than in females.

Data from US Department of Health and Human Services, US Department of Agriculture: *Nutrition monitoring in the United States: an update report on nutrition monitoring,* DHHS Pub No (PHS) 89-1255, Washington, DC, 1989, US Government Printing Office.

data were collected in 1977-1978, however, and may not represent current trends.

A recent report from the Georgia Centenarian Study[44] indicated that people age 100 or over, living in the community, had a mean energy intake of 1,581 kcal and obtained 42% of their kilocalories from fat. In comparison, individuals ages 60 to 69 and 80 to 89 from the same geographic area had caloric intakes of 1,605 and 1,423 kcal, respectively, and obtained 40% and 37% percent of their total energy from fat. Although the number of centenarians interviewed was small (22), it is interesting to note that all had stable body weights

throughout adulthood despite their rather high fat intakes.

Patterns of Food Intake

Older people decrease their energy intakes; however, they continue to select **nutrient-dense foods**. A survey of 372 Wisconsin households[90] found that the older households (individuals age 65 or older) used less milk, but the same amount of meat, more fruits and vegetables, and more breads and cereals than younger households. The 65 and older age group reported a mean of 0.8 servings a day from the dairy group, in contrast to the 1.2 servings indicated by the 25 to 34 age group. With respect to breads and cereals, the younger group reported an average of 2.7 servings a day, whereas the 65 and older group had an average of 3.2 servings. A similar pattern existed for fruits and vegetables; the younger households had a mean of 2.6 and the older households 3.1 servings a day. Members of the older households were also less likely to skip meals and ate more nutritious breakfasts.

Some older adults decrease their caloric intake by cutting back on all foods normally eaten rather than selectively reducing intake.[28] The detrimental effect of this practice on diet quality was apparent in two groups of women with mean ages of 72 and 81 and caloric intakes of 2,074 and 1,674 kcal, respectively.[28] Protein intake decreased from 53 to 48 g, calcium from 924 to 760 mg, and iron from 11.3 to 8 mg. Among the older subjects in the Georgia study,[44] protein intake was 66 g in the 60 to 69 age group, 58 g in the 80 to 89 group, and 52 g in those age 100 or older.

Milk and other dairy foods contribute 77% of the calcium in the U.S. food supply,[77] as well as protein, vitamin D, vitamin A, and riboflavin; hence, a decrease in consumption of dairy products, as was noted in the older Wisconsin households, affects not only calcium status but other nutrient levels as well. Selecting protein foods relatively low in fat allows a reduction in energy intake, yet ensures adequate B-complex vitamins, iron, and zinc. Whole-grain products add valuable vitamins and trace minerals to the diet as caloric needs decline.

Foods that contain primarily simple carbohydrates and fat (e.g., sweet baked items, soft drinks, crackers, alcoholic beverages) should be the first items to be deleted from the diet. Food preparation methods that add additional kilocalories in the form of fat or rich sauces should be avoided.

Food patterns also differ among the older and younger segments of the over-60 population. Fischer and coworkers[32] found that people age 60 to 70 made more healthful food selections than those in the 75 to 85 age group. The "young" seniors consumed more high-fiber breads, pasta, and rice and more fresh and frozen vegetables. The "older" seniors reported fewer low-fat milk products and more high-fat cheeses, pastries, pies, and cakes compared to the 60 to 70 age group. The "young" seniors also made healthy choices in their selection of more unsaturated fats and reduced-calorie or low-fat salad dressings. The one category in which the older group demonstrated a more favorable food selection pattern was in their preference for lean meat.

The influence of educational level and health beliefs on the food selection patterns of the very old warrants further investigation. Fischer and coworkers[32] found that the older seniors (age 75 to 85) believed that improved diet would result in improved health, although they tended to select less nutritious food items. It may be that health professionals who encourage dietary changes in the young-old do not make the same degree of effort toward nutrition education in the **old-old,** or those in the oldest age group may not have access to appropriate nutrition education materials.

Health Considerations

Medical advice or the belief that a particular food is good or bad for health can lead to changes in food preparation and consumption. Davies[22] reported that among 100 people over age 60, all had made some change in food choice in their recent past, and most of the changes were motivated by the belief that it would improve their health. **Perceived health benefit** was a stronger determinant of food choice than convenience, price, or prestige value for 194 older Canadians.[51] In a group of 244 healthy older people in New Mexico,[38] 18% reported that they were very concerned about eating foods that contained cholesterol, most often citing possible atherosclerosis as the basis for their concern. Eighty-one percent of those very concerned were restricting their intakes of certain foods, most notably foods containing animal fats.

Older people are also becoming increasingly interested in food components other than fat that may influence their health. A study of older people in Wales[105] reported that 7% of the men and 10% of the women age 65 to 74 had changed their diet for health reasons. Specific changes included increasing their consumption of fish and fiber and decreasing their consumption of meat, salt, fats, and sugar. Moreover, these older people indicated a desire for more information on food labels. These findings support the idea that nutrition education can be effective in helping older people modify their food patterns.[51,105] Such modifications could be significant, since research has demonstrated that improved nutrition helps offset the development of chronic diseases. Obesity, **atherosclerosis,** heart disease, colon cancer, diabetes, **osteoporosis,** and **periodontal disease** are all associated with long-term eating habits.[104]

Ethnic Food Patterns

Ethnic origin continues to exert an influence on food patterns in the later years. Elderly Mexican American women in Texas[6] consumed flour tortillas, legumes, poultry, eggs, and organ meats more frequently than non-Hispanic women of similar age. The Mexican American women were more likely to cook with saturated fats and had a higher sugar intake. Of concern was their low use of dairy foods and fruits and vegetables rich in vitamins A and C.

Tong[45] examined the food habits of 62 elderly Vietnamese who had lived in the United States for 15 years. Based on a 24-hour diet recall record, it was evident that many ethnic foods were still part of the meal pattern. Breakfast still consisted of the traditional "pho" (beef soup with rice noodles, bean sprouts, and fresh herbs), and both lunch and dinner usually consisted of a stir-fried item and rice. Typical American foods such as hamburgers, pancakes, and pizza were not particularly liked. Only 5% of those interviewed used milk or cheese regularly.

A study of 45 elderly Chinese women in California[14] revealed that 95% still consumed mainly Chinese staple foods, including rice, noodles, and dumplings, at lunch and dinner. Breakfast varied between American breakfast items, bread, rolls, pastries, hot cereal, cookies, and crackers, and traditional Chinese foods. There was no association between the length of time lived in the United States and their use of American foods. A problem for older ethnic groups may be the availability of ethnic food items. Buying them may require transportation to a particular market and when available, these items may be expensive.

Vegetarian Food Patterns

The NFCS[101] included 464 people who identified themselves as vegetarians. Of these, 25 men (5% of the total) and 47 women (10% of the total) were over age 65. As a group the vegetarians had higher intakes of calcium, magnesium, phosphorus, and vitamin A than did the nonvegetarians. Vitamin B_{12} was the nutrient consistently lower in those identifying themselves as vegetarians. Vitamin B_6 intakes were similar in both groups. In general, the fat intake of the vegetarians was lower, the carbohydrate intake higher, and the protein intake comparable to the nonvegetarians.

General Trends

Changes in food marketing. Changes in agriculture, food preservation, food processing, and food technology have multiplied the food items available to the older consumer. Forecasters[92] of food trends among the general population predict such things as:

- An increase in microwave cooking, some suggesting that even cars will be equipped with microwave ovens in the future
- An increase in the use of nontraditional meal sources (e.g., vending machines) and a decrease in the use of traditional groceries for meal preparation
- An increase in gourmet preprepared items
- An increase in home delivery of foods and meals

With respect to the elderly, forecasters believe that more foods will be specifically formulated for this age group, with an emphasis on their special nutritional needs, packages that are easy to open, and products that are easy to prepare. General trends such as increased availability of home-delivered meals and groceries, and food items that require only reheating, will also benefit older people and will allow the physically impaired to remain independent for a longer period.

Leveille and Cloutier[57] described the response of the food industry to the needs of elderly people with specific health problems. Low-sodium, low-fat products have begun to emerge to facilitate food preparation for people with heart disease; high-fiber foods are available to offset constipation and **diverticulosis,** and lactose-free dairy products provide an option for those with **lactose intolerance.** Programs that provide meals to the elderly are also responding to changes in food technology. In a random sample of 430 nutrition programs providing home-delivered meals to elderly people,[5] more than 30% offered frozen meals to be reheated and consumed at a later time as part of their meal service.

Food marketing and implications for nutrition. Although older people use staple foods that have been available throughout their lifetime (e.g., whole milk, white bread, potatoes, and tomatoes), they also routinely consume food items that have become available in recent decades through food technology or improved transportation. Frozen dinners and entrees appear in food records obtained from older adults, and egg substitutes, low-calorie mayonnaise, and diet margarine have gained acceptance.[86] The variety of foods consumed, however, is still lowest in the 75 and over age group.[30]

At one time it was assumed that food habits formed early in life and did not change; however, it is apparent that older adults are faced with changing living situations and resources, and food patterns are adapted accordingly. Any change in food habits has nutritional implications. Changes for health reasons would be expected to have a positive effect on nutrient intake. On the other hand, physical disability, economic problems, and social isolation can lead to changes that reduce dietary quality. The adoption of newly marketed food items by this age group does affirm that nutritious foods not used previously may be accepted if they are introduced in a positive way.

PSYCHOLOGIC ASPECTS OF FOOD SELECTION
Changing Roles in the Household

Just as advancing age leads to changes in personal roles, so it can also bring about changes in household roles. Although the woman in the household may have taken primary responsibility for meal planning and food preparation throughout the early and middle stages of the family life cycle, this pattern may change when both the husband and wife are retired and are at home. With retirement may come an increase in the husband's involvement in food decisions. This was observed in 82 retired Iowa couples who were compared with couples in other stages of the life cycle.[85] Not only did retired husbands participate to a greater extent in food-related decisions, their level of participation also had nutritional implications. The greater the husband's involvement in both meal planning and actual food purchasing, the better the diet. Women who expressed dissatisfaction with their traditional role consumed poorer diets and showed little interest in food-related activities. This finding has important implications for nutrition education. Although food programs are often directed toward women, leaders should make an effort to involve men, who may be more receptive to new information and who appear to strongly influence food decisions within a retired family.

Feelings of Self-Worth

Good food, well prepared, conveys the message that an individual is important and that someone cares.[74] Yet there are times when the presentation of food in a professional manner, following the food safety and sanitation requirements of an institutional setting, conveys a less positive message. Lesnoff-Caravaglia[55] describes the reaction of an older woman at a con-

gregate meal site being served by a plastic-gloved hand. "I know it looks odd to be served by that plastic hand. I know it is to make sure the food is germ free, but I sometimes get the feeling that it is not my food they are protecting, but themselves. I feel as though it is the plate of an old person they don't wish to touch." Food patterns are enmeshed in a psychosocial context, and changes in food patterns by their very nature challenge the cultural and personal values embodied in these patterns.[74] Feelings of worthlessness or rejection can lead to a loss of interest in food and subsequent changes in nutrient intake.

Level of Social Interaction

Throughout life eating is a social activity.[96] Typical examples are birthday parties, wedding breakfasts, or sharing a pizza. Losing a spouse or friends results in a loss of eating companions for the older adult, who may now be eating alone for the first time in his or her life. Loneliness contributes to malnutrition in some older individuals. Among 418 rural older people,[53] those with low morale scores had many problems with their diet. Morale was evaluated on the basis of personal well-being, degree of loneliness, and attitude toward aging. Health and economic problems were also common in this population and no doubt contributed to both low morale and diet problems.

Walker and Beauchene[106] conducted a study of 61 independently living older people age 60 to 94 and evaluated the effect of loneliness on dietary adequacy. Their findings indicated that loneliness was related to the number of social contacts reported—those who had more social contacts were less lonely. The mean number of social contacts over the 3-day evaluation period was 17.7 with a range of 3 to 48. It is interesting to note, however, that the length of time spent in contact with others was not related to the degree of loneliness. This suggests that even a short telephone call or visit to bring a home-delivered meal may add to an older individual's psychological or emotional well-being. Neither age nor physical health influenced the degree of loneliness, although the older blacks interviewed had higher loneliness scores than the older whites.

Loneliness, in turn, was significantly related to overall dietary adequacy in these older people; the greater the degree of loneliness reported, the lower the intake of protein, iron, riboflavin, niacin, ascorbic acid, and phosphorus. Social factors such as being married, having strong religious ties, and having close neighbors also have been associated with higher intakes of some nutrients.[66] Social interaction may be particularly important for the nutritional well-being of institutionalized or homebound older people.[45,85] Kim and others[45] provided a nutrition education program for older people in a nursing home. They observed increases in nutrient intake while the program was being conducted, but these increases were not sustained. These workers considered the positive changes in nutrient intake to be a result of the attention given to the elderly residents by the researchers and others participating in the program.

Within the context of social contact or isolation, Troll[96] maintains that it is important to differentiate between isolation and desolation. **Isolates** are those who are relatively content living alone and may have done so most of their lives. The **desolates,** on the other hand, live alone but experience a high degree of loneliness. Physical isolation may be far less important than the frequency of communication or exchange of messages. An individual who lives with other people but is ignored is far more lonely than the person who lives alone but has a daily telephone conversation with a friend or child.

Of the 1,809 people over age 64 and living alone who participated in a national health survey,[50] 73% reported an in-person contact with relatives, and 69% reported an in-person contact with friends or neighbors in the 2 weeks prior to the survey. In addition, 84% had at least one telephone conversation with relatives in the previous 2 weeks, and 81% had a telephone conversation with a friend or neighbor over the same period. Related to these data is the observation that older people who were satisfied with the degree of attention they received from family members in the form of visits or telephone calls had fewer complaints about food and were better able to adjust to a prescribed diet.[53]

These findings may also be relevant to the increasing numbers of older individuals who are homebound and need help with activities of daily living (ADLs) (see Chapter 1). That assistance provides a social contact that could have important nutritional ramifications. Also, the home care provider is in a unique position to monitor for signs of malnutrition and to initiate corrective action before the condition becomes advanced and further threatens the person's health.[35]

Food Preferences

Food preferences are molded by our ethnic, cultural, and religious backgrounds. Older people, like most people, prefer foods associated with pleasant experiences or related to their home or place of origin.[37] Preferred foods may have been given as special treats or served on holidays or special occasions.[74] For lonely older people, food cravings may arise from the need for emotional gratification. **Age-appropriate expectations** can sometimes influence food selection, although these are more likely to be the expectations of younger individuals as to what "older people should eat" rather than the expectations of older people themselves.

Mental Status

Mental disorders in an older adult can involve confusion, irritability, acute depression or, in extreme situations, true dementia. Dementia can have several causes, such as **senile dementia of the Alzheimer type (SDAT),** multiinfarct dementia arising from a stroke or other cerebrovascular incident, or dementia associated with excessive long-term alcohol intake. It has been estimated that 1% to 6% of those over age 65 have severe dementia, and 2% to 15% have mild dementia.[18,108] Whatever the cause, dementia is likely to pose nutritional problems. Those with severe **organic brain disease** or SDAT may forget to eat or may be unable to differentiate between breakfast, lunch, and dinner. If they are unable to prepare food, meals may consist totally of bread and jam or prepackaged foods, limiting nutrient intake both quantitatively and qualitatively. (The biologic aspects of SDAT are reviewed in Chapter 1.)

Stages of Dementia and Nutritional Implications

SDAT is a progressive disorder in which the older individual becomes increasingly unable to function, both mentally and physically. Complications associated with SDAT can include behavioral disorders (e.g., hostility, extreme agitation, or uncooperativeness), psychiatric problems (e.g., depression, anxiety, or paranoia), and metabolic disturbances (e.g., dehydration, infection, or drug toxicity).[12]

The development of SDAT usually is divided into three stages, although Butler[12] emphasizes that there is tremendous variability among individual patients.

The initial stage of SDAT is characterized by recent memory loss, the inability to retain new information, and problems in judgment. Difficulties in shopping and preparing and storing food are likely. Impaired memory and judgment can lead to such nutrition complications as forgetting to eat or eating the same meal twice.[69] SDAT patients have difficulty recognizing and detecting odors. This olfactory malfunction often is manifested as a greater preference for sweet and salty foods.[43,110]

In the intermediate stage of dementia, increased agitation becomes evident.[79] Energy requirements may escalate by as much as 600 kcal a day.[59] Patients seldom consume sufficient kilocalories to meet these increased energy needs and begin to lose weight. In this stage individuals may require some assistance with eating such as cutting food into bite-size pieces or spreading margarine or butter on bread.

During the final stage of SDAT, the individual may be unable to swallow and may require tube feeding. Some patients may simply refuse to open their mouths or swallow when spoon fed,[29] whereas others may become compulsive eaters or try to eat inedible objects.[59] Fischer and Johnson[33] indicate that dementia is a leading cause of weight loss in the elderly. Memory loss, disorientation, impaired judgment, apathy, **apraxia,** combative feeding behavior, and appetite disturbances are factors identified with the weight loss observed in demented patients.

Nutrient Intake in Dementia

Nutritional supplements are very important in meeting the needs of patients with advanced SDAT. In two reports describing SDAT patients in long-term care facilities, mean caloric intakes were 1,532[59] and 1,558 kcal,[93] although individual intakes ranged from 995 to 2,120 kcal. Nutritional supplements, including fortified beverages and puddings, provided 29% of total kilocalories and 41% of total protein in the patients studied by Suski and Nielson.[93] Without nutritional supplements the daily intakes of their 19 nonambulatory SDAT patients were deficient in kilocalories and all nutrients but vitamin C and iron. Among the 13 elderly SDAT patients studied by Litchford and Wakefield,[59] calcium and niacin fell below 25% of the recommended dietary allowances (RDAs) when supplements were not included. In SDAT patients classed as wanderers, daily caloric intake even with supplements fell 600 kcal below energy expenditure; in those who were sedentary, intake fell only 200 kcal below energy expenditure.[59]

Feeding of patients with dementia. It may help when feeding dementia patients to offer fewer selections and small portion sizes, with between-meal snacks provided as needed.[59] Distractions such as a television or ringing telephone should be kept to a minimum.[15] Food temperatures need to be checked, because patients may not recognize they have burned their mouths. Also, food consistency may need to be modified, and tough or crispy foods may need to be excluded. Pureed foods may be necessary to prevent choking. Providing major nutrient sources at the noon meal, when cognitive and attentive abilities are at their peak, may optimize nutrient intake.[93] (See Chapter 4 for guidelines for feeding individuals with swallowing disorders.)

Areas for further research. In a clinical situation the older patient with dementia who must be fed should be weighed regularly, since weight loss can be significant. It also appears that **nonambulatory** patients are more likely to lose weight than **ambulatory** patients. Whether ambulatory patients are more likely to receive food from visitors or other sources requires further study. Likewise the effect of other medical complications associated with dementia bears further investigation. Fifty percent of a group of 44 patients with SDAT or multiinfarct dementia were found to have energy or protein malnutrition.[84] This was in spite of the fact that their mean dietary intake (as determined by food weighings) met recommended levels for energy, protein, vitamins, and minerals. A noteworthy finding among the malnourished patients was their higher number of infections (over fourfold) that were being treated with antibiotics.[91]

PHYSIOLOGIC ASPECTS OF FOOD SELECTION

The physical changes that occur as a result of normal aging and degenerative disease influence food habits. Loss of appetite or diminished taste sensitivity makes eating less pleasurable. A physical disability that restricts food shopping and meal preparation limits food choices. Physiologic changes affect both psychologic outlook and level of social activity, making it difficult to identify the true cause of any observed changes in food patterns.

Sensory Aspects of Food Selection

Appetite. Research examining appetite in elderly people has been limited. It is known, however, that such factors as diminished taste acuity, drugs, and poor dental status, all issues of concern in older people, can adversely affect appetite. Nevertheless, in a Georgia study,[10] only 4% to 5% of older adults ranging in age from 60 to over 100 reported that a physical condition interfered with their appetite.

Older people with a number of health problems are more likely to have poor appetites. Anorexia is a common side effect of many prescription drugs.[69] For example, **digoxin** often causes nausea as well as anorexia. Common **psychotropic drugs,** including some tranquilizers, increase the appetite in younger patients but produce a disinterest in food in the elderly.[9] Appetite may be affected by psychological factors. In a study evaluating loneliness and dietary adequacy, the higher the loneliness score, the lower the caloric intake.[106]

Taste acuity. Altered taste sometimes occurs in older people. The sense of taste is controlled by the number and level of function of the taste buds on the tongue and pharynx, and the integrity of the nerve supply to this region. Early

workers reported a decrease in the number of taste buds as well as some **atrophy** of remaining taste buds in advanced age.[7] More recent work suggests that a loss of taste buds, if it does occur, is not necessarily of practical importance. Zallen and others,[112] who evaluated the **taste acuity** for salt of elderly people, contend that actual taste sensations do not diminish with age when concentrations fall within the normal continuum found in food. When people age 65 to 78, living in the community, were presented with various salt concentrations in the form of mashed potatoes and chicken broth, their taste acuity did not differ from others age 20 to 35.

On the basis of extensive work with groups of all ages, Bartoshuk[7] concluded that many older adults do have elevated taste thresholds to the basic modalities of sweet, salty, sour, and bitter. This means that older people are less able to detect a taste when it is present in a test solution at very low concentrations, but at the concentrations usually found in foods, taste is not altered. Tests of taste on various regions of the tongue and pharynx reveal discrete losses of taste buds, but taste buds for all modalities are repeated extensively, thus ensuring that some degree of taste perception will remain. Bartoshuk[7] suggests that the redundancy of taste buds is a protective mechanism, since sodium (salt) is essential for life, a sweet sensation encourages continued caloric intake, and a bitter flavor protects against ingestion of poisons or harmful substances.

Some older individuals do have **distorted taste perception.** Although an intense degree of sweetness becomes unpleasant in most younger people, this is not true for many older people. This may explain why some older people crave items high in sugar. For those who do experience diminished taste, one possible explanation may be the reduced saliva flow associated with aging, since only dissolved substances can be distinguished by the taste buds.[65] Wearing dentures or poor dental hygiene can form a residual taste in the mouth that masks or overpowers other tastes. Martin[65] suggests that the taste buds of the hard palate are more insensitive to taste when obstructed by dentures. Certain prescription drugs contribute to reduced taste or cause an interfering taste. Nutritional status may influence taste; poor zinc status, however, has not been shown to be a primary cause of decreased taste acuity in older people (see Chapter 7).

Olfactory acuity. Existing studies on **olfactory acuity** changes with age indicate large individual differences.[13] There are indications that olfactory function generally undergoes a blunting with age; however, these changes are very gradual and go largely unnoticed.[13] Martin[65] suggests that poor health and smoking may exert a greater negative effect on olfactory sensitivity than aging itself.

Individuals over age 60 with olfactory losses (anosmia) indicated that a lessened ability to smell decreased their enjoyment of food but did not influence their appetite.[31] Their nutrient intakes were notably low for vitamin B_6 and zinc; however, these nutrients are low in the diets of older people with a normal sense of smell. The older people with diminished olfactory function used several strategies to compensate for their loss of smell. They used more spices to strengthen flavor, enhanced the visual presentation of their food, and emphasized the social atmosphere at mealtime. Flavor enhancers such as simulated food odors that can be added to their respective food counterparts are being tested with older people who have severe loss of smell.

Dental Problems

In general, dental health in the United States has improved. Americans are seeing a dentist more regularly for preventive dental care, they are reducing **dental caries** through self-care, and they are keeping their teeth longer. Nevertheless, dental problems still exist in the older population. Data obtained from elderly people in Iowa and North Carolina and from a national survey[8,71] (Table 12-1) indicate that the older population has an unmet need for dental care. Most older people are not covered by dental insurance and may not be able to afford dental services to repair cavities, treat gum diseases, or prepare dentures. Serious periodontal disease and decayed teeth can be painful and can cause the person to avoid certain foods. Foods that are very hot or very cold can aggravate oral pain, as can very crisp or fibrous foods that require significant biting force.

The aging process leads to a thinning of the

TABLE 12-1   Oral Health Status of Older Adults

Condition	Occurrence (%)
Edentulous	40-62*
Need for denture replacement or repair	22
Denture-related mucosal lesions	32
Gingival bleeding (after probing)	47
Periodontal weakening (loosening of teeth)	95
No dental visit in past 2 years	44

*Forty percent among those ages 60 to 70; 62% among those over age 70.

oral tissues and increased vulnerability to oral injury. This makes the older individual more likely to suffer mucosal damage as a result of ill-fitting dentures.[72] Untreated periodontal disease and infection can cause loosening of tooth attachment and subsequent loss of even healthy teeth. **Gingivitis** and infection of the oral tissues detract from overall physical well-being. Despite its importance, oral health is sometimes neglected in long-term care facilities.

Loss of teeth and having no or ill-fitting dentures interfere with the pleasure associated with eating, although the influence of dental status on nutrient intake is controversial. Papas and coworkers[73] evaluated the nutrient intake of 181 independent-living older people in Boston with respect to their dental status. Three lifestyle characteristics were found to adversely influence dietary quality: low educational level, low income level, and wearing either partial or full dentures. Those who had one or two full dentures consumed almost 20% less of most nutrients than those who had their natural teeth. This finding was independent of all other demographic characteristics. It cannot be ascertained from these data, however, whether this difference in nutrient intake occurred as a result of tooth loss.

An on-going longitudinal study of 370 middle-age and older adults[73] has suggested that the development of dental caries is related to intake of fermentable carbohydrates in the form of cakes, cookies, and breakfast cereals. Those who remained free of root caries, to which older people are more susceptible, consumed fewer sugary items, 50% more milk, and 25% more cheese. It also appears that deficiencies of folic acid, ascorbic acid, and zinc contribute to the progression of periodontal disease. Inasmuch as many older people have marginal vitamin and mineral status, this relationship deserves further evaluation.

Providing quality nutrient sources requiring only limited chewing is a priority for older people with poor dental status. Dairy products, eggs, ground meat, well-cooked chicken and fish, and legumes are good sources of high-quality protein. Fruit juices, cooked green and yellow vegetables, and potatoes can provide vitamins A, C, and B_6. Many fresh fruits such as apples, melons, or bananas can be eaten by those who are partly or completely edentulous if the fruit is ripe, peeled, and cut into small pieces. Pureed foods should be considered only when all other possibilities have been exhausted.

Xerostomia

A related dental concern is **xerostomia,** which impairs the ability to lubricate, masticate, and swallow food (see Chapter 4). Xerostomia can result from a number of conditions, including mouth breathing and stress.[65] However, the side effects of medications are a primary cause of the condition in elderly people.[80] Clinical management of xerostomia may include avoiding the following: caffeinated drinks; dry, bulky, spicy, salty, or highly acidic foods; alcohol; and tobacco. Saliva stimulants such as sugarless hard candy or lozenges and sugarless gum may be helpful. Lubricating the lips and dentures with petroleum jelly may be beneficial. Small, frequent mouthfuls of water help moisten the mouth. (Guidelines for food selection for those with swallowing problems can be found in Chapter 4).

Physical Health

Physical disability. A significant number of older people living in the community have some limitation in activity that can affect both food procurement and preparation (see Chapter 1). If the older person has limited vision or movement, he or she may not be able to shop for groceries; consequently, all food supplies must be delivered. Preparing vegetables can be difficult for someone whose hands are crippled with arthritis; moving about the kitchen requires special effort for a person who must grasp a cane or walker for support. Poor eyesight can interfere with reading a nutrition label or package directions for food preparation.

Unfortunately, there has been little nutritional evaluation of people with physical disabilities who live at home. Lonergan and associates[60] observed that elderly British women with poor eyesight and **osteoarthritis** of the hands and joints had poor energy intakes (1,000 kcal or less) and low **skinfold thicknesses.** In a study of about 2,200 **frail elderly** in New York state,[81] the very-low-income people with reduced mobility had the highest nutritional risk. Poor financial resources, as indicated by an income below the poverty level or receiving food stamps, limits one's ability to buy appropriate quantities and types of food or to pay for home care services. Those who were homebound and lived alone indicated an unmet need for help with food preparation and had an increased risk of days without eating. About half of the individuals with both financial problems and restricted mobility had days with nothing to eat.

One measure of diet quality used in this study[81] was the frequency of consumption of green or yellow vegetables. Those who needed help with meal preparation consumed green and yellow vegetables infrequently. Recipients of home-delivered meals in Minnesota[4] indicated that meal preparation was more difficult for them than getting groceries. Those women had problems opening cellophane wrappers and cutting food, suggesting a lack of hand strength and coordination. This would influence the preparation of fresh or frozen vegetables.

The nutritional vulnerability associated with physical disability was also apparent in 53 homebound Boston elderly;[75] only 4% had diets that achieved the guidelines for the basic four food groups. Among patients in a long-term care facility,[64] poor protein status and below-normal skinfold thicknesses were the result of poor caloric intake before rather than after admission. **Undernutrition** was especially evident in those with severe arthritis. One fourth of all older people with limited activity require special services such as home-delivered meals or a homemaker aide (see Chapter 13).

Food items that can be prepared in the microwave oven offer an alternative for older people with limited movement. Individually portioned packages, although more expensive, prevent the problem of having to deal with leftovers. Nutrition education should focus on wise selection of preprepared foods that contain a minimum of sodium and fat and appropriate levels of protein, vitamins, minerals, and fiber. There should be a continuing effort on the part of food technologists to develop food items high in nutritional quality that require little preparation.

Prescribed diets. Chronic diseases such as diabetes mellitus, cardiovascular disease, or kidney disease frequently include a dietary prescription as part of their management. Older individuals following a prescribed diet may be restricted in sodium, fat, cholesterol, protein, carbohydrate, or energy. In the NFCS,[101] the proportion of individuals on physician-prescribed diets rose with age. Of the individuals 75 years or older who were following a special diet, 80% indicated that the diet was prescribed. The NFCS did not indicate the specific nature of these prescribed diets.

In the Georgia Centenarian Study,[44] 17% of those 100 years of age or older were following a low-salt diet, and 4% were following a low-cholesterol diet. Among the subjects age 60 to 69, 15% and 18%, respectively, were on low-salt or low-cholesterol diets. It was not indicated whether these special diets were prescribed by a physician. Race may be a factor in the adoption of low-sodium diets, since 25% of the older black participants in the Georgia study[44] were following low-salt diets, compared to only 11% of the older white participants. Of 75 frail elderly people attending an adult day care center,[63] (mean age = 76 years), 36% were on special diets. These diets included low-salt (16 respondents), diabetic (12 respondents), and low-calorie (5 respondents) versions. Nearly 61% of those placed on special diets were having difficulty following the diet as given.

A study should be done on the sources of the diets being followed by older people. In one outpatient geriatric clinic,[94] about 20% of those following special diets had obtained their diet information from someone other than a health professional. Nearly half of those trying to lose weight had planned their own diet, consulted a friend, or used another nonprofessional source. Among the NFCS participants,[101] older women were more likely to self-prescribe diets than were older men (Table 12-2). About the same proportion of men and women were following physician-prescribed diets or had obtained their diet at a group program (most likely a weight control program). Other diet sources included friends, neighbors, or relatives.

Diets believed to either prevent or alleviate arthritis, if continued for extended periods without professional supervision, can be dangerous to health. Some older people have eliminated milk, citrus fruit, or bread from their diets in the belief that these foods cause arthritis. Although new research suggests that particular dietary patterns may influence the severity and progression of arthritic symptoms, no such regimen should be attempted without professional supervision and follow-up (see Chapter 8). It is important to follow up on an older person who has been placed on a **modified diet.** Although

TABLE 12-2   Sources of Special Diets Followed by Older People*

Source	Men (%)	Women (%)
Physician	76	76
Group program	0	5
Heard or read about it	2	3
Self-prescribed	3	4
Other	14	11

*Not all reported diet source; percentages do not equal 100.
From US Department of Agriculture: Nutrient intakes: individuals in 48 states, year 1977-78, Nationwide Food Consumption Survey, Rep No 1-2, Washington, DC, 1984, US Government Printing Office.

the plan may be tentative or designed for short-term treatment, based on the patient's degree of improvement, the individual may continue to follow the diet for months or even years, even when it is no longer appropriate.

Prescribed diets have a positive influence on nutrient intake if foods high in kilocalories and low in nutrient density are limited or deleted.[54] Yet, deleting favorite foods or severely limiting the use of salt reduces the pleasure associated with eating. Boykin[11] recommends an individual approach in developing a diet for an older person, recognizing the need to consider favorite foods from the lifelong pattern even if they are somewhat inappropriate for the diet prescribed. How often and under what conditions such foods can be included should be based on a nutrition and health assessment in consultation with the patient's physician. Including the patient in the decision-making process allows development of a diet that will be accepted and followed.

SOCIOLOGIC ASPECTS OF FOOD SELECTION

Household Size

Although it is true that a person eating alone may be less motivated to prepare an adequate meal, many factors, including age, sex, economic situation, health status, and number of social contacts with family or friends, also influence the food intake of older people who live alone. Davis and coworkers[23,24] evaluated the influence of household size on dietary quality in the 4,402 adults age 55 and over who participated in the NFCS. Older men living alone were more likely to have poorer quality diets than older women living alone, and the proportion of single men with poor quality diets increased with age.[24] Fourteen percent of the single men age 55 to 64 had poor diets, but this rose to 25% among those age 75 or older. The pattern for single women was less consistent: 22% of those in the youngest age group (55 to 64) had poor diets, compared with 16% and 21% in the groups age 65 to 74 and 75 and over, respectively. In this evaluation a poor diet was defined as one with an intake below 67% of the RDA for at least five of the nine nutrients evaluated. These nutrients included vitamins A, C, B_6, and B_{12}, thiamin, riboflavin, iron, calcium, and magnesium.

As described in Table 12-3, poverty status, a lower weekly food expenditure, and poor health contributed to poor quality diets. However, the variable that was most important was the caloric intake. Individuals eating alone did not make poorer food choices, they consumed less food overall. Older people living alone are more likely to skip meals and consume a higher proportion of their total kilocalories away from home.[23] Meals consumed away from home could include congregate meals obtained at senior centers. Skipping meals may be an indication that food resources are inadequate.

Ryan and Bower[83] evaluated socioeconomic status and living arrangements in 268 older adults in South Carolina and found no signifi-

TABLE 12-3 *Factors Affecting Dietary Quality in Older People*

	Men		Women	
Quality of Diet	High	Low	High	Low
Quality of diet				
Energy intake (kcal)	2,136	1,222	1,593	934
Money spent for food (per week)	$19.42	$16.09	$19.02	$15.70
Poor health (% of group)	29	51	32	45
Income below poverty level (% of group)	9	15	15	26

Adapted from Davis MA and others: Living arrangements and dietary quality of older US adults, *J Am Diet Assoc* 90:1667, 1990.

cant differences in nutrient intake between those living alone and those living with someone. However, only 15% of these older adults were over age 75, the group most vulnerable to poor intake. Also, most of the individuals interviewed (89%) were found to have low nutrient intake (less than 67% of the RDA for four index nutrients: iron, vitamin B_6, calcium, and vitamin A).

Among 539 Dutch elderly,[109] nutritional status evaluated on the basis of blood and urine analyses (specific tests were not indicated) did not differ by household size. Total plasma **carotenoids** were lower in those living alone, although total fruit and vegetable consumption was similar in all households. Those living alone did tend to prepare their meat, potatoes, and vegetables for 2 or more days at a time. Reheating of vegetables could decrease the vitamin content. Preparing food ahead does ensure the availability of an appropriate meal to be reheated on days when physical illness precludes extensive meal preparation. If there is no one else in the household and a neighbor or support person is unavailable, the older person forced to remain in bed because of illness may have nothing to eat or drink. This can lead to dehydration and, over time, malnutrition.

People who continue to live in their own homes usually have adequate facilities for food storage and preparation, including a working stove, oven, and refrigerator, and if trends hold true, a microwave oven will not be uncommon. The type and size of an appliance affect its use. Older people may hesitate to heat their conventional oven for one item such as a baked potato. The ease, convenience, and lower utility cost of a microwave oven make it an acceptable alternative. An older style refrigerator or an apartment-size refrigerator with a small freezer compartment will be a problem for one who shops or has groceries delivered only infrequently. Food storage and preparation facilities are sometimes less than adequate in senior housing apartments that have little counter space, limited cabinet space, and a small refrigerator.

Individuals who rent a room and have no access to kitchen facilities are forced to eat in restaurants or elsewhere. They may heat some foods on a hotplate in their rooms or use a heating coil for hot water for soup or beverages. These people are likely to be at or below the poverty level and, consequently, at high risk for poor nutrition. This group includes the hidden elderly, who reside in rundown hotels in deteriorating inner city neighborhoods. These individuals need access to government nutrition programs, including congregate or home-delivered meals, and food stamps. Participation in these programs has been shown to reduce the nutritional risk of these older people (see Chapter 13).[34]

Food Shopping Patterns

Food shopping can be a recreational or leisure time activity for the healthy older person with available transportation, or a problem for the physically disadvantaged. Physical limitations, lack of transportation, and the changing locations of supermarkets can present problems in food shopping for some older people. In one report 70% of those interviewed reported problems with food shopping, whereas only 20% had difficulty with meal preparation after food was brought into the home.[37]

On the other hand, Senauer and coworkers[87] emphasize that the social contact afforded by shopping should not be underestimated. In rural America, more than 51% of the elderly go to the grocery store at least twice a week and usually spend at least half an hour there.[87] With the changing face of today's supermarket, older people actually may increase the time they spend shopping. Today's convenience-conscious consumer wants everything under one roof, from a traditional supermarket to a pharmacy, post office, in-store restaurant, and caterer.[41] In addition, it is predicted that home-delivery, order-ahead service and drive-through grocery pick-up will become available.[87] The supermarkets of the future are likely to respond to the growing elderly population with such services as benches to rest on, small-size packages, and help in handling groceries and carts.[2]

Although the young-old may look forward to shopping, the old-old or frail elderly can find food shopping somewhat difficult. Reported problems include lifting heavy items, difficulty in reaching or stooping for items on high or low shelves, and failing eyesight, which affects the ability to read labels. Dependence on a cane or walker interferes with pushing a market basket, although many larger supermarkets now provide motorized carts for shoppers who need them.

Transportation to a food store can be a problem for older people who no longer drive. In rural areas, if a store is within walking distance, it usually is a general store with a limited variety of items and package sizes, and prices tend to be higher. Urban elderly can have a similar problem, since inner city supermarkets are closing because of poor profit margins and the growth of suburban malls. Independently owned grocery markets are frequently replaced by self-service convenience stores with higher prices. Having no means of transportation to a food store was a problem for elderly women in a metropolitan community in Louisiana,[89] although many lived within a mile of a grocery store and likely were able to walk. In contrast, urban elderly people living in a senior housing complex in a Massachusetts city[17] had access to transportation services, and few walked to the grocery store.

Walking to the store and carrying heavy bags home present serious problems for those who must use a cane. In northern locations, sidewalks covered with ice and snow may preclude walking for several days at a time. Research evaluating the influence of shopping patterns on the nutritional adequacy of the diet is not currently available. Helping older people with shopping might be encouraged for those seeking worthwhile volunteer activities.

Life-style and Leisure Time

Meals consumed each day. Because the daily schedule is less rigid after retirement, older people sometimes move away from the traditional pattern of three meals a day. Breakfast, however, is a popular meal with older people. In the NFCS,[68,101] 16% to 18% of adults ages 50 to 61 skipped breakfast at least some of the time, whereas only 9% of those ages 62 or older ever skipped breakfast. The omission of breakfast has a major impact on overall dietary quality in older age groups. Use of a ready-to-eat cereal was found to increase the average daily intake of all vitamins and minerals, includ-

ing vitamin B_6, folacin, calcium, and magnesium, nutrients that tend to be low in the diets of older people.[68]

It is interesting to note that the centenarians interviewed in Georgia[44] were more likely to eat breakfast regularly than were those ages 60 to 69. Also, elderly whites interviewed in that study were more likely to eat breakfast than elderly blacks. According to Stanton and McNutt,[92] only a minority of the general population eat three meals a day. On the other hand, in older people eating three meals a day is the most common pattern.

Snacking. In recent years Americans have been moving away from the traditional three meals a day to a **grazing** pattern, with an increase in mini meals and snacks.[92] An issue among younger people has been the nutritional quality of the snacks being selected, which in some cases provide primarily kilocalories and fat. In contrast, Murphy and others[71] found that in older age groups, snacking increased caloric intake but did not decrease the overall quality of the diet. This suggests that foods of reasonable nutrient density were being selected as snacks.

Not all evidence, however, confirms the existence of widespread snacking in the older population. A Minneapolis daily newspaper reported a survey of 600 elderly people in which about half were classified as being concerned about their nutrition.[107] Those who were "nutrition concerned" cooked most of their meals at home and rarely snacked throughout the day. Snacking patterns may reflect ethnic patterns. Vietnamese elderly[95] were found to snack very infrequently. For those that reported snacking, snack foods included fruit, cake, cookies, soup with crackers, tea, or coffee. Among older Chinese women in California,[14] fresh fruit was likely to be the snack of choice.

Promoting appropriate snack items could be of particular importance to older people for whom television watching is a major pastime. For 47 older New Yorkers,[16] the more hours of television they watched daily, the greater was the percentage of their total kilocalories contributed by snacks. In those individuals the overall quality of the diet deteriorated as the proportion of kilocalories from snacks increased. Food items commonly used as snacks included sweet baked items, crackers, beverages high in sugar, potato chips, and candy. Snack choices such as fruit, a low-fat dairy food, or a whole-grain product will improve the nutrient intake of older adults.

Meals away from home. Eating away from home has been increasing in the general population, and older adults are also participating in this trend. The NFCS[101] found that 27% of people age 75 or older had a meal or snack away from home at least once during the 3-day diet record period. About one third of those age 65 to 74 ate away from home at least once. Fast food operations have begun to attract the older market.[87] In 1989, McDonald's restaurants did 30% of their business with people over age 50.[36] In an urban location one fast food chain is testing a delivery service similar to that available from many pizza restaurants.

Sex

Single older men tend to have poorer diets than single older women.[24,27,48] Davis and co-workers[24] found that in the United States, single men age 75 or older were at the highest risk for diets low in important nutrients; this parallels the finding of Exton-Smith[27] among older British men. In the British study, 41% of the single men over age 74 had low skinfold thicknesses, compared to only 22% of the men of similar age living with relatives.

The current generation of older men is less accustomed to food preparation and, if widowed, may have diets lacking in variety; other factors such as education, income, or food preferences also enter in. In a study of Dutch elderly,[109] the single men consumed fewer fresh fruits than the single women or the married couples, although their serum vitamin C and retinol levels were in the normal range. In general, older men are more likely than older women to consume sufficient levels of protein and vitamins and minerals, because overall they consume more food and have higher energy intakes.

Trends in Social Patterns

Socioeconomic status influences both social participation and nutrition in older people. For example, the 50 to 64 age group spends about 14% more money on food than do younger age groups.[87] Individuals between 40 and 60 years of age spend a greater proportion of their discretionary income on "catered experiences" such as travel tours and culinary events.[111] Over 80% of luxury travel is attributed to people over age 60.[36] Travel increases with age, income, and education, and with travel comes exposure to new foods.[36]

As the older population becomes more diverse, it will be increasingly important to evaluate the influence of social contact in all groups. For the older adult who travels extensively, social contacts may be primarily short-term acquaintances, whereas for the older adult in poor health who seldom leaves home, visits or calls from family members may be the usual source of social interaction. For elderly people whose children have moved to different geographic locations, neighbors or workers from social agencies may be the only visitors. Each of these groups will have different social patterns and expectations, as well as accessibility to food. Another area for further study is the food pattern of widowed versus older single people. The single person who is accustomed to eating alone may be less vulnerable to nutritional inadequacy in later years than the individual for whom eating alone is a new experience.

ECONOMIC ASPECTS OF FOOD SELECTION

Food Purchases in Older Households

Older households spend a larger proportion of their total income on food than younger households. Over the past 25 years, aggregate food expenditures have declined as the proportion of the population in older age groups has risen.[87] The average annual expenditure for food (in 1984 dollars) for older Americans age 55 to 64 was $3,602, compared to $1,865 for those age 75 or older. The decline in food expenditure included money spent for food at grocery stores and convenience stores, and money spent for food eaten away from home. Retirement and subsequent changes in total income are also a factor influencing the amount of money spent for food. Regardless of one's age at retirement, food expenditures still decline. For individuals who retired after age 62 and had income from Social Security, the decline in food expenditures was between 4% and 13%; for those under age 62 who had faced involuntary retirement, the decline was as high as 33%.[42] Across all age groups, individuals with incomes in the lowest quintile spent only 62% of the amount of money for food as those in the highest quintile.[87]

There are also differences in food consumption patterns between the older and younger segments of the population that may reflect economic or other factors. Shrimper found that individuals over age 74 tended to eat less beef and fewer citrus fruits, legumes, and nuts.[88] Others have reported a higher consumption of fruits, vegetables, whole-grain breads, breakfast cereals, milk, eggs, and desserts in individuals age 50 or older.[19] The higher consumption of flour and cereal products is a general finding among older population groups[99] and may reflect the fairly reasonable cost of these items.

Income Status and Nutritional Adequacy

Several studies suggest a relationship between income and nutrient intake. Posner and coworkers[75] found 53 homebound, low-income older people to be at nutritional risk. Depending on the individual nutrient (kilocalories, protein, vitamin A, vitamin C, thiamin, riboflavin, niacin, iron, or calcium), 40% to 80% failed to achieve the appropriate RDA. The decline in the nutritional quality of the diet with decreasing income was not the result of poor food choices but of a decrease in the amount of food available.

In their analysis of the factors influencing dietary adequacy in people over age 64, Murphy and coworkers[71] found a significant predictor of dietary quality to be money spent for food. People with better quality diets spent on the average $3.33 to $3.60 more for food a week. Money spent for food was significantly related to caloric intake. Individuals age 65 to 84 with better quality diets had higher incomes than those with lower quality diets. Surprisingly, income level was not a factor in dietary quality in those age 85 or older. Ryan and Bower[83] found a significant positive relationship between nutrient intake and socioeconomic status in 268 South Carolina residents age 55 or older. The two nutrients most likely to be deficient were calcium and vitamin B_6. Dairy foods, protein foods, bananas, and vegetables all tend to be relatively expensive foods. The energy intakes of the low-income elderly were also found to be 100 to 200 kcal a day below that of the more affluent.

It is difficult to separate the effects of income, education, and ethnic group on food intake. Kohrs and coworkers[49] found that dietary levels of total fat, protein, thiamin, and niacin were higher among older adults who completed more than 12 years of school. Older people with less education are likely to have lower incomes, but at the same time may have fewer sources of information. The individual with limited reading ability has less opportunity to learn about food selection.

Income and ethnic group influence food consumption in older people.[101,102] Caloric intake decreases with income but is lower in elderly blacks than in elderly whites regardless of income. Protein intake is adequate among all sex and income groups, confirming that older people recognize the importance of protein foods. Differences in the consumption of dairy foods based on ethnic preferences influence the intake of both calcium and magnesium (Fig. 12-2). Available iron will be reduced if less-expensive vegetable proteins are substituted for meat, fish, or poultry, or if enriched or whole-grain breads and cereals are replaced with sweet baked products. Vitamin B_6 levels are lower in people with lower incomes and less money to spend for food (Fig. 12-3).

In contrast to certain nutrients that decrease in the diet according to income or particular ethnic group, vitamin A intakes were higher among those with incomes below $6,000 a year (Fig. 12-3). The use of dark greens by older black adults very likely contributed to the high level of vitamin A activity calculated for these diets. Nevertheless, available data emphasize the nutritional vulnerability of low-income elderly. (For data on intakes of all nutrients based on

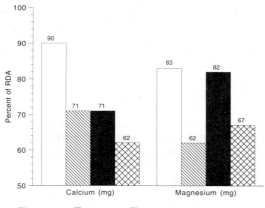

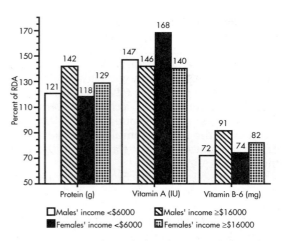

FIG. 12-2   Nutrient intakes can differ according to sex or ethnic group. Calcium intakes are higher in males than in females in white and black adults. Magnesium intakes are similar in males and females but lower in older black adults.

Data from US Department of Agriculture: *Nutrient intakes: individuals in 48 states, year 1977-78, nationwide food consumption survey 1977-78,* report no 1-2, Washington, DC, 1984, US Government Printing Office.

FIG. 12-3   Protein and vitamin B$_6$ intakes tend to be higher in older adults with higher incomes; in contrast, vitamin A intakes are similar or even higher in low-income versus high-income older adults.

Data from US Department of Agriculture: *Nutrient intakes: individuals in 48 states, year 1977-78, nationwide food consumption survey 1977-78,* report no 1-2, Washington, DC, 1984, US Government Printing Office.

the poverty ratio, see Tables 10-1, 10-2, 10-3, and 10-4).

Influence of Food Stamps

Food assistance programs that increase buying power can improve the quality of the diet. Unfortunately, eligible older people are less likely to participate in the food stamp program than eligible younger people; 40% of eligible nonparticipants are age 65 or older.[87] In 1983 only 7% of those over age 64 received food stamps,[98] although 14% had incomes below the poverty level.[97] In general, it is estimated that fewer than half of the elderly people eligible for food stamps actually participate in the program, and for those that do participate, benefits may be minimal (about $10 a month).[105] Older people may be less well informed about available programs, may lack transportation to the appropriate office, or may choose not to apply because of pride.

Efforts to ease these problems have included processing food stamp applications by mail or telephone and providing applications to outreach workers at senior centers and congregate meal sites. These methods also eliminate the embarrassment of having to appear at the local family assistance or welfare office. Although consideration has been given to providing cash payments rather than food stamps, the fact remains that cash could be used for pressing needs other than food, such as fuel, housing, or medical expenses.

For older people who do participate in the food stamp program, there appear to be some nutritional benefits.[40] Lopez and Habicht[61] examined food stamp participation and caloric intake among the elderly poor interviewed in NHANES I and NHANES II. Poor older women who participated in the food stamp program had higher body weights and greater skinfold thicknesses than nonparticipants similar in income. However, in a related study[62] iron status evaluated on the basis of hemoglobin and transferrin saturation levels was still a problem among the elderly poor regardless of food stamp participation. Other factors including race, sex, general health status, and the length of time receiving food stamps may have helped confound these results. Food stamp participants were consuming higher levels of dietary iron. In NHANES I,[62] elderly poor not receiving food stamps had mean iron intakes of only 6.8 mg, compared with the 9.6 mg reported by food stamp recipients and the 10.1 mg reported by the nonpoor of similar age. The food sources of iron in these diets were not defined.

A U.S. Department of Agriculture evaluation of 854 older people either receiving or eligible to receive food stamps[100] suggests that men age 65 to 74 and both sexes age 75 or older benefit most from food stamps. Intakes of protein, calcium, magnesium, and vitamin A did not differ between participating and nonparticipating women age 65 to 74; those receiving food stamps did have higher intakes of vitamin B_{12}, suggesting higher intakes of animal foods, although both groups exceeded the RDA. Men age 75 or over who were not receiving food stamps met less than 67% of the RDA for energy, magnesium, and vitamin B_6, and only 71% of the RDA for vitamin A. Men of similar age receiving food stamps met at least 75% of the RDA for all nutrients except vitamin B_6. Vitamin B_6 and magnesium were low in all diets. This could indicate the greater use of more highly processed bread and cereal products and less use of vegetables, meat, poultry, fish, and dairy products. Food selection patterns could also be improved by nutrition education programs directed toward these groups.

Community Meal Programs for the Poor

A New York state survey[78] of individuals eating at soup kitchens reported that 93% had household incomes in the previous month that were less than 100% of the poverty level, and more than half were less than 50% of the poverty level. One fifth of the meal recipients were men age 60 or older. In contrast, a national survey[34] found participation in soup kitchen and food pantry programs to be low among 3,602 older adults despite the fact that three fourths of these respondents had incomes below the poverty level. Of those who indicated they did not have enough money to buy food, 76% never used a soup kitchen, and 83% never used a food pantry. The low utilization of soup kitchens and food pantries by impoverished older people is interesting and largely unexplained. Pride, lack of transportation, or fear of personal harm in the neighborhood where the program is located may deter participation by needy older people. The nutritional impact of soup kitchens and other emergency food programs on the elderly population deserves further investigation.

NUTRITION FOR OLDER PEOPLE WITH SPECIAL NEEDS
Helping the Functionally Impaired

Older people who are seriously ill or recovering from illness are sometimes unable to feed themselves. This can be a temporary situation, with self-feeding resuming as strength is regained. In the case of a stroke, organic brain syndrome such as SDAT, or chronic neurologic disorder such as **parkinson's disease,** some degree of **paralysis** or loss of coordination can be permanent and can prohibit the usual motions involved in self-feeding. Data from the **National Medical Expenditure Survey**[103] indicate that assistance with meals is a common need among physically disabled older people. Of the various home services available for people with functional disabilities, help with meals was the most frequent type of assistance and was provided to 18.5% of the functionally impaired.

Problems in meal preparation and self-feeding can be caused by weaknesses of the hand and arm muscles, making it difficult to lift utensils such as a bowl, cup, or spoon. Partial paralysis can limit range of motion or make it difficult to flex the fingers and hand to grasp a plate or fork. If the affected tissue or muscle group has an adequate blood and nerve supply, weakened muscles often can be strengthened by appropriate exercises. If, however, the neuromuscular weakness resulted from actual wasting of the muscle tissue or denervation of the muscle because of brain damage or disease, it is less likely that normal function can be restored. The latter types of disorders include **myasthenia gravis,** organic brain disease, and **stroke.**

Utensils for Special Needs

Various devices have been developed to assist individuals with some degree of functional loss.[47] In many cases only a slight modification of existing utensils will facilitate food handling. Special aids often are available from local hospital supply companies or by mail order (see selected resources at the end of this chapter).

Cups. Lightweight plastic cups are easier to handle than glass or china. A cup with a partial lid or small opening (plastic travel cup) will prevent spills for those with abrupt movements and poor coordination. Sports drink containers with their wide base, plastic composition, and fitted lid and straw, are also good alternatives. A stretch-knit coaster slipped onto the bottom of a glass or an adhesive-backed bathtub safety tread attached around the sides provides a nonslippery surface for grasping.[47]

Forks and spoons. Utensils with extra-thick bamboo or plastic handles are easier to grasp if flexing the fingers is difficult. An inexpensive solution is placing a foam curler over the handle of a standard utensil, since the foam surface increases the friction and aids in holding. For those unable to grasp, a cuff with a pocket holding a standard utensil can be slipped over the hand to facilitate self-feeding. A swivel spoon or spoon with an extra long handle is helpful when motion is limited.[47]

Plates and bowls. A suction device to prevent a dish or bowl from moving will assist the older person attempting to prepare food with the use of only one hand. A plate with a broad edge to push food against when filling a spoon or fork will help those with limited motor skills. Because self-feeding can require considerable time for one who is slowly regaining skills, a plastic dish with a lower compartment filled with hot water is necessary to keep food at a palatable temperature.

When the older individual with some functional loss returns home, meal preparation must also be resumed. Use of a microwave oven can facilitate the transition, since it requires little dexterity of movement and can heat or reheat food in short periods of time. The major difficulty associated with preprepared microwavable foods can be opening or preparing the package for placement in the microwave oven. Many packages require use of a scissors and hand strength for cutting through a cardboard covering.

Regaining Self-Feeding Skills

Types of food for self-feeding. Relearning feeding skills can be a long and difficult process. Careful selection and preparation of the foods offered and a positive approach will facilitate progress and encourage effort. If chewing or swallowing is also a problem, a soft diet rather than pureed foods is not only more palatable but also requires less skill in eating. Avoid cutting foods into many small pieces; fewer motions are required to eat fewer medium-sized pieces. Finger foods are ideal, since they require less effort and energy to eat. Ideas for making difficult items into finger foods include putting ground meat or sandwich filling in a pita pocket, serving an egg hard cooked and peeled, or cutting raw fruits and vegetables into strips, flowerets, or quarters. An easy-to-eat meal might include a pita sandwich, soup served in a mug, apple slices (peeled and cored), and a carton of milk with a straw.

Environment for self-feeding. Attention and praise provide incentive for continuing what may be a painful and frustrating activity. Having the individuals in a self-feeding program sit at a table facing each other promotes both social interaction and mutual support as patients become helpful to each other.[20,21] Reducing the general noise level so that patients may more easily converse with staff members and each other contributes to a positive meal environment. Sensitizing staff members to avoid negative outbursts, such as scolding a self-feeding patient who has accidentally spilled food, is essential for a rehabilitation program to succeed.

The physical appearance of the dining area should also be considered. Elmstahl and co-workers[26] reported a situation in which the dining room of a long-term care facility was redecorated to more closely resemble a dining area of the 1940s. For these patients the 1940s were very active periods of their lives. Following the change in decor, food intake improved. It is interesting to note that these patients did not gain weight despite an increase in energy intake. This was attributed to the increase in physical activity that resulted from their improved psychologic outlook.

Feeding the Chronically Ill

A myriad of factors contributes to feeding difficulties and subsequent malnutrition in a chronically ill elderly patient. The older person may actively resist feeding, may have difficulty swallowing, or may have altered appetite and taste because of medications he or she is taking. Preserving the dignity of the individual who has to be fed will influence general receptivity to the food offered. The emotional empathy between the individual performing the feeding and the patient is critical to successful feeding and continuing nutritional intake. A caring, patient attitude on the part of the care-giver will encourage food intake in a frail older person for whom food mastication and swallowing require concentrated effort. Feeding the chronically ill older patient requires attention to the following:

The position of the patient: The individual should be sitting upright with the hips at a 90-degree angle. (Never feed an individual in a **supine** position, because this increases the danger of choking and **food aspiration.**)[3]

The presentation of the food: Only small amounts of food should be offered at a time; forcing food into the mouth too rapidly increases the fear of choking and the danger of food aspiration. Straws that may supply liquid more rapidly than it can be swallowed should not be used.[3] Infant rice cereal is a relatively inexpensive and effective thickener for thin liquids that are difficult to handle.[91]

The nutrient density of the food: Items rich in energy, protein, vitamins, and minerals should be emphasized,[58] since the patient may tire quickly and consume only limited amounts of food (see Chapter 5 for ideas on fortifying foods with protein supplements).

A Team Approach

Evaluating any loss in function and planning appropriate therapy to help the patient achieve the highest level of independence possible requires a cooperative effort by the nurse, physician, nutrition professional, **occupational therapist,** and physical therapist. Successful feeding of patients who cannot feed themselves requires attention to the type of food to be offered and the appropriate feeding techniques. The rehabilitation required to help a patient relearn self-feeding skills demands careful planning and supervision. The dietary intake of patients with feeding problems must be monitored carefully and adjustments made as may be necessary.

The needs of patients for disease-related nutrition intervention must also be considered from a team perspective. Lan and Justice[52] surveyed 212 medical charts of elderly patients in 11 long-term care facilities. Of the 120 patients with diagnosed coronary heart disease, 99% were not on a modified diet as generally prescribed for this condition; of the 38 diabetic patients, 18% were not on calorie-controlled diets nor was fiber intake encouraged; and of the 55 hypertensive patients, 44% were not on any level of sodium restriction. Modified diets have three major purposes: (1) to relieve the symptoms associated with the disease, (2) to delay the onset of complications, and (3) to reduce the need for required medications. Thus the large number of patients not being provided with modified diets is troublesome. Lan and Justice suggested that the relatively few hours that consulting dietitians spend in the facility may prevent them from establishing effective communication with the attending physician. In situations where the dietitian is not present on a daily basis, a special effort must be made to establish the effective team approach necessary to meet the nutritional needs of the impaired elderly adult.

DIETARY PATTERNS: IMPLICATIONS FOR NUTRITION EDUCATION

Most older adults have a varied diet that includes foods from all major food groups. Most older people regularly consume some protein foods (meat, fish, poultry, and eggs); more than 90% of low-income elderly had at least one serving of these foods on a 24-hour recall record.[100] Mean intake was about 6½ ounces daily. Among more than 2,650 people over age 64 interviewed as part of the **NHANES Epidemiologic Follow-Up Study (NHEFS)**,[70] servings from the protein group averaged 1.6 per day among white men and women but only 1.2 among black men and women.

Breads and cereals are popular in this age group and generally are consumed daily. In one report about one fifth of low-income people age 75 or over had a ready-to-eat cereal on the day of the interview.[100] Contrary to popular opinion, only one third had a sweet baked product. The NHEFS population[71] consumed 2½ servings of grains, bread, or cereal each day. Current recommendations suggest at least six servings a day.

Consumption of milk is low in older men and women. Although more than three fourths report using milk on a daily basis, total intake represents only 250 to 300 mg of calcium, or about 1 cup of milk a day.[100] Servings of dairy foods averaged 1.6 a day, for elderly whites in the NHEFS study,[71] but only 1.2 among elderly blacks. The recommended amount is two servings a day.

Vegetables and fruits were consumed in the recommended amounts by the NHEFS subjects.[71] They had 2.7 servings of fruit each day (two to four servings are recommended) and 3.2 servings of vegetables (three to five servings are recommended); however, use of vegetables was lower in elderly blacks, who had only 2.9 servings. On the average all had one serving a day of a citrus fruit, but the daily intake of vegetables supplying vitamin A precursor carotenoids was only about half a serving. Limited use of dark green and deep yellow vegetables was also observed in a U.S. Department of Agriculture[100] evaluation of low-income older people. Although three fourths had a least one vegetable daily, fewer than 10% of the men and 20% of the women had a good source of the carotenoids. With the exception of men age 75 or over, three fourths of the low-income group reported having citrus fruit or juice regularly.

Regardless of limited budgets, older people appear to consume foods from the meat group regularly. These items, coupled with increased servings of enriched or whole-grain bread and cereal, should provide adequate iron, although iron absorption in older people is not well understood. Encouraging the use of whole-grain products would add to intakes of trace minerals such as zinc, magnesium, and chromium. Although frankfurters and luncheon meats were reported by fewer than 20% of low-income older people on the day of record,[100] protein foods lower in sodium and fat that provide more protein for less cost (see Chapter 5) should be emphasized.

Incorporating dairy products into the daily meal pattern is essential if intakes of calcium and riboflavin are to be adequate. These items also contribute vitamins A and D and protein and should be a priority in nutrition education. The contribution of grain products to a healthy diet must be emphasized. Finally, many older people are not consuming adequate amounts of dark green or deep yellow vegetables. This may relate to cost or to problems in the preparation of fresh vegetables. Frozen vegetables with no added sodium are an alternative to fresh, particularly in the winter months.

Summary

Adaptation to changes in life-style, health, and economic status can bring about changes in eating patterns. Increasing age and decreasing energy requirements result in consumption of less food and can lead to nutritional inadequacy. Older people do change their food patterns according to general food trends and product availability and so can be receptive to nutrition education.

Social activity and social contact are positively related to the nutritional quality of the diet. Depression, loneliness, and diminished feelings of self-worth can lead to disinterest in food. Patients with organic brain syndrome who cannot feed themselves often show weight loss and should be monitored closely. Efforts at rehabilitating patients with loss of motor skills or partial paralysis should include self-feeding.

Changes in taste and smell, loss of teeth, and physical disability can adversely affect nutrient intake. A person who is homebound and dependent on others for food delivery or who cannot move about easily in the home to carry on meal preparation is forced to depend on preprepared food items and can have limited intakes of fresh produce and dairy products. Prescribed diets or drugs used to treat chronic disease can result in diminished appetite, xerostomia, and problems in food selection. Snacking, when it prevails, can either add to or detract from the quality of the diet, and nutrition education should emphasize healthy, nutrient-dense snack choices.

Low-income older people are likely to have diets poorer in nutritional quality than higher income older people. Food stamps can make a significant nutritional contribution to the diets of older recipients; eligible older people who do not participate in the program tend to have diets with inadequate levels of many nutrients. Although older people living alone may have poor diets, this is not always the case. Since such individuals are typically poor and advanced in age (75 or older), factors other than eating alone contribute to the problem. Men living alone and people over age 74 are at particular risk for dietary inadequacy.

REVIEW QUESTIONS

1. Do older people eat differently as they age? If yes, in what ways? If no, why not? Are older people "set in their ways" when it comes to food habits?
2. Does aging alter energy consumption and nutrient intakes? Does race or very old age influence energy intake? What is the Baltimore Longitudinal Study of Aging and what information about nutrition and aging is the study providing? What are nutrient-dense foods and why are they important in the diet of older persons?
3. What are some of the changes in the food marketplace that affect food choices of the elderly? What implications do these marketplace changes have for older persons with chronic diseases such as osteoarthritis, diverticulosis, and heart disease?
4. How do changes in roles within the family structure influence eating patterns? Does social interaction positively or negatively influence eating patterns in the elderly? What does "age-appropriate expectations" mean when it comes to food selection? How do mental disorders affect nutritional status?
5. Do taste and smell change as people age? What effect might these sensory changes have on food selection? What dental problems are common in

older persons and how do these influence food intake? How does household size influence eating habits?

SUGGESTED LEARNING ACTIVITIES

1. Go to the frozen food section of your grocery store and prepare a list of all frozen meals that would be acceptable meeting the following criteria: less than 300 mg of sodium and less than 30% of the kilocalories from fat. Type your list for use in education classes for older persons.
2. Prepare a recipe booklet with feeding hints for caregivers of persons with senile dementia of the Alzheimer type.
3. Visit a long-term care facility and ask the food service director if you can observe in the dining room at meal service times. Record your observations about the ambiance of the facility, the meals served, and the interaction of the staff and the residents. How does this compare with what you have learned in this chapter?
4. Interview an older relative about the foods eaten, household composition, mealtimes, and foods served for special holiday or religious meals. Give an oral report to your class on the differences and similarities that you found as compared with your meal pattern.
5. Ask your instructor to play a simulation game with the class, such as, "Into Aging." This will give you some insight into the social, psychologic, and physiologic difficulties experienced by many older people. After the game, conduct a group discussion about your feelings on "getting old." (Hoffman T, Reif S.: *Into aging*, Thorofare, NJ, 1968, Slack.)

Key Terms

Provided here for review is a list of the major terms in this chapter. The definitions can be found in the Glossary, which begins on p. 336. To help you understand how these terms are applied, the page number is given for the first mention of each term in the chapter.

age-appropriate expectations , 291

ambulatory, 292

anosmia, 294

apraxia, 292

atherosclerosis, 288

atrophy, 293

Baltimore Longitudinal Study of Aging (BLSA), 286

REFERENCES

1. Angulo JF: Foodways, ideology, and aging: a developmental dilemma, *Am Behavioral Scient* 32(1):41, 1988.
2. Anonymous: Helping elderly shoppers, *Supermarket Business* 44:53, 1989.
3. Anonymous: Practical solutions to eating problems of the elderly, *J Am Diet Assoc* 91:1417, 1991.
4. Asp EH, Darling ME: Home-delivered meals: food quality, nutrient content, and characteristics of recipients, *J Am Diet Assoc* 88:55, 1988.
5. Balsam AL: Frozen meals for the homebound elderly, *Catering and Health* 1:253, 1990.
6. Bartholomew AM and others: Food frequency intakes and sociodemographic factors of elderly Mexican Americans and non-Hispanic whites, *J Am Diet Assoc* 90:1693, 1990.
7. Bartoshuk LM: Taste: robust across the age span, *Ann NY Acad Sci* 561:65, 1989.
8. Beck JD, Hunt RJ: Oral health status in the United States: problems of special patients, *J Dental Educ* 49:407, 1985.
9. Blumberg JB, Suter P: Pharmacology, nutrition, and the elderly: interactions and implications. In Chernoff R, editor: *Geriatric nutrition: the health professional's handbook*, Gaithersburg, Md, 1991, Aspen Publishers.
10. Bowman BA, Rosenberg IH, Johnson MA: Gastrointestinal function in the elderly. In Munro H, Schlierf G, editors: *Nutrition of the elderly*, Nestle Nutrition Workshop Series vol 29, New York, 1992, Raven Press.
11. Boykin LS: Soul foods for some older Americans, *J Am Geriatr Soc* 23:380, 1975.
12. Butler RN: Senile dementia of the Alzheimer type. In Abrams WB, Berkow R, editors: *Merck manual of geriatrics*, Rahway, NJ, 1990, Merck, Sharp & Dohme Research Laboratories.
13. Cain WS, Stevens JC: Uniformity of olfactory loss in aging, *Ann NY Acad Sci* 561:29, 1989.
14. Chau P and others: Dietary habits, health beliefs, and food practices of elderly Chinese women, *J Am Diet Assoc* 90:1667, 1990.
15. Clagget MS: Nutritional factors relevant to Alzheimer's disease, *J Am Diet Assoc* 89:392, 1989.
16. Clancy KL: Preliminary observations on media use and food habits of the elderly, *Gerontologist* 15:529, 1975.
17. Cohen NL, Ralston PA: Factors affecting dietary quality of elderly blacks: final report, Washington, DC, 1992, AARP Andrus Foundation.

18. Council on Scientific Affairs, American Medical Association: Dementia, *JAMA* 256:2234, 1986.

19. Cronin FJ and others: Characterizing food usage by demographic variables, *J Am Diet Assoc* 81:661, 1982.

20. Davies ADM, Snaith PA: Mealtime problems in a continuing-care hospital for the elderly, *Age Ageing* 9:100, 1980.

21. Davies ADM, Snaith PA: The social behaviour of geriatric patients at mealtimes: an observational and intervention study, *Age Ageing* 9:93, 1980.

22. Davies L: Nutrition education of the elderly. In Prinsley DM, Sandstead HH, editors: *Nutrition and aging,* New York, 1990, Alan R Liss.

23. Davis MA and others: Living arrangements and dietary patterns of older adults in the United States, *J Gerontol* 40(4):434, 1985.

24. Davis MA and others: Living arrangements and dietary quality of older U.S. adults, *J Am Diet Assoc* 90:1667, 1990.

25. Elahi VK and others: A longitudinal study of nutritional intake in men, *J Gerontol* 38:162, 1983.

26. Elmstahl S and others: Hospital nutrition in geriatric long-term care medicine. I. Effects of a changed meal environment, *Compr Gerontol A* 1:29, 1987.

27. Exton-Smith AN: Panel on Nutrition of the Elderly: A nutrition survey of the elderly, Reports on Health and Social Subjects No 3, London, 1972, Her Majesty's Stationery Office.

28. Exton-Smith AN, Stanton BR: Report on an investigation into the dietary of elderly women living alone, London, 1965, King Edward's Hospital Fund for London.

29. Fabiszewski KJ and others: Management of advanced Alzheimer's disease. In Volcier L and others, editors: Clinical management of Alzheimer's disease, Rockville, Md, 1988, Aspen Publishers.

30. Fanelli MT, Stevenhagen KJ: Characterizing consumption patterns by food frequency methods: core foods and variety of foods in diets of older Americans, *J Am Diet Assoc* 85:1570, 1985.

31. Ferris AM, Duffy VB: Effect of olfactory deficits on nutritional status: does age predict persons at risk? *Ann NY Acad Sci* 561:113, 1989.

32. Fischer CA and others: Nutrition knowledge, attitudes, and practices of older and younger elderly in rural areas, *J Am Diet Assoc* 91:1398, 1991.

33. Fischer J, Johnson MA: Low body weight and weight loss in the aged, *J Am Diet Assoc* 90(12):1697, 1990.

34. Food Research and Action Center: A national survey of nutritional risk among the elderly, Washington, DC, 1987, Food Research and Action Center.

35. Gallagher-Allred C: Nutrition and the elderly, *Caring,* 5:68, 1991.

36. Gerber J: How the aging explosion will create new food trends, *Food Technol* 43:134, 1989.

37. Gibson MJ: Nutrition programs for the aging: how effective are they? *Aging Int* 9(4):17, 1982-1983.

38. Goodwin JS and others: Concern about cholesterol and its association with diet in a group of healthy elderly, *Nutr Res* 5:141, 1985.

39. Hallfrisch J and others: Continuing diet trends in men: the Baltimore Longitudinal Study of Aging (1961-1987), *J Gerontol* 45:M186, 1990.

40. Hama MY, Chern WS: Food expenditure and nutrient availability in elderly households, *J Con Affairs* 22:3, 1986.

41. Hamel R: Food fight, *Am Demogr* 11:37, 1989.

42. Hausman JA, Paquette L: Involuntary early retirement and consumption. In Burtless G, editor: *Work, health, and income among the elderly,* Washington, DC, 1987, Brookings Institute.

43. Hope RA, Fairburn CG, Goodwin GM: Increased eating in dementia, *Inter J Eating Dis* 8:111, 1989.

44. Johnson MA and others: Nutritional patterns of centenarians, *Int J Aging Hum Dev* 34(1):57, 1992.

45. Kim S, Schriver JE, Campbell KM: Nutrition education for nursing home residents, *J Am Diet Assoc* 78:362, 1981.

46. Kivett VR, Scott JP: The rural by-passed elderly: perspectives on status and needs (the Casewell Study), Technical Bull No 260, Raleigh, NC, 1979, North Carolina Agricultural Research Service.

47. Klinger JL, Frieden FH, Sullivan RA, editors: *Mealtime manual for the aged and handicapped,* Camden, NJ, 1978, Campbell Soup Co.

48. Kohrs MB, Czajka-Narins DC, Nordstrom JW: Factors affecting nutritional status of the elderly. In Munro HN, Danforth DE, *Nutrition, aging, and the elderly,* New York, 1989, Plenum Press.

49. Kohrs MB and others: Title VII—Nutrition

Program for the Elderly. II. Relationship of socioeconomic factors to one day's nutrient intake, *J Am Diet Assoc* 75:537, 1979.

50. Kovar MG: Aging in the eighties, age 65 years and over living alone, contacts with family, friends, and neighbors, Advance data No 116, National Center for Health Statistics, US Department of Health and Human Services, Hyattsville, MD, 1986.

51. Krondl M and others: Food use and perceived food meanings of the elderly, *J Am Diet Assoc* 80:523, 1982.

52. Lan S-J, Justice CL: Use of modified diets in nursing homes, *J Am Diet Assoc* 91:46, 1991.

53. Learner RM, Kivett VR: Discriminators of perceived dietary adequacy among the rural elderly, *J Am Diet Assoc* 78:330, 1981.

54. LeBovit C, Baker DA: Food consumption and dietary levels of older households in Rochester, New York, *Home Econ Res Rep* No 25, Washington, DC, 1965, US Department of Agriculture.

55. Lesnoff-Caravaglia G: The aesthetic attitude and common experience. In Lesnoff-Caravaglia G, editor: *Values, ethics, and aging,* New York, 1985, Human Sciences Press.

56. Letsou AP, Price LS: Health, aging and nutrition, *Clin Geriatr Med* 3(2):253, 1987.

57. Leveille GA, Cloutier PF: Role of the food industry in meeting the nutritional needs of the elderly, *Food Technol* 40:82, 1986.

58. Lipschitz DA, Mitchell CO: The correctability of the nutritional, immune, and hematopoietic manifestations of protein-calorie malnutrition in the elderly, *J Am Coll Nutr* 1:17, 1982.

59. Litchford MD, Wakefield LM: Nutrient intakes and energy expenditures of residents with senile dementia of the Alzheimer's type, *J Am Diet Assoc* 87:211, 1987.

60. Lonergan ME and others: A dietary survey of older people in Edinburgh, *Br J Nutr* 34:517, 1975.

61. Lopez LM, Habicht JP: Food stamps and the energy status of the US elderly poor, *J Am Diet Assoc* 87:1020, 1987.

62. Lopez LM, Habicht JP: Food stamps and the iron status of the US elderly poor, *J Am Diet Assoc* 87:598, 1987.

63. Ludman EK, Nieman JM: Frail elderly: assessment of nutrition needs, Gerontologist 26:198, 1986.

64. MacLennan WJ, Martin P, Mason BJ: Energy intake, disability, disease, and skinfold thickness in a long-stay hospital, *Gerontol Clin* 17:173, 1975.

65. Martin W: Oral health in the elderly. In Chernoff R, editor: *Geriatric nutrition: the health professional's handbook,* Gaithersburg, Md, 1991, Aspen Publishers.

66. McIntosh WA, Shifflet P: Influence of social support systems on dietary intake of the elderly, *J Nutr Elderly* 4(1):579, 1984.

67. McIntosh WA and others: The relationship between beliefs about nutrition and dietary practices of the elderly, *J Am Diet Assoc* 90:671, 1990.

68. Morgan KJ, Zabik ME, Stampley GL: Breakfast consumption patterns of older Americans, *J Nutr Elderly* 5(4):19, 1986.

69. Morley JE, Silver AJ: Anorexia in the elderly, *Neurobiol Aging* 9:9, 1988.

70. Murphy SP, Everett DF, Dresser CM: Food group consumption reported by the elderly during the NHANES I Epidemiologic Followup Study, *J Nutr Educ* 21:214, 1989.

71. Murphy SP and others: Factors influencing the dietary adequacy and energy intake of older Americans, *J Nutr Educ* 22:284, 1990.

72. Palmer CA, Papas AS: Nutrition and oral health of the elderly, *World Rev Nutr Diet* 59:71, 1989.

73. Papas AS and others: Longitudinal relationships between nutrition and oral health, *Ann NY Acad Sci* 561:124, 1989.

74. Peters GR, Rappoport L: Aging and the psychosocial problematics of food, *Am Behavioral Scient* 32:31, 1988.

75. Posner BEM, Smigelski CG, Krachenfels MM: Dietary characteristics and nutrient intake in an urban homebound population, *J Am Diet Assoc* 87:452, 1987.

76. Rammohan M, Juan D, Jung D: Hypophagia among hospitalized elderly, *J Am Diet Assoc* 89:1774, 1989.

77. Raper N, Marston R: Nutrient content of the US food supply and tables of nutrients provided by the US food supply, HNIS Administrative Rep No 299-21, Hyattsville, Md, 1988, US Department of Agriculture.

78. Rauschenback BS and others: Dependency on soup kitchens in urban areas of New York state, *Am J Public Health* 80:57, 1990.

79. Rheaume Y, Riley ME, Volcier L: Meeting nutritional needs of Alzheimer patients who pace constantly, *J Nutr Elderly* 7:43, 1987.

80. Rhodus N, Brown J: The association of xerostomia and inadequate intake of older adults, *J Am Diet Assoc* 90:1688, 1990.

81. Roe DA: In-home nutritional assessment of inner city elderly, *J Nutr* 120:1538, 1990.

82. Rounds TQ: Where in the world have you been? *Am Demogr* 10:30, 1988.
83. Ryan VC, Bower ME: Relationship of socioeconomic status and living arrangements to nutritional intake of the older person, *J Am Diet Assoc* 89:1805, 1989.
84. Sandman P and others: Nutritional status and dietary intake in institutionalized patients with Alzheimer's disease and multiinfarct dementia, *J Am Geriatr Soc* 35:31, 1987.
85. Schafer RB, Keith PM: Social-psychological factors in the dietary quality of married and single elderly, *J Am Diet Assoc* 81:30, 1982.
86. Sellery SB: New product opportunities: diet food for older Americans, *J Nutr Elderly* 4:31, 1984.
87. Senauer BH, Asp E, Kinsey J: Food trends and the changing consumer, St Paul, Minn, 1991, Eagen Press.
88. Shrimper R: Effects of increasing elderly population on future food demands and consumption. In Capps O, Senauer B, editors: Food demand analysis, Blacksburg, Va, 1986, Southern Regional Research Committee and Farm Foundation.
89. Singleton N, Overstreet MH, Schilling PE: Dietary intakes and characteristics of two groups of elderly females, *J Nutr Elderly* 1(1):77, 1980.
90. Slesinger DP, McDivitt M, O'Donnell FM: Food patterns in an urban population: age and sociodemographic correlates, *J Gerontol* 35(1):432, 1980.
91. Stanek K, Hensley MS, Van Riper MS: Factors affecting use of food and commercial agents to thicken liquids for individuals with swallowing disorders, *J Am Diet Assoc* 92:488, 1992.
92. Stanton JL, McNutt K: Future food for Americans, *Food and Nutrition News* 62(5):1, 1990.
93. Suski NS, Nielson CC: Factors affecting food intake of women with Alzheimer's type dementia in long-term care, *J Am Diet Assoc* 89:1770, 1989.
94. Templeton CL: Nutritional counseling needs in a geriatric population, *Geriatrics* 33:59, 1978.
95. Tong A: Eating habits of elderly Vietnamese in the United States, *J Nutr Elderly* 10:35, 1991.
96. Troll LE: Eating and aging, *J Am Diet Assoc* 59:456, 1971.
97. US Bureau of the Census: Poverty in the United States: 1990, Curr Pop Rep Series P-60, No 175, Washington, DC, 1991, US Government Printing Office.
98. US Congressional Budget Office: Trends in family income: 1970-1986, Washington, DC, 1988, US Government Printing Office.
99. US Department of Agriculture: A decade in review, *Nat Food Review* 13(3):1, 1990.
100. US Department of Agriculture: Food and nutrient intakes of individuals in 1 day, low-income households, November 1977 - March 1978, Nationwide Food Consumption Survey 1977-1978, Preliminary Rep No 11, Washington, DC, 1982, US Government Printing Office.
101. US Department of Agriculture: Nutrient intakes: individuals in 48 states, year 1977-78, Nationwide Food Consumption Survey 1977-1978, Rep No 1-2, Washington, DC, 1984, US Government Printing Office.
102. US Department of Health and Human Services, US Department of Agriculture: Nutrition monitoring in the United States: an update report on nutrition monitoring, DHHS Pub No (PHS) 89-1255, Washington, DC, 1989, US Government Printing Office.
103. US Department of Health and Human Services: Americans needing home care: data from the National Health Survey, DHHS Pub No (PHS) 86-1581, Hyattsville, Md, 1986, US Government Printing Office.
104. US Department of Health and Human Services: Healthy People 2000: national health promotion and disease prevention objectives, DHHS Pub No (PHS) 91-50213, Washington, DC, 1991, US Government Printing Office.
105. Vetter NJ and others: The relationship between dietary habits and beliefs in elderly people compared with younger people, *J Nutr Elderly* 9(4):3, 1990.
106. Walker D, Beauchene RE: The relationship of loneliness, social isolation, and physical health to dietary adequacy of independently living elderly, *J Am Diet Assoc* 91:300, 1991.
107. Wascoe Jr D: Survey studies elderly in all shades of grey, *Minneapolis Star Tribune*, Dec 6, 1989.
108. Weiler PG: The public health impact of Alzheimer's disease, *Am J Public Health* 77:1169, 1987.
109. Westenbrink S and others: Effect of household size on nutritional patterns among the Dutch elderly, *J Am Diet Assoc* 89:793, 1989.
110. Williams TF: Research and care: essential partners in aging, *Gerontologist* 28:579, 1988.
111. Wolf D: The ageless market, *Am Demogr* 9:26, 1987.
112. Zallen EM, Hooks LB, O'Brien K: Salt taste

preferences and perceptions of elderly and young adults, *J Am Diet Assoc* 90:947, 1990.

SELECTED RESOURCES

Conacher G: *Kitchen sense for disabled people,* Dover, NH, 1986, Croom Helm (on behalf of the Disabled Living Foundation).

Institute of Rehabilitation Medicine, New York University Medical Center and Campbell Soup Co: *Mealtime management for people with disabilities and the aging,* ed 2, New York, 1978, Campbell Soup Co.

Klinger JL: *Self-help manual for arthritis patients,* New York, 1980, Arthritis Foundation.

Sargent JV: *An easier way: handbook for the elderly and handicapped,* Ames, Ia, 1981, Iowa State University Press.

13

Nutrition and the Continuum of Health Care in Older Adults

Marsha Read
Eleanor D. Schlenker

Objectives

****

After studying the chapter, the student should:

✔ *Understand why there is a need to provide health and nutrition services to older Americans.*

✔ *Recognize the types of nutrition services provided by the federal, state, and local governments.*

✔ *List the types of long-term care facilities available for adults and discuss types of nutrition services that must be provided.*

✔ *Apply the principles of food management and food safety to delivery of home meals for the elderly.*

✔ *Identify the effect of federally funded nutrition programs on nutrient intakes of older people.*

Introduction

Providing food for older people at home is an activity described in early folklore. In the well-known fairy tale, Little Red Riding Hood was visiting her grandmother and taking a basket of food. When the extended family was the general rule, older people had relatives nearby who provided any assistance that was needed. With the current nuclear family and increased mobility, many older people now live at great distances from other family members. Services developed by community organizations and government agencies now help meet the need for meal, shopping, or transportation services. A health professional working with older people must be knowledgeable regarding the food and nutrition services available in the community, the nutrient contribution of the food provided, and the system for client referral.

CONCEPT OF LONG-TERM CARE
The Continuum of Care

The **continuum of care** refers to the range of health, nutrition, social, and personal services required to support independent living and personal well-being at the highest possible level. An individual may require one service or a range of services. For the older person who can no longer drive or handle bundles of groceries, grocery delivery or assistance with grocery shopping may be the only service required. If the individual is unable to prepare meals, homemaker services or **home-delivered meals** may solve the problem. When help is needed with **activities of daily living (ADLs)** such as eating, dressing, or bathing, personal services will be required. This implies a need for a continuum of nutrition and health services ranging from preventive health services such as regular physical examinations, nutrition education, or **congregate meals** for the healthy older person, to home delivery of meals to the frail elderly individual, to the skilled nursing facility required for the aged adult with numerous medical problems who is confined to bed.[45]

Home and Community Services

Types of services. Support services may be formal or informal.[60] Formal services are provided by **home health agencies,** government agencies, or for-profit agencies, and in most instances payment is required. The formal services provided by government agencies funded under the **Older Americans Act** are an exception. Those services are available to all people age 60 or older at no charge, although voluntary donations are encouraged. Typical formal services include congregate meals, home-delivered meals, transportation, homemaker services (may involve shopping, meal preparation, or housekeeping), senior center services (social, educational, or referral), telephone checks, personal care (assistance with ADLs), and health care (visit of home health nurse).[52]

Short and Leon[52] reported that in-home meal and housekeeping services were used by 1.4 million people over age 65. Services used to a lesser extent included telephone checks and transportation.

The use of formal home and community services is influenced by age; living arrangement; and functional status, which is defined by limitations in ADLs and **instrumental activities of daily living (IADLs).**[66] Recent statistics suggest that of all people age 65 to 74 who have difficulty walking or have at least one ADL or IADL limitation, 32% use at least one formal service; this increases to 43% in those age 85 or older. Among older adults with at least three ADL limitations, 47% use formal services. The help received from others in the household should not be underestimated, since only 24% of those with two ADL limitations who live with others use formal services, compared to 56% of those who live alone.[66]

Informal services are provided by family members, friends, or neighbors, usually at no cost. More than 60% of functionally dependent older people are cared for by family members.[59] Family care may continue for an extended period until an acute illness or other crisis makes home care impossible. An older individual with impaired mobility may be cared for by a spouse or adult child who handles meal preparation and household chores. Debilitating illness requiring confinement to bed can result in short-term or permanent institutionalization if formal services by a home health nurse or supervised home health aide cannot be arranged or are not sufficient to meet the person's needs. Unfortunately, formal services are not always available to assist a family attempting to care for an older person. Providing meals on weekends and delivering supplemental groceries might be easily handled by family members if home-delivered meals or homemaker services are available Monday through Friday.

Nutrition-related services such as homemaker services or home-delivered meals do not exist in some localities, and costs are not reimbursed under most existing insurance plans.[67] When such services do exist and are financially accessible, older people may not know about them. A survey of elderly adults in the Chicago area[12] revealed that residents of public housing were more likely to be aware of a local home-delivered meals program than suburban homeowners.

Current issues in home care. A major development that has strained the resources of agencies providing home care services was the implementation of the **prospective payment system** based on **diagnosis-related groups (DRGs)**.[68] Because payment rates are fixed according to the DRG into which the older patient is assigned, hospitals limit costs by reducing the length of the hospital stay. Consequently, Medicare patients are being discharged earlier and "sicker" and in greater need of home services. In a survey of 35 home health agencies,[68] 83% reported an increasing severity of illness in the patients they were serving. Patients were also more likely to be readmitted to the hospital and more frequent home health visits were required. The increasing home care needs of the acutely ill older population have limited the availability of services to the frail elderly.

This trend of an increased need for services after discharge from the hospital has also been reported by nutrition programs.[3] In one location 44% of those requesting home-delivered meals were early releases from area hospitals, and many were in need of special diets such as restricted sodium or renal diets.[3] Older people requesting home-delivered meals to support continued independent living often were bypassed and available funds used for emergency services. An Ohio study[40] emphasized that case management of the acutely ill older person being cared for at home requires the services of a nutrition professional who can assess nutrition needs, assist in the planning of appropriate meal services, and monitor the patient's progress. Unfortunately, nutrition services are seldom reimbursed by insurance and thus are not available to those with a low income. Nutrition services are also critical to the support of patients and families served by hospice programs.[4]

The demands for nutrition services for acutely ill older individuals are competing for dollars now allocated to nutrition programs providing meals, nutrition screening, and nutrition education important for maintaining frail elderly people and preventing debilitating disease.[5] The needs are increasing, but funding strategies are lagging behind.

A new community-based service to assist older people and their families is the **adult day care center**.[39] This facility provides supervision, personal care, and appropriate activities in a structured environment. Older people spend the day in the facility and return to their homes in the evening. Services are directed toward maintaining the physically or mentally impaired older adult and, to the extent possible, restoring physical and communication skills through directed activities or therapy. The adult day care center offers an ideal setting for nutrition screening and intervention with the older patient and family members.

Resident Facilities for Long-Term Care

Several types of resident facilities accommodate older people with physical or mental disabilities, serious illness, or a need for supervision or personal care. Facilities differ as to the level of nursing or personal care provided and the availability of services by a nutrition professional. In resident facilities, patients are assigned to a level of care based on confinement to a bed or wheelchair, mental state, ability to perform ADLs, and need for medical and nursing care. About 91% of institutionalized people need help with bathing, and 40% need some assistance with eating.[28] About 1.5 million people over age 64 are being cared for in nursing homes.[67] There are three main types of resident facilities:

- A *skilled nursing facility* provides 24-hour professional nursing care under the supervision of a physician. Most patients are confined to a bed or wheelchair and require skilled nursing procedures and supervised medications. A nutrition professional must be available on a consultant basis to provide specialized nutrition care.[4]
- An *intermediate-care facility* is not required to have registered nurses present at all times, since patients do not require constant nursing care but do need services be-

yond the level of room and board. Patients are more likely to be ambulatory and able to handle their medications without direct supervision. A nutrition professional must be available on a consultant basis to provide appropriate nutrition care.[4]

- A *personal care home* provides only room, board, and supervision with no medical services. This type of facility does not qualify for Medicaid or Medicare reimbursement. In many states there is no requirement for the services of a nutrition professional.

A new concept in resident long-term care is the **continuing-care retirement community,** which provides all options of care ranging from meal services only, to assisted living facilities offering personal care, to skilled nursing care.[68] Older people usually join the community while in good health and live independently, although options for meal services in a community dining room are available. As the need for personal or nursing care arises, the resident moves from one level of care to another. Such communities place a strong emphasis on promoting health, and nutrition services directed toward both preventive health and acute care are likely to be available.

Home Versus Institutional Care

The relative benefits and cost effectiveness of home versus institutional care remain controversial.[17,59,63,68] However, rising institutional costs have stimulated new interest in more sophisticated levels of home care. For example, elderly individuals requiring tube feeding or who have serious illnesses such as chronic obstructive pulmonary disease are now cared for at home.[40] Cost containment measures tend to favor home care over institutional care, yet few data are available on the true cost of home care. Homebound elderly in Minnesota[71] who were dropped from a home care program because of financial exigency had subsequent hospitalization rates that were twice as high as those for individuals who remained in the program. Older people in New York[49] receiving home-delivered meals had half the risk of institutionalization of those similar in age and health who were without services.

Comparing the cost of institutionalization (nursing home, group home, or other extended-care facility) versus home care services is not appropriate unless the relative quality of the services can be evaluated.[63] Community-based services do appear to serve a different clientele, people with less severe disabilities and fewer medical problems than those in nursing homes. Nevertheless, it has been estimated that 10% to 40% of those confined to long-term care facilities who do not require assistance with the ADLs could have remained in the community if in-home services had been available.[63]

NUTRITION PROGRAM FOR THE ELDERLY (TITLE III-C)
Pertinent Legislation

The amended version of the Older Americans Act of 1965 is the major piece of federal legislation providing nutrition programs for people age 60 and over. When establishing the **Nutrition Program for the Elderly** in 1972, Congress pointed to the fact that many elderly people do not eat adequately because (1) they cannot afford to do so; (2) they lack the skills to select and prepare nourishing, well-balanced meals; (3) they have limited mobility, which may impair their capacity to shop and cook for themselves; and (4) many feel rejected and lonely, feelings that can obliterate the incentive to prepare and eat a meal alone.[42] Although these factors remain important, the continued aging of the elderly population and the increased prevalence of **functional disability** have added to the complexity of the services needed.

The nutrition program, designed to provide nourishing meals in a social setting, was originally established under Title VII of the Older Americans Act. In 1978 it was reorganized under Title III-C and is still often referred to as the **Title III-C nutrition program.** The 1978 amendments provided for the integration of nutrition and social services, including (1) transportation services, and (2) the establishment of a home-delivered meals component with separate funding.[26] Previous guidelines restricted the number of meals that could be home delivered and emphasized meals served in a congregate setting.

The increasing number of **frail** and home-bound elderly has supported an ever-growing demand for meals delivered to the home. In recent years home-delivered meals have increased at the rate of 12% a year.[5] The total budget for the nutrition program, including federal, state, and local funds and participant contributions, is about $1 billion annually.[5] More than 250 million meals are served each year, and about 40% of these are home delivered.[42] More than 2.7 million older Americans participate in congregate meals, and nearly 800,000 receive home-delivered meals.[42]

General Organization

Under the Older Americans Act, each state is required to establish **area agencies on aging**, which are responsible for planning, organizing, and implementing nutrition and social services in a given geographic area. A nutrition project serving a designated area administers a variable number of congregate meal sites and home-delivered meals services, depending on the size of the area and its population density. Funds are appropriated by the federal government according to the number of people age 60 or over residing in the state. A small percentage of total operating funds (15%) must be contributed from state or local sources. Many programs have expanded their funding base through local fund-raising efforts and grants secured from charitable foundations. Meal recipients are also encouraged to make a donation toward the cost of the meal received.

Under federal guidelines a hot or cold meal is served or delivered 5 days a week, usually at noon. In rural and sparsely populated areas, meals may be served only 1 to 4 days a week. Generally neither meal sites nor home-delivery services operate on weekends.

Nutrient Content of Meals

Nutrient requirements. Regulations developed for the Nutrition Program for the Elderly when it was initiated required that each meal provide one third of the recommended dietary allowance (RDA) for this age group.[5,48,54]

The Title III-C Meal Pattern (Table 13-1), which indicates both the types and amounts of food to be included in each meal, was developed to assist in meal planning and is still used by many programs. Based on the RDAs for men and women over age 50, a meal providing approximately one third of the daily energy needs should contain about 600 to 800 kcal.[48]

Since 1972 our nutrition knowledge has expanded, with an emphasis on dietary patterns for preventing disease as well as ensuring nutritional adequacy. Some programs recommend limiting fat to no more than 30% of total kilocalories, although a recent review[48] mentions several reasons why the fat content could be somewhat higher. First, most Title III-C programs provide only one meal each day, and for some participants, especially the homebound, this may be their only major meal; thus providing a higher level of all nutrients can be justified. Also, for older individuals with chronic disease for whom unintended weight loss is a serious threat, a low-fat diet is inappropriate. Finally, gravies and sauces are often necessary to maintain temperature and moisture in meals that are transported and held for an extended period of time. At the same time, a meal containing only 30% fat will benefit the healthy young-old who participate in these programs.[48] The vast differences in health status between

TABLE 13-1   Title III-C Meal Pattern

Food Type	Recommended Portion Size
Meat or meat alternate	3 ounces of cooked edible portion
Vegetables and fruits	Two ½-cup servings
Enriched whole-grain bread or alternate	One serving (one slice of bread or equivalent)
Butter or margarine	1 teaspoon
Dessert	½ cup
Milk	½ pint (1 cup)

From the US Department of Health, Education, and Welfare: *Guide to effective project operations: the Nutrition Program for the Elderly,* Corvallis, Ore, 1973, Oregon State University.

older adults who attend congregate meals and some chronically ill adults who receive home-delivered meals accentuate the complexity associated with menu planning and management in Title III-C programs.

Emphasis on nutrient density. Because the Title III-C meal is the major source of nutrients for many participants, maximizing **nutrient density** provided is critical. Fruits and vegetables are important sources of the carotenoids, vitamins B_6 and C, folic acid, potassium, magnesium, and fiber, and are likely to be consumed only infrequently at other meals. Dark green, deep yellow, and citrus items and potatoes are particularly good nutrient sources. The nutrient content of meals can be enhanced by selecting dessert options from this group, such as a citrus fruit, banana, or pumpkin pudding.

Although bread and cereal products prepared from enriched grains are acceptable, whole-grain items will improve the intake of fiber, vitamins, and trace minerals such as manganese and chromium. Whole-grain foods may be particularly important for physically impaired older people who consume mostly preprepared foods at other meals. Whole-grain breads and pasta can be introduced gradually to improve acceptance among those less accustomed to these items.

Because rising food costs limit the size and frequency of servings of meat, fish, liver, or poultry, other sources of high-quality protein, vitamin B_6, iron, and zinc need to be considered. Legumes, lentils, peanut butter, or tofu (if well accepted) are possible alternatives. If cheese or other milk-based items are the primary protein source, iron and zinc must be provided elsewhere in the meal. Whole-grain items and a dessert containing eggs, peanut butter, or iron-rich fruits could contribute the other nutrients needed. Vegetable protein products made from soybeans are low in fat and relatively inexpensive, and as meat extenders contribute high-quality protein.[48] It is wise, however, to monitor the sodium content of these products.

Older people generally consume less than the recommended level of calcium (see Chapter 7), suggesting that milk-based menu items be emphasized. The fluid milk provided with the meal is more likely to be consumed if low-fat milk and buttermilk are available; buttermilk was preferred by black and Spanish American adults attending a Title III-C program in Texas (see Chapter 4). Milk and dairy products can also be used in cooking. Nonfat dry milk or grated lower fat cheeses can fortify soups, sauces, or mashed potatoes, increasing the calcium, protein, and riboflavin content. (Cheese is sometimes available to Title III-C programs as a government commodity item.)

Dessert should be a significant source of nutrients as well as a pleasant climax to the meal. Plain fruit or a baked fruit dessert made with whole grains contributes important vitamins and minerals. Pudding, custard, or ice cream provides calcium and high-quality protein for those who do not drink milk. In a home-delivered meals program, meals containing milk-based desserts fortified with nonfat dry milk had twice the calcium content of meals with desserts consisting of canned fruit or baked products prepared from a mix. Moist, flavorful baked products prepared with whole grains, oatmeal, raisins, applesauce, pumpkin, sweet potato, or banana will contain iron, B-complex vitamins, and trace minerals. Recipes contributing primarily sugar and fat should be avoided.

Special diets. At one time it was proposed that all nutrition programs offer a special diet option. It has been recognized, however, that this may not be possible because of related food costs, limitations of the caterer or other meal provider, or lack of an appropriate nutrition professional to supervise and implement the service.[11,48] Rather strict, physician-ordered regimens used in the treatment of specific medical problems (e.g., low-protein diets for **renal insufficiency**) usually are not available. Alternatively, special dietary options such as a meal somewhat lower in fat, sodium, or simple carbohydrates involve rather simple modifications and are easily accommodated. Implementation of the DRGs and use of home-delivered meals by acutely ill elderly people have intensified the need for home delivery of therapeutic diets.[3] Some programs have arranged to purchase such meals from hospital food service departments; however, the cost of these meals, if available, far exceeds the cost of the usual meals bought or produced by the nutrition program.[3]

A survey of 430 Title III-C nutrition programs[11] found that 67% offered a special dietary option. An earlier study of 91 meal programs[62] reported that 42% were making some effort to provide special diets, but for about one third this involved only limited changes such as no added salt or no added sugar. Special diets for reasonably healthy older people usually involve limiting kilocalories, sodium, or fat. For patients with diabetes mellitus or for others who must limit their caloric intake, the Title III-C meal pattern is likely to be acceptable if portion size is controlled, skim or low-fat milk is available, and fruit is offered as an alternative to a high-sugar, high-fat dessert. No salt should be added in meal preparation; those wishing to add salt may do so at the table. Preprepared entrees and soup or gravy mixes high in sodium should be avoided.

Serving procedures can influence the adaptability of meals to a variety of diets. At congregate meal sites it may be possible to ask participants if they wish to have added gravy or sauce when the item is served. Salad dressing can be provided in a small plastic cup when meals are home delivered. Margarine or butter, if added to vegetables, should be limited.

Limiting fat, sugar, and salt and increasing fiber and nutrient-dense carbohydrate foods should be goals in menu planning. Frozen or fresh vegetables are preferable to canned vegetables that contain added sodium. Unfortunately, cost or availability of a government commodity food often must take precedence over nutrient content, since funding has not kept pace with the increasing need for meals.

Food Service Management in Meal Programs

Nutrition projects may choose to prepare their own food or buy food from a caterer. This decision will depend on (1) the availability of food preparation facilities, (2) the proximity of meal sites to one another, and (3) the availability of potential caterers.[65] When there are several meal sites in a particular locality, meals may be prepared in a central kitchen operated by the nutrition project or a caterer and distributed to nearby sites. In rural areas, where meal sites are

at some distance from one another, each meal site may prepare its own meals, or meals may be purchased from a local vendor. In any given area the savings accrued through volume buying or large-scale food production must be evaluated in terms of the cost of transporting the prepared food to the serving locations. In a survey of 430 nutrition programs,[10] about 25% had their meals prepared by a caterer, 14% prepared meals on site, 16% prepared meals in their own central kitchen, and the remainder used some combination of these methods.

A major consideration in selecting a food service option is **total meal cost**, which includes food, labor, transportation, and administration costs. Cost control studies of nutrition projects that bought meals from a caterer and those that prepared their own food either on site or in a central kitchen indicated that meal cost was not related to the number of people served, whether the location was urban or rural, or the food preparation system.[65] The studies showed that selecting one system over another will not necessarily reduce costs. Projects with lower costs had (1) reduced labor and administrative costs by using personnel more efficiently, (2) sought better buys in food and supplies, and (3) shared facilities with other programs to decrease overhead. Larger nutrition projects with a greater number of meal sites had reduced costs compared to projects with fewer sites as a result of lower administrative costs per site. Other projects successfully used volunteers and elderly participants to reduce labor costs.

Balsam and Carlin[7] pointed out that regional cooperation among several nutrition projects can result in a lower contract price for catered meals from food service companies and for paper and other supplies. Being a member of a food bank offers the potential for lower cost food purchasing. Also, large-scale preparation of frozen meals for use at a later time offers cost control benefits.[8] Management practices that reduce or stabilize costs need to be emphasized in both project research and staff training.

Transportation of Prepared Food

Holding time. When food is prepared at a central location and transported either to meal sites for congregate meals or to individual homes, loss of nutrients, microbial growth, and deterioration in appearance, texture, and flavor are potential problems. The total length of time that food is held at serving temperature after final heating includes the time at the preparation site before or after packaging, the transportation time to the serving location, and the time food is held at the meal site or in the home before being eaten.[35] McCool and Posner[35] recommend that food be held less than 2 hours after final heating. Total holding time is influenced by the size of the geographic area served by the nutrition project or the length of the delivery route for home-delivered meals. Heavy traffic, poor roads in rural areas, and adverse weather conditions significantly increase holding time. Transportation time can be reduced by increasing the number of delivery vehicles, thereby shortening delivery routes. If existing constraints result in holding times beyond the 2-hour limit, prepared meals should be discontinued and frozen or shelf-stable items used in their place. Losses in food quality as a result of extended holding time may have influenced the reported preference of congregate meal participants for meals cooked on-site.[31]

Losses of ascorbic acid and the B-complex vitamins accelerate when food is held at serving temperature for long periods. A British evaluation of six home-delivered meals programs serving 4,200 meals daily[61] reported that cooked vegetables were held about 24 minutes before being placed in insulated delivery containers, and an additional 23 minutes transpired before the first meal was delivered. The time between delivery of the first and last meal was about 90 minutes. In this situation total holding time for the meals delivered last was 137 minutes, or 17 minutes beyond the recommended time. Losses of vitamin C averaged 31% to 54% during the holding period before delivery and up to 19% during delivery.[61] Because of the substantial losses of ascorbic acid from hot vegetables, a citrus juice or fruit in which the ascorbic acid is more stable may be a better menu choice. Nutrient losses through holding time should be considered when developing menus for meal programs.

Packaging of food. Packaging materials for transporting hot and cold foods must maintain the food at safe and acceptable temperatures, prevent contamination, be reasonable in cost, and be easily handled by both staff and older recipients. Desirable characteristics of meal delivery packaging are listed in the box below.[38,48,55]

Food served at meal sites usually is transported in bulk containers and portioned on-site. Bulk containers with an electrical power source that can be preheated and thermally controlled are available, although expensive. Home-delivered meals are individually packaged, keeping hot and cold items separate. The need for long-term investment and appropriate technology is particularly pertinent in relation to temperature control; hot and cold items are delivered under weather conditions ranging from 100° F in summer to −30° F in winter.

❖

IDEAL MEAL DELIVERY PACKAGING

• *Food containers*
Impervious to moisture
Firm (will not bend easily)
Easily stacked
Deep enough so that liquids do not spill
Resistant to heat transfer
Safe for reheating of food in conventional or microwave oven
Easily sealed
Environmentally safe for disposal
No sharp edges
No transfer of odor, flavor, or residue to food
Easily opened by older recipient or volunteer
• *Carrying case*
Easily cleaned with water and detergent
Stain and grease resistant
Impervious to moisture
Lightweight and easy to handle
Easily stacked
High degree of insulation
Tight-fitting latches or doors
Appropriate size and shape for delivery vehicle
Side bars or rails to prevent bulk food containers from tilting

To prevent microbial growth, cold items must be maintained at a temperature below 45° F and hot items at a temperature above 140° F.[35]

An English study[61] suggests that even electrically preheated carrying cases may not maintain hot foods at the appropriate temperature when holding time extends beyond 2 hours. The temperature of the last hot meals delivered was 106° F. However, the hot food may not have been heated to 165° F, the recommended temperature before being placed in the container. A manual developed for nutrition program managers[48] emphasizes the importance of preheating or precooling carrying containers before filling with bulk food or portioned meals. Because hot air rises, it is wise when transporting bulk food to put the foods with greater density on the bottom, to maximize heat transfer to foods of lesser density.

As innovations in food technology expand the types and methods of packaging and preservation, including more aseptic packaged goods, irradiated foods, and controlled- and modified-atmosphere packages, the holding properties of delivered foods probably will improve.[21, 53] Ultrapasteurized fluid milk that can be safely stored without refrigeration is available in both bulk and 1-cup containers. Frozen meals also diminish the potential of foodborne illness resulting from inappropriate handling of hot food.[8] The introduction of such foods will continue to have an impact on both congregate and meal delivery programs.

Congregate Meal Programs

Establishment of meal sites. Congregate meal sites have been established in community or recreation centers, municipal buildings, public housing, senior citizens centers, and churches. Important criteria in selecting a location for a congregate meal site are accessibility and familiarity to older people in the community.[55] Programs located in senior centers with on-going activities are more likely to be well attended.[62] An appropriate location has a major concentration of elderly people within walking distance or accessible public transportation. **Title III-B social service funds** are used to provide transportation to congregate meal sites[26];

however, the need is greater than can be accommodated with existing funds.

Importance of social component. The opportunity for **socialization** is one of the reasons given for participation in Title III-C meal programs[14,62]; in fact, in a nationwide survey Kirschner and associates[32] found that elements of socialization were as important as the meal itself to many participants. Older focus-group members commented that, "It's fellowship that's important."[44] Involving meal participants as volunteers or paid employees at the meal site also promotes self-esteem and a sense of being needed. The Title III-C nutrition program may be particularly important to older people living alone, since 58% of those who attended for at least 18 months lived alone, compared to only 43% of their nonparticipating neighbors similar in socioeconomic status.[62] In a national survey[62] about one fourth of older adults indicated they had no one to ask for help in a time of sickness or need. Friends from the meal site could provide this support.

Social support and referral to appropriate services can be critical for homeless or other disadvantaged older people. Unfortunately, these individuals, who are most in need of services, may not be welcome at congregate meal sites if they are unkempt or unclean in appearance or somewhat eccentric in behavior.[11] Reaching this target population may require innovative programs in the neighborhoods where these older people are found.

Home-Delivered Meals

Early history. The concept of home-delivered meals began early in this century. In 1905 the invalid kitchens of London began sending hot meals to housebound patients. The first meal delivery program in the United States began in Philadelphia in 1954. The program operated through a settlement house serving an area of about 5 square miles and delivered meals to 50 homebound clients each day.[38] Since that time the number of programs in the United States has expanded rapidly. Currently about 1,350 programs provide home meals.[11]

Program development. Meal delivery programs were first organized by community nonprofit organizations and health and social service agencies such as hospitals, churches, nursing homes, and visiting nurses associations. In many community-sponsored programs meals are delivered by volunteers who pay their own transportation costs, whereas in some Title III-C programs those who deliver meals are paid for both their time and mileage.

Meal delivery programs operate Monday through Friday. A hot meal is delivered at noon, and sometimes a cold meal is included to be eaten later. Some programs include additional frozen or cold meals before the weekend or a holiday. About half of all programs offer the option of weekend meals, but only 22% offer supper meals.[11] Delivery of cold or frozen meals requires that the recipient have appropriate storage facilities and a means of reheating a frozen meal. No program provides meals on all days or for all meals of the day.

Financial resources. Meal delivery programs differ in their funding sources and community affiliations.[66] Some programs receive no Title III-C funds and rely completely on private contributions, community funds, and fees from recipients. These programs depend heavily on volunteer help and are not subject to any federal regulations regarding program eligibility or the nutritional content of meals. Other programs combine both voluntary contributions and funds received from the local Title III-C agency, which contracts for meals to eligible recipients. Acceptance of Title III-C funds requires adherence to federal regulations regarding client eligibility and meal content. In some locations Title III-C programs deliver meals from a central kitchen or congregate meal sites. Title III-C funds have allowed the expansion of meal delivery to low-income elderly who cannot afford to pay.[50] Cooperation between established community meal delivery programs and Title III-C programs maximizes the use of resources and avoids duplication of effort.[50]

Eligibility requirements. Older people can request meal delivery or be referred by a family member, physician, visiting nurse, outreach worker, or social worker. Under Title III-C there are two requirements[50]: the recipient must be age 60 or over (spouses under age 60 can also be served), and the recipient must be confined to the home because of disability or other extenuating circumstances; eligibility must be documented by Title III-C or health personnel and recertified every 6 months.

All prospective clients should be visited and evaluated before meal delivery is initiated. If the individual can leave home, transportation to a Title III-C meal site provides an opportunity for social interaction as well as a meal. A two-person household may need home-delivered meals if one person is caring for an invalid partner and has little time to prepare meals. Home-delivered meals should not perpetuate an inappropriate situation as with an older person whose physical or mental condition has deteriorated to the point that living alone is hazardous.

Profile of recipients. Although home-delivered meals programs have been in existence for many years, descriptive information about recipients is limited. In a survey of nearly 600 recipients of Title III-C home-delivered meals,[64] the typical client was an older woman living alone. Nearly half were age 80 or older, despite the fact that this age group accounts for only about one fifth of the over-65 population. Although all income levels were represented, most recipients were considered low income. Of 16 home-delivered meal recipients in Alabama,[69] 12 were women and 4 were men; none were able to shop for food. The age range of 32 homebound meal recipients in North Carolina[56] was 60 to 96 years, with a mean of 78 years. About 45% of the group were black, which represented the approximate proportion of older black adults in that community. Twenty-two older adults between the ages of 65 and 86 were on a waiting list for meals.

Overall health status is a primary factor in determining the length of time an individual will receive meals at home. In an evaluation conducted in New York state,[23] about one third of all clients received meals for less than 6 months. This included individuals who depended on home-delivered meals after early release from the hospital or during general convalescence. Short-term users also included seriously ill older people who either died (these were most frequently cancer patients) or were moved to long-term care facilities. Older adults who continued to receive meals over a period of years were more likely to have chronic conditions that affected their mobility and level of activity.

Meal delivery procedures. For homebound elderly people, the social interaction with the individual delivering the meal is very important. This may be the only person they see that day, and the visit, although brief, reinforces the fact that someone cares about them. The success of a program depends to a great extent on the reliability and personal qualities of those delivering the meals, and their selection and training are critical.[70] Because they will be entering the homes of older people who are vulnerable both physically and emotionally, all must be carefully screened. Those who deliver meals must be trained to handle any irregular situation. If a recipient does not answer the door, they should know the person or agency to call, since this could indicate an emergency. The need for referral is particularly important if the recipient lives alone. Delivery staff should be alert to any physical or mental change in the older client and relay this information to the appropriate individual.

Food preferences of recipients. Recipients of home-delivered meals who were interviewed as part of a national evaluation of Title III-C services indicated general satisfaction with the meals.[44] An important finding was that they enjoyed a greater variety of food with meal delivery than would be possible if they were forced to manage for themselves. General concerns were entrees that were too greasy or too bland and vegetables that were overcooked. (These concerns were also expressed by congregate meal participants.) Another concern related to the meal pattern; one participant noted that on some days there was no meat, or no slice of bread, or no dessert.[44] It is difficult to know whether an entire meal component was omitted or if it was perceived to be missing because the meal included a meatless entree such as macaroni and cheese, or fruit for dessert rather than a more traditional item.

In a Minnesota study,[6] about two thirds of those receiving meals at home had problems chewing the meat that was served. Program managers must also be alert to the possible limitations in hand and finger motions of physically impaired older clients. Some meal recipients reported problems with cutting meat, opening cellophane wrappers, or spreading items on their bread.

Nutritional Impact of Meal Programs

Meal nutrient content. Title III-C meals are expected to provide one third of the RDA, but in many cases meals provide more than this amount for some nutrients. Biochemical analysis of meals collected from 119 different sites[65] revealed that more than three fourths contained at least 50% of the RDA for men of protein, calcium, phosphorus, vitamin A, and riboflavin; at least 40% of the RDA for iron and vitamin C; and about 33% of the RDA for energy, thiamin, and niacin. Half of the meals provided at least 67% of the day's requirement for protein and vitamin A. Zinc was the nutrient most frequently below 33% of the RDA. Energy, vitamin A, thiamin, and niacin were more likely to be low for men than for women because men's allowances are higher.

Although national evaluations suggest that meals often contain well above one third of the RDA, meals in a particular locality may fall below this level. In home-delivered meals obtained from a caterer over a 5-day period,[6] nutrients below one third of the RDA were energy (32%), calcium (23%), thiamin (29%), and riboflavin (30%). The meals did contain more than half the daily allowance for protein, vitamin A, and niacin. The marginal levels of several important nutrients were related to the meal supplier's failure to follow the Title III-C Meal Pattern. Evaluation of 30 meals collected over a 6-year period (Table 13-2) indicated that only the requirements for a serving of bread or grain and a serving of butter or margarine were met in all meals. The requirement for 1 cup of milk was not met in any of the meals evaluated. Program managers responsible for **quality assurance** must regularly evaluate the meals actually supplied by caterers and enforce contract specifications.

Nutrient intakes of congregate meal participants. Title III-C congregate meal participants consume better diets on the days that include a site meal and consume better diets than nonparticipating neighbors of similar age and socioeconomic background (Fig 13-1). A na-

TABLE 13-2   *Adherence of Catered Home-Delivered Meals to the Title III-C Guidelines**

Food Item	Number of Meals (%)
Meat (3 ounces) or alternate	9 (30%)
Fruits and vegetables (two, ½-cup servings)	20 (67%)
Bread or alternate (one slice)	30 (100%)
Whole-grain bread or alternate (optional)	10 (33%)
Butter or margarine (1 teaspoon)	30 (100%)
Dessert (½ cup)	20 (67%)
Milk (1 cup)	0 (0)

*Based on evaluation of 30 meals over 6 years.
Modified from Asp EH, Darling ME: Home-delivered meals: food quality, nutrient content, and characteristics of recipients, *J Am Diet Assoc* 88:55, 1988.

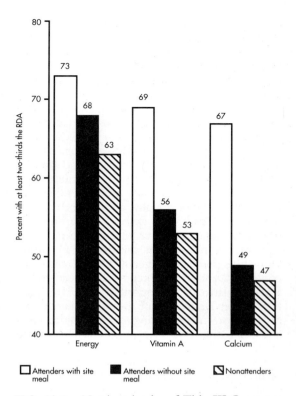

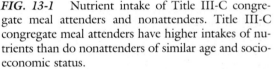

FIG. 13-1   Nutrient intake of Title III-C congregate meal attenders and nonattenders. Title III-C congregate meal attenders have higher intakes of nutrients than do nonattenders of similar age and socioeconomic status.

(Data from US Department of Health and Human Services: Longitudinal evaluation of the national Nutrition Program for the Elderly: report on first-wave findings, DHEW Pub No (OHDS) 80-20249, Washington, DC, 1979, US Government Printing Office.)

tionwide evaluation of Title III-C programs[62] found that the total daily intake of older adults who consumed a congregate meal was higher in virtually all nutrients compared to nonparticipants, former participants, and current participants who did not eat a program meal 24 hours before the survey. Calcium and vitamin A were most influenced by participation.

Among 68 older Mississippians,[37] those who regularly attended a congregate meal site had a mean calcium intake of 829 mg, compared to only 591 mg reported by nonparticipating neighbors. Ascorbic acid intakes fell below the RDA for 23% of the nonparticipants versus only 3% of the participants. These data suggest that older people consume limited amounts of milk and fewer citrus fruits or dark green vegetables at home. A participant in a focus group evaluating congregate meals[44] reported eating plenty of foods not eaten before, such as green vegetables. The importance of fruits and vegetables consumed at the meal site is further emphasized by the Missouri finding that 43% of nonparticipants had less-than-acceptable levels

of serum vitamin A compared to only 4% of those who attended a congregate meal 2 to 5 days a week.[18] Hemoglobin levels were also higher among men age 75 and over who had at least two congregate meals per week.

Kohrs and coworkers[33,34] evaluated the impact of Title III-C meals on the nutritional status of 466 rural older people in central Missouri. In that region menus provided from 40% to 80% of the RDA for most nutrients, and both men and women consumed nearly half of their daily intakes at the meal site. Socioeconomic factors influenced the Title III-C contribution to daily nutrient intake. Individuals with less education or who were previously employed as unskilled workers consumed a greater share of their nutrients at the congregate meal than those with more schooling and a technical or professional occupation. Since education and occupation are closely related to income, this finding suggests that the program helped the economically disadvantaged. Those benefiting most were women over age 75 who lived alone. It is interesting to note that in a Nebraska study,[72] 56% of meal site attenders were between 70 and 79, and 55% lived alone.

Nutrient intakes of recipients of home-delivered meals. The dietary adequacy of homebound older people depends not only on the nutrient content of the meals delivered but also on the food resources available on nondelivery days and for meals not included on delivery days. In two British studies both energy and vitamin intakes[20,54] were improved by meal delivery. The home-delivered meal supplied 70% of the vitamin A and 82% of the ascorbic acid consumed on that day.[54] Delivered meals contained only about 1,100 mg of potassium, and the diets of recipients generally were low in this nutrient.[19]

Little is known about the food intake of meal recipients on weekends. Although it is assumed that family members or neighbors provide assistance, this is likely not true for all. Individuals who lack other resources may save items from the noon meal for the evening meal or for weekend days. Home health nurses who visited older clients receiving home-delivered meals have reported finding food stockpiled in the refrigerator or even stored at room temperature.[6] In one survey,[54] about 50% of recipients saved food to eat at a later time. For an older individual dependent on food delivery, building a food reserve may represent a need for food security. The saving of food emphasizes the importance of available refrigeration for those receiving home-delivered meals and the need for nutrition education about meal storage. When refrigeration is not available, perishable items not consumed immediately must be discarded.

Evaluation of 3-day dietary records, including delivery and nondelivery days, obtained from 95 rural and urban home-meal recipients in California[57] indicated that many had low nutrient intakes. Seventy percent fell below two thirds of the RDA for three nutrients, and 25% fell below this level for up to 12 nutrients. The rural men were significantly underweight compared to the urban men (**body mass index [BMI]** of 21 versus 24), but the rural and urban women had a similar BMI, 25 versus 26. The rural elderly were more dependent on family members for assistance with shopping and cooking, whereas the urban elderly were more likely to have help from neighbors or paid workers.

An evaluation of home-meal recipients versus nonrecipients in North Carolina[56] indicated that more than half of both groups consumed less than the recommended level of vitamin A, riboflavin, calcium, phosphorus, and iron. Only 3% of recipients and 14% of nonrecipients met the RDA for all nutrients evaluated. It is surprising that nonrecipients (who were on the waiting list for home-delivered meals) had in some cases better diets. It may be that family members or neighbors made a special effort to provide meals or groceries to those still waiting for home-delivered meals. Conversely, it could have been assumed that recipients of home-delivered meals had sufficient food even though they received only five meals a week.

A pilot study of 16 home-meal recipients in Alabama[69] indicated that the home-delivered meal provided 40% to 50% of the daily nutrient intake on weekdays. A significantly higher proportion of recipients fell below 67% of the RDA for thiamin, riboflavin, calcium, and iron on weekend days. Despite the small number of subjects and the limitations of 24-hour dietary recall records used for dietary evaluation, this study does support the need for weekend meals.

Innovative Approaches for Target Populations

Success in reaching target populations. Despite the success of the Title III-C program, there continue to be unmet needs among the clientele to be served.[11] The original legislation creating the nutrition program emphasized the needs of poor elderly and disadvantaged minority elderly. A recent report to Congress[42] indicated that 51% of congregate meal attenders and 59% of home-meal recipients were poor. Others have estimated that 22% of the elderly poor nationwide are reached by congregate meal programs.[44] The general participation of low-income older people is related to the relative number living in the immediate area served. Poor individuals are also more likely to attend daily.[62]

Minority participation in Title III-C programs has been less than would be expected based on the number of black and Hispanic elderly people with incomes below the poverty level. Only about 17% of all meals are served to minority elderly.[42] Greater effort is needed to target services to these groups by creating additional meal sites and delivery programs in areas with large minority populations and providing culturally appropriate meals within existing programs. Participation in congregate meals by mobility-impaired older people is extremely low (2% to 3% of participants), and recruitment efforts have been relatively unsuccessful.[62] This could relate to the physical characteristics or locations of meal sites or the need for help among frail or physically impaired individuals, such as service at the table if the meal is handled buffet style.

Programs directed toward target populations. The usual 5-day pattern of meal service by both congregate and home-delivered meals programs does not supply the nutritional needs of older people with no other food resources. A survey of 594 home-delivered meals programs nationwide[69] indicated that 32% provided some weekend meals. Balsam and Rogers[11] reported that weekend meals were provided by 50% of home-delivered meals programs but only 17% of congregate meal programs. Sixty-one percent of the programs surveyed offered shopping assistance in the form of an escort service or grocery delivery. A new idea is the **luncheon club**,[9] in which frail elderly meet every day for a meal in the home of a member or in the social room of their housing complex. Food is delivered daily in bulk or preportioned, depending upon the program.

✤
POSSIBLE SUBSTITUTIONS IN THE TITLE III-C MEAL PATTERN

Meat or meat alternate (3 ounces)—
  substitutions for 1 ounce cooked meat:
    1 ounce cooked fish or poultry
    1 egg
    1 ounce cheddar cheese
    ½ cup cooked dried beans, peas, or
      lentils
    ¼ cup cottage cheese
Examples of combinations that meet the
  standard of 3 ounces of meat or equivalent:
    Cheeseburger made with 2 ounces of
      cooked beef plus a 1-ounce slice of
      cheese
    Italian lasagna (2 ounces meat, 2
      tablespoons cottage cheese, and ½ egg
      per serving)
    Cheese enchilada (1 ounce cheese and 1
      cup refried beans)
Fruits and vegetables (two ½-cup
  servings)—substitutions for ½ cup
  vegetable or fruit:
    ½ cup vegetable juice
    ½ cup fruit juice
Bread (one serving)—substitutions for one
  slice of bread or one roll:
    ½ cup cooked spaghetti, macaroni, or
      noodles (enriched)
    ½ cup cooked rice (enriched or whole
      grain)
    5 saltine crackers (enriched) or 2 graham
      crackers
    1 cornmeal muffin
    1 tortilla
Dessert (½ cup)—suggestions for one serving
  of dessert:
    ½ cup fruit (fresh, canned, frozen)
    ½ cup pudding
    ½ cup ice cream, sherbet, or ice milk
    1 serving cake or cobbler
    2 cookies

Adapted from Staton M and others: *Handbook for site operations: the Nutrition Program for the Elderly,* Corvallis, OR, 1975, Oregon State University.

Currently relatively few nutrition programs regularly serve ethnic meals.[44] Federal guidelines do offer suggestions for substitutions basic to various ethnic tastes (see box). The paucity of programs offering meals appropriate for specific ethnic groups no doubt contributes to the low Title III-C participation by minority and non-English-speaking older people.

Of concern is the relationship between the number of service innovations and the proportion of minority and low-income elderly in the area served. Contrary to expectations, supper or weekend meals, meals for homeless older people, or food pantry assistance are less likely to be found in those regions serving the people in greatest need.[11]

A group that continues to increase in number but receives limited support from Title III-C programs is defined as the **socially impaired elderly**—the homeless, those who live in **single-room occupancy,** those who are physically abused or neglected, alcoholics, or those recently deinstitutionalized.[11] Intensive outreach efforts to seek those in need coupled with the development of geographically accessible programs in which the socially impaired older person is made to feel welcome should be a priority in the years ahead.

Future Directions of the Nutrition Program for the Elderly

The Title III-C program has significant implications for health promotion and prevention of malnutrition and debilitating illness in the older population. Several issues relating to meal nutrient content, program management, and funding will influence its future effectiveness.

Nutrient content of meals. The nutrition standards for meal planning should be expanded to address sodium, fat, and other food components related to disease prevention. Professional groups[5] continue to recommend that meals provide an averaged intake over 5 days that meets one third of the RDA. If two or three meals a day are provided, 5-day averaged intakes should equal two thirds or 100% of the recommended level. Opinions differ as to whether programs should provide only the minimum level of nutrients required per meal

(33% of the RDA) rather than a higher level.[5] Providing the minimum amounts of food makes it possible to serve the maximum number of meals with the funds available. On the other hand, if the Title III-C meal at noon is the person's major food source, an increased level of nutrients is mandated. Providing more than one meal a day for those with limited resources may be the appropriate response.

Level of funding. Currently home-delivered and congregate meals compete for funds. The growing demand for home care has led to an on-going transfer of funds from congregate to home-delivered meals.[5] This shift in funds reflects attention to immediate versus long-term needs. Congregate meals have a long-term role in maintaining nutritional status and reducing future disability and dependency. Both programs require an adequate level of funding to offset future health care costs.[27] Funding problems also result in increased emphasis on suggested donations from congregate and home-delivered meal recipients. This approach can result in reduced participation of low-income and homeless older adults who are most in need of nutritious food.[11,42,44]

Leadership by nutrition professionals. Current federal regulations do not require the services of nutritional professionals within the Title III-C program. A survey of 430 nutrition programs found that only 9% had project directors who were nutrition professionals.[11] A project director may be responsible for the overall supervision of as many as 145 meal sites.[62] To maximize nutrient content, meal planners must recognize not only the nutritional contributions of particular foods but also the overall nutrient requirements of older individuals as related to both physiologic and socioeconomic factors. The nutrition professional also can address program cost containment, food safety, and overall meal quality.[5]

Nutrition education and referral. Title III-C programs offer a model for providing nutrition education and health promotion services. On-going nutrition assessment (see Chapter 11) could identify what other nutrition or support services are necessary to allow the individual to remain independent.[15] Interestingly, a recent expert panel[22] concluded that congestive heart disease, hypertension, and the adverse effects of drugs were areas with high potential for intervention as related to older adults. Each of these conditions can benefit from nutrition intervention.

Food and meal services. The reduction in cost associated with weekly delivery of five or more frozen meals is estimated to range from 16% to as much as 50%.[8,43] As frozen meals continue to grow in popularity, it will be necessary to seek ways to provide daily social contact, either in person or by telephone, for the homebound adult who no longer receives daily meal delivery. It will also be important to monitor food freezing practices. Individual meal sites with freezers that were not intended for freezing large quantities of food at one time need guidelines as to the number of frozen meals that can be safely produced.[60]

For homebound older people who are able to cook, groceries can supplement either frozen or hot meals. In one study with rural elderly,[30] groceries were delivered weekly to supplement two home-delivered hot meals. Recipes and preparation suggestions were included. Fresh vegetables and fruits, dairy products, and high-protein foods were emphasized. The weekly delivery of perishable food items allowed these homebound elderly to manage with only one major food delivery a month by a relative or neighbor to supply staple items. Canned, dehydrated, irradiated, and freeze-dried foods that can be stored at room temperature for a year or more may replace meal delivery or provide a food reserve for weekends or emergencies.

MEAL SERVICES IN LONG-TERM CARE FACILITIES
Nutritional Adequacy and Food Service Management

Federal regulations governing food service in skilled nursing and intermediate-care facilities eligible for Medicare and Medicaid reimbursement address both the nutritional quality of the food to be provided and the scheduling of meals[16]:

- Meals and snacks must provide 100% of the RDA.

- Meals and snacks must adhere to the physician's diet order.
- At least three meals must be served.
- Bedtime nourishment must be offered unless prohibited by the physician's diet order.
- No more than 14 hours may elapse between the evening meal and breakfast.

To facilitate implementation states have developed menu patterns expected to provide the level of kilocalories and nutrients required. As pointed out by Coulston,[16] however, fiscal restraints influence the quality of both the food and nutrition services provided. Although the financial reimbursement to long-term care facilities is increased periodically as the costs of patient care increase, an individual facility decides how these funds are allocated, and food budgets may not be increased. In fact, if other costs exceed the reimbursement level, the food budget may actually be decreased, resulting in food of lesser quality and nutrient content.

An important consideration in planning meals in a long-term care facility is nutrient density. In 14 nursing homes in Wisconsin,[51] the RDAs for calcium, iron, thiamin, riboflavin, and niacin were not met unless individuals consumed more than 2,000 kcal. At the median energy intake (1,620 kcal for men; 1,361 kcal for women) only protein and vitamins A, C, and B_{12} met the RDAs for both sexes. At caloric intakes of 2,000 kcal, menus still contained less than the recommended levels of magnesium, zinc, pyridoxine, and folic acid. More than half of the 108 women studied consumed less than 55% of the RDAs for those four nutrients.

Caloric intakes varied widely within the Wisconsin population.[51] Men consumed from 983 to 3,007 kcal and women from 513 to 2,613 kcal. Other workers[58] have reported mean caloric intakes of 1,720 and 1,330 kcal for institutionalized men and women, respectively. Sempos and coworkers[51] concluded that nursing home menus should be planned to meet the RDAs on low energy intakes and suggested that 1,400 kcal be used as a base. Obviously, patients who are ambulatory and active should not be limited to 1,400 kcal.

Allington and coworkers[1,2] developed a

model food plan based on 16 food groups that defines the number of pounds from each food category that must be used per month per 100 patients if the RDA is to be met for all nutrients without exceeding 110% of the RDA for energy. To remain within the caloric requirement, cake and pastry desserts were reduced. Food items that were increased included meat, fish, and poultry; dried peas, beans, and nuts; green, leafy vegetables; bananas; and dry cereals, including wheat germ and bran flakes. Such changes, however, also increase costs.

Patient Satisfaction With Meals Served

Addressing food issues in long-term care facilities, Gallagher[24] emphasized that "above all, we want the residents to eat." This requires that food tastes good, looks attractive, and is served in a pleasant environment. Tablecloths or tray liners in soft colors not only increase the appeal of the food served but also help those with impaired vision to distinguish plates and cups from the table surface. A glass of milk can be difficult to see placed on a white tablecloth.

Special attention to recipe development can turn inexpensive food items and even pureed dishes into popular menu additions. Experimenting with a pastry bag and thickening agents will improve the quality and appeal of such items as pureed tuna on pumpernickel or angel food cake with pureed strawberry sauce.[24] The current trend away from special diets may also encourage greater food intake among older patients. Using seasonings other than salt and avoiding high-sodium mixes will enable most patients to follow the regular diet even if sodium must be reduced. With the exception of concentrated sweets, diabetic patients can enjoy a regular diet if the exchanges are defined. These innovations likely will result in higher costs; thus the advantages for patients and the positive impressions that will be created among family members must be carefully presented to administrators.[24] Consortium food purchasing by several nursing homes can effect cost savings, as was the case for Title III-C programs.

Food acceptance by residents in long-term care facilities is also influenced by the timing of meals. When the three major meals were scheduled close together (e.g., at 8:15 AM, 12 PM, and 4:45 PM), residents were not hungry when the next meal arrived. An associated problem is the extended time between the evening snack and breakfast (often 10 to 12 hours). Items such as sandwiches, milk, crackers and cheese, fruit, and juice should be available as evening snacks, particularly for frail elderly people who consume only a small amount of food at a time.

NUTRITION EDUCATION FOR OLDER ADULTS

Appropriate food intake is a powerful influence for maintaining health and preventing chronic disease. Thus nutrition education should be an important component of on-going health promotion services for older people and their care-givers.

Food and Nutrition Knowledge of Older People

Dietary intake is influenced by nutrition knowledge and the ability to select a nutritionally adequate diet from the food choices available. People develop a food pattern and acquire food knowledge through a lifetime of experience. For adults with few years of formal schooling, nutrition knowledge generally is acquired through informal sources such as newspapers or magazines and friends or acquaintances. Nutrition education should build on the nutrition knowledge clients may already have and provide appropriate information useful in daily food selection.

According to the results of formal knowledge tests, many older adults have only a limited knowledge of the foods required for good health. In a study of 165 people over age 64 living in Oregon,[46] participants were asked to name the four groups of foods required for a balanced diet. Fewer than 5% failed to mention protein foods or the need for fruits and vegetables, but 27% to 28% did not name the grain or dairy groups. It should not be assumed, however, that failure to name these food groups reflects a failure to consume the foods involved. Although younger individuals are willing to learn facts regardless of the relevance to their personal situation, older people want to make immediate use of any information presented. From this standpoint it would be of value to focus on the types of food to be included in a meal or in the daily food pattern rather than on food groups per se.

Older Arizona adults interviewed at 15 Title III-C congregate meal sites[29] demonstrated applied food and nutrition knowledge. Although they tended to have incorrect information about weight control and the need for nutritional supplements, the majority were correct as to alternative sources of protein (77%); the relationship of appropriate cooking and storage methods to nutrient retention (92%); the importance of green, leafy vegetables as good sources of vitamin A (88%); the use of calcium supplements as an alternative when dairy foods are not consumed (80%); and the fact that the nutritional value of meat is not determined by its cost (70%).

The formal education of these older people was limited (40% finished only grade school), emphasizing the need for visual rather than technical nutrition education materials.

Older people are particularly concerned about maintaining their health and independence, and this makes them especially vulnerable to claims of renewed vitality or relief from chronic complaints with use of nutritional supplements. The money needed to buy costly vitamin or mineral supplements might better be used to buy wholesome food. Among 102 Iowa elderly,[41] 49% used vitamin and mineral supplements regularly, and about one fourth were following recommendations from health magazines. Of the 20 individuals who were taking supplements on their physician's advice, eight were taking an inappropriate amount (more than 150% of the RDA) plus additional individual supplements not prescribed by the physician.

In a random sample of 424 older people in Texas,[36] about two thirds were taking supplements, with vitamin C (25%), calcium (23%), and multivitamins with minerals (19%) most commonly used. Elderly women were more

likely to believe in nutritional supplements, whereas elderly men were more likely to trust the nutritional value of ordinary foods. Older people with higher incomes and higher educational levels were less likely to use supplements or "health foods," although they also had doubts about the nutrient content of ordinary foods. Surprisingly, supplement users had higher nutrient intakes per 1,000 kcal of vitamin B_6, magnesium, and fiber than nonusers, indicating more appropriate food choices. Vitamin C intake from food among both users and nonusers of supplements exceeded the RDA, yet 25% of those interviewed consumed additional vitamin C in supplement form. McIntosh and coworkers[36] concluded that even inaccurate information about nutrition and health can in some cases create an increased awareness that leads to a more nutritious diet.

Nutrition educators must be sensitive to older individuals who are most likely to overuse nutritional supplements. Older Iowa women classified as users, nonusers, or overusers of supplements (consumed 200% or more of the RDA) did not differ on the basis of age, education, income, or perceived dietary adequacy.[47] Overusers of supplements were more likely to live alone and have medically diagnosed health problems. Overuse of particular supplements among these women included vitamin B_6 (more than 10 times the RDA); thiamin, riboflavin, and vitamin C (more than 40 times the RDA), iron (400 mg a day); vitamin D (25,000 IU a day); and calcium (3 g a day). Reasons given by older people for using vitamin and mineral supplements often include the ideas that most elderly people need supplements and that supplements will make them feel better physically.[29,36]

Sources of Nutrition Information

The appropriateness of nutrition-related decisions made by older people may relate to their source of nutrition information. In general, older people rely on less formal sources of nutrition information, including magazines, newspapers, cookbooks, television, and physicians.[13] Older women are more likely to use food labels for nutrition information than older men. In one report[13] 78% of older respondents reported reading labels, and energy, sodium, cholesterol, and fat content were among the particular ingredients evaluated. Sources of information differ between urban and rural elderly people. Cookbooks were more popular among rural older adults (25% versus 16%), and dietitians were more commonly consulted by urban older adults (20% versus 3%). The increased availability of dietitians in urban areas likely influenced this finding. About 21% of older people use their physician as their source of nutrition information.

Older adults do express an interest in nutrition and health information. Among participants at 15 Title III-C congregate meal sites,[29] 90% indicated a wish for nutrition education programs at least once a month. About half were receiving nutrition education at their meal site, and the others were not. Older people prefer a verbal and visual format for nutrition education, including talks, filmstrips, demonstrations, or movies rather than lectures or written materials. The limited formal education of some older people can present problems in their use of health-related written materials. Topics for nutrition education suggested by Title III-C participants[29] were vitamins, weight control, special diets (e.g., low fat or diabetic), cholesterol issues, and the nutritional value of foods. Among older Boston residents,[25] food safety in the home and in industry food processing were the topics of greatest importance. Older people need reassurance as to the safety and nutritional adequacy of the food supply.

The Title III-C nutrition program offers tremendous potential for disseminating food and nutrition information, both in programs at congregate sites and through written materials distributed with home-delivered meals. Perhaps the most obvious nutrition education activity is the meal itself, which should reinforce positive principles of menu planning. Through both educational and recreational activities, senior centers can promote health and well-being. The degree of misinformation among older people about weight control, the nutrient content of available foods, and the need for costly and potentially toxic doses of vitamin and mineral supplements underscores the need for appropriate and relevant activities.

Summary

Food and nutrition services are important components of long-term care for both healthy and impaired older people. Long-term care can involve community-based services to support independent living or resident care for those requiring skilled nursing care, personal care, or supervision. Food-related formal services can include congregate or home-delivered meals or homemaker services providing food shopping or meal preparation. Informal services by family members or neighbors may involve grocery shopping or bringing meals on weekends when formal services are not available. Use of formal services increases with age, the number of ADL limitations, and living alone.

The Nutrition Program for the Elderly, funded under the Older Americans Act (Title III-C), provides a hot meal at noon, either in a congregate setting or home delivered, that is planned to contain at least one third of the RDA. Title III-C participants tend to receive about half of their daily nutrient intake from the noon meal and have better diets than neighbors of similar age and socioeconomic background who do not participate, and better diets on days that include a Title III-C meal.

Increasing amounts of Title III-C funds are being directed toward providing home-delivered meals. Problems with food safety, acceptability, and nutrient content arise with food delivery to both congregate meal sites and homebound recipients when holding and transportation time extend beyond 2 hours and ideal food temperatures are not maintained. Another critical issue associated with Title III-C programs is that food is not provided on weekend days or for all meals of the day. Unmet needs are most obvious among the homeless, minority, and non-English–speaking older populations, and innovative services to address these needs are less likely to exist in areas serving the disadvantaged.

A major consideration in both community-based and resident care programs is nutrient density. In resident facilities where food intake may be extremely low, it is best to plan menus providing the required levels of nutrients within 1,400 kcal. All programs should provide opportunities for nutrition education and health promotion activities for the clients being served.

REVIEW QUESTIONS

1. What is meant by the phrase "continuum of care?" What is the Older Americans Act and what types of nutrition and social services are provided through this congressional act? Why are nutrition services not used by all elderly who are eligible for them?
2. What is the difference between a skilled nursing facility (SNF), an intermediate care facility (ICF), and a personal care home? What types of services are provided by nutrition professionals in each of the three facilities? What is a continuing care retirement community?
3. What are the nutrition requirements for the Nutrition Program for the Elderly? Given the emphasis on lower fat diets, why do some meals for the elderly contain a slightly higher level of fat? Why is nutrient density an important concept in meal planning for older people? What types of meals can be offered to homebound clients who need a special therapeutic diet?
4. What factors influence whether a nutrition project will prepare its own meals or contract with a caterer? What factors should be considered when choosing a food service option? How are meal sites selected for nutrition programs? How can someone become eligible to receive a home-delivered meal?
5. What is the nutritional impact of the Title III-C program? Do people who attend a nutrition site have better nutrient intakes on attendance days than on days when they do not eat at the site? Do they have better nutritional intakes than those who do not attend? Are there any groups of elderly not being well-served by the current nutrition programs?

SUGGESTED LEARNING ACTIVITIES

1. Go through the telephone book in your community and identify one skilled nursing facility, an intermediate care facility, and a personal care home. Call each and ask who provides the nutrition services. Set up a telephone interview with the person responsible for nutrition services and ask her or him what type of nutrition services are provided. Write a short paper on the results of your interviews.
2. Make arrangements to go with a volunteer on a home-delivered meal route for 2 weeks. During this time, note holding times for food before delivery and note how foods are packed. Also, note if the volunteer delivering meals has much time to socialize with the clients. Give an oral report to the class about your observations.
3. Obtain a copy of *Effective Menu Planning for the Elderly Nutrition Program* from the Gerontological Nutrition Practice Group of The American Dietetic Association (1991). Using this manual as a guide, write an outline of the steps you would take if you were a nutrition project manager responsible for opening a new nutrition center.
4. Design a recipe contest with your classmates to see who can come up with the healthiest, most nutrient-dense, and best-tasting dessert that would be appropriate to serve at a congregate meal site. After selecting three finalists, prepare each dessert and take it to a senior center and have it taste-tested by participants at the center. Choose a winner and provide the participants and the center director with a copy of the recipe.
5. Write a lesson plan to present the USDA Food Guide Pyramid to a group of healthy older adults. What would you emphasize in your education session that would be different if you were making the presentation to a younger audience?

Key Terms

Provided here for review is a list of the major terms in this chapter. The definitions can be found in the Glossary, which begins on p. 336. To help you understand how these terms are applied, the page number is given for the first mention of each term in the chapter.

adult day care center, 315
activities of daily living (ADLs), 314
area agency on aging, 317
body mass index (BMI), 325
congregate meals, 314
continuing care retirement community, 316
continuum of care, 314
diagnosis related groups (DRGs), 315
disability, 316
frail, 317
functional, 316
home-delivered meals, 314
home health agency, 314
instrumental activities of daily living (IADLs), 314

REFERENCES

1. Allington JK and others: A short method to ensure nutritional adequacy of food served in nursing homes. I. Identification of need, *J Am Diet Assoc* 76:458, 1980.
2. Allington JK and others: A short method to ensure nutritional adequacy of food served in nursing homes. II. Development of a model food plan, *J Am Diet Assoc* 76:465, 1980.
3. American Dietetic Association: DPGs collect data for ADA testimony: effect of DRGs on demand for home-delivered meals, *J Am Diet Assoc* 85:1638, 1985.
4. American Dietetic Association: Nutrition, aging, and the continuum of health care: technical support paper, *J Am Diet Assoc* 87:345, 1987.
5. American Dietetic Association: ADA's testimony on reauthorization of the Older Americans Act, *J Am Diet Assoc* 91:849, 1991.
6. Asp EH, Darling ME: Home-delivered meals: food quality, nutrient content, and characteristics of recipients, *J Am Diet Assoc* 88:55, 1988.
7. Balsam A, Carlin JM: Consortium contracting, *Community Nutritionist* 2:9, 1983.
8. Balsam AL, Carlin JM: Frozen meals for the homebound elderly, *Catering and Health* 1:253, 1990.
9. Balsam A, Osteraas G: Developing a continuum of community nutrition services: Massachusetts elderly nutrition programs, *J Nutr Elderly* 6(4):51, 1987.
10. Balsam A, Rogers B: Food service trends in the elderly nutrition program, *J Nutr Elderly* 9(1):19, 1989.
11. Balsam A, Rogers BL: *Service innovations in the elderly nutrition program: strategies for meeting unmet needs,* Medford, MA, 1988, Tufts University School of Nutrition.
12. Bild BR, Havighurst RJ: Senior citizens in great cities: the case of Chicago, *Gerontologist* 16:76, 1976.
13. Briley ME and others: Sources of nutrition information for rural and urban elderly adults, *J Am Diet Assoc* 90:986, 1990.
14. Carlin JM: Response: letters from readers: sharing meals, sharing moments. *Food Management* 23(7):10, 1988.
15. Chapman N, Sorenson A: Health promotion and aging: nutrition, Background papers, Surgeon General's Workshop on Health Promotion and Aging, Menlo Park, Calif, 1988, Henry J Kaiser Family Foundation.
16. Coulston AM: Nutrition management in nursing homes. In Morley JE, Glick Z, and Rubenstein LZ, editors: *Geriatric nutrition: a comprehensive review,* New York, 1990, Raven Press.
17. Council on Scientific Affairs, American Medical Association: Home care in the 1990s, *JAMA* 263(9):1241, 1990.
18. Czajka-Narins DM and others: Nutritional and biochemical effects of nutrition programs in the elderly, *Clin Geriatr Med* 3:275, 1987.
19. Davies L, Hastrop K, Bender AE: Potassium intake of the elderly, *Mod Geriatr* 3:482, 1973.
20. Davies L, Hastrop K, Bender AE: The energy benefit of meals on wheels, *Mod Geriatr* 4:220, 1974.
21. Downes TW: Food packaging in the IFT era: five decades of unprecedented growth and change, *Food Technol* 43(9):228, 1989.
22. Fink A and others: Assuring the quality of health care for older persons: an expert panel's priorities, JAMA 258:1905, 1987.
23. Frongillo EA and others: Continuance of elderly on home-delivered meals programs, *Am J Public Health* 77:1176, 1987.
24. Gallagher A: Elegance adds appeal to nursing home food service, *J Am Diet Assoc* 90:1663, 1990.
25. Goldberg JP, Gershoff SN, McGandy RB: Appropriate topics for nutrition education for the elderly, *J Nutr Educ* 22:303, 1990.
26. Greene J: Coordination of Older Americans Act programs, *J Am Diet Assoc* 78:617, 1981.
27. Hess MA: President's page: ADA as an advocate

for older Americans, *J Am Diet Assoc* 91(7):847, 1991.

28. Hing E: Use of nursing homes by elderly: preliminary data from the 1985 National Nursing Home Survey, US Department of Health and Human Services, National Center for Health Statistics, Advance data 135, May 14, 1987.

29. Hutchings LL, Tinsley AM: Nutrition education for older adults: how Title III-C program participants perceive their needs, *J Nutr Educ* 22:53, 1990.

30. Keeney DB and others: Nutrition evaluation of a grocery delivery program for rural homebound elderly, *Fed Proc* 48:829, 1983.

31. Kendrick OW, Slezak D: Nutrition program for the elderly: participants' perception of food quality by type of food service system, *J Nutr Elderly* 9(1):27, 1989.

32. Kirschner and Associates: An evaluation of nutrition services for the elderly (executive summary), Administration on Aging, US Department of Health and Human Services, Washington, DC, 1983, US Government Printing Office.

33. Kohrs MB, O'Hanlon P, Eklund D: Title VII Nutrition Program for the Elderly. I. Contribution to one day's dietary intake, *J Am Diet Assoc* 72:487, 1978.

34. Kohrs MB and others: Title VII Nutrition Program for the Elderly. II. Relationship of socioeconomic factors to one day's nutrient intake, *J Am Diet Assoc* 75:537, 1979.

35. McCool AC, Posner BM: *Nutrition services for older Americans: food service systems and technologies, program management strategies,* Chicago, 1982, The American Dietetic Association.

36. McIntosh WA and others: The relationship between beliefs about nutrition and dietary practices of the elderly, *J Am Diet Assoc* 90:671, 1990.

37. McNaughton JP, Kilgore CT: Impact of Title III–funded feeding program on nutrient intake and blood profiles of elderly in Mississippi, *J Nutr Elderly* 5(2):35, Winter, 1985-86.

38. National Council on the Aging: Home-delivered meals for the ill, handicapped, and elderly, *Am J Public Health* 55(suppl):1, 1965.

39. National Institute on Adult Daycare: *Standards and guidelines for adult day care,* Washington, DC, 1990, National Council on the Aging.

40. Nutrition Strategic Study Committee: *Nutrition strategic study: a report to the director of the Ohio Department of Aging,* 1989, Columbus, Ohio, Ohio Department of Aging.

41. Oakland MJ, Thomsen PA: Beliefs about and usage of vitamin/mineral supplements by elderly

42. O'Shaughnessy C: Older Americans Act nutrition program: CRS report for Congress, Congressional Research Service, Washington, DC, January 19, 1990.

43. Osteraas G and others: Developing new options in home-delivered meals: the SMOC demonstration elderly nutrition project, *J Am Diet Assoc* 82:524, 1983.

44. Ponza M, Wray L: Final results of the elderly programs study, Alexandria, Va, 1990, Food and Nutrition Service, US Department of Agriculture.

45. Posner BM, Krachenfels MM: Nutrition services in the continuum of health care, *Clin Geriatr Med* 3:261, 1987.

46. Probart CK and others: Factors that influence the elderly to use traditional or nontraditional nutrition information sources, *J Am Diet Assoc* 89:1758, 1989.

47. Ranno BS, Wardlaw GM, Geiger CJ: What characterizes elderly women who overuse vitamin and mineral supplements? *J Am Diet Assoc* 88:347, 1988.

48. Rhodes SS, editor: *Effective menu planning for the elderly nutrition program,* Chicago, 1991, The American Dietetic Association.

49. Roe DA: Nutritional surveillance of the elderly: methods to determine program impact and unmet need, *Nutr Today* 24:24, 1989.

50. Rosenzweig L: Coordination of private and public home-delivered meals programs, Annual Meeting of the National Association of Meals Programs, Syracuse, NY, April 19, 1982.

51. Sempos CT and others: A dietary survey of 14 Wisconsin nursing homes, *J Am Diet Assoc* 81:35, 1982.

52. Short P, Leon J: Use of home and community services by persons ages 65 and older with functional difficulties, National Medical Expenditure Survey Research Findings 5, DHHS Pub No (PHS) 90-3466, Rockville, Md, 1990, US Department of Health and Human Services.

53. Sills-Levy E: US food trends leading to the year 2000, *Food Technol* 43(4):128, 1989.

54. Stanton BR: Feeding the elderly: meals on wheels in London, *J NZ Diet Assoc* 26:11, 1972.

55. Staton M and others: *Handbook for site operations: the Nutrition Program for the Elderly,* Corvallis, Ore, 1975, Oregon State University.

56. Steele MF, Bryan JD: Dietary intake of homebound elderly recipients and nonrecipients of home-delivered meals, *J Nutr Elderly* 5(2):23, 1985-86.

57. Stevens DA, Grivetti LE, McDonald RB: Nutrient intake of urban and rural elderly receiving home-delivered meals, *J Am Diet Assoc* 92:714, 1992.

58. Stiedmann M, Jansen C, Harrill I: Nutritional status of elderly men and women, *J Am Diet Assoc* 73:132, 1978.

59. Stone RI, Murtaugh CM: The elderly population with chronic functional disability: implications for home care eligibility, *Gerontologist* 30(4):491, 1990.

60. Thole C, Gregoire MB: Time-temperature relationships during freezing of packaged meals in feeding programs for the elderly, *J Am Diet Assoc* 92:350, 1992.

61. Turner J, Glew G: Home-delivered meals for the elderly, *Food Technol* 36:46, 1982.

62. US Department of Health and Human Services: Longitudinal evaluation of the national Nutrition Program for the Elderly: report on first-wave findings, DHEW Pub No (OHDS) 80-20249, Washington, DC, 1979, US Government Printing Office.

63. US Department of Health and Human Services: Long-term care: background and future directions, HCFA 81-20047, Washington, DC, 1981, US Government Printing Office.

64. US Department of Health and Human Services: The home-delivered meals program: a service delivery assessment, Washington, DC, 1981, US Government Printing Office.

65. US Department of Health and Human Services: Analysis of food service delivery systems used in providing nutrition services to the elderly (executive summary), Washington, DC, 1982, US Government Printing Office.

66. US Department of Health and Human Services: Long-term care for the functionally dependent elderly, Vital and Health Statistics Series 13, No 104, Washington, DC, 1990, US Government Printing Office.

67. US House of Representatives Select Committee on Aging, US Senate Special Committee on Aging: Legislative agenda for an aging society: 1988 and beyond, House Select Committee on Aging Pub No 100-664, Senate Special Committee on Aging Pub No 100-J, Washington, DC, 1988, US Government Printing Office.

68. US Senate Special Committee on Aging: Home care at the crossroads: an information paper, Serial No 100-H, Washington, DC, 1988, US Government Printing Office.

69. Walden O and others: The provision of weekend home-delivered meals by state and a pilot study indicating the need for weekend home-delivered meals, *J Nutr Elderly* 8(1):31, 1988.

70. Wolgamot I: *Mobile meals,* Washington DC, (no date given), National Council on the Aging.

71. Woodworth DL: Ramsey County Alternative Care Grants Study, St Paul, Minn, Wilder Research Center, November 1986 (revised March 1987).

72. Zandt SV, Fox H: Nutritional impact of congregate meals programs, *J Nutr Elderly* 5(3):31, 1986.

Glossary

acetaminophen drug used to relieve pain and reduce fever

acetylcholine a neurotransmitter; acts as a vasodilator and depresses cardiac function

achlorhydria absence of hydrochloric acid in the gastric juice

acromial process bony projection of the upper arm where the shoulder blade connects with the clavicle

Activities of Daily Living (ADLs) list of activities used to measure the ability of an individual to handle self-care; includes eating, dressing, bathing, transfer from bed to chair, walking, and toileting

acute sharp or intense; disease or illness that begins suddenly, reaches a peak rapidly, and then subsides after a short period

ad libitum fed allowed to eat as much as desired

adenosine triphosphate molecule that stores energy in the cell

adhesion a band of scar tissue that binds together two tissue surfaces that are normally separate from each other; when it occurs in the abdomen or intestine it can result in an obstruction

adiposity relative amount of body fat

adrenergic inhibitors drugs that block the effects of the sympathetic nervous system that are mediated by norepinephrine

adult day care center facility that provides personal assistance and physical and social activities to frail or physically or mentally impaired older people who live in the community but require care throughout the day

adverse drug reaction a harmful, unintended effect of a drug

aerobic capacity the maximum amount of air that can be moved in and out of the lungs in a given amount of time

aerobic exercise exercise that increases oxygen uptake and improves cardiovascular fitness, such as jogging, brisk walking, or cycling

age-appropriate expectations patterns of behavior considered by the general public to be appropriate for or associated with older people

albumin a protein in the blood which serves as an indicator of protein status; contributes to maintenance of appropriate osmotic pressure and fluid balance between extracellular and intracellular fluids

aldosterone a hormone produced in the adrenal cortex that acts on the kidney to cause sodium reabsorption and, in turn, water reabsorption

alkalosis a situation in which the pH of extracellular fluids rises above 7.44; can be caused by an excess of bicarbonate ions or an abnormally low level of hydrogen ions

alpha islets groups of cells in the pancreas that synthesize and release glucagon

alpha tocopherol the form of vitamin E having the highest biologic activity

aluminum hydroxide a compound in many antacids that binds phosphates and prevents their absorption

alveoli small air sacs in the lungs where gases are exchanged

ambulatory able to walk

American Academy of Family Physicians a national organization of physicians specializing in family and general medicine

American Dietetic Association a national organization of registered dietitians and other nutrition and dietetic professionals specializing in providing nutritional care and foods and nutrition information to individuals and groups

amitriptyline hydrochloride drug used to treat depression

amylase enzyme that breaks down starch to dextrins and maltose

analgesic drug that relieves pain

anemia a decrease in the number of or hemoglobin content of red blood cells

anemia of chronic disease an anemia resulting from the effects of inflammation, liver disease, heart disease, or kidney disease on erythropoiesis and not from a lack of dietary iron

angular stomatitis inflammation at the corners of the mouth

anorexigenic (anorectic) drugs drugs that decrease appetite

anosmia loss or impaired sense of smell

antacid drug that neutralizes the HCl in the stomach

antagonist a drug or agent that exerts an opposite action to that of another or competes for the same receptor site

anthropometric relating to body measurements, such as height, weight, and skinfold measurements, used to estimate body composition

antiarrhythmic drug prevents or alleviates abnormal heart rhythm

antibiotic drug that destroys microorganisms; used to treat infections

anticholinergic agent blocks the effects of the parasympathetic nervous system that are mediated by acetylcholine

anticoagulant agent prevents or delays blood clotting

antidiabetic agent drug used to control diabetes; lowers blood glucose levels

antidiuretic hormone (ADH) hormone formed in the hypothalamus and released from the posterior pituitary that increases the reabsorption of water by the renal tubule and decreases the formation of urine

antigenic causing the production of antibodies

antihypertensive agent reduces high blood pressure

antineoplastic agent controls the proliferation or kills cancer cells

antioxidant a chemical substance that prevents or retards the oxidation of the double bonds in unsaturated fatty acids; this reaction occurs in the body and in foods containing fats and oils

antipsychotic drug diminishes psychotic symptoms associated with mental disorders

antipyretic agent reduces fever

antirheumatic agent reduces or prevents the chronic inflammation of a joint, ligament, or muscle

antivitamin a substance that inactivates a vitamin

apo-1-lipoprotein activates the enzyme necessary to release cholesterol from the peripheral tissues and allow its removal by high-density lipoproteins

apraxia a psychomotor disorder in which the ability to program muscle movements and control voluntary motions necessary to carry out tasks is impaired

arachidonic acid an omega-6 fatty acid composed of 20 carbons and 4 double bonds that can be synthesized from linoleic acid

area agency on aging local agency established by a state government to administer and implement social and nutrition services to older adults in a given geographic area

arterial pressure the stress exerted on the arterial walls by the circulating blood

aspartate aminotransferase an enzyme required for the transfer of an amino group for the formation of glutamic acid; serum levels increase following myocardial infarction or liver damage

aspiration pneumonia pneumonia caused by the inhalation of food or fluid into the lungs; can be caused by swallowing disorders or feeding an older person when lying down

ataxia an inability to coordinate movement, resulting in a staggering gait and imbalance; caused by a brain injury such as a stroke

atherosclerotic related to the deposition of yellowish fatty plaque on the inner walls of the large arteries; sometimes referred to as hardening of the arteries

atrial fibrillation rapid random contractions of the atrial compartments of the heart

atrial natriuretic peptide hormone that increases the excretion of sodium and water

atrophic gastritis chronic inflammation of the stomach lining with loss of mucosal cells and reduced secretion of HCl

atrophy wasting away of body tissue

autoimmune developing antibodies to one's own tissues

avidin a substance in raw egg white that binds with biotin and prevents its absorption

B-cells cells of the immune system that produce antibodies (immunoglobulins) that defend against virus and bacteria

bacterial overgrowth extensive proliferation of bacteria in the upper duodenum as a result of low acid secretion in the stomach; bacteria can bind with vitamins and prevent their absorption and break down bile salts

bacteriocidal able to destroy bacteria

balance method method used to determine the requirement for protein or a mineral; the requirement is the level of intake at which equilibrium is reached (intake equals losses in urine, feces, and sweat)

Baltimore Longitudinal Study of Aging (BLSA) a longitudinal study of men and women ranging in age from young adults to 100 years and over being carried on by the National Institute on Aging; participants' nutrient intake and physiologic and psychologic function are evaluated every 2 years

baroreceptors nerve endings in the major blood vessels that are sensitive to changes in blood pressure

basal metabolism the amount of energy required to maintain essential body processes when an individual is awake, at rest, and has not eaten for at least 14 hours

Beck Depression Inventory a questionnaire including psychologic and physiologic symptoms, used to diagnose depression in older adults

beriberi the deficiency disease resulting from a lack of thiamin and characterized by changes in the peripheral nerves and the heart

beta carotene a precursor of vitamin A found in plant foods, especially dark green and deep yellow vegetables and fruits

beta islets groups of cells in the pancreas that synthesize and release insulin

beta tocopherol a form of vitamin E with reduced biologic activity

bicarbonate an ion (HCO_3-) resulting from the dissociation of carbonic acid; acts in the acid-base buffering system

bile acid sequestrant substance that binds with bile acids in the intestine and prevents their reabsorption

bile salts emulsifiers synthesized by the liver and released by the gallbladder to aid in the digestion of fat

biliary colic pain resulting from the passage of a stone through the bile duct

bioavailable able to be absorbed

bioelectrical impedance a method of determining body fat content based on the electrical resistance of particular tissues

biopsy the removal of a small piece of tissue from a body part for microscopic examination

biphosphates a group of compounds that inhibit activity of the osteoclasts and bone resorption

body mass index (BMI) Quetelet index; body weight divided by body height squared (kg/m^2)

bone marrow soft tissue found in the center of the long bones where hematopoiesis takes place

bradykinesia a condition in which all voluntary movements and speech are slowed

branched-chain essential amino acids isoleucine, leucine, and valine; these amino acids are active in muscle metabolism

breath hydrogen expired hydrogen used to measure the completeness of digestion of disaccharides, particularly lactose

bronchiole small airway within the lungs that transports inspired air and waste gases

bronchodilator drug that relaxes the smooth muscle lining the bronchioles, allowing them to expand in diameter

cachexia general wasting and emaciation associated with serious diseases, such as cancer

calcitonin a hormone that opposes the action of parathyroid hormone in regulating blood calcium levels and bone mineralization

calcitriol term used for 1,25-dihydroxycholecalciferol, the active metabolite of vitamin D

calcium carbonate a form of calcium used as a calcium supplement

calcium channel blockers drugs that inhibit the flow of calcium ions across muscle membranes, thereby relaxing muscle tone and reducing muscle spasms

calcium-citrate-malate compound a form of calcium added to orange juice as a calcium supplement

calculi small stones formed by the precipitation of mineral salts; can block the bile duct or urinary tract

calibration to standardize an instrument using a reference weight or solution

cancellous bone porous, spongy bone with a lattice-like structure

carbamazepine drug used to relieve pain and prevent convulsions

cardiac arrhythmia an abnormal rate or rhythm of contraction of the heart muscle

cardiac glycosides drugs that increase the force of the contraction of the cardiac muscle and decrease the heart rate

cardiac output quantity of blood pumped per minute (average value is approximately 5 liters)

carotenoids type of yellow, red, and orange pigments found in plant foods; some are precursors of vitamin A and some appear to be protective against cancer

cataract (senile) degenerative change in the lens of the eye that results in a loss of transparency and, if untreated, loss of vision

catharsis purging or violent emptying of the bowel

celiac disease condition resulting from lack of the enzyme necessary to break down the protein in gluten present in wheat and some other grains; results in diarrhea, steatorrhea, and general malabsorption unless gluten is eliminated from the diet

centenarian a person age 100 years or over

cerebral hemorrhage rupture of a blood vessel in the brain

cerebrovascular accident stroke; interruption of blood flow to an area of the brain because of blockage or breakage of the blood vessel supplying blood to that region

cerebrovascular disease pathologic changes in the blood vessels in the brain

ceruloplasmin a plasma transport protein for copper

chelating agent a substance that combines with a mineral ion in a ringlike structure

chemotherapy the use of chemicals to destroy cancer cells

chlorpromazine drug used to control psychotic symptoms and vomiting

chlorpropamide an oral antidiabetic drug

cholecalciferol vitamin D_3

cholecystokinin a hormone produced by the upper intestinal mucosa that stimulates contraction of the gallbladder and secretion of pancreatic digestive enzymes

cholestyramine drug used to lower blood cholesterol or lipid levels

cholinesterase enzyme that breaks down acetylcholine to choline and acetate

chronic prolonged; a disease that develops slowly and persists for a long time, possibly for the remaining years of life

chronic obstructive pulmonary disease (COPD) a progressive and irreversible lung disease in which the airways are decreased in size and the passage of air is reduced

chronologic age a person's age in years

cimetidine drug that inhibits the production and secretion of acid in the stomach

cinchonism condition of headache, deafness, and ringing in the ears caused by excessive intake of quinine

clavicle the long curved horizontal bone above the ribs that joins the shoulder blade at the acromial process

clofibrate drug used to lower high blood cholesterol or triglyceride levels

cobalamin the cobalt-containing portion of the vitamin B_{12} molecule

cognitive related to the mental processes of acquiring knowledge, judgment, reasoning, and memory

cohort a group of individuals in a scientific study who share a common characteristic such as age, sex, or health status

colchicine drug used to treat gout

colestipol drug used to lower high blood cholesterol levels

collagen a protein consisting of small bundles of fibers; found in tendons, ligaments, and bone matrix

computerized tomography an x-ray technique used to determine body composition

condyle a rounded projection at the end of a bone that forms a joint with other bones and holds muscle ligaments in place

congestive heart failure condition caused by the inability of the heart to pump all the blood returned to it; associated with retention of sodium and water by the kidney and development of edema

congregate meal program program funded under the Older Americans Act that provides a hot meal at noon Monday through Friday in a social setting for persons age 60 and over

constipation difficulty in passing stools

continuing care retirement community a retirement community designed to provide a range of living situations and services to support independent living for healthy older people and provide skilled nursing care for those who may come to require more specialized care with advancing age

continuum of care the range of health and nutrition services that will allow an individual to maintain the highest level of independence and personal well-being possible

core foods foods eaten daily; staple foods in the dietary pattern

cortical bone compact, dense bone found in the shafts of the long bones

coumarin a drug that prevents blood clotting

creatinine a product of muscle metabolism; urinary creatinine excretion can be used to estimate body muscle mass

cross-sectional a comparison of data from two or more groups of people evaluated at the same time

cyanocobalamin vitamin B_{12}

D-xylose a pentose used to measure the completeness of carbohydrate absorption; substance is not metabolized, so the total amount absorbed will be excreted in the urine

7-dehydrocholesterol compound in the skin that on exposure to sunlight is synthesized into vitamin D

dementia a progressive loss of mental function caused by physiologic changes or disease

demographic relating to the size, geographic distribution, and general characteristics of human populations, including age, sex, income, race, and health

dendrite a treelike branch of a nerve cell that conducts impulses toward the nerve cell body

dental caries tooth decay

depletion the situation in which body tissue levels and stores of a nutrient are being lost as a result of poor intake, poor absorption, or excessive metabolism or excretion

desolates term applied to older persons living alone who are discontented and long for their spouses or other family members who have died or moved away

desquamation the shedding of the outer layer of cells

Determine Your Nutritional Health Checklist a list of health, socioeconomic, and food intake criteria used to assess the nutritional risk of an older person

diabetes mellitus a disorder of carbohydrate, fat, and protein metabolism resulting from a lack of insulin secretion by the pancreas

diabetic neuropathy damage to the peripheral nerves caused by high blood glucose levels in poorly controlled diabetes

diagnosis related groups (DRGs) classifications of patients based on primary and secondary diagnoses and procedures; used to determine the level and extent of care eligible for Medicare reimbursement

diastolic blood pressure the blood pressure when the heart muscle is relaxed and blood is entering the heart chambers

diazoxide a drug used to lower blood pressure

diet history a method of dietary assessment that evaluates past and present food intake and related factors, including food preparation and shopping habits, use of vitamin or mineral supplements, health factors, cultural and ethnic food patterns, and economic factors influencing food selection

Dietary Guidelines for Americans a set of general goals for nutrient intake and diet pattern established by the United States Departments of Agriculture and Health and Human Services in an effort to promote health and reduce chronic disease

dietary status the relative adequacy of the diet as compared with the Recommended Dietary Allowances for an individual of that age, sex, or condition

digitalis intoxication excessive intake of digitalis leading to drug poisoning

digoxin a drug that increases the strength of the contraction of the cardiac muscle and slows the heart rate

1,25-dihydroxyvitamin D the active form of vitamin D; also called *calcitriol*

disability loss or impairment of physical or mental fitness

distorted taste perception changes in the degree of recognition of the basic tastes, or changes in taste (e.g., bitter taste with many foods; unpleasant taste with sweet items)

diuretic a drug that decreases the reabsorption of water in the renal tubule and increases urine output

diurnal variation a change in level or secretion of a substance over a 24-hour period

divalent cation an atom with a positive valence of 2

diverticulitis inflammation and infection of the pouchlike projections (diverticuli) found in the colon in advanced age

diverticulosis pouchlike projections in the colon common among older people; may be related to low fiber intake

docosahexaenoic acid an omega-3 fatty acid found in fish; has 22 carbon atoms and 6 double bonds

dolomite a naturally occurring mineral containing calcium that is unsuitable as a calcium supplement because it may contain toxic minerals such as lead or mercury

dopamine a neurotransmitter and precursor of norepinephrine

dowager's hump spinal deformity resulting in kyphosis (or a hunchback appearance) caused by fractures of the vertebrae of the upper back

dual photon absorption an x-ray technique used to determine body composition

dyspepsia discomfort in the abdominal region following eating

dysphagia difficulty in swallowing

edema the abnormal accumulation of fluid in the extracellular spaces of tissues

edentulous without teeth

eicosapentaenoic acid an omega-3 fatty acid found in fish; has 20 carbon atoms and 5 double bonds

electrolyte an element or compound that forms ions when placed in water (e.g., potassium, sodium chloride)

emollient substance that softens the skin or mucous membranes

endometrial relating to the inner lining of the uterus

envelope measurements circumference measurements of the waist or hip

epidemiologic study of the factors or conditions associated with the incidence, prevalence, or control of a particular disease

erythrocyte a red blood cell

erythrocyte aspartate transaminase enzyme requiring vitamin B_6 as a coenzyme; enzyme activity used as an indicator of vitamin B_6 status

erythrocyte glutathione reductase enzyme requiring riboflavin as a coenzyme; enzyme activity used as an indicator of riboflavin status

erythrocyte protoporphyrin a component necessary for the formation of the hemoglobin molecule; used as an indicator of iron status and a developing anemia

erythrocyte transketolase enzyme requiring thiamin as a coenzyme; enzyme activity used as an indicator of thiamin status

erythropoiesis production of red blood cells

erythropoietin hormone secreted by the kidney that stimulates the production of red blood cells

estrogen female sex hormone produced by the ovaries

ethacrynic acid a diuretic

etidronate biphosphate compound used in treatment of osteoporosis

factorial method method for determining the requirement for protein by adding all routes of obligatory nitrogen loss and calculating the level of dietary protein required to replace those losses

fasting to refrain from eating for a specific period of time

fat free mass (FFM) the body mass with all fat removed, including the fatty acids found in cell membranes and essential structures

fecal fat undigested fat appearing in the feces

femur bone in the leg that extends from the hip to the knee

ferric iron trivalent form of iron that occurs naturally in foods but cannot be absorbed

ferritin a protein-iron complex that serves as a storage form of iron; serum ferritin is highly correlated with liver iron stores

ferritin model a method for establishing the existence of anemia based on serum ferritin levels, transferrin saturation, and erythrocyte protoporphyrin levels

ferrous iron divalent form of iron; form in which iron is absorbed

flatulence an excessive amount of gas or air in the stomach and intestinal tract that can result in distention and discomfort

fluorapatite a bone mineral crystal composed of calcium, phosphate, hydroxyl, and fluoride ions that is highly resistant to bone resorption

Focused Drug Therapy Review Program a patient education program that uses a systematic approach to affect prescriber and patient behavior change to reduce error and promote appropriate drug use

folylmonoglutamate the form of folate that is absorbed

folylpolyglutamate the form of folate occurring naturally in foods

folylpolyglutamate hydrolase enzyme breaks down folylpolyglutamates, the form of folate naturally occurring in foods. to folylmonoglutamates, which can be absorbed

Folstein Mini Mental State Examination a series of questions used to determine the mental alertness and cognitive function of an older person

food aspiration the accidental inhalation of food into the lungs

food assistance programs government-supported programs that provide food or meals or increased income to purchase food; includes congregate or home-delivered meal programs, commodity food distribution programs, and food stamps

food diary a means of assessing nutrient intake by asking an individual to record the types and amounts of all foods, liquids, and supplements consumed over a certain number of days

food frequency questionnaire a means of assessing nutrient intake in which individuals are asked to indicate how frequently they consume particular foods; may also include the amount of each food consumed

Food Guide Pyramid a tool for planning a daily diet developed by the United States Department of Agriculture that emphasizes higher numbers of servings per day of breads, cereals, fruits, and vegetables and fewer numbers of servings per day of meats, fish, poultry, and dairy foods

food idiosyncracy a food habit or pattern that is unique to a particular individual

food insecurity the limited availability or uncertainty of adequate food as related to income, inability to shop for groceries, no one to assist with food preparation, or limited ability to feed oneself

food intolerance an adverse reaction to a particular food resulting in discomfort or physical symptoms; may relate to a problem in digestion or absorption or metabolism of a nutrient

frail physically weak; requiring assistance with heavy household chores or when going outside the home

Framingham Heart Study a long-term prospective epidemiologic study being carried on in the community of Framingham, Mass. to evaluate risk factors associated with cardiovascular and other chronic diseases

free radical an unstable high-energy compound with an unpaired election that causes oxidation reactions in unsaturated fatty acids

functional related to the special work or activity of an organ or body part

furosemide a diuretic drug

gallstone a small stone formed by the accumulation of bile salts; it can block the bile duct

gangrene death of tissue resulting from bacterial invasion and a loss of blood flow

gastrectomy removal of all or part of the stomach

gastric emptying time amount of time required for a test meal to completely pass out of the stomach and into the duodenum

gastric motility the spontaneous peristaltic movements in the stomach that mix food and gastric secretions and move food through the stomach and into the duodenum

gastric phytobezoar a solid mass of vegetable fiber or seeds forming in the stomach; a food ball

gastritis inflammation of the stomach lining with loss of mucosal secretory cells

gastroesophageal reflux the backflow of stomach contents into the esophagus as a result of poor function of the lower esophageal sphincter

Georgia Centenarian Study an on-going longitudinal study of community-living persons age 100 and over in Georgia

Geriatric Depression Scale a series of questions designed to determine the existence or extent of depression in an older individual and its effect on daily activities or self-care

geriatrics the branch of medicine dealing with changes in physiologic function, diseases, and care of older people

gerontology the scientific study of the aging process, including biologic, sociologic, psychologic, and clinical aspects

gingivitis red, swollen, or bleeding gums

glomerular filtrate the fluid portion of the blood that is filtered by the kidney

glomerular filtration rate (GFR) the amount of blood plasma that can be filtered in a given amount of time (GFR of a young adult is about 125 ml/min)

glossitis inflammation of the tongue

glucagon a hormone produced by the alpha islets of the pancreas that stimulates the conversion of glycogen to glucose and gluconeogenesis in the liver to bring about a rise in plasma glucose levels

glucocorticoid hormones steroid hormones secreted by the adrenal cortex that promote the release of amino acids from muscle for gluconeogenesis and exert an antiinflammatory effect

gluconeogenesis the formation of glucose from other compounds, usually amino acids from which the amino group has been removed

glucose tolerance the ability of the body to metabolize a load of glucose; is measured by administering a standard dose of glucose by mouth and measuring blood glucose levels for 2 to 3 hours thereafter

glucose tolerance factor a chromium amino acid complex that facilitates the binding of insulin to its cell receptor

glutamine a nonessential amino acid that serves as an amino group donor in synthetic reactions

glutathione peroxidase enzyme that participates in antioxidant reactions and protects tissues against damage from free radicals

gluteal relating to the buttocks

gluten a protein found in wheat and some other grains

glycemic control an effort to control blood glucose levels in persons with diabetes mellitus through defined treatment involving diet, injection of insulin, or use of other drugs

glycosuria an abnormally high level of glucose in the urine occurring in diabetes mellitus

glycosylated hemoglobin compound formed by the combining of glucose with the end amino group of a hemoglobin chain; used to monitor blood glucose control in diabetes mellitus

glycosylation the joining of glucose with the end amino group of a protein molecule

glycyrrhizic acid a substance found in licorice root that mimics the action of aldosterone

granulocyte a type of white blood cell having granules in the cytoplasm

grazing food pattern in which an individual eats many small meals or snacks throughout the day rather than several large meals

H₂-receptor antagonist drug that prevents the secretion of acid in the stomach

half life the time required for a substance to lose half of its activity or for half of it to be metabolized or excreted

Healthy People 2000: National Health Promotion and Disease Prevention Objectives a national strategy to promote health and prevent unnecessary disease and disability in Americans of all ages by the year 2000

heartburn a burning pain in the esophagus caused by the backflow of gastric contents and acid

helicobacter pylori the pathogenic microorganism associated with the development of atrophic gastritis

hematopoiesis the formation of blood cells in the bone marrow

heme the iron-containing complex of the hemoglobin molecule

heme iron iron complexed in the hemoglobin molecule; found in animal tissues

hemochromatosis condition involving excess deposition of iron in the tissues as a result of inappropriately high iron absorption; may have a genetic basis

hemoglobin the protein-iron complex in erythrocytes that binds and transports oxygen to the tissues and removes carbon dioxide

hepatic retinyl ester hydrolase enzyme in the liver that breaks down retinyl esters and releases retinol for transport to body tissues

hepatotoxicity the situation in which a drug or alcohol is harmful to the liver

heterogeneous dissimilar; not uniform throughout

hiatus hernia a protrusion of the stomach upward toward the diaphragm, which can result in backflow of stomach acid into the esophagus

high-density lipoprotein (HDL) a plasma lipoprotein complex relatively high in protein and low in cholesterol and believed to slow the development of atherosclerosis by assisting in the transport of cholesterol to the liver where it is excreted in the bile

hippuric acid (see paraaminohippuric acid)

Hispanic Health and Nutrition Examination Sur-

vey (HHANES) a survey conducted by the United States government to determine the nutritional status and chronic disease risk of the Hispanic population

Hodgkin's disease a type of malignancy that causes enlargement of the lymph tissue and production of abnormal macrophages and other white blood cells

home health agency an agency that provides and supervises health-related services in the home, ranging from personal care and homemaking services to skilled nursing care

home-delivered meals meals prepared and delivered by a government or community agency to home-bound older people

homocysteine an intermediate compound in the synthesis of cysteine that accumulates in the blood in vitamin B_{12} deficiency

hydralazine drug used to lower blood pressure

hydrochloric acid HCl; secreted in the stomach by the parietal cells as a part of gastric juice

hydroxyapatite the major mineral crystal found in bone; contains calcium, phosphate, and hydroxyl ions

25-hydroxyvitamin D metabolite of vitamin D formed in the liver

hypercalcemia abnormally high blood calcium level

hypercalciuria abnormally high level of calcium in the urine

hypercapnia abnormally high level of carbon dioxide in the blood

hyperfiltration situation in which the kidney increases the amount of blood plasma filtered in response to a high flow of blood to the kidney

hyperglycemia abnormally high blood glucose level

hyperinsulinemia excessively high blood insulin level

hyperkalemia abnormally high level of potassium in the blood

hyperkeratosis overgrowth of the dry, cornified layer of the epidermis

hyperlipidemia an excess of lipids or fat substances, including lipoproteins and phospholipids, in the plasma

hypermagnesemia abnormally high level of magnesium in the blood

hypernatremia abnormally high level of sodium in the blood

hyperparathyroidism excessive secretion of parathyroid hormone

hyperperfusion situation in which an abnormally large quantity of blood is delivered to the kidney for filtration

hyperphagic to overeat, excessive appetite

hypertension blood pressure that is above normal; often defined as systolic pressure ≥ 140 mm Hg and diastolic pressure > 90 mm Hg

hyperthyroidism above-normal secretion of thyroid hormones

hypervitaminosis A condition resulting from excessive intakes of preformed vitamin A over an extended period; leads to liver damage

hypnotic agent substance with a calming effect; reduces anxiety

hypoalbuminemia abnormally low blood albumin level

hypochlorhydria secretion of an abnormally low level of HCl in the gastric juice

hypocholesterolemia an abnormally low level of cholesterol in the plasma

hypochromic having less than normal color; used to describe a red blood cell with a below-normal hemoglobin content

hypoferremia an abnormally low level of iron in the blood

hypoglycemic agent a drug that lowers blood glucose levels used in the treatment of diabetes mellitus

hypokalemia abnormally low level of potassium in the blood

hyponatremia abnormally low level of sodium in the blood

hypophagic poor appetite, anorexia

hypoprothrombinemia abnormally low level of prothrombin in the blood resulting from vitamin K deficiency

hypothalamic-neurohypophyseal relating to the hormonal pathway existing between the hypothalamus and the posterior lobe of the pituitary gland (neurohypophysis); controls release of antidiuretic hormone

hypothyroidism below-normal secretion of thyroid hormones

hypoxia lack of sufficient oxygen for the tissues

iatrogenic disorder caused by a drug, treatment procedure, or diagnostic procedure

imipramine drug used to treat depression

immunocompetence the ability of the immune system to respond to stimulation by an antigen; may be decreased in older people with reduced T-cell function

immunoglobulins group of humoral antibodies that defend against microorganisms or environmental toxins

incontinence loss of ability to control urination or defecation

inflammatory bowel disease chronic inflammation and infection of the colon and rectum resulting in watery diarrhea containing blood and pus

initiation the first step in the development of cancer; a carcinogen acts on a cell to produce an irreversible genetic mutation

insensible water loss unnoticed loss of fluid from the body through expired air, feces, and continual loss from the skin

insoluble will not dissolve in water or other solvent

insoluble fiber indigestible cellulose, hemicellulose, and lignin found in cereal grains and vegetables that increase fecal bulk

Instrumental Activities of Daily Living (IADLs) a list of activities used to determine an individual's ability to live independently; activities include shopping, preparing meals, managing money, using the telephone, doing housework, and going outside unassisted

insulin-dependent diabetes mellitus (IDDM) form of diabetes mellitus in which the beta cells are incapable of producing any insulin; patient is prone to ketoacidosis

intermediate care facility (ICF) a health facility that provides services to people with physical or emotional conditions that require constant care but do not require skilled nursing care or highly specialized procedures

intestinal motility the rhythmic contractions of the intestinal muscle layer that move the intestinal contents along the passageway

intravascular occurring inside a blood vessel

intrinsic factor substance secreted by the gastric mucosa that is necessary for the normal absorption of vitamin B_{12}

irritable bowel syndrome abnormally increased motility in the small and large intestines resulting in diarrhea and pain; appears to be caused by emotional stress and not disease

ischemic heart disease damage to the heart from a decreased blood supply and insufficient oxygen

isolates term used to describe older people who live alone and lead fairly solitary lives but are content with their level of social interaction

isoniazid drug used to treat tuberculosis

isotope a form of a chemical element that differs in molecular weight from the standard and can be used to track metabolic processes in the body

jaundice a yellowing of the skin caused by abnormally high levels of bilirubin in the blood; may indicate liver disease or obstruction of the bile duct

Joint Commission on Accreditation of Healthcare Organizations a private nongovernment agency that establishes standards for the operation of hospitals and other healthcare facilities and conducts an accreditation program

ketoacidosis complication of diabetes mellitus in which ketones accumulate in the blood, resulting in acidosis, mental confusion, dyspnea, and, if untreated, coma

ketone bodies products arising from incomplete oxidation of fatty acids that accumulate in the blood and urine in uncontrolled diabetes mellitus (e.g., beta-hydroxy-butyric acid, acetoacetic acid, and acetone)

koilonychia a condition in which the nails are thin and concave from side to side (spoon nails); may occur in iron-deficiency anemia

Kupffer cells specialized liver cells that remove bacteria from the blood delivered to the liver from the gastrointestinal tract through the portal vein

kyphosis abnormal curvature of the spine resulting in a hunchback appearance; caused by osteoporosis in the vertebrae

labeled amino acid an amino acid containing a radioactive atom and used to study amino acid and protein metabolism

lactase enzyme that breaks down lactose into glucose and galactose

lactobacilli a nonpathogenic bacteria normally found in the intestine that ferments lactose to lactic acid

lactose intolerance inability to break down lactose because of a deficiency of the enzyme lactase

laxative drug causing emptying of the bowel

lean body mass compartment of the body that includes all tissues with the exception of the fat contained in the adipose tissue; lean body mass does include the "essential fat," fatty acids contained in membranes and other structural tissues

leukocyte a white blood cell that defends against bacteria and toxic substances

leukotrienes compounds found in white blood cells that produce allergic and inflammatory reactions and are associated with development of rheumatoid arthritis

levodopa drug used to treat Parkinson's disease

life expectancy the number of years a person of a given age, sex, and race can be expected to live

lingual lipase lipase secreted by the serous glands in the mouth

linoleic acid an omega-6 fatty acid with 18 carbon atoms and 2 double bonds that cannot be synthesized by the body; the essential fatty acid

linolenic acid an omega-3 fatty acid with 18 carbon atoms and 3 double bonds that is a substrate for the synthesis of eicosapentaenoic and docosahexaenoic acids

lipase enzyme that breaks down triglycerides into fatty acids and glycerol

lipoprotein a molecule composed of protein and lipid; the form in which lipids are transported in the plasma

lipoprotein lipase enzyme located on the inner surface of the blood vessels that hydrolyzes triglycerides in the chylomicrons and very-low-density lipoproteins and allows the fatty acids to enter the cells

longevity a long life (beyond that normally expected for a particular species)

longitudinal a scientific study of changes occurring within the same individuals over time

loop diuretic type of diuretic causing loss of potassium

lordosis an increased curvature of the back; individual appears to be bent over

low-density lipoprotein (LDL) a plasma lipoprotein complex high in cholesterol content and believed to contribute to the development of atherosclerosis

lymphocyte a type of white blood cell; includes the B cells and T cells

macrocytic anemia blood disorder with impaired production of normal red blood cells and the presence of abnormally large red blood cells; usually related to vitamin B_{12} or folic acid deficiency

macromineral a mineral present in the body in substantial amounts (e.g., calcium, phosphorus)

malabsorption impaired absorption of one or more nutrients as a result of incomplete digestion, changes in the cells of the mucosa, pattern of nutrient intake, or disease

malnutrition any nutrition-related disorder; may relate to an inappropriately high or low nutrient intake, an imbalanced nutrient intake, or impaired absorption or assimilation of nutrients in food

mandible the lower jaw bone

marginal nutritional status condition in which body nutrient stores have been depleted but impaired health or function is not yet evident

maximum oxygen consumption the greatest amount of oxygen that the cardiovascular system can transport from the lungs to the exercising muscles at any given time

MCV model method for diagnosis of anemia based on mean cell volume, transferrin saturation, and erythrocyte protoporphyrin levels

mean corpuscular volume (MCV) the average size of the red blood cells; used to diagnose anemia

median the middle value in a distribution, with half of the values falling above and half of the values falling below

metabolic alkalosis abnormal condition in which blood pH rises above 7.45; caused by an abnormal loss of acid or an increased level of bicarbonate or other basic compound

metabolic efficiency relative gain in weight per unit of energy intake

metabolic rate oxygen consumption per unit of body weight in a given period

metalloenzyme enzyme with a mineral element as part of its structure

metastasis the spread of cancer cells from one organ to another

methotrexate drug used to treat cancer

3-methylhistidine an amino acid synthesized in the muscle; urinary 3-methylhistidine excretion is used to estimate total muscle mass

methylmalonic acid a metabolite that accumulates in blood and urine in vitamin B_{12} deficiency

Metropolitan height and weight table a table defining the appropriate body weight for a person of a given height and sex compiled by the Metropolitan Life Insurance Company based on the body weights of policyholders with the longest lifespans

micelle a particle containing lipids and bile salts that moves fatty acids from the intestinal lumen to the intestinal mucosa for absorption

microcytic smaller than normal

microvascular relating to the capillaries

milk-alkali syndrome a condition of alkalosis brought about by very excessive consumption of milk, calcium-containing antacids, or other alkaline substances; most likely to occur in older people with peptic ulcer

modified diet diet developed for the alleviation or treatment of a physiologic or medical problem that requires or restricts certain foods

monoamine oxidase (MAO) inhibitor drug used to treat depression and anxiety; has a potentially dangerous interaction with foods high in tyramine (e.g., red wine, aged cheeses)

monounsaturated fatty acid a fatty acid containing only 1 double bond (e.g., oleic acid)

morbidity illness or disease

mortality rate the number of deaths per unit of population for a specific region, age group, or disease and usually expressed as deaths per 1000, 10,000, or 100,000

mortality ratio the total number of deaths among persons of a given sex or condition divided by the total number of individuals in the population

mucopolysaccharide a compound comprising protein and carbohydrate found in connective tissue, collagen, and bone matrix

mucosal block an early theory developed to explain the regulation of iron absorption; it was suggested that an increased concentration of ferritin in the mucosal cell inhibited further uptake of iron

myasthenia gravis a nerve condition resulting in chronic fatigue and weakness of the muscles of the face and throat

myelin sheath a lipid-containing substance that forms a covering for the major nerves

myocardial contractility the degree of strength of the heart contraction

myocardial infarction heart attack; condition resulting from the occlusion of a coronary artery and interruption of the blood supply to cardiac tissue

myocardium the muscle layer of the heart

myoglobin the iron-protein molecule in the muscle that stores oxygen

National Cholesterol Education Program (NCEP) a program developed and implemented by the U.S. government to develop public awareness of the cardiovascular disease risk associated with elevated blood cholesterol levels and to implement intervention strategies

National Council on the Aging an organization whose membership comprises both professionals and the lay public and that promotes research and services related to older people

National Food Consumption Survey (NFCS) A survey conducted by the United States Department of Agriculture to determine the types and quantities of foods consumed and the nutrient intakes of the general population

National Health Interview Survey an on-going survey conducted by the U.S. government to determine the health habits, utilization of health and medical services and facilities, extent of chronic and acute illnesses, prevalence of disability, and unmet needs for health care in the general population

National Medical Expenditure Survey an on-going survey conducted by the U.S. government to determine out-of-pocket expenses for health care and public and private insurance reimbursement for physicians' visits, hospital services, drugs, and related expenses

negative nitrogen balance situation in which the amount of nitrogen consumed is less than the amount of nitrogen lost through all excretory routes, resulting in a net loss of body nitrogen

neomycin a drug used to treat infection

neoplasia the abnormal development or division of cells, leading to tumors

nephritis kidney disease resulting in some loss of function

nephron the functional unit of the kidney that filters the blood plasma

neuroendocrine relating to the functional interaction between the nervous system and the endocrine glands

neuroleptic agent a drug that leads to an altered degree of consciousness with reduced anxiety and motor activity and indifference to surroundings

neutron activation analysis an irradiation technique to determine body composition based on body content of particular mineral elements

neutrophil a type of white blood cell that engulfs and destroys bacteria

NHANES (National Health and Nutrition Examination Survey) a survey conducted by the United States government at regular intervals to determine the nutritional status and chronic disease risk of the general population

NHANES Epidemiologic Follow-Up Study (NHEFS) a study conducted by the U.S. government to reinterview NHANES participants and determine any changes in their nutrient intake, health status, and chronic disease risk factors

nicotinamide form of niacin

nicotinic acid a form of niacin

nightblindness poor vision in dim light or at night as a result of vitamin A deficiency

nonambulatory unable to walk

nonheme iron iron found in plant foods and in animal tissues other than hemoglobin or myoglobin

noninsulin-dependent diabetes mellitus (NIDDM) type of diabetes mellitus resulting from a reduced output of insulin by the beta islets of the pancreas and the reduced effectiveness of insulin in moving glucose into muscle and adipose cells

nonsteroidal antiinflammatory drug (NSAID) type of drug used to treat osteoarthritis and rheumatoid arthritis; available over the counter as ibuprofen

norepinephrine hormone produced by the adrenal medulla that increases blood pressure by constricting the blood vessels

normotensive having normal blood pressure

nutrient-dense foods foods that contain protein, vitamins, or minerals in a percentage of the RDA equal to or above the percentage of kilocalories provided

nutrition monitoring an ongoing program of the United States government or other agency to continually assess the nutritional status of the population to determine the existence or development of any nutrition problems

Nutrition Program for the Elderly a program funded by the Older Americans Act that provides congregate or home-delivered meals to persons age 60 and over

nutrition screening strategies to identify individuals who have nutrition-related problems or are at risk for development of nutrition-related problems

Nutrition Screening Initiative a program developed to promote routine nutrition screening and improved nutritional care in the health care system, with a current emphasis on older people

nutrition surveillance on-going observation or evaluation of the nutritional well-being of a population group for the purpose of detecting changes that would indicate a need for intervention or for evaluating an on-going intervention program

nutritional anemia anemia caused by a lack of a particular nutrient such as iron, vitamin B_{12}, or folate

nutritional assessment an evaluation of the nutritional condition and health of an individual based on dietary records, clinical examination, and biochemical and anthropometric measurements

nutritional imbalance an inappropriate intake of one or more nutrients as related to overall nutrient intake or energy expenditure

Nutritional Risk Index (NRI) a set of criteria for identifying individuals who are likely to have a less-than-adequate nutrient intake or poor nutritional status

nutritional status the nutritional health of an individual as determined by past and present intakes of protein, fat, carbohydrate, vitamins, and minerals, and related health and physiologic factors; evaluation must be based on dietary, clinical, biochemical, and anthropometric measurements

obligatory nitrogen loss the lowest level of nitrogen excretion that can be reached by an individual on a protein-free diet

occult concealed or hidden; not easily observed

occupational therapist a certified professional who plans activities to assist the impaired individual (who may have experienced illness or injury) in regaining self-feeding, food preparation, or other motor skills

Older Americans Act the major piece of federal legislation providing nutrition and social services for noninstitutionalized persons age 60 and over

old-old United States census designation for persons age 75 to 84

olfactory acuity sharpness of the sense of smell

omega-3 fatty acid a type of polyunsaturated fatty acid found in fish that is believed to prevent blood platelet aggregation and retard the progression of vascular disease

omnivore an individual who consumes both plant and animal foods

oophorectomy surgical removal of the ovaries

oral consumed by mouth

oral glucose tolerance test test to evaluate the body's ability to metabolize carbohydrate and diagnose the presence of diabetes mellitus; a standard amount of glucose is given by mouth, and blood glucose levels are measured for 2 to 3 hours following

organic brain disease brain disorder related to a physiologic change or injury in brain cells

organic brain syndrome change in behavior or cognitive function caused by a physiologic alteration

such as loss of brain cells, cerebral arteriosclerosis, or decreased synthesis of neurotransmitters

orthostatic hypotension abnormally low blood pressure that occurs when a person stands up

osmolality the osmotic pressure exerted by a solution expressed on the basis of the number of ions or particles per kg of water or solvent

osmoreceptors nerve cells in the hypothalamus that are sensitive to the concentration of electrolytes or molecules in the blood

osmotic diuresis increased excretion of water resulting from a substance present in the renal tubule at a level that is too high to be effectively reabsorbed (e.g., glucose or urea)

osteoarthritis localized degenerative changes in the joints resulting in pain, swelling, and often some degree of disability

osteoblast a cell that synthesizes bone matrix and assists in the deposit of mineral to form new bone

osteoclast a cell that dissolves bone mineral and removes remaining matrix in the resorption of bone

osteomalacia adult rickets; bone disorder in which mineral but not matrix is lost from the bone

osteoporosis a bone disorder occurring in older individuals leading to loss of bone mineral and matrix, loss of bone strength, and increased risk of bone fracture

overload excessive tissue levels or stores of a nutrient as a result of abnormally high intake and absorption and limited ability for excretion; occurs with iron

overnutrition the situation in which the level of nutrient intake exceeds the body needs

over-the-counter (OTC) drug available without a prescription

oxalate compounds found in spinach and various other vegetables that bind divalent cations such as calcium and iron and prevent their absorption

pancreatic insufficiency inadequate secretion of pancreatic hormones or enzymes as a result of physiologic deterioration or disease

papophagia ingestion of large quantities of ice

paraaminohippuric acid substance actively secreted into the urine by the kidney; used to measure total plasma flow through the kidney

paraaminosalicylic acid drug used to treat tuberculosis

paralysis loss of muscle function

parathyroid hormone (PTH) controls the calcium level in the blood

parietal cell cells lining the stomach that produce hydrochloric acid

parkinson's disease a neurologic disorder occurring in persons above age 60 characterized by tremors, muscle weakness and rigidity, and a shuffling gait

parotid glands the largest pair of the salivary glands

passive absorption/reabsorption absorption occurring by diffusion; does not require energy

patella the flat bone in front of the knee joint; also called the kneecap

penicillamine drug that binds with and removes minerals from the blood; acts as an antiinflammatory agent and is used to treat rheumatoid arthritis

pepsinogen protein secreted by the chief cells in the gastric mucosa that is converted to pepsin in the presence of gastric acid

peptic ulcer a loss of the protective mucous membrane in an area of the stomach or duodenum as a result of excessive acid production, stress, or certain drugs

perceived health benefit an individual's impression of the value of a particular behavior in developing or maintaining good health

periodontal disease inflammation of tissues around the teeth; can result in loosening and loss of teeth and damage to the jaw bone

peripheral relating to the areas of the body outside of the viscera

peristalsis the rhythmic contractions of the muscle in the wall of the gastrointestinal tract that propel the food through the tract

pernicious anemia an anemia characterized by immature macrocytic red blood cells and accompanied by the deterioration of neural tissues; caused by a lack of intrinsic factor necessary for normal absorption of vitamin B_{12}

peroxidation the addition of an oxygen atom at a double bond in an unsaturated fatty acid; can occur in the body or in a foodstuff

personal care home a facility that provides room, board, and supervision for older persons but no medical or health services

phagocytosis process by which cells of the immune system surround, enclose, and digest microorganisms, cell debris, or foreign matter

pharmacodynamics the study of how drugs act in a living person and the relationship between drug dosage and the observed response

pharmacokinetics the study of the absorption, metabolism, and excretion of drugs and the duration of activity

phenolphthalein a laxative that increases the motor activity of the lower intestinal tract

phenothiazine drugs a family of drugs used to control psychotic behavior

phenytoin drug used to prevent seizures or convulsions

phylloquinone vitamin K

physical signs an objective observation that is made by a qualified examiner, such as noting a rash or condition of the tongue

Physician's Desk Reference (P.D.R.) a reference book published annually containing information supplied by manufacturers regarding drugs used in the United States

phytate phosphoric acid compounds found in grains that bind iron, magnesium, and other divalent cations and prevent their absorption

plasma the fluid portion of the blood

plasma amino acid response curve a method for determining the requirement for a specific amino acid

platelet aggregation the joining together of blood platelets in response to an injury in the blood vessel; the first step in forming a blood clot

pneumonia infectious disease of the lungs in which the airways and alveoli fill with fluid, making breathing and gas exchange difficult

polypharmacy use of a number of drugs at one time

polyphenols a group of substances that occur in tea and interfere with the absorption of iron and possibly other minerals

positive nitrogen balance situation in which the amount of dietary nitrogen consumed exceeds the amount of nitrogen excreted by all routes, leading to a net gain in body nitrogen

postprandial after eating

potassium-sparing diuretics type of diuretic that does not increase loss of body potassium

poverty income ratio a measure of the income status of an individual or family relative to the minimum income needed to meet basic needs as determined by the federal government; a value of <1 indicates poverty status

poverty level the minimum income required to provide the basic necessities of food, clothing, and shelter as determined by the federal government

prealbumin a plasma transport protein with a short half life used as an indicator of protein status

preformed vitamin A form of vitamin A present in animal foods

premenopausal prior to menopause

presbyesophagus loss of elasticity of the esophagus, which interferes with the movement of food down the passageway

pro re nata (PRN) Latin term used in prescription writing that means "as the occasion arises"

proliferative capacity the ability of cells to multiply

promotion the second step in the development of cancer; a carcinogen or chemical agent acts on a genetically altered cell to stimulate uncontrolled growth

propranolol drug used to lower blood pressure and control cardiac arrhythmias

prospective a study designed to examine the relationship between a particular illness or disease and a particular habit or environmental factor such as diet or smoking; healthy subjects are recruited for study and observed over time to determine the rate at which the disease develops

prospective payment system payment system based on the diagnostic-related groups (DRGs) in which hospitals are reimbursed by Medicare according to the procedures and days of care considered to be necessary for the treatment of a particular condition

protease enzyme that breaks peptide bonds

protein turnover the continuous process of protein breakdown and synthesis occurring in the body

protein-energy malnutrition (PEM) a condition resulting from a deficiency in both kilocalories and protein

protein-losing enteropathy excessive loss of visceral proteins in the feces as a result of an intestinal disease

psychotropic agents drugs that affect behavior or mental activity

pteroylglutamic acid folic acid

pulmonary embolism blockage of an artery in the lung by air, a blood clot, or an atherosclerotic particle

purpura small red or purple spots under the skin resulting from hemorrhages of the capillaries

pyridoxal kinase enzyme that transfers a phosphate group to the pyridoxine molecule to form pyridoxal phosphate

pyridoxal phosphate (PLP) a coenzyme containing vitamin B_6 that is necessary for transamination reactions; plasma PLP levels are used as an indicator of vitamin B_6 status

quality assurance an evaluation of nutrition and health services provided and the results achieved as compared with accepted standards

quinidine drug used to prevent fibrillation of the atria and rapid heart beat

receptor site a chemical structure on the cell membrane where a hormone or antigen binds

Recommended Dietary Allowances (RDAs) the level of intake of an essential nutrient considered to be adequate to meet the daily needs of practically all healthy persons of a particular age, sex, or condition

recumbent lying down

red cell folate highly correlated with liver folate stores and used as an indicator of folate status

reference standards a set of values derived from normal, healthy individuals with which values obtained from clients, patients, or other population groups are compared

relative weight the body weight of an individual divided by the average or desirable body weight of persons of the same height, sex, and age

renal 1-α-hydroxylase enzyme in the kidney that converts 25-hydroxyvitamin D to 1,25-dihydroxyvitamin D

renal insufficiency inability of the kidney to excrete waste materials and conserve water, electrolytes, and other important molecules to the extent needed

renal tubular reabsorption the reabsorption by the kidney of water, glucose, vitamins, and electrolytes from the glomerular filtrate

renal tubular secretion the energy-requiring elimination of ions or molecules by the kidney (e.g., H^+, drug metabolites)

renin an enzyme produced in the kidney in response to low blood pressure; it causes the formation of angiotensin

renin-angiotensin-aldosterone system enzyme-hormonal feedback system that controls blood pressure through the reabsorption and excretion of water and sodium

reserve capacity the ability of an organ system to adjust to an increased need that may arise from physiologic stress or disease

residual volume air remaining in the lungs after the individual has exhaled

resorption (bone) the loss of bone matrix and mineral

respondent a person who agrees to provide requested information in a dietary or health study

resting energy expenditure the amount of energy required to maintain essential body processes when the individual is at rest and neither perspiring nor shivering; differs from basal metabolism in that the individual has not fasted and the measurement may include the thermic effect of food

reticuloendothelial cells cells lining the blood vessels that attack virus and bacteria and produce antibodies against foreign molecules

retinol the form of vitamin A with the highest biologic activity

retinol-binding protein a protein that transports retinol in the plasma and is sometimes used as an indicator of protein status

retinyl ester form in which vitamin A is stored in the liver

retrospective study a study which examines relationships between a current condition or state of health and practices or occurrences in the past

rheumatoid arthritis a chronic, systemic, inflammatory disease resulting in swelling of the joints, destruction of the cartilage, and muscle atrophy

rickets a bone disorder occurring in growing children in which bone matrix is not mineralized because of a lack of vitamin D and failure to absorb calcium

salicylic acid precursor for a family of drugs used to relieve pain, reduce fever, and control inflammation

scoliosis abnormal curvature of the spine to the right or the left

sebaceous glands glands in the skin that secrete the oil that prevents drying of the skin

Second National Health and Nutrition Examination Survey (NHANES II) a survey conducted by the U.S. government to determine the nutritional status and chronic disease risk of the general population

secondary not the major or usual cause of a disorder, but the result of an associated factor or disorder

secular changes changes related to the passage of time

senescence the process of growing old

senile dementia of the Alzheimer type (SDAT) degenerative brain disease occurring beyond middle age and resulting in changes in behavior and in loss of memory, cognitive function, and speech

senna extract a type of cathartic that increases motor activity in the lower intestine

sepsis infection

serotonin a neurotransmitter derived from tryptophan

single-room occupancy situation of older persons living in inner city hotels that provide a small sleeping area but no other services or supervision

skilled nursing facility (SNF) a facility providing health and personal care under the supervision of a physician to patients requiring a high level of skilled nursing care

skinfold calipers an instrument used to measure the thickness of a skinfold as an indicator of the level of body fat

skinfold compressibility the degree to which the skinfold is pressed together when grasped with the skinfold caliper; an increase in connective tissue will decrease compressibility

skinfold thickness the width of a skinfold as measured with a skinfold caliper

Social Security a national government insurance system that provides income payments to retired persons age 65 and over based on their income while still employed; is the major source of income for retired persons in the United States

socially impaired individuals with behavioral or psychologic problems relating to alcoholism, mental illness, organic brain disease, or the mental and emotional stress related to homelessness

sodium-induced hypertension sensitivity of some individuals to develop hypertension as a result of excessive sodium intake

soluble fiber components of pectins and gums found in fruits, oats, and legumes that reduce the rate of gastric emptying, have water-holding properties, increase fecal bulk, and contribute to the lowering of serum cholesterol levels

somatomedin C substance synthesized by the liver that is believed to bring about the anabolic effects associated with growth hormone

spastic colon increased or uncontrolled contractions of the colon; irritable bowel syndrome

splanchnic blood perfusion blood flow to the visceral organs, including the liver, heart, lungs, kidneys, and digestive organs

stadiometer an apparatus for measuring sitting or standing height

steatorrhea appearance of higher-than-normal levels of fat in the feces

stem cell an immature cell that has the potential to develop into one of several different mature cells

stomatitis inflammation or soreness of the mouth

stroke loss of blood supply to a part of the brain caused by a blockage or rupture of a blood vessel

stroke volume the amount of blood ejected from the heart with each contraction

styloid process the bony, peglike projection in the region of the temple

subcutaneous fat fat located directly under the skin

sulfonylurea an oral antidiabetic agent that stimulates production of insulin by the pancreas

supine lying on the back

symptoms manifestations reported by the patient, such as fatigue or headache

systemic circulation movement of the blood throughout the arteries and veins of the entire body and back to the heart

systolic blood pressure the blood pressure when the heart muscle contracts and blood is being ejected from the heart; systolic pressure is usually higher than diastolic pressure

tachycardia rapid heart beat (over 100 beats/min)

taste acuity the sharpness of perception of the basic tastes: sweet, salty, bitter, sour

T-cells activated white blood cells that attack fungi, viruses, and tumors; responsible for cell-mediated immunity

testosterone the male sex hormone secreted by the testes

tetracycline drug used to treat infections

theophylline (xanthine derivative bronchodilator) increases the diameter of the bronchi; used in the treatment of asthma and emphysema

therapeutic index the difference between the minimum therapeutic dose and the minimum toxic dose of a drug

thermal buffer physiologic mechanism to avoid fluctuations in body temperature (e.g., body fluids can absorb or give off heat)

thermic effect of food (TEF) energy expended in the digestion, absorption, and metabolism of ingested food

thiazide diuretic type of diuretic associated with urinary loss of potassium and sodium and urinary conservation of calcium

thioridazine hydrochloride used to treat mental disorders and depression in the elderly

thrombosis a blood clot attached to the wall of a blood vessel that may occlude the flow of blood

thyroid-stimulating hormone (TSH) a substance released by the anterior lobe of the pituitary that causes the thyroid gland to release thyroid hormones

thyroxin (T_4) hormone produced by the thyroid gland that controls the metabolic rate of body cells

tinnitus ringing in the ears

Title III-B social service program the program funded by the Older Americans Act that provides transportation services to congregate meal sites, medical appointments, or grocery stores for persons age 60 and over

Title III-C nutrition program the program funded by the Older Americans Act that provides for the implementation of congregate and home-delivered meals for persons age 60 and over

tocopherol equivalent basis for expressing the vitamin E activity of compounds as compared to the activity of 1 mg of alpha tocopherol

tolbutamide an oral antidiabetic agent used in management of noninsulin-dependent diabetes mellitus

total body respiratory chamber a chamber with a controlled temperature and air flow in which a person can live for 24 hours and total oxygen consumption and energy metabolism can be determined

total body water (TBW) includes all the water in the intracellular and extracellular body compartments

total iron-binding capacity the total concentration of transferrin available for iron uptake or saturation

total meal cost the total cost of providing a congregate or home-delivered meal, including food, packaging, labor, delivery, and administrative costs

trabecular bone spongy bone with a latticelike structure found in the ends of the long bones and the vertebrae

trace elements minerals present in the body in very small amounts

transaminase enzyme that transfers amino groups and requires vitamin B_6 as a coenzyme

transferrin the transport protein for iron

transferrin saturation the relative proportion of transferrin in the blood that is combined with an iron molecule

transketolase an enzyme essential in carbohydrate metabolism that requires thiamin as a coenzyme; red blood cell transketolase activity is used as a measure of thiamin status

triceps skinfold skinfold thickness measurement taken at the triceps muscle in the upper arm

truncal relating to the body trunk rather than to the arms or legs

tryptophan load test test used to evaluate vitamin B_6 status

tuberculosis chronic infection of the lungs, with accumulation of cell masses and connective tissue that interferes with air passage and gas exchange

tyramine an amino acid that can be synthesized in the body from tyrosine and stimulates the release of epinephrine and norepinephrine; also found in various food products, including aged cheeses and red wine

undernutrition condition characterized by an insufficient level of kilocalories and/or protein, vitamins, and minerals

unintentional weight loss loss of weight occurring without a deliberate dietary or exercise modification; unwanted weight loss

United States Pharmacopeia Dispensing Information (U.S.P.D.I.) a reference recognized officially by the Food and Drug Administration that contains descriptions, uses, strengths, and standards of purity for selected drugs

validity the extent to which a measurement or instrument accurately measures what it is intended to measure

vasoconstrictor agent that causes the blood vessels to decrease in diameter

vasodilator agent that causes blood vessels to increase in diameter

vegan an individual who consumes no food of animal origin

very-low-calorie diet diet used for weight loss that contains only 400 to 800 kcal; should be used only under strict medical supervision

very-low-carbohydrate diet popular but dangerous diet for weight loss that leads to high losses of body fluids, protein, and electrolytes; contains little (<50 g) or no carbohydrate

very-low-density lipoprotein (VLDL) a plasma lipoprotein with a high content of triglycerides

visceral organs organs found in the abdominal cavity (e.g., heart, liver, kidney, spleen, digestive organs)

visceral proteins the proteins synthesized in the liver, including albumin, transferrin, and retinol-binding proteins

vital capacity the maximal amount of air that can be moved in and out of the lungs in one breath

waist-to-hip ratio waist circumference divided by the hip circumference; a higher ratio is associated with greater abdominal fat (male pattern) and higher risk of chronic disease; a lower ratio is associated with greater fat in the hip region (female pattern) and lower disease risk

warfarin drug that prevents blood clotting

Wernicke-Korsakoff syndrome a condition characterized by double vision, involuntary eye movements, and decreased muscular coordination and mental function as a result of degenerative brain changes; associated with alcoholism and thiamin deficiency

xanthurenic acid a metabolite of tryptophan that is present at high levels in the urine of vitamin B_6–deficient persons

xerostomia dry mouth; abnormally low secretion of salivary fluids

x-ray absorptiometry method used to evaluate bone density

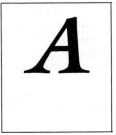

Recommended Dietary Allowances

TABLE A-1   Recommended Dietary Allowances for Persons Ages 51 and Over (Revised 1989)

	Males	Females
Weight*		
(kg)	77	65
(lb)	170	143
Height*		
(cm)	173	160
(in)	68	63
Protein (g)	63	50
Vitamin A (μg RE)†	1000	800
Vitamin D (μg)‡	5	5
Vitamin E (mg α-TE)§	10	8
Vitamin K (μg)	80	65
Vitamin C (mg)	60	60
Thiamin (mg)	1.2	1.0
Riboflavin (mg)	1.4	1.2
Niacin (mg NE)‖	15	13
Vitamin B_6 (mg)	2.0	1.6
Folate (μg)	200	180
Vitamin B_{12} (μg)	2.0	2.0
Calcium (mg)	800	800
Phosphorus (mg)	800	800
Magnesium (mg)	350	280
Iron (mg)	10	10
Zinc (mg)	15	12
Iodine (μg)	150	150
Selenium (μg)	70	55

*Weights and heights given are actual median values for the U.S. population ages 51 and over as reported by NHANES II. These height-to-weight ratios may not be ideal.

†Retinol equivalents: 1 retinol equivalent = 1 μg retinol or 6 μg β-carotene.

‡As cholecalciferol: 10 μg cholecalciferol = 400 IU of vitamin D.

§α-Tocopherol equivalents: 1 mg d-α tocopherol = 1α-TE.

‖1 NE (niacin equivalent) = 1 mg niacin or 60 mg dietary tryptophan.

TABLE A-2   Estimated Safe and Adequate Daily Dietary Intakes of Selected Vitamins and Minerals for Adults

Vitamin/Mineral	Intake*
Biotin	30-100 μg
Pantothenic acid	4.0-7.0 mg
Copper	1.5-3.0 mg†
Manganese	2.0-5.0 mg†
Fluoride	1.5-4.0 mg†
Chromium	50-200 μg†
Molybdenum	75-250 μg†

*Because there is less information on which to base allowances, these figures are provided in the form of ranges of recommended intakes.

†Because the toxic levels for many trace minerals may be only several times usual intakes, the upper levels given in this table should not be habitually exceeded.

TABLE A-3   Estimated Sodium, Chloride, and Potassium Minimum Requirements of Healthy Adults

Mineral	Intake
Sodium*	500 mg
Chloride*	750 mg
Potassium†	2000 mg

Adapted from Food and Nutrition Board: *Recommended dietary allowances,* ed 10, Washington, DC, 1989, National Academy Press.

*No evidence suggests that higher intakes confer any health benefit.

†Desirable intake may considerably exceed this value (about 3500 mg for adults).

B

Government Agencies and Professional and Voluntary Organizations Serving the Aged

AGENCIES—UNITED STATES GOVERNMENT

ACTION
1100 Vermont Ave., N.W.
Washington, DC 20525
(Administers programs serving the aged, including RSVP and Foster Grandparents Program)

Administration on Aging
Wilbur J. Cohen Bldg.
330 Independence Ave., S.W.
Washington, DC 20201

Arthritis and Musculoskeletal Interagency Coordinating Committee
National Institutes of Health
Bldg. 31, Room 4C32
Bethesda, MD 20892

Department of Agriculture
Office of Information
14th Street and Independence Ave., S.W.
Washington, DC 20250

Gerontology Research Center—National Institute on Aging
Baltimore City Hospitals
4940 Eastern Ave.
Baltimore, MD 21224

National Institute on Aging
National Institutes of Health, Bldg. 31
9000 Rockville Pike
Bethesda, MD 20205

Social Security Administration
6401 Security Blvd.
Baltimore, MD 21235

United States House of Representatives
Select Committee on Aging
H1-A712 O'Neill House Office Bldg.
Washington, DC 20515-6361

United States Senate
Special Committee on Aging
Dirkson Senate Office Bldg.
Room G-31
Washington, DC 20510-6400

Veterans Administration
810 Vermont Ave., N.W.
Washington, DC 20420

PROFESSIONAL AND VOLUNTARY ORGANIZATIONS

General Aspects of Aging

Aging in America
1500 Pelham Parkway, S.
Bronx, NY 10461

American Aging Association
c/o Denham Harman, M.D.
College of Medicine
University of Nebraska
Omaha, NE 68105

American Bar Association
Commission on Legal Problems of the Elderly
1800 M Street, N.W.
Washington, DC 20036

American Society on Aging
833 Market Street
Room 516
San Francisco, CA 94103

Asian and Pacific Coalition on Aging
1102 Crenshaw Blvd.
Room 43
Los Angeles, CA 90019

Association for Adult Development and Aging
c/o American Association for Counseling and Development
5999 Stevenson Ave.
Alexandria, VA 22304

Association for Gerontology in Higher Education
600 Maryland Ave., S.W.
West Wing 204
Washington, DC 20024

Gerontological Society of America
1275 K Street, N.W.
Suite 350
Washington, DC 20005-4006

Institute of Retired Professionals
The New School of Social Research
66 W. 12th Street
New York, NY 10011

International Center for Social Gerontology
117 N. First Street
Suite 204
Ann Arbor, MI 48104

International Federation on Aging
449 Swanston Street, 1st Floor
Melbourne 3000, Australia

International Federation on Aging
1909 K Street, N.W.
Washington, DC 20049

Legal Services for the Elderly
132 W. 43rd Street, 3rd Floor
New York, NY 10036

Little Brothers—Friends of the Elderly
1658 W. Belmont Ave.
Chicago, IL 60657

National Association of Counties
Aging Program
440 First Street, N.W.
Washington, DC 20001

National Association of Foster Grandparents
Program Directors
195 East San Fernando Street
San Jose, CA 95112

National Caucus and Center on Black Aged
1424 K Street, N.W.
Suite 500
Washington, DC 20005

National Center on Arts and the Aging
c/o National Council on the Aging
600 Maryland Ave., S.W.
West Wing, Suite 100
Washington, DC 20024

National Committee for Senior Americans
P.O. Box 9009
Valley Forge, PA 19485

National Council on the Aging
600 Maryland Ave., S.W.
West Wing 100, Suite 208
Washington, DC 20024

National Hispanic Council on Aging
2713 Ontario Rd., N.W.
Suite 200
Washington, DC 20009

National Indian Council on Aging, Inc.
P.O. Box 2088
Albuquerque, NM 87103

National Institute on Age, Work, and Retirement
c/o National Council on the Aging
600 Maryland Ave., S.W.
West Wing, Suite 100
Washington, DC 20024

National Interfaith Coalition on Aging
P.O. Box 1924
Athens, GA 30605

National Pacific/Asian Resource Center on Aging
2033 6th Ave.
Suite 410
Seattle, WA 98121

National Retired Teachers Association (NRTA)
1909 K Street, N.W.
Washington, DC 20049

National Senior Citizens Law Center
2025 M Street, N.W.
Suite 400
Washington, DC 20036

Service Corps of Retired Executives Association
1825 Connecticut Ave., N.W.
Suite 503
Washington, DC 20009

Southern Gerontological Society
c/o Gerontology Center
Georgia State University
Atlanta, GA 30303

U.S. Conference on Mayors
Task Force on Aging
1620 I Street, N.W.
Washington, DC 20006

Physical and Mental Health

Alzheimer's Association
551 5th Ave.
Suite 601
New York, NY 10176

American Cancer Society
1599 Clifton Road, N.E.
Atlanta, GA 30329

American Diabetes Association
National Service Center
P.O. Box 25757
1660 Duke Street
Alexandria, VA 22314

American Geriatrics Society
770 Lexington Ave.
Suite 400
New York, NY 10021

American Heart Association
7320 Greenville Ave.
Dallas, TX 75231

American Lung Association
1740 Broadway
New York, NY 10019

American Medical Association
  Committee on Aging
  515 N. State Street
  Chicago, IL 60610
American Nurses' Association, Inc.
  Council of Nursing Home Nurses
  Division on Gerontological Nursing Practice
  2420 Pershing Rd.
  Kansas City, MO 64108
American Osteopathic Association
  142 E. Ontario Street
  Chicago, IL 60611-2864
American Parkinson Disease Association
  116 John Street
  Suite 417
  New York, NY 10038
American Psychiatric Association
  Council on Aging
  1400 K Street, N.W.
  Washington, DC 20005
American Psychological Association
  Division of Adult Development and Aging
  1200 17th Street, N.W.
  Washington, DC 20036
American Public Health Association
  Section of Gerontological Health
  1015 15th Street, N.W.
  Washington, DC 20005
American Society for Geriatric Dentistry
  211 E. Chicago Ave.
  Suite 1616
  Chicago, IL 60611
Arthritis Foundation
  1314 Spring Street, N.W.
  Atlanta, GA 30309
Huntington's Disease Society of America
  140 W. 22nd Street
  6th Floor
  New York, NY 10011-2420
National Center for Health Promotion and Aging
  c/o National Council on the Aging
  600 Maryland Ave., S.W.
  West Wing, Suite 100
  Washington, DC 20024
National Geriatrics Society
  212 W. Wisconsin Ave.
  Milwaukee, WI 53202

National Health Services
  1200 18th Street
  Suite 602
  Washington, DC 20036
National Safety Council
  444 North Michigan Ave.
  Chicago, IL 60611
National Therapeutic Recreation Society
  National Recreation and Park Association
  3101 Park Center Dr.
  Alexandria, VA 22302

Long-Term Care Facilities and Services

American Association of Homes for the Aging
  1129 20th Street, N.W.
  Suite 400
  Washington, DC 20036
American College of Health Care Administrators (Nursing Homes)
  325 S. Patrick Street
  Alexandria, VA 22314
American Health Care Association
  1201 L Street, N.W.
  Washington, DC 20005
Council of Home Health Agencies and Community Health Services
  National League for Nursing
  10 Columbus Circle
  New York, NY 10019
Health Insurance Association of America
  1025 Connecticut Ave., N.W.
  Suite 1200
  Washington, DC 20036
National Association for Families Caring for Their Elders, Inc.
  1141 Loxford Terrace
  Silver Spring, MD 20901
National Association for Home Care
  519 C Street, N.E.
  Washington, DC 20002
National Citizens' Coalition for Nursing Home Reform
  1424 16th Street, N.W.
  Suite L2
  Washington, DC 20036
National Hospice Organization
  1901 N. Moore Street
  Suite 901
  Arlington, VA 22209

National Institute on Adult Daycare
  c/o National Council on the Aging
  600 Maryland Ave., S.W.
  West Wing, Suite 100
  Washington, DC 20024
National Voluntary Organizations for Independent Living for the Aging
  c/o National Council on the Aging
  600 Maryland Ave., S.W.
  West Wing, Suite 100
  Washington, DC 20024
North American Association of Jewish Homes and Housing
  2525 Centerville Road
  Dallas, TX 75228
Special Constituency Section on Aging and Long-Term Care Services
  c/o American Hospital Association
  840 N. Lake Shore Drive
  Chicago, IL 60611

Physical Rehabilitation Services

American Dance Therapy Association
  2000 Century Plaza
  Suite 108
  Columbia, MD 21044
American Foundation for the Blind
  15 W. 16th Street
  New York, NY 10011
American Occupational Therapy Association
  1383 Piccard Drive
  Rockville, MD 20850
American Physical Therapy Association
  200 S. Service Rd.
  Roslyn Heights, NY 11577
American Speech-Language-Hearing Association
  10801 Rockville Pike
  Rockville, MD 20852
Association for Education and Rehabilitation of the Blind and Visually Impaired
  206 N. Washington Street
  Suite 320
  Alexandria, VA 22314
Institute for Rehabilitation and Research
  1333 Moursund Ave.
  Houston, TX 77030
National Hearing Aid Society
  20361 Middlebelt Road
  Livonia, MI 48152

National Information Center for Deafness
  Gallaudet University
  800 Florida Ave., N.E.
  Washington, DC 20002-3625
National Rehabilitation Association
  633 S. Washington Street
  Alexandria, VA 22314
National Society to Prevent Blindness
  500 E. Remington Road
  Schaumburg, IL 60173

Nutrition Information and Research

American Dietetic Association
  216 W. Jackson Blvd.
  Suite 800
  Chicago, IL 60606
American Institute of Nutrition
  9650 Rockville Pike
  Bethesda, MD 20814
American Society for Clinical Nutrition
  9650 Rockville Pike
  Bethesda, MD 20814
Society for Nutrition Education
  1700 Broadway
  Suite 300
  Oakland, CA 94612

Nutrition and Social Services

Catholic Golden Age
  1012 14th Street, N.W.
  Suite 1003
  Washington, DC 20005
Jewish Association for Services for the Aged
  40 W. 68th Street
  New York, NY 10023
National Association of Area Agencies on Aging
  600 Maryland Ave., S.W.
  West Wing, Suite 208
  Washington, DC 20024
National Association of Meals Programs
  204 E Street, N.E.
  Washington, DC 20002
National Association of Nutrition and Aging Services Programs
  2675 44th Street, S.W.
  Suite 305
  Grand Rapids, MI 49509

National Association of Older American Volunteer Program Directors
    1148 Bingham Terrace
    Reston, VA 22091
National Association of RSVP Directors, Inc.
    RSVP of El Paso
    Two Civic Center Plaza
    El Paso, TX 79999
National Association of Senior Companion Project Directors
    Street Landry Parish Community Action Agency
    P.O. Box 1510
    Opelousas, LA 70570
National Association of State Units on Aging
    2033 K Street, S.W.
    Suite 304
    Washington, DC 20006
National Institute of Senior Centers
    National Council on the Aging
    600 Maryland Ave., S.W.
    West Wing 100, Suite 208
    Washington, DC 20024

Research on Aging

American Federation for Aging Research
    725 Park Ave.
    New York, NY 10021
Center for Research on Aging
    Purdue University
    1365 Stone Hall
    West Lafayette, IN 47907-1365
Center for Studies in Aging
    University of North Texas
    P.O. Box 13438
    Denton, TX 76203-3438
Center for Study of Aging and Human Development
    Duke University Medical Center
    Box 3003
    Durham, NC 27710
Center for the Study of Aging
    University of Alabama
    Box 870326
    University, AL 35487-0326
Center for the Study of Aging
    706 Madison Ave.
    Albany, NY 12208

Center on Adult Development and Aging
    University of Miami Medical School (D-101)
    1425 10th Ave., N.W.
    Suite 200
    Miami, FL 33136
Institute for Health and Aging
    University of California, San Francisco
    School of Nursing
    San Francisco, CA 94143-0612
Institute for Health, Health Care Policy, and Aging Research
    Rutgers University
    30 College Ave.
    New Brunswick, NJ 08903
Institute on Aging
    Portland State University
    Box 751
    Portland, OR 97207
Institute on Aging
    Temple University
    1601 N. Broad Street
    Philadelphia, PA 19122
Policy Center on Aging
    Brandeis University
    Heller Graduate School
    Waltham, MA 02254
USDA Human Nutrition Research Center on Aging
    Tufts University
    711 Washington Street
    Boston, MA 02111

ADVOCACY GROUPS-GENERAL MEMBERSHIP

American Association of Retired Persons
    1909 K Street, N.W.
    Washington, DC 20049
American Senior Citizens Association
    P.O. Box 41
    Fayetteville, NC 28302
Association of Informed Senior Citizens
    560 Herndon Parkway
    Suite 110
    Herndon, VA 22070
Children of Aging Parents
    2761 Trenton Road
    Levittown, PA 19056

Gray Panthers
311 S. Juniper Street
Philadelphia, PA 19107
Gray Panthers' National Task Force on Older Women
6407 Maiden Lane
Bethesda, MD 20034
International Senior Citizens Association
1102 S. Crenshaw Blvd.
Los Angeles, CA 90019

National Alliance of Senior Citizens
2525 Wilson Blvd.
Arlington, VA 22201
National Council of Senior Citizens
925 15th Street, N.W.
Washington, DC 20005
Villers Advocacy Associates
1334 G Street, N.W.
Washington, DC 20005

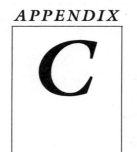

APPENDIX

C

Tools for Evaluating Dietary Status

DIET HISTORY FORM FOR OLDER ADULTS

• *Name* _____ *Address* _____ *Age* _____

1. What type of housing do you live in?
   Public housing for senior citizens _____ Single family house _____ Rented apartment _____
      Rented room—kitchen privileges _____ Rented room—no kitchen privileges _____
      No home _____ (If older person is homeless, skip to question 7)
2. What type of household do you live in?
   Alone _____ With spouse _____ With other family members _____ With friends _____
3. Do you prepare your own meals? Yes _____ No _____ Partially _____
   If not, who does? _____
4. What kind of facilities are available for cooking your food? (Check all that apply)
   None _____ Conventional range _____ Conventional oven _____ Microwave oven _____
   A hotplate only _____ Small appliances only _____
   Is this a satisfactory arrangement for you? Yes _____ No _____
   If not, why not? _____
5. Do you have a refrigerator in working condition?
   Yes _____ No _____
6. Do you have adequate storage area for food supplies?
   Adequate refrigerator space Yes _____ No _____
   Adequate freezer space Yes _____ No _____
   Adequate cabinet space Yes _____ No _____
7. Some people have problems with shopping. How do you usually get to the food store?
   Walk to and back _____ Walk to, public transit back _____ Walk to, taxi back _____
      Public transit both ways _____ Ride from friend/neighbor/relative _____
      Use own car _____ Ride from senior center or community services _____
      Do not shop _____
   Is this arrangement satisfactory for you? Yes _____ No _____
   If not, why not? _____

8. Where do you do your major food shopping? Neighborhood grocery _____
      Supermarket _____ Food cooperative _____ Convenience store (24-hour store) _____
      Health food store _____ Food pantry _____ Do not shop _____
9. Is there any other store in which you would rather shop?
   Yes _____ No _____
   If yes, why? _____
10. What keeps you from shopping there? _____
11. Are groceries delivered to your home? Yes _____ No _____
    If yes, how frequently are they delivered? _____
    What types of food items are delivered? _____
12. With whom do you usually eat your meals?
    Alone _____ Spouse _____ Friends _____ Other _____
13. Is your choice of food restricted because of problems with chewing?
    Yes _____ No _____
    If yes, what foods can't you eat? _____

Adapted from Christakis G, ed: *Nutritional assessment in health programs,* Washington, DC, 1973, American Public Health Association and Dietary Interview Questionnaire, Agricultural Experiment Station, Burlington, University of Vermont.
Continued.

❖

DIET HISTORY FORM FOR OLDER ADULTS-cont'd

14. What is your present dental status?
    Edentulous, no dentures _____ Edentulous, single denture _____
    Edentulous, upper and lower dentures _____ Painful or missing teeth _____
    Own teeth satisfactory _____
15. How would you describe your appetite? Excellent _____ Good _____ Poor _____
    Varies _____ Never get hungry _____
16. Is your physical activity restricted in any way? Yes _____ No _____
    If yes, type of restriction _____
    Does this interfere with food preparation? Yes _____ No _____
    Does this interfere with food shopping? Yes _____ No _____
17. Has the amount of food you eat regularly changed in the last 12 months? Yes _____ No _____
    If yes, how has it changed? _____
    Why has it changed? _____
18. Have the types of food you eat regularly changed in the last 12 months? Yes _____ No _____
    If yes, what foods have you started to eat? _____
    What foods have you stopped eating? _____
       Why? _____
19. Has your weight changed in the last year? No change _____
    Approximate number of pounds gained _____ Approximate number of pounds lost _____
    Explanation for weight change, if known _____
20. Have you been following a special diet of some kind in the past 12 months?
    None _____ Low residue _____ Low sodium _____ Low cholesterol _____ Low fat _____
    Diabetic _____ Bland _____ Weight reduction _____ High fiber _____ Other _____
21. Did a doctor put you on this diet? Yes _____ No _____
    If no, how did you decide to follow this diet? _____
22. Some people have problems following their diet. Do you find your diet difficult to follow?
    No problem—easy to follow _____ Moderately difficult _____ Very difficult _____
    If difficult to follow, why?
       Don't understand the diet and what foods I should or should not eat _____
       Recommended foods too expensive _____
       Recommended foods difficult to prepare _____
       Recommended foods not familiar to me _____
       Recommended foods don't taste good _____
       Recommended foods not available where I get my meals _____
23. Do you participate in any of the following nutrition programs?
    Congregate meal program _____
    If yes, how frequently do you attend per week? _____
    Home-delivered meals program _____
    If yes, how many meals are delivered per week? _____
    Homeless shelter _____
    How many meals do you receive per week? _____
    Commodity food distribution _____
    If yes, what food do you receive? _____
    Food stamps _____
    If not participating now, would you like to participate in any of these nutrition programs?
    Yes _____ Program(s) _____

DIET HISTORY FORM FOR OLDER ADULTS- *cont'd*

24. Do the nutrition programs in which you now participate adequately meet your food needs?
    Yes _____ No _____
        If not, what are your unmet food needs? _____

25. Do you regularly skip meals? Yes _____ No _____
    If yes, about how many meals per week do you skip? _____
    Why do you usually skip meals? _____

26. Do you have enough money to buy the foods you need? Yes _____ No _____

27. What is your biggest problem regarding food and meals? _____

28. Do you smoke? Yes _____ No _____

29. Do you use alcoholic beverages? Yes _____ No _____
    If yes, about how often do you use these beverages?
    Every day _____ A few times each week _____ A few times each month _____

30. Do you take any vitamin, mineral, or protein supplements? Yes _____ No _____
    If yes, what do you take? _____
    (Ask to see container if possible.)
    How frequently do you take them? _____
    Were these supplements recommended by your doctor? Yes _____ No _____

31. Do you use any of the following over-the-counter drugs on a regular basis?
    Aspirin _____ Antacids _____ Laxatives _____ "Water" pills _____ Pain pills _____
    Sleeping pills _____ Antidiarrhea preparations _____ Other (describe) _____
    If yes, were these drugs recommended by your doctor? Yes _____ No _____

32. Do you take any prescription drugs regularly? Yes _____ No _____
    If so, what drugs? (Ask to see container if possible.)
    Drug _____
    Drug _____

33. About how many glasses or cups of the following liquids do you drink each day?
    Water _____ Soft drinks _____ Tea or coffee _____ Fruit juices or drinks _____ Milk _____
    Soup or broth _____ Alcoholic beverages _____

34. Do you eat at regular times each day? Yes _____ No _____
    Describe a typical daily pattern of when and where you eat _____
    _____
    What types of food do you usually eat at those times? _____
    _____

35. What specific kinds of the following foods do you eat most often?
    Deep yellow or orange fruits _____ About how often _____ Never eat _____
    Citrus fruits or juice _____ About how often _____ Never eat _____
    Other fruits or juice _____ About how often _____ Never eat _____
    Dark green or deep yellow vegetables _____ About how often _____ Never eat _____
    Potatoes _____ About how often _____ Never eat _____
    Cruciferous vegetables (broccoli, cauli-
    flower, Brussels sprouts, cabbage) _____ About how often _____ Never eat _____
    Other vegetables _____ About how often _____ Never eat _____
    Meat _____ About how often _____ Never eat _____

Continued.

DIET HISTORY FORM FOR OLDER ADULTS- *cont'd*

Fish _____ About how often _____ Never eat _____
Poultry _____ About how often _____ Never eat _____
Eggs _____ About how often _____ Never eat _____
Milk _____ About how often _____ Never eat _____
Cheese _____ About how often _____ Never eat _____
Other dairy foods _____ About how often _____ Never eat _____
Whole-grain bread, rolls, muffins, or tortillas _____ About how often _____ Never eat _____
Enriched bread, rolls, or muffins _____ About how often _____ Never eat _____
Whole-grain cereal _____ About how often _____ Never eat _____
Enriched cereal _____ About how often _____ Never eat _____
Dried peas or beans _____ About how often _____ Never eat _____
Peanut butter or nuts _____ About how often _____ Never eat _____
Cookies, cake, or pie _____ About how often _____ Never eat _____
Crackers, corn chips, pretzels,
or similar snack foods _____ About how often _____ Never eat _____

Hints for Dietary Interviews

Check carefully for the following information:
- *Additions to foods already recorded such as*

Fats: butter, margarine, honey-butter, peanut butter, mayonnaise, lard, meat drippings, cheese spreads, or 'lite' spreads.
   Used on toast, bread, rolls, buns, cookies, crackers, sandwiches, nachos.
   Used on vegetables.
   Used on potatoes, rice, pasta.
Sugars: jam, jelly, honey, syrup, or other natural sweeteners.
   Used on bread, sandwiches, vegetables, fruit, cereal, coffee, tea.
Milk: cream, half-and-half, whole, low-fat (% fat), skim.
   Used with cereal, coffee, tea, desserts, soups.
Gravy: used on bread, biscuits, meat, potatoes, rice, noodles.
Salad dressings: used on vegetables, salads, sandwiches.
Other spreads: catsup, mustard, relish, salsa.
Chocolate or other flavoring to milk.

- *Aspects of food preparation*

Preparation of eggs (e.g., fried, scrambled, hard-cooked, poached, yolk removed).
Preparation of meat, poultry, fish (e.g., deep fat-fried, stir-fried, boiled, stewed, roasted, baked, broiled).
Preparation of mixed dishes—major ingredients used (e.g., tuna fish and noodles, macaroni and cheese, bean burrito).

- *Special detail about food items*

Type of milk (whole, low-fat (% fat), skim, powdered, low-fat chocolate).
Type of carbonated beverage (naturally sweetened, artificially sweetened).
Type of fruit (canned in syrup, canned in juice, frozen, fresh, dried, cooked with sugar added).
Type of fruit juice, fruit drink (naturally or artificially sweetened), or juice substitute.

Adapted from Fomon SJ: *Nutritional disorders of children. Prevention, screening and follow-up,* DHEW Pub No (HSA) 77-5104, Washington, DC, 1977, US Government Printing Office.

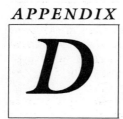

D *Selected Resources*

FOR PROFESSIONAL USE
Nutrition Education and Health Promotion

American Association of Retired Persons: All available from Health Advocacy Services, AARP, 601 E Street, N.W., #B5, Washington, DC 20049.

Activities with impact: innovative program ideas for adult housing residences, 1987.

Health risks and preventive care among older blacks (#D13741), no date given.

Health risks and preventive care among older Pacific Asian Americans (#D13743), no date given.

Health risks and preventive care among older Hispanics (#D13740, English; #D13742, Spanish), no date given.

Health risks and preventive care among older American Indians and Alaskan natives (#D13744), no date given.

Healthy older adults 2000: healthy people 2000 national health promotion and disease prevention objectives for older adults (series of pamphlets), no date given.

AARP health promotion publications list, no date given.

Perspectives in health promotion and aging (bimonthly newsletter).

American Dietetic Association: All available from American Dietetic Association, 216 W. Jackson Blvd., Suite 800, Chicago, IL 60606-6995.

Cardiovascular disease: nutrition for prevention and treatment, 1990.

Chinese American food practices, customs, and holidays, 1990.

Hmong American food practices, customs, and holidays, 1992.

Jewish food practices, customs, and holidays, 1990.

Meal planning with Jewish foods, 1990.

Meal planning with Mexican American foods, 1989.

Mexican American food practices, customs, and holidays, 1989.

Navaho food practices, customs, and holidays, 1992.

Planificacion de comidas con alimentos Mexicanoamericanos, 1990.

American Society on Aging: *Generations special issue on alcohol and drugs: abuse and misuse,* 1988. Available from American Society on Aging, 833 Market Street, Suite 516, San Francisco, CA 94103.

Anonymous: *Medicine is no mystery* (program kit for group sessions on medication management), 1991. Available from National Council on the Aging, Dept. 5087, Washington, DC 20061-5087.

Anonymous: Posters featuring older persons eating meals in a variety of settings. Available from Phoenix Systems, 601 S. Minnesota Ave., Ste. L-102, Sioux Falls, SD 57104.

Campbell-Lindzey S, Monoco M: *Elderly nutrition: resource packet for educators,* 1988. Available from Nutrition Center, Pennsylvania State University, Benedict House, University Park, PA 16802.

Corbin DE, Metal-Corbin J: *Reach for it! A handbook of exercise and dance activities for older adults,* 1983. Available from Eddie Bowers Publishing Co., 2600 Jackson St., Dubuque, IA 52001.

Donavin DP: *Aging with style and savvy: books and films on challenges facing adults of all ages,* 1990. Available from American Library Association, ALA Books, 50 East Huron St., Chicago, IL 60611-2795.

Franklin BA and others: *On the ball: innovative activities for adult fitness and cardiac rehabilitation programs,* 1990. Available from Brown and Benchmark, 25 Kessel Court, Madison, WI 53711.

Harveywebster MJ, Usinger-Lesquereux J: *Nutrition information for people who receive home-delivered meals,* 1988. Available from University of Nevada-Reno, College of Agriculture, Nevada Cooperative Extension Service, Reno, NV 89557.

Helgeson EM, Willis SC: *Handbook of group activities for impaired older adults,* 1987. Available from Haworth Press, 10 Alice St., Binghamton, NY 13904-1580.

Horn BJ: *Facilitating self care practices in the elderly,* 1990. Available from Haworth Press, 10 Alice St., Binghamton, NY 13904-1580.

Hurly O: *Safe therapeutic exercise for the frail elderly: an introduction,* 1988. Available from Center for the Study of Aging, 706 Madison Ave., Albany, NY 12208.

Institute of Health and Aging: *A resource guide for fitness programs for older persons,* Pub No 85-G5, no date given. Available from Institute of Health and Aging, University of California at San Francisco, 201 Filbert St., Suite 500, San Francisco, CA 94133.

Kantor M: *Nutrition for older Americans—more questions than answers,* 1987. Available from University of Maryland, Cooperative Extension Service, Computer Science Bldg. 2100, College Park, MD 20742-2451.

Lincoln Area Agency on Aging, Lincoln-Lancaster County Health Department: *Lifetime health program: a comprehensive approach to health data collection, health contracting, and health education intervention sessions for older adults.* Available from Lincoln-Lancaster County Health Department, 2200 St. Mary's Ave., Lincoln, NE 68502.

Massachusetts Office of Elder Affairs: *Nutrition and health education for older adults at home,* no date given. Available from Executive Office of Elder Affairs, 38 Chauncy St., Boston, MA 02111.

National Agricultural Library: *Nutrition and the elderly: resource listing,* no date given. Available from U.S. Dept. of Agriculture Food and Nutrition Information Center, Room 111, Beltsville, MD 20705.

National Arthritis and Muscoskeletal and Skin Diseases Information Clearinghouse: *Osteoporosis patient education materials: an annotated bibliography,* 1988. Available from NAMSIC, Box AMS, Bethesda, MD 20892.

National Audiovisual Center: *Media for health and behavior* (listing of health promotion films), 1990. Available from National Audiovisual Center, National Archives and Records Administration, Customer Services Section, 8700 Edgeworth Drive, Capitol Heights, MD 20743-1300.

National High Blood Pressure Education Program: All available from the National Heart, Lung, and Blood Institute Information Center, 4733 Bethesda Ave., Suite 530, Bethesda, MD 20814-4820.

The working group report on ambulatory blood pressure monitoring, 1991.

The working group report on management of patients with hypertension and high blood cholesterol, 1991.

A selected listing of audiovisual materials on heart health, 1990.

National Institute of Senior Centers: *Program ideas book,* no date given. Available from North Shore Senior Center, 620 Lincoln Ave., Winnetka, IL 60093.

Newman JM: *The melting pot: an annotated bibliography and guide to food and nutrition information for ethnic groups in America,* 1986. Available from Garland Publishing Company, 717 Fifth Ave., Suite 2500, New York, NY 10022.

North Dakota State University: *Harvest health at home—eating for the second fifty years (series of newsletters and implementation guide),* 1990. Available from Home Economics Extension, Box 5016, 219 Family Life Center, North Dakota State University, Fargo, ND 58105.

Price G, Fitz PA: *Cultural diversity and the allied health curriculum: issues in aging,* 1990. Available from Dean's Office, School of Allied Health Professions, University of Connecticut, Box U-101, 358 Mansfield Road, Storrs, CT 06268.

Pynoos J, Cohen E: *Home safety guide for older people: check it out, fix it up,* 1990. Available from Serif Press, 1331 H St., N.W., Suite 110LL, Washington, DC 20005.

Smiley J: *Creative recreation and socialization for senior citizen centers,* 1988. Available from Community Nutrition Institute, 2001 S St., N.W., Suite 530, Washington, DC 20009.

Weiss JC: *The feeling great wellness program for older adults,* 1988. Available from Haworth Press, 10 Alice St., Binghamton, NY 13904-1580.

Long-Term Care Programs and Facilities

Alta Bates-Herrick Rehabilitation Center: *Dysphagia dining* (handbook for people with swallowing disorders). Available from Alta Bates-Herrick Rehabilitation Center, Dept. of Nutrition and Food Services, 2001 Dwight Way, Berkeley, CA 94704.

American Dietetic Association Consulting Dietitians in Health Care Facilities: *Dining skills: practical interventions for the caregivers of eating-disabled older adults,* Chicago, 1992. Available from CD-HCF, P.O. Box 2067, Pensacola, FL 32513.

Gerwick CL: *Nutrition care in nursing facilities,*

1991. Chicago, Available from American Dietetic Association, 216 W. Jackson Blvd., Suite 800, Chicago, IL 60606-6995.

Healthcare Nutrition Services, ARA Services: *Geriatric nutrition care manual for long-term care,* 1988. Available from Healthcare Nutrition Services Marketing Dept., P.O. Box 8018, Philadelphia, PA 19101.

Hermann-Zaidins, M, Touger-Decker R: *Nutrition support in home health,* 1989. Available from Aspen Publishers, 200 Orchard Ridge Dr., Gaithersburg, MD 20878.

Program Planning, Implementation, and Management

Allegheny County Health Department: *The menu planning teaching kit* (designed for facilities serving 25 people or less), no date available. Available from Allegheny County Health Department Nutrition Services, 239 Fourth Ave., Investment Bldg., Pittsburgh, PA 15222.

American Association of Retired Persons: *Celebrating diversity: a learning tool for working with people of different cultures* (#D14078), no date available. Available from AARP Fulfillment, 1909 K St., N.W., Washington, DC 20049.

Anonymous: *How to start a respite service for people with Alzheimer's and their families. A guide for community-based organizations,* 1987. Available from Brookdale Center, Hunter College, 425 East 25th St., New York, NY 10010.

Anonymous: *Meals-On-Wheels America* (resource guide for funding and managing home delivered meals programs), no date available. Available from Meals-on-Wheels America, 280 Broadway, New York, NY 10007.

Department of Nutrition and Dietetics: *Collection of recipes: home and quantity recipes.* Available from Indiana University School of Medicine, University Hospital, Room D132, 1100 W. Michigan St., Indianapolis, IN 46223.

Gray M, and others: *Neighbor helping neighbor volunteer program,* 1981. Available from Publications, Institute on Aging, JM-20, University of Washington, 3935 University Way N.E., Seattle, WA 98195.

Jones LM, Fischer BR: *Simplified recipes for adult care centers,* 1990. Available from Van Nostrand Reinhold, 7625 Empire Dr., Florence, KY 41022.

Maine Bureau of Mental Health: *Topics in aging and mental health* (training manual on normal aging, depression, dementia, dysfunctional behavior and communication for nursing home and boarding home staff), no date available. Available from Bureau of Mental Health, State House Station #40, Augusta, ME 04330.

National Association of Nutrition and Aging Services Programs (NANASP): *Many hats (newsletter for congregate meal site managers),* no date available. Available from NANASP, 2675 44th St., S.W., Suite 305, Wyoming, MN 49509.

New York State Office for the Aging: Available from State Office for the Aging, Agency Building 2, Empire State Plaza, Albany, NY 12223-0001.
Menu manual, 1988.
Food service policy and procedure manual, 1988.

Pettit J, Weinstein J: *Programs to help older people eat better,* 1989. Available from Community Nutrition Institute, 2001 S St., N.W., Suite 530, Washington, DC 20036.

Philadelphia Health Management Corporation: *Eating the low-fat way. A nutrition program for older adults with home and quantity size recipes,* 1987. Available from Thomas Jefferson University Hospital, 111 S. 11th St., Philadelphia, PA 19107-5099.

Puerto Rican Dietetic Association: *Recipe manual.* Available from Regional Nutrition Specialist, Administration on Aging, Region II Office, 26 Federal Plaza, Rm 4149, New York, 10278.

Rhodes, S.S.: *Effective menu planning for the elderly nutrition program,* 1991. Available from American Dietetic Association, 216 W. Jackson Blvd., Chicago, IL 60606-6995.

Shugart GS, Molt MK, Wilson ME: *Food for Fifty,* ed 8, 1989. Available from MacMillan Company, 100 Front St., Box 500, Riverside, NJ 08075.

Stewart A: *Cooking for elderly people,* 1988. Available from Winslow Press, Telford Road, Bicester, Oxon OX6 OTS, England.

Turner S, Aronowitz V: *Healthwise quantity cookbook,* 1990. Available from Center for Science in the Public Interest, 1875 Connecticut Ave., N.W., Suite 300, Washington, DC 20009-5728.

United States Department of Agriculture: *Quick and easy commodity recipes for the food distribution program on Indian reservations* (70 traditional and nontraditional recipes for Native Americans), no date available. Available from Food and Nutrition Service, Nutrition Science and Education Branch, 3101 Park Center Drive, Room 607, Alexandria, VA 22302.

United States Department of Agriculture, Food and Nutrition Service: *Quantity recipes for school food service*, Program Aid 1371, 1988. Available from Superintendent of Documents, Washington, DC 20402-9325.

United States Department of Transportation: *Financing and Sustaining Mobility Programs in Rural Areas* (No. DOT-1-87-2), 1987. Available from Technology Sharing Program, DRT-1, 400 7th St., S.W., Washington, DC 20590.

Wood, M., and Harris, K.: *Quantity Recipes, New York College of Human Ecology*, no date available. Available from Cornell University, Savage Hall, Ithaca, NY, 14853.

Nutrition Screening Initiative

Nutrition Screening Initiative. Available from Nutrition Screening Initiative, P.O. Box 1960, Maple Grove, MN 55364-0058.
Screening older Americans' nutritional health: current practices and future possibilities, full report, 1991.
Nutrition screening I: toward a common view, full report, 1991.
Nutrition screening manual for professionals caring for older Americans, 1991.

FOR THE LAY PUBLIC
Nutrition Education and Health Promotion

American Association of Retired Persons. Available from American Association of Retired Persons, 1909 K St., N.W., Washington, DC 20049.
Action for a healthier life: a guide for mid-life and older women, 1988,

Eating for your health: a guide to food for healthy diets, 1991.
How does your nutrition measure up? 1991.
Pep up your life: a fitness book for seniors, 1987.
Staying well, 1991.
Strategies for good health, 1986.

American Diabetes Association: *Take charge of your health—be alert to what you eat and do*, 1990. Available from local American Diabetes Association chapters.

American Dietetic Association. Available from American Dietetic Association, 216 W. Jackson Blvd., Suite 800, Chicago, IL 60606-6995.
Alphabet soup: nutrients from food and supplements, 1990.
Diabetes and food: a guide for people with non-insulin dependent diabetes mellitus, 1991.
Eat healthy, stay fit: tips on nutrition for the mature adult, 1989.
Lowfat living: a guide to enjoying a healthy diet, 1988.
Pocket supermarket guide, 1989.
Staying healthy—a guide for elder Americans, 1990.

American Foundation for the Blind. Available from American Foundation for the Blind, 15 West 16th St., New York, NY 10011.
Environmental modifications for the visually impaired: a handbook, no date given.
Low vision questions and answers: definitions, devices, services, no date given.

American Heart Association. Available from American Heart Association, 7320 Greenville Ave., Dallas, TX 75231.
Cholesterol and your heart, 1988.
How to have your cake and eat it too: a painless guide to low-fat, low-cholesterol eating, 1988.

American Heart Association: *Low fat, low cholesterol cookbook*, 1989. Available from Random House, 400 Hahn Rd., Westminster, MD 21157.

American Institute for Cancer Research. Available from American Institute for Cancer Research, Dept. HP, 1759 R St., N.W., Washington, DC 20009.
Cooking solo—healthful eating for one or two, 1990.
Be your best: nutrition after fifty, 1990.

Anderson, J.A.: *Be heart smart . . . the H C F*

way to a healthy heart, 1989. Available from HCF Nutrition Research Foundation, P.O. Box 22124, Lexington, KY 40522.

Anonymous: *Guide to good nutrition (for persons with common gastrointestinal problems),* no date given. Available from Gastro-Intestinal Research Foundation, 70 East Lake St., Suite 1015, Chicago, IL 60601.

Anonymous: *Health after 50* (monthly newsletter). Available from Johns Hopkins Medical Letter, Subscription Dept., P.O. Box 420176, Palm Coast, FL 32142.

Anonymous. Available from Growers of Washington State Apples, Box 550-Dietitians, Wenatchee, WA 98807.
Healthy choices for people with diabetes, 1991.
Healthy choices for people with high blood pressure, 1991.

Anonymous: *Resources for elders with disabilities,* 1990. Available from Resources for Rehabilitation, 33 Bedford St., Suite 19A, Lexington, MA 02173.

Belsky JK: *Here tomorrow: making the most of life after fifty,* 1990. Available from Johns Hopkins University Press, 701 W. 40th St., Suite 275, Baltimore, MD 21211.

California Dietetic Association, Los Angeles District: *La dieta diabetica* (English-Spanish booklet of exchange lists for meal planning), no date given. Available from CDA-Los Angeles District, P.O. Box 3506, Santa Monica, CA 90403.

Center on Aging: *Health tips for the Latino elderly,* 1990. Available from Center on Aging, Weber State College, 3750 Harrison Blvd., Ogden, UT 84408-1212.

D'Urso-Fischer E: *Growing older . . . eating better; the white crane cookbook,* 1989. Available from White Crane Wellness Center, 929 West Belmont St., Ann Sather 2nd Floor, Chicago, IL 60657.

Gershoff S: *Tufts University guide to total nutrition,* 1990. Available from Harper-Collins, Publisher, 1000 Keystone Industrial Park, Scranton, PA 18512-4621.

Gillian J, Kirkpatrick J: *Guiltless gourmet,* 1988. Available from Diabetes Center, Inc., Suite 250, 13911 Ridgedale Drive, Minnetonka, MN 55343.

Gordon M: *Old enough to feel better,* 1989. Available from Johns Hopkins University Press, 701 W. 40th St., Suite 275, Baltimore, MD 21211.

HCA Wesley Medical Center: *Taste the good life. More than just a cookbook,* 1989. Available from Health Strategies, HCA Wesley Medical Center, P.O. Box 47826, Wichita, KS 67214.

Kreschollek M, Bentivegna B: *The guaranteed goof-proof healthy microwave cookbook,* 1990. Available from Bantam Books, 414 E. Golf Rd., Des Plaines, IL 60016.

Langholz E, and others. Available from Bristol Publishing Enterprises, Inc., P.O. Box 1737, San Leandro, CA 94577.
The Nutrition Game. The Right Moves If You're Over 50. 1990.
Over 50 and Still Cooking: Recipes for Good Health and Long Life, 1990.

Mankato Heart Health Program: *Cooking a la heart cookbook,* ed 2, 1991. Available from Appletree Press, 151 Good Counsel Drive, Suite 125, Mankato, MN 56001.

Marks, B.: *Microwave diabetes cookbook,* 1991. Available from Surrey Books, Suite D120, 230 East Ohio St., Chicago, IL 60611.

National Center for Nutrition and Dietetics: *New LEAN toward health* (brochure on low-fat foods), 1991. Available from National Center for Nutrition and Dietetics, 216 W. Jackson Blvd., Suite 800, Chicago, IL 60606-6995.

National Consumers League: *Food and drug interactions* (English or Spanish), no date given. Available from National Consumers League, Publications Coordinator, 815 15th St., N.W., Suite 928-N, Washington, DC 20005.

National Council on Patient Information and Education. Available from NCPIE, 666 Eleventh St., N.W., Suite 810, Washington, DC 20001.
Priorities and approaches for improving prescription medicine use by older Americans, no date given.
Medicines, what every woman should know, no date given.

National Council on the Aging. Available from NCOA, Dept. 5087, Washington, DC 20061-5087.
Senior wellness calendar, 1992.
Eating well to stay well, 1987.

National Dairy Council. Available from National Dairy Council, 6300 North River Road, Rosemont, IL 60018-4233.
Calcium: you never outgrow your need for it, no date given.
For mature eaters only: guidelines for good nutrition, no date given.
Getting along with milk: for people with lactose intolerance, no date given.
Healthy dividends: a plan for balancing your fat budget, no date given.
Osteoporosis: Are you at risk? (also available in Spanish), 1990.

National Fisheries Institute: *Eat fish twice a week,* 1991. From National Fisheries Institute, Communications Department, 1525 Wilson Blvd., Suite 500, Arlington, VA 22209.

National Institute on Aging: single copies available free from NIA Information Center, P.O. Box 8057, Gaithersburg, MD 20898-8057.
The resource directory for older people, 1991.
Age page (series of fact sheets covering a variety of health topics, including food shopping, nutrition, drugs, alcohol).

National Institutes of Health: *Noninsulin dependent diabetes,* 1990. Available from Consumer Information Center, Dept. 424-V, Pueblo, CO 81009.

National Livestock and Meat Board. Available from Education Department, National Livestock and Meat Board, 444 N. Michigan Ave., Chicago, IL 60611.
50+: a growing force, 1989.
Sterling advice for the silver years, 1991.

National Osteoporosis Foundation. From National Osteoporosis Foundation, 2100 M St., N.W., Suite 602, Washington, DC 20037.
Boning up on osteoporosis, 1991.
Bone wise (education kit for older adults), 1991.
Facts about osteoporosis, arthritis, and osteoarthritis, 1991.
Living with osteoporosis, 1991.
Osteoporosis: a woman's guide, 1988.

Reader D, Franz M: *Pass the pepper please: healthy meal planning for people on sodium restricted diets,* 1988. Available from Diabetes Center, Inc., Suite 250, 13911 Ridgedale Drive, Minnetonka, MN 55343.

Rippe JM, Ward A: *Complete book of fitness walking,* 1989. Available from Prentice Hall, 15 Columbus Circle, New York, NY 10023.

Ross Laboratories: *Eating to make the most of maturity,* 1991. Available from Ross Laboratories, Columbus, OH 43216.

Stare F, Aronson V: *Food for fitness after fifty: a menu for good health in later years,* 1987. Available from Lippincott, 227 E. Washington Square, Philadelphia, PA 19106-3780.

TJ Lipton Company: *Food facts for senior citizens.* From The Lipton Kitchens, 800 Sylvan Ave., Englewood Cliffs, NJ 07632.

United States Department of Agriculture. From U.S. Department of Agriculture Human Nutrition Information Service, 6505 Belcest Road, Hyattsville, MD 20782.
Calories and weight: the USDA pocket guide, 1990.
Dietary guidelines and your diet: eating better when eating out, HG 232-11, 1989.
Dietary guidelines and your diet: making bag lunches, snacks, and desserts, HG 232-9, 1989.
Dietary guidelines and your diet: preparing foods and planning menus, HG 232-8, 1989.
Dietary guidelines and your diet: shopping for food and making meals in minutes, HG 232-10, 1989.
Plan ahead to make your food dollars count, Program Aid No. 1347, 1984.
The food guide pyramid, Home and Garden Bulletin No. 252, 1992.
Using less sugar, fat, and salt, Program Aid No. 1388, 1986.

United States Department of Agriculture and United States Department of Health and Human Services: *Nutrition and your health: dietary guidelines for Americans,* HG 232, Third ed., 1990, U.S. Government Printing Office, Washington, DC 20402.

United States Department of Health and Human Services. From U.S. Government Printing Office, Washington, DC 20402.
Eating to lower your high blood cholesterol, NIH Publication No. 87-2920, 1987.
Test your healthy heart I.Q., NIH Publication No. 88-2724, 1988.
The Baltimore Longitudinal Study of Aging: older and wiser, NIH Publication No. 89-2797, 1989.
The fight against heart disease: diet, exercise, and other keys to a healthy heart, HHS Publication No. (FDA) 86-1126, 1988.

AUDIOVISUAL RESOURCES
Nutrition Education and Health Promotion

American Dietetic Association, American Heart Association, and National Cholesterol Education Program. Available from ADA Controlling Cholesterol Video Offer, c/o Zadox Inc., 5420 N.W. Foxhill St., Kansas City, MO 64152.

Controlling cholesterol: through diet and nutrition (30-minute video).

Controlling cholesterol: guidelines for eating out (30-minute video).

Controlling cholesterol: introduction to a healthy lifestyle (30-minute video).

Anonymous: *Alcohol, drugs and seniors: tarnished dreams* (23-minute video). Available from AIMS Media, 6901 Woodley Ave., Van Nuys, CA 91406-4878.

Anonymous: *Making life a little easier: self-help tools for the home* (slide/tape or video and brochure). Available from AARP A/V Programs, Program Resources Dept., 601 E St., N.W., Washington, DC 20049.

Anonymous: *Put away your frying pan* (10-minute videotape on healthy cooking techniques for Black Americans). Available from Health Promotion Council of Southeastern Pennsylvania, 311 S. Juniper St., Philadelphia, PA 19197-5803.

National Dairy Council: *Spice of life* (15-minute videotape giving practical suggestions for healthy eating for older adults). Available from National Dairy Council, 6300 North River Road, Rosemont, IL 60018-4233.

Pawtucket Heart Health Program: *After fifty* (30-minute videotape in the Controlling Cholesterol series). Available from Pawtucket Heart Health Program, Memorial Hospital of Rhode Island, 111 Brewster St., Pawtucket, RI 02860.

Texas Agricultural Extension Service. Available from Minority Peer Education Project, Texas A&M University, College Station, TX.

Reverend Jones (an educational kit including video and users guide focusing on high blood pressure for black elderly), 1990.

Fanny (an educational kit including video and users guide focusing on late onset diabetes for black elderly), 1990.

Turner Educational Services (CNN): user's guide and videos available from Turner Broadcasting, 1 CNN Center, P.O. Box 105366, Atlanta, GA 30348.

Eating healthy for life (20-minute video),

Eating healthy for heart health (20-minute video),

Eating healthy when dining out (20-minute video),

Eating healthy for weight control (20-minute video),

Nutrition Program Development

American Association of Retired Persons: *Healthy aging: model health promotion programs for minority elders* (45-minute video and companion booklet). Available from National Resource Center on Health Promotion and Aging, AARP, 1909 K St., N.W., 5th Floor, Washington, DC 20049.

Beverly Foundation: *Geriatric nutrition, patient assessment, and care planning reconsidered* (51-minute video). Available from Beverly Foundation, 70 South Lake Ave., Suite 750, Pasadena, CA 91101.

San Francisco Commission on Aging: *Getting it right* (45-minute video developed for in-service training of congregate meals site staff and volunteers); series available in Chinese, English, Japanese, Spanish, and Tagalog. Available from Spot 52 Productions, P.O. Box 460903, San Francisco, CA 94146-0903.

San Jose State University Instructional Resources Center. Available from Instructional Resources Center, San Jose State University, San Jose, CA 95192-0026.

Family counseling with an older Afro-American family (film).

Family counseling with an older Hispanic family (film).

United States Department of Agriculture: *Food safety is no mystery* (34-minute training video in English or Spanish). Available from Modern Talking Picture Service, 5000 Park St., N., St. Petersburg, FL 33709.

This resource list is provided for reader information and does not imply endorsement by the author.

Index